Pathophysiology
of Renal
Disease

Pathophysiology of Renal Disease
Second Edition

BURTON DAVID ROSE, M.D.
Director, Clinical Nephrology
Brigham and Women's Hospital
Associate Professor of Medicine
Harvard Medical School
Boston, Massachusetts

McGRAW-HILL BOOK COMPANY

New York St. Louis San Francisco Auckland Bogotá Hamburg
Johannesburg Lisbon London Madrid Mexico Milan Montreal New Delhi
Panama Paris San Juan São Paulo Singapore Sydney Tokyo Toronto

PATHOPHYSIOLOGY OF RENAL DISEASE

Copyright © 1987, 1981 by McGraw-Hill, Inc. All rights reserved. Printed in the United States of America. Except as permitted under the United States Copyright Act of 1976, no part of this publication may be reproduced or distributed in any form or by any means, or stored in a data base or retrieval system, without the prior written permission of the publisher.

1 2 3 4 5 6 7 8 9 0 DOCDOC 8 9 4 3 2 1 0 9 8 7

ISBN 0-07-053629-5

This book was set in Meridien by McFarland Graphics and Design; the editors were William Day and Muza Navrozov; the production supervisor was Avé McCracken; the designer was Maria Karkucinski; the cover was designed by Edward R. Schultheis. Front cover illustration was adapted from A. Vander, *Renal Physiology, 2d ed.,* McGraw-Hill, New York, 1980.
R. R. Donnelley & Sons Company was printer and binder.

Library of Congress Cataloging-in-Publication Data

Rose, Burton David, date
   Pathophysiology of renal disease.

   Includes bibliographies and index.
   1. Kidneys—Diseases.   I. Title.   [DNLM: 1. Kidney
Diseases—physiopathology.   WJ 300 R795p]
RC903.9.R67   1987   616.6'1   86-33710
ISBN 0-07-053629-5

For Gloria, Emily, Anne, and Daniel

CONTENTS

4 MECHANISMS OF PROGRESSION OF RENAL DISEASE

BURTON D. ROSE
BARRY M. BRENNER

5 PATHOGENESIS, CLINICAL MANIFESTATIONS, AND DIAGNOSIS OF GLOMERULAR DISEASE

BURTON D. ROSE

6 NEPHROTIC SYNDROME AND GLOMERULONEPHRITIS

BURTON D. ROSE
JEROME B. JACOBS

7 VASCULAR DISEASES OF THE KIDNEY

ROBERT M. BLACK

CONTRIBUTORS

WILLIAM M. BENNETT, M.D.

Head, Division of Nephrology
Professor of Medicine, University of Oregon Health Sciences Center
Portland, Oregon

ROBERT M. BLACK, M.D.

Nephrologist, Fallon Clinic
Assistant Professor of Medicine, University of Massachusetts Medical School
Worcester, Massachusetts

BARRY M. BRENNER, M.D.

Director, Division of Nephrology, Brigham and Women's Hospital
Professor of Medicine, Harvard Medical School
Boston, Massachusetts

JEROME B. JACOBS, Ph.D.

Director of Electron Microscopy Laboratory, The Saint Vincent Hospital
Instructor in Pathology, University of Massachusetts Medical School
Worcester, Massachusetts

LAURENCE A. TURKA, M.D.

Fellow in Nephrology, Brigham and Women's Hospital
Boston, Massachusetts

PREFACE

The aim of this book is to teach medical students, house officers, and practicing physicians the basic aspects of intrinsic renal disease and hypertension. Although the basic outline is similar to that of the first edition, so many new advances have been made in the past six years in both pathophysiology and clinical management that the text has essentially been completely rewritten. As an example, Chapter 4 is new, dealing with the mechanisms responsible for the progression of renal disease. This exciting area offers hope in the therapy of many disorders, such as diabetic nephropathy, in which reduction of the intraglomerular pressure may prevent progressive glomerular injury, even in the absence of strict glycemic control.

The material that is presented reflects the core of information that I believe the clinician should possess. I have tried, wherever possible, to include discussions both of the mechanisms of disease and of how to derive a differential diagnosis based upon the findings present at initial evaluation. Thus, there are separate chapters reviewing the pathogenesis and approach to glomerular disease and to essential hypertension. In addition, the first two chapters present a broad overview of renal disease, including the common laboratory tests used to assess renal function (creatinine clearance, urinalysis, and urine sodium and osmolality) and a general diagnostic approach to help determine what kind of renal disease is present.

There are also certain areas that are not covered. Renal physiology and fluid and electrolyte disorders are presented in my other book, *Clinical Physiology of Acid-Base and Electrolyte Disorders, 2d. ed.* (McGraw-Hill, 1984). Space limitations and a desire to emphasize those problems that are most commonly seen by the nonnephrologist have led to the omission of chapters on urinary tract infections (other than chronic pyelonephritis), chronic renal failure, dialysis and transplantation, renal stones, and renal neoplasms.

ACKNOWLEDGMENTS

Many people made important contributions to bring this book to completion. I would particularly like to thank Bob Black, Rick Lifton, Bob Stanton, Tom Moore, and many students and residents at the Harvard Medical School and the Brigham and Women's Hospital for reviewing parts of the text; Beth Kaufman Barry and Muza Navrozov at McGraw-Hill for their continuing support and attention to detail; Sheila Putnam, Michelle Herry, and Donna McDermott for their secretarial assistance; and finally (but not least) my daughters—Emily, for her diligence in preparing and editing the references, and Anne, for help in checking the reference citations.

Pathophysiology of Renal Disease

1

CLINICAL ASSESSMENT OF RENAL FUNCTION

Burton D. Rose

The evaluation of the patient with kidney disease involves two basic steps: (1) establishing the correct diagnosis and (2) estimating the degree of renal dysfunction. Although the history and physical examination are frequently helpful, laboratory tests play a central role in this process. The most important of these tests are estimation of the glomerular filtration rate (GFR), examination of the urine, radiologic studies, and renal biopsy. This chapter reviews in some detail the meaning of these tests and the kinds of information that they can provide. The following chapter then discusses their specific use in the patient with renal disease.

MEASUREMENT OF GFR

The GFR is the best clinical estimate of functioning renal mass. To appreciate why this relationship is true, it is first necessary to briefly review normal renal physiology.

The basic unit of the kidney is the nephron, with each kidney in humans containing approximately 1.0 to 1.3 million nephrons. Each nephron consists of a glomerulus, which is a tuft of capillaries interposed between two arterioles (the afferent and efferent arterioles), and a series of tubules lined by epithelial cells (Fig. 1–1). As with other capillaries, an ultrafiltrate of plasma is formed across the glomer-

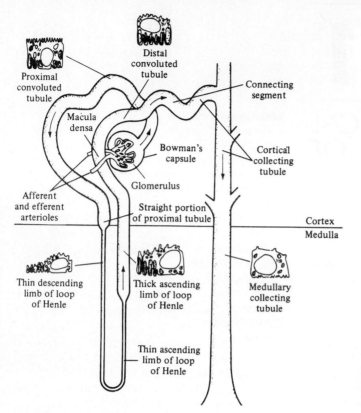

FIG. 1–1. Relationships of the component parts of the nephron. (*Adapted from R. Vander, Renal Physiology, 2d ed., McGraw-Hill, New York, 1980.*)

ulus. The filtrate is then altered by the tubules which reabsorb and, to a lesser degree, secrete solutes and water. The normal GFR is 135 to 180 L/day, an amount roughly equal to 10 times the extracellular volume. To prevent excessive fluid losses, 98 to 99 percent of the filtrate undergoes net reabsorption, resulting in a urine output of only 1 to 2 L/day.

These nephrons perform a variety of essential functions*,[1]:

1. They participate in the maintenance of the constant extracellular environment that is required for adequate functioning of the cells. This is achieved by excretion

of some of the waste products of metabolism (such as urea, creatinine, and uric acid, as well as many drugs) and by specific adjustment of the urinary excretion of water and electrolytes to match intake and endogenous production. To attain the latter goal, the kidney is able to regulate individually the excretion of solutes (such as sodium, potassium, and hydrogen) and water, largely by changes in tubular reabsorption or secretion. For example, water excretion appropriately increases after a water load. This change is mediated by reduced secretion of antidiuretic hormone (ADH) from the posterior lobe of the pituitary. The relative absence of ADH diminishes the permeability of the collecting tubules to water, thereby lowering water reabsorption and promoting water excretion.

*The specific mechanisms by which these functions are performed, including the role of hemodynamic and neurohumoral factors in the regulation of the GFR, are generally beyond the scope of this discussion but are reviewed in detail in Ref. 1.

2. The nephrons secrete hormones that participate in the regulation of systemic and renal hemodynamics (renin, prostaglandins, and bradykinin), red blood cell production (erythropoietin), and calcium, phosphorus, and bone metabolism (1,25-dihydroxycholecalciferol, the most active form of vitamin D).

3. The nephrons perform such miscellaneous functions as catabolism of peptide hormones and synthesis of glucose (gluconeogenesis) in fasting conditions.

When renal disease is present, one or more of these functions may be impaired. For example, the kidney is resistant to the effects of ADH in patients with nephrogenic diabetes insipidus, resulting in an inappropriate increase in water excretion. However, all other renal functions are normal in this disorder. In contrast, there is a generalized decrease in all kidney functions in patients with advanced renal failure. Waste product excretion is reduced, producing elevations in the concentrations of urea and creatinine in the blood; edema, hyperkalemia, and acidemia may result from decreased excretion of water and electrolytes; and anemia and bone disease may occur because of diminished production of erythropoietin and the active form of vitamin D.

However, not all renal functions are impaired with lesser degrees of renal disease. Even if two-thirds of the nephrons are not functioning, clinically significant changes in electrolyte and water balance usually do not occur because of a series of specific adaptations that result in increased solute and water excretion in each of the remaining nephrons. For example, although less sodium is filtered (owing to the decrease in the number of functioning nephrons), sodium excretion remains equal to intake because of an appropriate reduction in tubular reabsorption. Similarly, renal hormone secretion also may be relatively well maintained. In this setting, determination of the GFR and examination of the urine may be the only ways to detect the presence of kidney disease, such as a reduction in functioning renal mass. Since the total GFR is equal to the sum of the filtration rates from each of the functioning nephrons, the loss of two-thirds of the nephrons will lead to a decrease in total GFR, although the net reduction will be less than two-thirds, due to compensatory hyperfiltration in the remaining nephrons (see "Compensatory Glomerular Hyperfiltration," below). Thus, *the GFR can be used to document the presence, estimate the severity, and follow the course of kidney disease.* A decrease in GFR implies either progression of the underlying disease or the development of a superimposed problem such as volume depletion or urinary tract obstruction.

Estimation of the GFR is also helpful in determining the proper dosage of those drugs that are excreted by the kidney. For example, digoxin, used in the treatment of heart failure, and the antibiotic gentamicin are excreted in the urine, primarily by glomerular filtration. When the GFR is reduced, drug excretion will decrease. If the dosage is not appropriately diminished, the drug will accumulate in the body, reaching potentially toxic levels (see Chap. 13).

CREATININE CLEARANCE

The clinical determination of the GFR involves measurement of the rate of urinary excretion of certain compounds. For example, the exogenously administered polysaccharide inulin has the following properties:

1. It is freely filtered at the glomerulus.
2. It is able to achieve a stable plasma concentration.
3. It is not reabsorbed, secreted, or metabolized by the kidney.

In this situation,

$$\text{Filtered inulin} = \text{excreted inulin}$$

The filtered inulin is equal to the GFR times the plasma inulin concentration (P_{in}), and the excreted inulin is equal to the product of the urine inulin concentration (U_{in}) and the urine flow rate (V, in milliliters per minute or liters per day). Therefore,

$$GFR \times P_{in} = U_{in} \times V$$

$$GFR = \frac{U_{in} \times V}{P_{in}}$$

The term $(U_{in} \times V)/P_{in}$ is called the clearance of inulin and is an accurate estimate of the GFR. The inulin clearance, in milliliters per minute, refers to that volume of plasma cleared of inulin by renal excretion. For example, if 1 mg of inulin is excreted per minute ($U_{in} \times V$) and the P_{in} is 1.0 mg/dL (or to keep the units consistent, 0.01 mg/mL), then the clearance of inulin is 100 mL/min; that is, 100 mL of plasma has been cleared of the 1 mg of inulin that it contained.

Despite its accuracy, the inulin clearance is rarely performed clinically because it involves both an intravenous infusion of inulin and an assay for inulin that is not available in most laboratories. Similar technical considerations limit the use of radiolabeled compounds such as iothalamate.[2]

The most widely used method to estimate the GFR is the endogenous creatinine clearance.[3-5] Creatinine is derived from the metabolism of creatine in skeletal muscle and is released into the plasma at a relatively constant rate. As a result, the plasma creatinine concentration (P_{cr}) is very stable, varying less than 10 percent per day in serial observations in normal subjects, even with marked variations in dietary intake.[6] Like inulin, creatinine is freely filtered across the glomerulus and is neither reabsorbed nor metabolized by the kidney. However, a small amount of creatinine enters the urine by tubular secretion in the proximal tubule.[3] Because of this tubular secretion, the amount of creatinine excreted exceeds the amount filtered by 10 to 20 percent in patients with relatively normal renal function. Therefore, the creatinine clearance (C_{cr}),

$$C_{cr} = \frac{U_{cr} \times V}{P_{cr}}$$

will tend to exceed the inulin clearance by 10 to 20 percent. Fortuitously, this is balanced by an error of almost equal magnitude in the measurement of the P_{cr}. The most commonly used method involves a colorimetric reaction after the addition of alkaline picrate. The plasma, but not the urine, contains noncreatinine chromagens (acetone, proteins, ascorbic acid, pyruvate), which account for approximately 10 to 20 percent of the normal P_{cr}.[3] Since both the U_{cr} and P_{cr} are elevated to roughly the same degree, the errors tend to cancel and the C_{cr} is a reasonably accurate estimate of the GFR, particularly if the GFR is greater than 40 mL/min (normal in adults is 95 to 120 mL/min).

However, as renal failure progresses and the total GFR falls, less creatinine is filtered and proportionately more of the urinary creatinine is derived from tubular secretion. As a result, urinary creatinine excretion is much higher than it would be if creatinine were excreted only by glomerular filtration, and the C_{cr} can exceed that of inulin by 10 to 40 percent or more.[3] This error, however, does not substantially detract from the clinical usefulness of the C_{cr}. For example, a C_{cr} of 35 mL/min indicates the presence of moderately severe renal disease. The fact that the GFR (as measured by the inulin clearance) may actually be only 20 to 25 mL/min is not so important since knowledge of the exact GFR is usually not necessary.

The normal values for the creatinine clearance are[3,5]:

1. In men, 120 ± 25 mL/min (about 175 L/day).
2. In women, 95 ± 20 mL/min (about 135 L/day).
3. The creatinine clearance normally declines with age, falling almost 1 mL/min per year over the age of 40.[7]
4. In infants, 17 mL/min per 1.73 m^2 body surface area (the size of the average adult) at birth, increasing to 50 mL/min per 1.73 m^2 by 4 weeks, and to adult levels by 1 year of age (about 100 mL/min per 1.73 m^2).[8,9]

The C_{cr} is usually determined in the following way. Venous blood is used for the P_{cr}. Urinary excretion ($U_{cr} \times V$) is concomitantly measured on a 24-h collection since shorter collections tend to give less reliable results.[10] For example, a 30-year-old woman who weighs 60 kg is being evaluated for possible kidney disease and the following results are obtained:

$$P_{cr} = 1.5 \text{ mg/dL}$$
$$U_{cr} = 100 \text{ mg/dL}$$
$$V = 1080 \text{ mL/day}$$

and

$$\frac{1080 \text{ mL/day}}{1440 \text{ min/day}} = 0.75 \text{ mL/min}$$

Thus

$$C_{cr} = \frac{U_{cr} \times V}{P_{cr}}$$
$$= \frac{100 \times 0.75}{1.5} = 50 \text{ mL/min}$$

Since this is roughly one-half the normal C_{cr}, this patient has lost approximately one-half of her GFR.

The major error involved in the determination of the C_{cr} is an incomplete urine collection. For this reason, it is important to know the normal values for creatinine excretion. In adults under the age of 60, daily creatinine excretion should be 20 to 25 mg/kg lean body weight in males and 15 to 20 mg/kg

in females.[3,11] From the ages of 60 to 90, there is a progressive 50 percent reduction in creatinine excretion (from 20 to 10 mg/kg in males), probably due to a decrease in skeletal muscle mass.[11] If creatinine excretion is found to be much less than these values, an incomplete collection should be suspected. In the patient described above, creatinine excretion was 18 mg/kg per day (1080 mg/60 kg), suggesting that a complete collection was obtained.

P_{cr} AND GFR

Changes in, and estimation of, the GFR also can be ascertained from measurement of the P_{cr}, a simpler test to perform than the C_{cr}. In a subject in the steady state,

Creatinine excretion
$$= \text{creatinine production}$$

Creatinine excretion is roughly equal to the amount of creatinine filtered (GFR $\times$ P_{cr}), whereas the rate of creatinine production is relatively constant. If these substitutions are made in the above equation,

$$\text{GFR} \times P_{cr} = \text{constant}$$

Thus, *the P_{cr} varies inversely with the GFR.* If, for example, the GFR falls by 50 percent, creatinine excretion also will be reduced. As a result, newly produced creatinine will accumulate in the plasma until the filtered load again equals the rate of production. This will occur when the P_{cr} has doubled,

$$\tfrac{1}{2} \text{ GFR} \times 2P_{cr} = \text{GFR} \times P_{cr} = \text{constant}$$

In adults, the normal P_{cr} is 0.8 to 1.3 mg/dL in men and 0.6 to 1.0 mg/dL in women.*,[3]

---

*Since children are growing and have an increasing muscle mass, the P_{cr} increases with age. From the ages of 1 to 20, the normal P_{cr} can be estimated from the following formulas[12]:

$$P_{cr} = 0.35 + \text{age (years)}/40 \quad \text{(boys)}$$
$$= 0.35 + \text{age (years)}/55 \quad \text{(girls)}$$

The reciprocal relationship between the GFR and the P_{cr} is depicted in Fig. 1–2. There are three important points to note about this relationship. First, this curve is valid *only in the steady state.* If a patient develops acute renal failure with a sudden drop in the GFR from 120 to 12 mL/min, the P_{cr} on day 1 will still be normal since there will not have been time for creatinine to accumulate in the plasma. After 7 to 10 days, the P_{cr} will stabilize roughly at 10 mg/dL, a level consistent with the reduced GFR. A clinical application of this concept is seen with the use of drugs that are excreted in the urine. When given to patients with renal insufficiency, they should be administered in reduced dosage (see Chap. 13). Nomograms have been devised which relate drug dosage, e.g., for gentamicin, to the P_{cr} on the assumption that the latter is a reflection of the GFR.[13] However, this is true *only* in the steady state. If the above patient with acute renal failure were given gentamicin in full dosage because of the normal P_{cr}, toxic levels would ensue.

It should be remembered that the steady state can be disturbed by changes in creatinine production as well as in GFR. When creatinine production is acutely increased, as with severe muscle breakdown, the P_{cr} can increase out of proportion to any change in GFR.[14] For similar reasons, the P_{cr} should be measured when the patient is fasting, since cooked meat and its broth contain enough creatinine to transiently raise the P_{cr} by as much as 1.0 mg/dL.[15] This can result in a doubling of the P_{cr} and an apparent 50 percent reduction in GFR in a subject with normal renal function.

Second, it is important to note the *shape* of the curve. In a patient with normal renal function, *an apparently minor increase in the* P_{cr} *from 1.0 to 2.0 mg/dL can represent a marked fall in the GFR from 120 to 60 mL/min.* In contrast, in a patient with advanced renal failure, a marked increase in the P_{cr} from 6.0 to 12.0 mg/dL reflects a relatively small reduction in the GFR from 20 to 10 mL/min. Thus, the initial elevation of the P_{cr} represents the major loss in GFR.

Third, the relationship between the GFR and the P_{cr} is dependent upon the rate of creatinine production, which is largely a function of muscle mass. In Fig. 1–2, a normal GFR of 120 mL/min is associated with a P_{cr} of 1.0 g/dL. Although this may be true for a 70-kg man, a similar GFR in a 50-kg woman

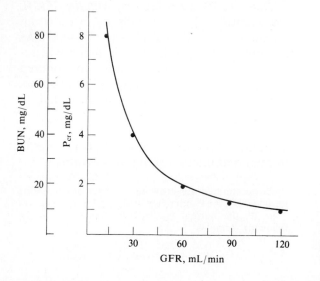

FIG. 1–2. Steady-state relationship between the plasma creatinine concentration (P_{cr}), blood urea nitrogen (BUN), and GFR.

might be associated with a P_{cr} of only 0.6 mg/dL. In this setting, a P_{cr} of 1.0 mg/dL is not normal and reflects a 40 percent fall in GFR.

To account for the effects of body weight, age, and sex on muscle mass, the following formula has been derived to estimate the C_{cr} from the P_{cr} in the steady state in adult men[16]:

$$C_{cr} \cong \frac{(140 - age) \times lean\ body\ weight}{P_{cr} \times 72}$$

This value should be multiplied by 0.85 in women since a lower fraction of the body weight is composed of muscle. The units of measure used in this formula are: C_{cr}, mL/min; age, years; lean body weight, kg; and P_{cr}, mg/dL.

The results obtained with this formula appear to correlate fairly well with a simultaneously measured C_{cr}. Its usefulness can be illustrated by the observation that a P_{cr} of 1.4 mg/dL represents a C_{cr} of 101 mL/min in an 85-kg, 20-year-old man,

$$C_{cr} \cong \frac{(140 - 20) \times 85}{1.4 \times 72}$$

but a C_{cr} of only 20 mL/min in a 40-kg, 80-year-old woman,

$$C_{cr} \cong \frac{(140 - 80) \times 40}{1.4 \times 72} \times 0.85$$

This example calls attention to the danger of overdosing elderly patients who have seriously impaired renal function despite a relatively normal P_{cr}. The use of this simple formula, while not absolutely accurate, will help to avoid this problem.

In summary, the P_{cr} varies inversely with the GFR in the steady state. Because of this relationship, serial measurements of the P_{cr} can be used to look for disease progression in patients with kidney dysfunction. The loss of functioning nephrons usually is associated with a reduction in the GFR and should result in an increase in the P_{cr}

PREDICTING THE COURSE OF RENAL FAILURE

In many patients with progressive renal disease, the rate of progression is relatively constant. As a result, the GFR should decrease linearly with time. Since the GFR varies inversely with the P_{cr}, the reciprocal of the P_{cr} ($1/P_{cr}$) should also decline at a relatively uniform rate. This prediction has been verified in patients with a variety of chronic renal diseases.[6,17] The manner in which this relationship can be used clinically is illustrated in Fig. 1–3. During the first 2 years of observation, this patient had a progressive reduction in renal function. Maintenance dialysis is usually required shortly after the P_{cr} reaches 10 mg/dL ($1/P_{cr} = 0.1$). By extrapolation, this should have occurred within

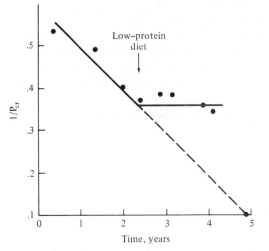

FIG. 1–3. Plot of the reciprocal of the P_{cr} versus time in a man with chronic pyelonephritis. There was a progressive and uniform decline in renal function during the first 2 years of observation. If this course had continued (dashed line), end-stage renal disease ($P_{cr} = 10$ mg/dL, $1/P_{cr} = 0.1$) would have occurred within the next 3 years. However, the institution of a low-protein diet (see "Compensatory Glomerular Hyperfiltration," below) resulted in stabilization of the P_{cr} and, since muscle mass was constant, the total GFR.

the ensuing 2 to 3 years. However, effective therapy was begun at this time, resulting in prolonged stabilization of the P_{cr}.

POTENTIAL ERRORS IN INTERPRETATION OF THE P_{cr}

In a variety of circumstances, the P_{cr} may be elevated without change in the GFR. This can result from increased creatinine production, decreased creatinine secretion, or the presence of compounds in the plasma, which may be measured as creatinine in certain assays (Table 1-1).[14,15,18-23]

Acetoacetic acid, for example, is measured as a noncreatinine chromagen by the alkaline picrate method. This can raise the measured P_{cr} by 0.5 to 2 mg/dL or more in patients with ketoacidosis.[20,21] This effect is rapidly reversed with correction of the ketoacidosis.

Cimetidine and trimethoprim, on the other hand, are organic bases which can competitively inhibit creatinine secretion by the organic base secretory pump in the proximal tubule. The net effect is a mild elevation in the P_{cr} (usually less than 0.5 mg/dL).[18,19] Ranitidine, a histamine (H_2)-receptor antagonist like cimetidine, does not appear to raise the P_{cr}.[24] Although ranitidine is also an organic base, it is generally given in much smaller doses (300 versus 1200 mg/day). The net result is much less tubular secretion of raniti-

dine and little interference with that of creatinine.[24]

BLOOD UREA NITROGEN AND GFR

Changes in the GFR also can be detected by changes in the concentration of urea in the blood, measured as the blood urea nitrogen (BUN). Like creatinine, urea is excreted primarily by glomerular filtration and the BUN tends to vary inversely with the GFR (Fig. 1-2).

However, two factors can alter the BUN without change in the GFR or P_{cr}. First, urea production may not be constant. Urea is formed by the hepatic metabolism of amino acids not utilized for protein synthesis. As amino acids are deaminated, ammonia is produced. The development of toxic levels of ammonia in the blood is prevented by the conversion of ammonia (NH_3) into urea in a reaction that can be summarized by the following equation:

$$2NH_3 + CO_2 \rightarrow H_2N - \overset{\displaystyle O}{\overset{\displaystyle \|}{C}} - NH_2 + H_2O$$
$$\text{Urea}$$

Thus, urea production and the BUN are increased when more amino acids are metabolized in the liver. This may occur with a high-protein diet, enhanced tissue breakdown (due to trauma, gastrointestinal bleeding, or the administration of corticosteroids), or decreased protein synthesis (due to tetracycline).[25] On the other hand, urea production and the BUN are reduced by severe liver disease or a low protein intake.

Second, urea excretion is not determined solely by glomerular filtration. Approximately 40 to 50 percent of the filtered urea is normally reabsorbed by the tubules. The reabsorption of urea tends to follow passively that of sodium and water. Thus, in states of volume depletion in which proximal sodium reabsorption is increased, urea reabsorption

---

TABLE 1-1. Factors Which Can Increase the P_{cr} without Change in the GFR

Increased creatinine production
  Massive rhabdomyolysis[14]
  Ingestion of cooked meat and its broth[15]
Compounds which decrease creatinine excretion
  by competing for secretion by organic base secretory
  pump
    Cimetidine[18]
    Trimethoprim[19]
Compounds measured as creatinine in certain assays
  Acetoacetic acid in ketoacidosis[20,21]
  Cefoxitin[22]
  Flucytosine[23]

also is enhanced. The net result is reduced urea excretion and an elevation in the BUN that is not due to a fall in GFR.[25] Under most conditions, the ratio of the BUN (normal value equals 10 to 20 mg/dL) to the P_{cr} is 10 to 15:1. When this ratio exceeds 20:1, one of the conditions associated with enhanced urea production or tubular reabsorption should be suspected (see p. 66).[25]

In summary, a reduction in the GFR results in elevation in both the BUN and P_{cr}. Because of the variability in urea production and reabsorption, the P_{cr} is a more reliable reflection of the GFR. For similar reasons, the urea clearance is not an accurate estimate of the GFR. Since urea is reabsorbed and the degree of reabsorption is variable, the quantity of urea excreted is much less than the amount filtered. As a result, the urea clearance is only 50 to 70 percent that of inulin.[26] Thus, the C_{cr} is the preferred clinical method for measuring the GFR with one exception. As described above, renal failure is associated with an increase in the percent of excreted creatinine derived from tubular secretion.[3,5] Thus, the C_{cr} can substantially exceed, whereas the urea clearance will continue to be less than, the inulin clearance. Consequently, in patients with advanced renal failure (P_{cr} greater than 4 mg/dL), the GFR is best estimated by taking the average of the creatinine and urea clearances[27]:

$$GFR \cong \frac{C_{cr} + C_{urea}}{2}$$

COMPENSATORY GLOMERULAR HYPERFILTRATION

The relationship between the total GFR and functioning renal mass frequently is altered with *mild renal disease*. As some nephrons are initially damaged, the remaining nephrons compensate by increasing their filtration rate.[28] The net effect is that the total GFR may be unchanged despite substantial renal damage. Thus, a patient with glomerulonephritis who has a stable P_{cr} of 1.1 mg/dL over a 1-year period may actually have significant disease progression during this time. More prominent urinary abnormalities or the development of hypertension may be the only clinical clues that this sequence has occurred. Specific confirmation would require a renal biopsy.

The adaptive hyperfiltration per functioning nephron reaches a maximum after about one-quarter to one-third of the nephrons have been destroyed. Any further loss of renal tissue is now accompanied by a reduction in the total GFR and an elevation in the P_{cr}. A simple example of this phenomenon occurs in a patient who donates a kidney for renal transplantation. Compensatory hyperfiltration returns the total GFR to 70 to 80 (not 100) percent of the previous baseline, even though one-half of the renal mass has been removed.

The mechanism underlying this adaptive response is incompletely understood. Afferent and, to a lesser degree, efferent arteriolar dilations result in increased glomerular pressure and flow that seem to account for the enhanced nephron GFR.[28] The observation that these hemodynamic changes can be prevented by a low-protein diet[29] suggests that they may be driven by amino acids or possibly protein metabolites that initially accumulate because of the reduction in total GFR.[30] It is known, for example, that a high-protein diet or the acute administration of amino acids can raise renal blood flow and the GFR.[30,31] How this occurs is uncertain, but humoral factors seem to have an important role since the increment in GFR can be prevented by the administration of somatostatin.[32,33]

Although beneficial initially, the high nephron filtration rate (or more likely the increase in intraglomerular pressure and flow) appears to damage the glomeruli in the long term, leading to proteinuria and glomerular sclerosis (see Chap. 4).[30,34] This deleterious effect of the hyperfiltration response is thought to contribute to the progression of renal failure in many patients, particularly those in whom the disease that produced the original renal damage is inactive or corrected (such as chronic pyelonephritis).[30,34] Prevention of these hemodynamic changes with a low-protein diet and/or correction of systemic hypertension (which will also tend to reduce intrarenal pressures) may be an effective way to preserve renal function.[6,34-36] For example, the patient with chronic pyelonephritis in Fig. 1–3 had progressive renal failure until the institution of a low-protein diet led to stabilization of renal function.

EXAMINATION OF THE URINE

A careful examination of the urine is the most important, noninvasive *diagnostic* tool available to the clinician. In contrast to the GFR, the findings on the urinalysis tell little about the severity of the disease, although they may point toward a specific diagnosis.

The urinalysis should be performed on a fresh specimen that is examined within 30 to 60 min of voiding. In males, a midstream specimen is usually satisfactory. However, in females, the external genitalia should first be cleaned to avoid contamination with vaginal secretions. The urine should be centrifuged at 3000 r/min for 3 to 5 min. Next, the supernatant should be carefully poured into a separate tube and the sediment completely resuspended by gently flicking the side of the tube. (When a large amount of sediment is present, 0.5 mL of urine can be added.) The sediment should be poured or transferred with a Pasteur pipette onto a slide and covered with a cover slip. Both the supernatant and sediment are then ready for detailed analysis.

COLOR

Normal urine is clear and has a light yellow color due to the presence of urochrome and other pigments. The urine will have a paler color when the urine output is high, as occurs after a water load or the administration of diuretics. Conversely, when the urine is concentrated, as after overnight water restriction, the color will be a darker yellow.

In addition to these physiologic variations, the urine color may, in certain conditions, be white (e.g., due to pyuria or phosphate crystals), green (e.g., due to the administration of methylene blue or amitriptyline), black (e.g., due to malignancy of the melanin-producing cells or ochronosis), or various shades of red or brown.[37-39] Although a complete review of these color phenomena is beyond the scope of this discussion, the finding of red or brown urine is not rare, and the workup of a patient with this abnormality should proceed in the following manner (Fig. 1–4). The urine should first be centrifuged. If the sediment is red* but the supernatant is clear, then hematuria is responsible for the red urine. However, if the supernatant is red to brown, it should be tested with a tablet (Hematest) or dipstick (Hemastix), both of which contain a dye, orthotolidine, which turns blue in the presence of heme. Red urine that is negative for heme can be produced by a variety of conditions including porphyria, the use of the bladder analgesic phenazopyridine, or the ingestion of beets in genetically susceptible subjects.[37] More commonly, the supernatant will be positive for heme, indicating the presence of hemoglobinuria or myoglobinuria.

Hemoglobinuria and myoglobinuria can

---

*Oxyhemoglobin is red but may be converted in an acid urine to methemoglobin which is brown.[40] Thus, hematuria or hemoglobinuria may be associated with red or brown urine. The urine color can also range from red to brown with myoglobinuria.

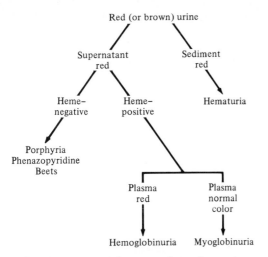

FIG. 1-4. Sequential approach to the patient with red or brown urine.

usually be distinguished by looking at the plasma which will be red with the former but will retain its normal color with the latter. Molecular size and plasma protein binding are responsible for this difference. Hemoglobin is released in states of intravascular hemolysis. It is rapidly bound to specific proteins (predominantly haptoglobin), and free hemoglobin appears in the plasma only when the protein binding capacity is exceeded. Hemoglobin is a tetramer ($\alpha_2\beta_2$) with a relatively high molecular weight (MW) of 68,000. Both free and protein-bound hemoglobin are too large to be significantly filtered across the glomerulus (see Fig. 1–6).[40,41] However, hemoglobin also exists as a smaller dimer ($\alpha_2\beta_2 \rightarrow \alpha\beta$, MW 34,000), a form in which it is more easily filtered.[40] The filtered dimer undergoes some reabsorption in the proximal tubule[42]; hemoglobinuria does not occur until the filtered load exceeds this reabsorptive capacity. Although this does not require a high plasma concentration of the dimer, the total hemoglobin concentration (protein-bound + tetramer + dimer) at this time generally exceeds 100 to 150 mg/dL[40,41] and the plasma will be red.

In contrast, myoglobin is released from damaged muscle. It has a molecular weight of only 17,000 and is not protein-bound. As a result, all the plasma myoglobin is freely filtered and rapidly excreted in the urine. Because of this rapid excretion, significant myoglobinemia does not occur (in the absence of renal failure) and the plasma retains its normal color.

PROTEINURIA

MECHANISMS

To understand how proteinuria occurs, it is first necessary to review the permeability characteristics of the glomerular capillary wall. This wall consists of three layers (Fig. 1–5): the fenestrated endothelium, the basement membrane, and the epithelial cells which are attached to the basement membrane by foot processes. The pores between the foot processes (slit pores) are closed by a thin membrane called the *slit diaphragm.*

The glomerular capillary wall is highly permeable to small solutes and water but shows a differential permeability to larger molecules (Fig. 1–6). Inulin, with MW 5200, is completely filtered, whereas albumin (MW 69,000) and ions (such as calcium) or drugs bound to albumin are filtered only to a limited degree. Below MW 60,000, there is a progressive increase in filtration. Thus, myoglobin (MW 17,000) is filtered more than albumin but less completely than inulin. The lack of albumin filtration is physiologically important since it prevents albumin loss in the urine, thereby preserving the plasma oncotic pressure.

The basement membrane appears to be the primary barrier to filtration, although the slit diaphragms between the foot processes may play a contributory role.[43,44] Nonfiltered

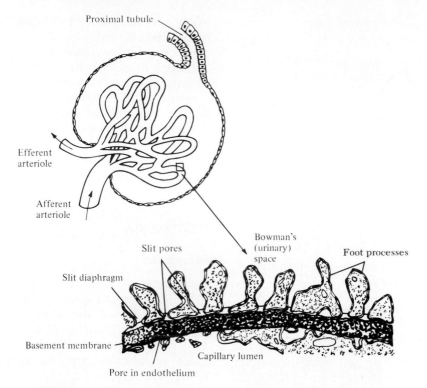

FIG. 1–5. Anatomy of the glomerulus. Bottom drawing shows the glomerular capillary wall which is composed of three layers: the epithelial cell (only the foot processes are shown), the basement membrane, and the capillary endothelium (*Adapted from R. Vander, Renal Physiology, 2d ed., McGraw-Hill, New York, 1980.*)

macromolecules that accumulate in the basement membrane are normally removed by phagocytosis by infiltrating both macrophages and the mesangial cells in the central part of the glomerular tuft.[45]

The inverse relationship between molecular size and the degree of filtration suggests that pores may exist within the basement membrane through which only molecules of a certain size can pass. However, pores have never been demonstrated by electron microscopy, suggesting that the size limitation to filtration may be a function of the molecular organization of the proteins in the basement membrane.

In addition to molecular size, molecular charge is the other major determinant of filtration.[43] The glomerular capillary wall contains sialoproteins and proteoglycans (such as heparan sulfate) that are negatively charged.[43,46] Most circulating macromolecules also are anionic within the physiologic pH range. Thus, it is possible that the limited filtration of albumin and other large proteins is due in part to electrostatic repulsion. Experiments using macromolecules such as dextran have confirmed this hypothesis. Anionic dextran sulfates of varying sizes are filtered to the same limited degree as endogenous proteins (Fig. 1–7). In comparison, there is markedly en-

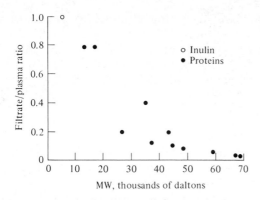

FIG. 1–6. Glomerular permeability to proteins. As the molecular weight falls below 70,000, there is a progressive increase in the ratio of the protein concentration in the filtrate to that in the plasma. The ratio of 1.0 for inulin indicates complete filtration of this substance. (*Adapted from F. Renkin and R. Robinson, N. Engl. J. Med., 290:785, 1974. Reprinted by permission from the New England Journal of Medicine.*)

constrict the efferent glomerular arteriole and tend to raise intraglomerular hydrostatic pressure.[50,51] The latter change could augment protein filtration by increasing effective pore size or by a direct hemodynamic effect.[48,49]

With these principles in mind, there are three mechanisms that have been shown in humans to be responsible for proteinuria resulting from increased glomerular permeability (see Chap. 5): (1) loss of the negative charges in the basement membrane[52,53]; (2) an increase in effective pore size or number due to direct damage to the basement membrane or possibly a change in the structure of the basement membrane resulting from the loss of anionic proteins[53,54]; or (3) the hemodynamic effects of angiotensin II and norepi-

hanced filtration of neutral and cationic dextrans: at the molecular size of albumin (36 Å), filtration is increased almost twentyfold with neutral and forty-five-fold with cationic dextran (Fig. 1–7). These results indicate that charge interaction with basement membrane proteins is an important factor in the limited filtration of macromolecules.*

The movement of macromolecules across the glomerular capillary wall is also influenced by vasoactive hormones such as angiotensin II and norepinephrine. Infusion of these hormones leads to mildly increased protein filtration and excretion.[48,49] The mechanism by which this occurs is incompletely understood. These hormones preferentially

*This charge limitation also is important in peripheral capillaries. The plasma oncotic pressure (determined primarily by albumin) acts to hold fluid in the vascular space. This effect is dependent upon the albumin concentration being high in the vascular space but low in the surrounding interstitium. The restricted movement of albumin across the capillary wall is due to its negative charge as well as its relatively large size.[47]

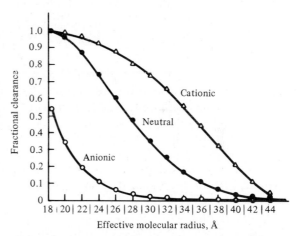

FIG. 1–7. Fractional clearances (the ratio of the filtration of a substance to that of inulin, which is freely filtered) of anionic, neutral, and cationic dextrans as a function of effective molecular radius. Both molecular size and charge are important as smaller or cationic molecules are more easily filtered. As a reference, the effective molecular radius of albumin is about 36 Å. (*From M. P. Bohrer, C. Baylis, H. D. Humes, R. J. Glassock, C. R. Robertson, and B. M. Brenner, J. Clin Invest., 61:72, 1978, by copyright permission of the American Society for Clinical Investigation.*)

nephrine, which may explain the mild proteinuria that may be seen in heart failure.[55] Glomerular proteinuria is characterized primarily by albuminuria although globulin excretion also may be increased.

Another type of proteinuria, called *tubular proteinuria* occurs when there is enhanced excretion of the normally filtered low-molecular-weight proteins, such as immunoglobulin light chains and β_2-microglobulin (MW less than 50,000).[56,57] Tubular proteinuria occurs in two settings: when proximal tubular reabsorption is impaired, as in the Fanconi syndrome; or when the production and subsequent filtration of low-molecular-weight proteins is increased to a level exceeding tubular reabsorptive capacity. The latter is most often seen in multiple myeloma with immunoglobulin light chains being excreted in the urine[58] but may also occur in acute monomyelocytic leukemia with lysozymuria.[59]

NORMAL VALUES

In normal subjects, low-molecular-weight proteins and small amounts of albumin are filtered. These proteins enter the proximal tubule where they are almost completely reabsorbed and then catabolized by the proximal tubular cells.[60] The net result is the daily protein excretion of less than 150 mg (usually 40 to 80 mg), of which approximately 10 mg is albumin.*[,56]

Abnormal proteinuria is generally defined as the excretion of more than 150 mg of protein per day. This definition is based on conventional methods used to measure total protein excretion. More sensitive assays that are not widely available can detect early renal disease with lesser degrees of proteinuria. In diabetic patients, for example, an

increase in resting albumin excretion to a rate exceeding 25 to 50 mg/day (with total protein excretion remaining in the normal range) is strongly predictive of the ultimate development of diabetic nephropathy (see p. 205).[61,62]

DETECTION

Analysis of a random urine specimen for protein should be performed on the supernatant since marked hematuria, pyuria, or uricosuria can result in a positive reading for protein if the unspun urine is used.[63] In most laboratories, the urine is tested for protein in one of two ways. The first method involves a dipstick (Albustix) impregnated with a dye, tetrabromophenol blue, which changes color according to the quantity of protein present. In the second method, 2.5 mL of supernatant is mixed with 7.5 mL of 3% sulfosalicylic acid. The degree of turbidity that ensues is proportional to the protein concentration (Table 1–2). False-positive results may occasionally be seen with either method (Table 1–3).[64] For example, patients with no kidney disease who take tolmetin (a nonsteroidal anti-inflammatory drug) may appear to have marked proteinuria when the urine is tested with sulfosalicylic acid.[65]

In general, the results obtained with the dipstick and sulfosalicylic acid correlate fairly well with each other and with exact measurement of the urinary protein concentration by immunoelectrophoresis.[63,66] However, there is one clinical situation in which the two methods give different results. The dipstick is most sensitive to albumin, whereas sulfosalicylic acid detects all proteins. Thus, the dipstick may be negative when low-molecular-weight proteins are in the urine, a finding that is often due to multiple myeloma with immunoglobulin light chain excretion.[63,67] In this setting, proteinuria could be missed if sulfosalicylic acid were not used. The presence of immunoglobulin light chains (Bence

---

*Not all the protein excreted in the urine is derived from glomerular filtration. Approximately 30 to 50 mg consists of Tamm-Horsfall mucoprotein, which is secreted by the cells in the loop of Henle (see "Sediment: Casts," below).

TABLE 1-2. Comparison of Methods of Measuring Urinary Protein Concentration

Protein Concentration, mg/dL	Dipstick*	Sulfosalicylic Acid
0	0	No turbidity
1–10	Trace	Slight turbidity
15–30	1^+	Turbidity through which print can be read
40–100	2^+	White cloud without precipitate through which heavy black lines on white background can be seen
150–350	3^+	White cloud with fine precipitate through which heavy black lines cannot be seen
>500	4^+	Flocculent precipitate

*The dipstick readings are graded from 0 to 4^+ depending on the color change produced.

Jones proteins) in the urine can be confirmed either by immunoelectrophoresis or by gradually heating the urine. Bence Jones proteins characteristically precipitate at 45 to 55°C and then redissolve when the temperature reaches 100°C.[68]

Thus, both the dipstick and sulfosalicylic acid should be used in testing the urine for protein. A more positive response with sulfosalicylic acid suggests the presence of nonalbumin proteins, whereas an equal response suggests that albumin is the principal urinary protein and that the primary disorder is an increase in glomerular permeability.

Although these tests are useful in documenting the presence of proteinuria, they may not be very accurate in assessing severity since the protein concentration is a function of urine volume as well as the quantity of protein present. For example, suppose a patient excretes 500 mg of protein per day. If the urine volume is 2 L, the protein concentration will be 25 mg/dL, resulting in a trace to 1^+ finding on the dipstick. However, if the urine volume is only 500 mL, the protein concentration will be 100 mg/dL and the dipstick will read 2^+. Thus the urine protein concentration should be correlated with the urine osmolality or specific gravity, measures of urinary concentration that tend to vary with the urine volume (see "Osmolality and Specific Gravity," below).

An accurate assessment of protein excretion is best achieved with a 24-h urine collection. This is diagnostically important since some renal disorders are associated with heavy proteinuria (greater than 3.5 g/day) and others with no or minimal proteinuria (see Chap. 2).

An alternative to a 24-h urine collection is to compare the concentrations (in milligrams per deciliter) of protein and creatinine (U_{prot}/U_{cr}) on a random daytime urine specimen.[69] Since

TABLE 1-3. False-Positive Results in Measurement of Urinary Protein Concentration

Condition	Dipstick	Sulfosalicylic Acid
Macroscopic hematuria	+	+
Urine pH > 8	+	−
Phenazopyridine	+	−
Radiocontrast media	−	+
High levels of penicillin or cephalosporin	−	+
Tolbutamide	−	+
Tolmetin	−	+
Sulfonamide	−	+

creatinine excretion is relatively constant, an increase in the U_{prot}/U_{cr} ratio represents an increase in protein excretion. (Changes in urinary concentration affect both parameters and do not change the ratio.)

The U_{prot}/U_{cr} ratio correlates closely with total protein excretion (in g/day per 1.73 m^2 body surface area). The normal value is less than 0.2 (or less than 200 mg per day); values of 1.0 and 3.5 represent total protein excretion of approximately 1.0 and 3.5 g/day per 1.73 m^2, respectively,[69] the latter being virtually diagnostic of glomerular disease. Since knowledge of the exact level of protein excretion is rarely necessary, the U_{prot}/U_{cr} ratio on a random urine specimen can be used to estimate the severity and follow the course of proteinuric patients.

pH

The urine pH reflects the degree of acidification of the urine and normally varies with systemic acid-base balance. In humans, the urine pH can range from 4.5 to 8.0 but usually is between 5.0 and 6.5. It is easily measured with a dipstick or paper containing dyes that change color according to the pH.

In certain conditions, the urine pH provides valuable clinical information.* A value above 7.0 to 7.5 suggests the possibility of a urinary tract infection with a urease-producing organism such as *Proteus mirabilis*. In this setting, the generation of ammonia (NH$_3$) from urinary urea directly raises the pH according to the Henderson-Hasselbalch equation:

$$pH = 9.3 + \log \frac{[NH_3]}{[NH_4^+]}$$

*The urine pH, osmolality, and sodium excretion are useful in the differential diagnosis of a variety of acid-base and electrolyte disorders. These principles are discussed in detail in Ref. 70. This section is primarily limited to the use of these parameters in the patient with renal disease.

The urine pH can also affect the urine sediment and possibly the development of kidney stones because of its effects on cast and crystal solubility (see "Sediment," below).

OSMOLALITY AND SPECIFIC GRAVITY

OSMOLALITY

The solute concentration of a solution is a function of the number of solute particles per unit volume and is most accurately measured by the osmolality of the solution.[71] In the plasma, where sodium salts are the primary solutes, the normal osmolality is roughly 285 mosmol/kg. Despite variations in solute and water intake, the plasma osmolality is normally maintained within very narrow limits because the kidney is able to excrete urine with an osmolality markedly different from that of the plasma.

These variations in the urine osmolality (U_{osm}) are mediated primarily by osmoreceptors in the hypothalamus that influence the secretion of antidiuretic hormone (ADH).[72] After a water load, for example, there is a transient reduction in the P_{osm}, which lowers ADH release. This diminishes water reabsorption in the collecting tubules, resulting in the excretion of the excess water in a dilute urine ($U_{osm} < P_{osm}$) in which the U_{osm} may fall to as low as 40 to 100 mosmol/kg.[73] Water restriction, on the other hand, sequentially raises the P_{osm}, ADH secretion, and renal water reabsorption, resulting in water retention and the excretion of a concentrated urine ($U_{osm} > P_{osm}$). The maximum U_{osm} that can be achieved in normal subjects is 900 to 1400 mosmol/kg.*,[74,75]

Antidiuretic hormone secretion also is stim-

*Maximum concentrating ability tends to fall with age. Thus, in a 70-year-old, the maximum urine osmolality may be only 650 mosmol/kg. This decrease in concentrating ability tends to be proportional to the decrease in the GFR that occurs with aging.[76]

ulated by effective circulating volume depletion.*,[72] This response, which is mediated primarily by the carotid sinus baroreceptors, is appropriate since the ensuing water retention will tend to restore normovolemia.

Because of the variation in urinary concentration with hydration and volume, a random U_{osm} has little diagnostic value unless correlated with the clinical state. Measurement of the U_{osm} is useful in patients with hyponatremia, hypernatremia, or polyuria[77] and in those with acute renal failure. The two most common causes of the latter disorder are effective volume depletion and acute tubular necrosis (see Chap. 3). Since volume depletion is a potent stimulus to the release of ADH, the U_{osm} may exceed 500 mosmol/kg in hypovolemic patients with otherwise well-preserved renal function.[78] In contrast, tubular dysfunction in acute tubular necrosis impairs concentrating ability, resulting in the excretion of urine with an osmolality between 1.0 and 1.2 times that of the plasma (the U_{osm} usually being between 300 and 350 mosmol/kg).[78,79] Thus, a high U_{osm} essentially *excludes* the diagnosis of acute tubular necrosis. The finding of a urine roughly isosmotic to plasma, however, is less useful diagnostically. It is consistent with acute tubular necrosis but does not rule out volume depletion if there is a concomitant impairment in concentrating ability, a common finding in the elderly or patients with underlying chronic renal disease.[76,80]

SPECIFIC GRAVITY

If an osmometer is not available, the concentration of the urine can be estimated by measuring the specific gravity. The *specific gravity* of a solution is defined as the weight of a given volume of the solution compared to that of an equal volume of distilled water.

*The definition of the effective circulating volume is discussed in Chap. 3.

For example, plasma is 0.8 to 1.0 percent heavier than water and therefore has a specific gravity of 1.008 to 1.010. In contrast to osmolality, which is dependent only on the number of particles in the solution, specific gravity is proportional to both the number and weight of the particles present.

In normal urine, in which the primary solutes are sodium and potassium salts, ammonium, and urea, the specific gravity varies in a reasonably predictable fashion with the osmolality (Fig. 1–8). However, when larger molecules, such as glucose, are present, there will be a disproportionate increase in the specific gravity, making it difficult to use this parameter to estimate urinary concentration. A frequent clinical example occurs after the administration of radiocontrast agents (MW

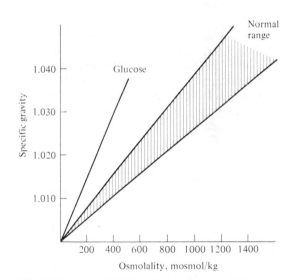

FIG. 1–8. Relationship between the specific gravity and osmolality of the urine from normal subjects who have neither glucose nor protein in the urine. For comparison, the relationship between the specific gravity and osmolality for glucose solutions is included. (*Adapted from B. Miles, A. Paton, and H. deWardener, Br. Med. J. 2:901, 1954. By permission of the British Medical Journal.*)

approximately 550). As these agents are excreted in the urine, the specific gravity can exceed 1.040, even though the osmolality may be similar to that of the plasma. The same effect can be produced by the antibiotic carbenicillin, which is given intravenously in large doses of 24 to 36 g/day.[81]

SODIUM EXCRETION

Urinary sodium excretion is normally determined by the extracellular fluid volume.[82] This relationship is based on the fact that body sodium is largely restricted to the extracellular space and acts osmotically to hold water in that space. Therefore, extracellular sodium stores are a main determinant of the volume of the extracellular fluid; this volume is maintained at a relatively constant level by appropriately varying sodium and water excretion in the urine.

In normal subjects, urinary sodium excretion roughly equals average dietary intake.[83] If volume expansion occurs after a salt load, normovolemia is restored by increasing sodium excretion in the urine. In this setting, the urine sodium concentration (U_{Na}) can exceed 100 meq/L. On the other hand, if vomiting or diarrhea results in volume depletion, further volume loss is minimized by markedly reducing sodium excretion. In normal subjects who become hypovolemic, the U_{Na} usually is less than 20 meq/L and may be as low as 1 meq/L.

These physiologic changes in sodium excretion are primarily mediated by alterations in tubular reabsorption, although changes in the GFR may play a contributory role. For example, a decrease in GFR and an increase in reabsorption in the proximal tubule, loop of Henle, and distal nephron all have been demonstrated in hypovolemic states.[82] A variety of factors participate in this response, including activation of the renin-angiotensin-aldosterone and sympathetic nervous systems and a reduction in systemic blood pressure.[82] These changes are reversed with volume expansion.[82,84]

Measuring the U_{Na} is useful in several clinical settings in which abnormal renal function may be present.[70] In particular, the U_{Na} (with the U_{osm}) is frequently helpful in distinguishing between effective volume depletion and acute tubular necrosis in patients with acute renal failure (see Chap. 3).[78,79,85] The U_{Na} generally exceeds 40 meq/L in the latter, in part because of the associated tubular damage and a consequent impairment in sodium reabsorption. In contrast, the U_{Na} is usually below 20 meq/L with volume depletion.

Since sodium excretion roughly reflects dietary intake, measurement of urinary sodium excretion (by obtaining a 24-h collection) can also be used to check dietary compliance in patients with essential hypertension. Restriction of sodium intake is frequently an important component of the therapeutic regimen (see p. 522), and adequate adherence should result in the excretion of less than 100 meq/day. The concurrent use of diuretics *does not interfere* with the utility of this test. For example, a thiazide diuretic initially increases sodium and water excretion by reducing sodium reabsorption in the distal tubule. However, the ensuing volume depletion enhances sodium reabsorption both in the distal nephron (via aldosterone) and the proximal tubule to prevent progressive fluid loss.[82] The net effect is the establishment (usually within 1 week) or a new steady state in which the plasma volume is somewhat diminished but sodium excretion is again equal to intake.[86]

Despite its usefulness, there are some pitfalls to relying upon the measurement of sodium excretion as an index of volume status. A low U_{Na}, for example, may be seen in *normovolemic patients* who have selective renal or glomerular ischemia due to bilateral renal artery stenosis or acute glomerulonephritis.[78,85,87] On the other hand, the U_{Na} may be inappropriately high in the presence of volume depletion if there is a defect in tubular sodium reabsorption. This may occur with the use of diuretics,* in aldosterone deficiency, or in advanced renal failure.[88]

The U_{Na} can also be influenced by the rate of water reabsorption. If there is a selective decrease in water reabsorption due to the absence of ADH (called diabetes insipidus), the urine output can exceed 10 L/day. In this setting, the daily excretion of 100 meq of sodium will be associated with a U_{Na} of 10 meq/L or less, incorrectly suggesting the presence of volume depletion. Conversely, a high rate of water reabsorption can raise the U_{Na} and mask the presence of hypovolemia. To correct for the effect of water reabsorption, the renal handling of sodium can be evaluated directly by calculating the fractional excretion of sodium (FE_{Na}).

FRACTIONAL EXCRETION OF SODIUM

The FE_{Na} can be calculated from a random urine specimen:

$$FE_{Na} \ (\%) = \frac{\text{quantity of Na excreted}}{\text{quantity of Na filtered}} \times 100$$

The quantity of sodium excreted is equal to the product of the U_{Na} and the urine flow rate (V); the quantity of sodium filtered is equal to the product of the plasma Na concentration (P_{Na}) and the glomerular filtration rate (or creatinine clearance = $U_{cr} \times V/P_{cr}$). Therefore,

$$FE_{Na} \ (\%) = \frac{U_{Na} \times V}{P_{Na} \ (U_{cr} \times V/P_{cr})} \times 100$$

$$= \frac{U_{Na} \times P_{cr}}{P_{Na} \times U_{cr}} \times 100$$

---

*Although chronic diuretic use does not prevent the attainment of a new steady state, a relatively high rate of sodium excretion, even if equal to intake, is still inappropriate in a hypovolemic patient.

The primary use of the FE_{Na} is in patients with acute renal failure. As described above, a low U_{Na} favors the diagnosis of volume depletion, whereas a high value points toward acute tubular necrosis. However, there is substantial overlap, particularly with a U_{Na} between 20 and 40 meq/L which may be seen with either disorder.[78,79,85] This overlap, which is due in part to variations in the rate of water reabsorption, can be minimized by calculating the FE_{Na}. Sodium reabsorption is appropriately enhanced in hypovolemic states, and the FE_{Na} is usually less than 1 percent; i.e., more than 99 percent of the filtered sodium is reabsorbed.[78,79,85] In contrast, tubular damage generally leads to an FE_{Na} in excess of 2 to 3 percent in acute tubular necrosis.[78,85,89] Exceptions to this rule do occur, however, as a low FE_{Na} may be seen in the latter disorder (see Chap. 3).[90]

The FE_{Na} is much less useful in patients with normal renal function. If the GFR is 180 L/day and the P_{Na} is 150 meq/L, then 27,000 meq of sodium will be filtered each day. Thus, the FE_{Na} will be under 1 percent if daily sodium intake is in the normal range of 125 to 250 meq, even if the patient is normovolemic. As a result, the U_{Na} is more helpful in diagnosing volume depletion unless a very low FE_{Na} is obtained, e.g., less than 0.2 percent.

CHLORIDE EXCRETION

Chloride is reabsorbed with sodium throughout the nephron. As a result, the rate of excretion of these ions is usually similar, and measurement of the urine chloride concentration (U_{Cl}) generally adds little to the information obtained from the more routinely measured U_{Na}. However, experimental studies employing a high-sodium, low-chloride diet indicate that chloride can be conserved independent of sodium, a response that appears to be mediated in part by active chloride reabsorption in the inner medullary collecting tubule.[91]

Similar findings may be seen in humans. As many as 30 percent of hypovolemic patients will have more than a 15 meq/L difference between the urine sodium and chloride concentrations.[92] This is due to the excretion of sodium with another anion (bicarbonate, carbenicillin) or chloride with another cation (ammonium, calcium). Thus it may be helpful to measure the U_{Cl} in a patient who seems to be volume-depleted but has a somewhat elevated U_{Na}. This most often occurs in metabolic alkalosis in which the urinary excretion of some of the excess bicarbonate as $NaHCO_3$ can elevate the U_{Na} (occasionally to over 100 meq/L), but the U_{Cl} will remain appropriately low.[93]

SEDIMENT

The urine sediment may contain cells, casts, crystals, and bacteria. From a diagnostic point of view, the presence or absence of certain findings is important. Of lesser concern is the quantity of cells or casts that are present. For example, 10 to 15 red cells per high power field (HPF) is just as significant as 50 to 60 red cells per HPF. Thus, measuring the total number of cells and casts excreted in a 24-h urine collection[94] is of no particular diagnostic value.

The sediment should first be inspected under a low-power objective with reduced light. The high, dry objective (400×) can then be used to identify the cells and casts that are present.*

*Newer dipsticks can detect white blood cells and bacteria as well as protein and heme with a high degree of accuracy.[95] Although useful as a screening test, they cannot replace examination of the urine sediment in patients with renal disease. The sediment in acute tubular necrosis, for example, characteristically shows epithelial cells and epithelial cell and granular casts, none of which would be detected by the dipstick.

RED CELLS

Red cells may be excreted in the urine from any site in the urinary tract. Careful examination of red cell morphology on a fresh urine specimen (particularly if viewed under phase contrast) may be very helpful in determining the site of bleeding.[96-98] In patients with extraglomerular lesions (such as stones or tumors), the red cells have a relatively uniform shape, being small, circular, and frequently orange-red, although the color may be leached out (Plate 1a). In comparison, the majority of red cells are *dysmorphic* with blebs, budding, and segmental loss of membrane in the presence of glomerular disease (Plate 1b). These changes could result from trauma to the cells as they pass through the damaged glomerular capillary wall or, possibly, to incomplete phagocytosis by tubular cells in the distal nephron.[96,99] If present, red cell casts and significant proteinuria (greater than 500 mg/day) also are characteristic of glomerular disease (see Chap. 2).

Yeast may occasionally be confused with red cells. However, yeasts are ovoid (not round), show budding, and frequently appear in chains.

WHITE CELLS

White cells are slightly larger than red cells and can be identified by their characteristic granular cytoplasm and multilobed nuclei (Plate 1c). When pyuria is the primary abnormality, particularly if the white cells are in clumps and bacteria are seen, infection at some site in the urinary tract should be strongly suspected. In this setting, the finding of white cell casts localizes the infection to the kidney. Tubulointerstitial diseases of the kidney, other than pyelonephritis, also are commonly characterized by pyuria and white cell casts (see Chap. 8). These findings may also be seen in other renal disorders such as acute glomerulonephritis and the

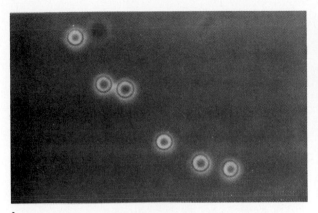

1a

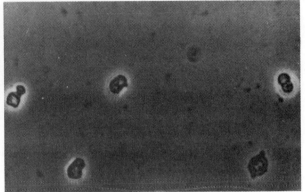

1b

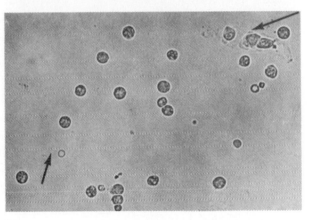

1c

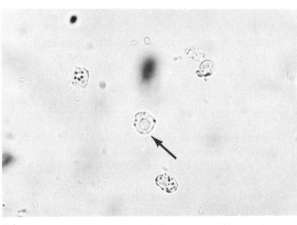

1d

PLATE 1. Cells in the urine sediment (*a*). Red blood cells with characteristic round appearance and no nucleus. Red cells may occasionally be confused with free fat droplets (see 1*f*) or yeast cells. The latter can be distinguished from red cells since they are ovoid, not round, and frequently show budding forms. (*b*) Dysmorphic "glomerular" red cells with varying shapes. (*c*) White blood cells with granular cytoplasm and multilobed nuclei. Red cells, which are smaller and have no nucleus (small arrow), and a white cell cast (large arrow) are also present. (*d*) Renal tubular epithelial cell (arrow) which is 1.5 to 3 times larger in diameter than a white cell and has a round nucleus. (*Plates 1, 2, and 3 prepared with the assistance of Drs. John Burton, Cecil Coggins, Andrew Cohen, and Allen Shuster; Plates 1a and 1b from R. G. Fassett, B. A. Horgan, and T. H. Mathew, Lancet, 1:1432, 1982; Plates 1f, 1g, and 2f from R. M. Kark, J. R. Lawrence, V. E. Pollak, C. L. Pirani, R. C. Muehrcke, and H. Silva: A Primer of Urinalysis, 2d ed., Harper & Row, New York, 1963. Reprinted by permission.*)

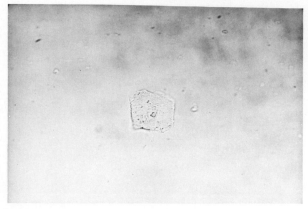

1e

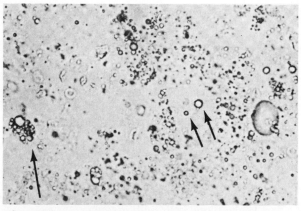

1f

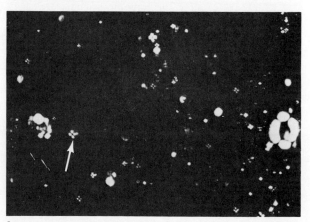

1g

PLATE 1 (Continued). (e) Large squamous epithelial cell with small nucleus. (f) Free fat droplets (small arrows) and an oval fat body (large arrow). Although they may appear similar to red cells, fat droplets have a dark outline, vary in size, and display anisotropism when viewed under polarized light. (g) The same field in 1e viewed under polarized light revealing "Maltese cross" appearance (as best exemplified by the arrow) of both the fat droplets and the oval fat body.

nephrotic syndrome. In these conditions, however, red cells, red cell casts, and/or proteinuria usually are the most prominent abnormalities.

In most diseases associated with pyuria, neutrophils are the primary leukocyte present. However, other white cells occasionally appear in the urine. Eosinophils may be seen in acute interstitial nephritis,[100] and lymphocytes may be found during a rejection episode in a patient with a renal transplant[101] or in those cases of interstitial nephritis[102] that are primarily due to the infiltration of lymphocytes.[103] When these diagnoses are suspected, eosinophils or lymphocytes can be identified by a Wright's stain of the urine sediment.

EPITHELIAL CELLS

Although epithelial cells may appear in the urine from the renal tubules, pelvis, ureters, bladder, urethra, or vagina, only tubular cells are of diagnostic importance. Renal tubular cells are 1.5 to 3 times the size of a white cell with a round, large nucleus (Plate 1*d*). Although cells from the lower urinary tract tend to be larger with a small nucleus (Plate 1*e*), they may look similar to those from the renal tubules. Thus, the presence of epithelial cells in casts is the only way to be certain of their renal origin. Occasional renal epithelial cells may be seen in the normal sediment and presumably reflect wear and tear. Increased numbers of epithelial cells may be shed in the urine in many renal diseases including acute tubular necrosis, glomerulonephritis, pyelonephritis, and the nephrotic syndrome.

In glomerular diseases associated with proteinuria, the tubular cells may undergo fatty degeneration with droplets appearing in the cytoplasm (Plate 1*f*).[104,105] These droplets are composed primarily of cholesterol esters and, to a lesser degree, cholesterol. When viewed under polarized light, they are doubly refractile (anisotropic) and reveal a characteristic "Maltese cross" appearance (Plate 1*g*). These cells are referred to as *oval fat bodies.* The fat droplets also may be free in the urine where they are circular and the same size as or smaller than a red cell. They can be differentiated from red cells by their variable size, dark outline, and the appearance of the Maltese crosses under polarized light.

The origin of this lipid is unclear.[105] It seems likely that lipoprotein-bound chlolesterol is filtered (a process that occurs only when glomerular permeability is increased) and then partially taken up by the tubular cells. The cholesterol appears in the sediment as an oval fat body when the cell is desquamated or as free fat droplets if the lipid is extruded from the cell.

CASTS

Many different kinds of casts may be observed in the sediment. In contrast to clumps of cells, true casts are cylindrical and have regular margins, since they conform to the shape of the tubular lumen in which they are formed. *The intrarenal origin of casts is central to their diagnostic value.* For example, red cell casts indicate a renal source of bleeding.

A simple classification of urinary casts is presented in Table 1–4. All casts have an organic matrix composed primarily of Tamm-Horsfall mucoprotein,[106,107] a protein that is secreted by the tubular cells in the thick ascending limb of the loop of Henle.[108,109] Approximately 30 to 50 mg of Tamm-Horsfall mucoprotein is excreted per day.[110]

The chemical characteristics of this protein tend to define the conditions in which casts are seen. Tamm-Horsfall mucoprotein becomes less soluble in the presence of an acid urine or a high electrolyte concentration or in conditions associated with tubular stasis or proteinuria.[111] Since the urine is most concentrated and acidic in the collecting tubules, casts form primarily in these seg-

TABLE 1–4. Classification of Urinary Casts

Type of Cast	Clinical Significance
Hyaline	Not indicative of renal disease. Seen primarily with small volume of concentrated urine or after diuretics.
Cellular	
Red cell	Virtually diagnostic of glomerulonephritis or vasculitis.
White cell	With pyuria alone, suggests a tubulointerstitial disorder such as pyelonephritis. Also may be one of findings in glomerular diseases.
Epithelial cell	Seen with tubular damage in acute tubular necrosis, other tubulointerstitial diseases, or exudative glomerulonephritis.
Fatty	Found in glomerular diseases associated with moderate to heavy proteinuria.
Granular	May represent degenerating cellular cast or aggregated proteins. Seen in many diseases.
Waxy and broad	Indicative of advanced renal failure.
Mixed and degenerating	Same meaning as the pure cellular casts if cellular constituents can be identified.

ments.[108] The relation to urinary stasis favors cast formation in oliguric nephrons or in collecting tubules into which poorly functioning nephrons drain. On the other hand, casts usually are not seen when the urine is very dilute (osmolality less than 150 mosmol/kg or specific gravity less than 1.004) or when the urine pH is greater than 6.5.[112,113]

When conditions favor protein precipitation, a process that has been likened to the setting of gelatin, any cells within the lumen will be trapped in the cast, resulting in a cellular cast. When the lumen is clear, the cast will be composed primarily of mucoprotein. These casts are called *hyaline casts* and have an optical density only slightly greater than that of the urine. Consequently, they are best seen under reduced light or particularly under phase contrast (Plate 2*a* and *b*).[114]

Hyaline casts are not indicative of renal disease. Since effective circulating volume depletion, e.g., due to gastrointestinal losses, results in the excretion of a small volume of an acidic, concentrated urine, it can be associated with more than 10 hyaline casts per HPF. Similarly, diuretics such as ethacrynic acid or furosemide produce an acid urine with a relatively high sodium chloride concentration. Since these conditions promote muco-

protein precipitation, hyaline cast excretion is markedly increased by these agents.[110]

In contrast to hyaline casts, cellular casts are associated with renal diseases characterized by increased excretion of cells. *Red cell* casts are identified by the characteristic shape of red cells within the cast (Plate 2*c*). Their color can range from orange-red to pale if the hemoglobin has been lost from the cells. Red cell casts almost always indicate glomerulonephritis or vasculitis, although an occasional red cell cast can rarely be seen in other conditions such as renal atheroemboli or interstitial nephritis.[115,116]

White cell and *epithelial cell casts* are identified by finding the respective cells within casts (Plate 2*d* and *e*). White cell casts may be found in tubulointerstitial diseases, acute glomerulonephritis, or the nephrotic syndrome. The latter two disorders, however, are characterized by many other findings in the urine such as moderate to heavy proteinuria, hematuria, and red cell casts. Epithelial cell casts can be seen in those conditions associated with increased desquamation of epithelial cells such as acute tubular necrosis or acute glomerulonephritis. *Fatty casts* are epithelial cell or granular casts in which doubly refractile fat droplets are observed

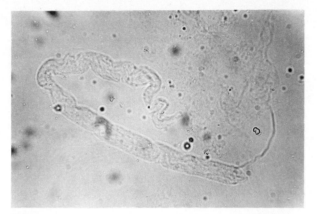

2*a*

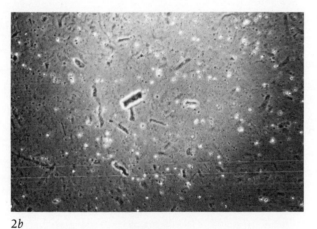

2*b*

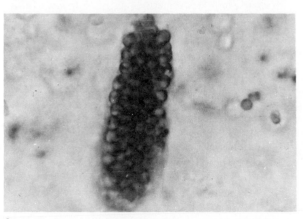

2*c*

PLATE 2. Casts in the urine sediment. (*a*) Hyaline cast, which is only slightly more refractile than water. (*b*) Multiple small hyaline casts can be easily visualized when viewed under phase-contrast. A large granular cast is present in the center of the field. (*c*) Red blood cell cast. Although this cast contains tightly packed red cells, it is more common to see fewer red cells trapped within a hyaline or granular cast.

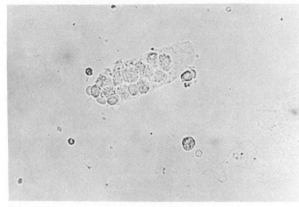

2*d*

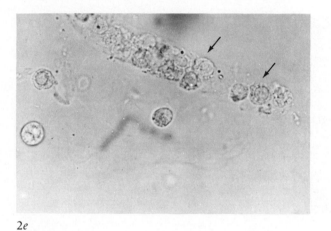

2*e*

2*f*

PLATE 2 (Continued). (*d*) White cell cast. (*e*) Renal tubular epithelial cell cast. Discrete tubular cells (arrows) can be identified within the matrix of a hyaline cast. (*f*) Fatty cast. The fat droplets within the cast can be differentiated from red cells by their dark outlines, variable size, and "Maltese cross" appearance under polarized light (see Plate 1*g*).

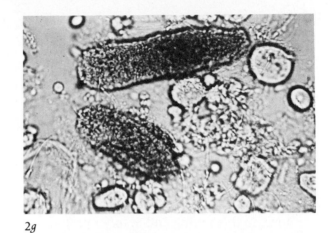

2*g*

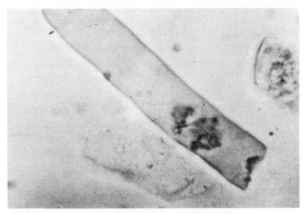

2*h*

PLATE 2 (Continued). (*g*) Granular casts. (*h*) Waxy cast, which may represent a degenerated granular cast. (*i*) Broad granular cast, which is wider than other casts and is usually seen only with advanced renal failure.

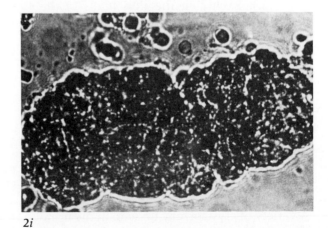

2*i*

(Plate 2*f*). These casts are seen primarily in diseases associated with heavy proteinuria (greater than 3 g/day).

Granular and *waxy casts* are thought to represent successive stages in the degeneration of cellular casts as they course through the nephron (Plate 2*g* and *h*).[111] This theory is based on the observation of cellular, combined cellular and granular, and combined granular and waxy casts in the same urine. However, the finding of granular casts in the urine of normal subjects after exercise suggests that they can on occasion be formed de novo. In this setting and in other proteinuric states as well, the granules may represent aggregated serum proteins that are trapped within the cast, rather than degenerated cells.[107,117] Granular casts are homogeneous with fine or coarse stippling. In contrast, waxy casts have an amorphous appearance. They can be differentiated from hyaline casts by their high optical density, which allows them to be seen even under bright light. Since the degeneration of a cast from cellular to granular to waxy is relatively slow, waxy casts are thought to occur in nephrons with markedly diminished flow and therefore are seen primarily in advanced renal failure.[118]

Broad casts are wider than other casts and tend to have a granular or waxy appearance (Plate 2*i*). Excluding the thin limbs of the loop of Henle, the tubular diameter is relatively uniform up to the collecting tubules into which many nephrons drain. Thus, broad casts are thought to form in these wider tubules when urinary stasis occurs because of the presence of large numbers of nonfunctioning or poorly functioning nephrons. Consequently, broad casts appear in the urine only in severe acute or chronic renal insufficiency and have been called "renal failure" casts.[118]

CRYSTALS

A variety of crystals may be seen in the urine (Plate 3). Their presence is determined by the relationship between three factors: (1) the degree of supersaturation which is primarily a function of the molar concentrations of the reactants, e.g., of calcium and oxalate for calcium oxalate crystals; (2) the presence or absence of inhibitors of crystallization; and (3) the urine pH which can affect the solubility and ionic composition of crystal-forming substances. For example, uric acid crystals and amorphous urates are seen in an acid urine (urine pH less than 6.0), whereas calcium phosphate crystals and amorphous phosphates are found in a relatively alkaline urine (urine pH greater than 7.0), which is usually due to infection with an urease-producing organism. In contrast, calcium oxalate and cystine crystallization are relatively independent of physiologic variations in pH. (Cystine does become much more soluble when the urine pH is greater than 7.4, an unusual occurrence in the absence of infection.)

The presence of crystals in the urine is of little diagnostic importance unless seen in the following settings. First, cystine crystals with their characteristic hexagonal shape are diagnostic of cystinuria.[120] Second, acute renal failure with calcium oxalate deposition in the tubules and calcium oxalate crystals in the urine may occur when oxalate production is markedly increased as with ethylene glycol ingestion (see p. 429).[121] Third, many uric acid crystals may be seen with acute renal failure due to uric acid deposition in the tubules. This usually occurs after an acute massive increase in uric acid production, which may follow the use of cytotoxic agents in malignant lymphoma.[122]

THE NORMAL URINALYSIS

Studies by Addis on 24-h urine collections showed that normal subjects excrete up to 1 million red cells, 3 million white and epithelial cells, and 10,000 casts (almost all hyaline) per day.[94] When examining a random

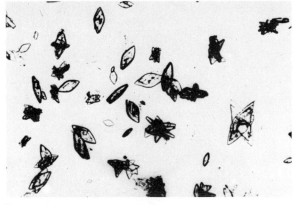

3a

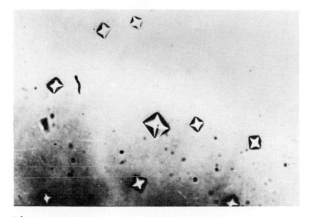

3b

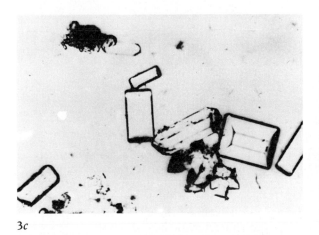

3c

PLATE 3. Crystals in the urine sediment. (*a*) Uric acid crystals, which are yellow or reddish-brown and are seen only in an acid urine. These crystals are pleomorphic, most often appearing as rhombic plates or rosettes. (*b*) Calcium oxalate crystals with "envelope" appearance. These crystals may also assume a dumbbell shape. (*c*) "Coffin-lid" ammonium magnesium phosphate crystals which form only in an alkaline urine.

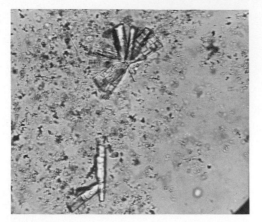

3d

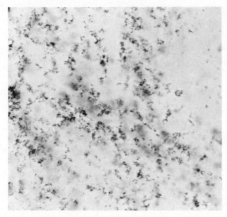

3e

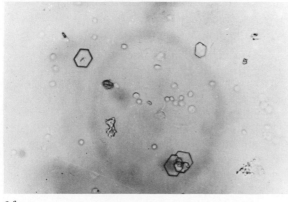

3f

PLATE 3 (Continued). (*d*) Calcium phosphate crystals with wedge-shaped stellate appearance. (*e*) Amorphous sludge, which usually represents either urates (acid urine) or phosphates (alkaline urine). (*f*) Cystine crystals with characteristic hexagonal shape.

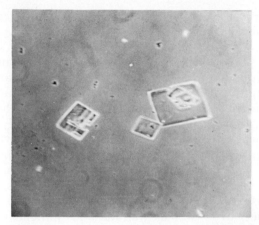

3*g*

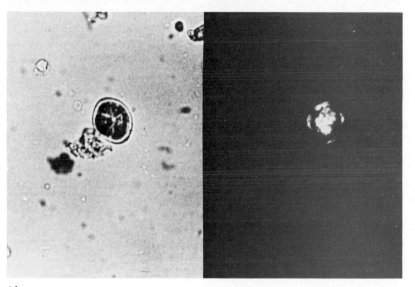

3*h*

PLATE 3 (Continued). (*g*) Cholesterol plates which may rarely be seen with atheroemboli to the kidney. (*h*) In some cases, extraneous material may contaminate the urine. Here, the appearance of talc crystals under both regular and polarized light is shown. The diuretic triamterene can form similar crystals in the urine.[119]

urine, this translates into 0 to 4 white cells and 0 to 2 red cells per HPF*,[123,124] and one cast every 10 to 20 low-power fields. Occasional uric acid, calcium oxalate, or phosphate crystals may also be present, depending in part on the urine pH. In addition, up to 150 mg of protein per day is considered normal. If the urine volume is 1 L, this represents a protein concentration of 15 mg/dL. Thus, either the dipstick or sulfosalicylic acid may register a trace to 1+ reaction.

Although the excretion of more cells, casts, or protein may be indicative of renal disease, it is important to be aware that a variety of stimuli such as severe exercise, fever, heart failure, and standing erect can produce transient changes in the urine in normal subjects.[125-132]

For example, mild proteinuria (usually less than 1 g/day), hyaline and granular casts, and some cells may be found in patients with heart failure or infection.[55,127-132] The mechanism by which these changes occur is incompletely understood. The above conditions tend to be associated with increased circulating levels of angiotensin II and/or norepinephrine. These hormones can produce proteinuria by their hemodynamic effects and possibly by increasing glomerular pore size.[48,49,133] Tubular damage, due to ischemia or infection, also may contribute since some patients have a preferential increase in the excretion of low-molecular-weight proteins ("tubular proteinuria").[132]

A second example occurs in runners who may have hematuria after completing a long race.[125,126] Although bladder trauma was thought to contribute to this problem, the concurrent findings of hyaline and granular casts, mild proteinuria, and dysmorphic changes in

the red cells (see Plate 1b) suggest a glomerular origin.[125,134] However, short-term intense exercise can induce proteinuria that has both glomerular and tubular components, indicating that some element of tubular dysfunction also contributes.[135] As with heart failure and infection, humoral factors may be responsible for these changes in the urinalysis.[135]

Another clinical disorder in which urinary abnormalities can be seen without apparent kidney disease is jaundice. In many patients with jaundice due to hepatitis, cirrhosis, or biliary obstruction, free renal tubular cells as well as granular and epithelial cell casts may be observed.[136] The mechanism by which these changes occur is not known. Marked hyperbilirubinemia is associated with decreased vascular resistance and impaired responsiveness to pressors such as angiotensin II and norepinephrine.[137] Thus, it is possible that ischemic tubular damage is responsible for the urinary abnormalities which disappear with recovery from the underlying disease.

In summary, because of the variety of conditions that can induce functional changes in the urinalysis, it is important to know the clinical status of the patient before assuming that urinary abnormalities indicate the presence of renal disease.

RADIOLOGIC STUDIES

A variety of radiologic studies are also used in the evaluation of patients with kidney disease. Table 1–5 depicts the general kinds of information that can be obtained from these tests. The characteristic findings seen in specific diseases are discussed in the following chapters.

RENAL BIOPSY

A renal biopsy is performed in patients with intrinsic renal disease when less invasive pro-

---

*The number of cells observed per HPF obviously can be influenced by the volume of supernatant in which the sediment is resuspended after centrifugation. To minimize excessive dilution, which can result in mild degrees of hematuria or pyuria being missed, the supernatant should be poured off as completely as possible unless a large amount of sediment is present.

TABLE 1-5. Major Uses of Radiologic Studies in Renal Disease

Test	Uses
Plain film of the abdomen	Kidney size and shape Evaluation of patients with radioopaque kidney stones
Intravenous pyelogram	Kidney size, shape, and caliceal anatomy Detection of site and, in many cases, cause of obstruction (Ultrasound or CT scan is preferred to document presence of obstruction.) Diagnosis of diseases with characteristic anatomic changes such as chronic pyelonephritis, medullary sponge kidney, and papillary necrosis Screening for renovascular hypertension (Renal scan or renal angiography is preferred.) In renal trauma, detection of renal arterial occlusion (by nonvisualization) or extravasation
Ultrasonography and CT scanning	Evaluation for urinary tract obstruction Evaluation of renal mass (cyst versus tumor) Early diagnosis of polycystic kidney disease Detection of nonopaque kidney stones
Radionuclide studies	Screening for renovascular hypertension Screening for renal thromboembolic disease Prognosis of acute renal failure Detection of vesicoureteral reflux
Renal arteriography	Direct visualization of renal arterial system for renovascular hypertension, polyarteritis nodosa, thromboembolic disease, or diagnosis of renal mass which is suspicious of tumor on ultrasound or CT scanning
Voiding cystourethrogram	Detection of vesicoureteral reflux (can be done noninvasively with radionuclide sudy)
Retrograde pyelography	Determination of site of obstruction Relief of obstruction (catheters inserted)
Percutaneous nephrostomy	Determination of site of obstruction Relief of obstruction (catheters inserted) Extract or pulverize renal calculi Instill drugs for dissolution of renal calculi

cedures such as the urinalysis and radiologic studies are not able to establish the correct diagnosis. Statistically, most biopsies are done in patients with glomerular disease or vasculitis. Although these disorders usually have characteristic urinary findings such as proteinuria, hematuria, and red cell casts, a biopsy is performed because there are many different types of glomerular disease and vasculitis with differing prognoses and responses to therapy (see Chaps. 6 and 7).

A percutaneous renal biopsy is the most common technique employed. In this pro-

cedure, the kidney is localized, usually by ultrasonography, although CT scanning or fluoroscopy can also be used.[138] A biopsy needle is then inserted into the kidney through a posterior approach and tissue obtained for examination by light, electron, and immunofluorescent microscopy (see Chaps. 5 and 6).

Bleeding is the major complication of a percutaneous biopsy. In most patients, the amount of blood lost is relatively small, with little change in hematocrit or blood pressure.[139] However, since more severe bleeding may occur requiring transfusions or, rarely, surgical intervention, general contraindications to percutaneous biopsy are a bleeding disorder, diastolic blood pressure greater than 110 mmHg (which usually can be controlled with antihypertensive medications), a renal mass (which can be avoided by biopsying the opposite kidney), or a single functioning kidney. In the latter circumstance or if a percutaneous biopsy has been unsuccessful, renal tissue can be obtained surgically. Although a larger specimen of tissue is obtained, open renal biopsy has the added potential problems of wound healing and infection and should be performed only when necessary.

Formation of a renal arteriovenous fistula is another complication that occurs in up to 5 to 15 percent of percutaneous biopsies. Although most patients remain asymptomatic, hematuria (which may be grossly visible), hypertension, abdominal or flank pain, or high-output heart failure may occur.[140] The diagnosis is established by renal arteriography. Specific treatment is usually not necessary since most fistulas close spontaneously within 1 to 18 months. In some patients, however, invasive radiologic techniques or surgery is required to close the fistula.[140]

SUMMARY

Measurement of the GFR and careful examination of the urine are essential parts of the evaluation of any patient with renal disease. Since the GFR is a rough index of the functioning renal mass, it can be used both to estimate the severity and to follow the course of known kidney disease. The clinical deter-mination of the GFR is most easily performed by measuring the endogenous C_{cr}. Once this has been done, changes in the GFR can be detected by serial measurements of the P_{cr}, which varies inversely with the GFR in the steady state. An increase in the P_{cr} suggests either progression of the underlying disease or a superimposed problem such as volume depletion. Because of the variability in urea production and tubular reabsorption, the BUN is a less accurate measure of the GFR than the P_{cr}.

When examining the urine, the finding of cells, casts, or crystals in the sediment or proteinuria may be of diagnostic importance. In contrast to the GFR, the urinalysis does not correlate well with disease severity, and, in certain conditions, the urinalysis may become less abnormal as the disease progresses.[112,113] In glomerulonephritis, for example, the progression from active inflammation to glomerular scarring typically results in a less active urinary sediment, with fewer cells and casts. Similarly, the associated fall in GFR decreases the quantity of albumin filtered and usually the amount excreted. Thus, following only the urinalysis would lead to the erroneous conclusion that the disease process had improved.

Radiologic studies and renal biopsy also may provide important diagnostic information. The former are particularly important in disorders with anatomic abnormalities such as urinary tract obstruction, chronic pyelonephritis, or polycystic kidney disease. A renal biopsy is performed in patients with intrinsic kidney disease when the specific diagnosis cannot be established by less invasive procedures.

REFERENCES

1. Rose, B. D.: *Clinical Physiology of Acid-Base and Electrolyte Disorders,* 2d ed., McGraw-Hill, New York, 1984.

2. Barbour, G. L., C. K. Crumb, C. M. Boyd, R. D. Reeves, S. P. Rastogil, and R. M. Patterson: Comparison of inulin, iothalamate, and ^{99m}Tc-DTPA

for measurement of glomerular filtration rate, *J. Nucl. Med.,* 17:317, 1976.

3. Doolan, P. D., E. L. Alpen, and G. B. Theil: A clinical appraisal of the plasma concentration and endogenous clearance of creatinine, *Am. J. Med.,* 32: 65, 1962.

4. Tobias, G. J., R. F. McLaughlin, Jr., and J. Hopper, Jr.: Endogenous creatinine clearance: A valuable clinical test of glomerular filtration and prognostic guide in chronic renal disease, *N. Engl. J. Med.,* 266:317, 1962.

5. Bennett, W. M., and G. A. Porter: Endogenous creatinine clearance as a clinical measure of glomerular filtration rate, *Br. Med. J.,* 4:84, 1971.

6. Mitch, W. E., M. Walser, T. I. Steinman, S. Hill, S. Zeger, and K. Tungsanga: The effect of a keto acid-amino acid supplement to a restricted diet on the progression of chronic renal failure, *N. Engl. J. Med.,* 311:623, 1984.

7. Hollenberg, N. K., D. F. Adams, H. S. Solomon, A. Rashid, H. L. Abrams, and J. P. Merrill: Senescence and renal vasculature in normal man, *Circ. Res.,* 34:309, 1974.

8. Guignard, J. P., A. Torrado, O. DaCumba, and E. Gautier: Glomerular filtration rate in the first three weeks of life, *J. Pediatr.,* 87:268, 1975.

9. Loggie, J. M., L. I. Kleinman, and E. F. VanMaanen: Renal function and diuretic therapy in infants and children, *J. Pediatr.,* 86:485, 1975.

10. Dodge, W. F., L. B. Travio, and C. W. Daeschner: Comparison of endogenous creatinine clearance with inulin clearance, *Am. J. Dis. Child.,* 113:683, 1967.

11. Siersbaek-Nielsen, K., J. M. Hansen, J. Kampmann, and M. Kristensen: Rapid evaluation of creatinine clearance, *Lancet,* 1:1133, 1971.

12. Schwartz, G. J., G. B. Haycock, and A. Spitzer: Plasma creatinine and urea concentration in children: Normal values for age and sex, *J. Pediatr.,* 88:828, 1976.

13. Cutler, R. E., A. M. Gyselynck, P. Fleet, and A. W. Forrey: Correlation of serum creatinine concentration and gentamicin half life, *J. Am. Med. Assoc.,* 219:1037, 1972.

14. Hamilton, R. W., L. B. Gardner, A. S. Penn, and M. Goldberg: Acute tubular necrosis caused by exercise-induced myoglobinuria, *Ann. Intern. Med.,* 77: 77, 1972.

15. Jacobsen, F. K., C. K. Christensen, C. E. Mogensen, F. Andreasen, and N. S. C. Heilskov: Pronounced increase in serum creatinine after eating cooked meat, *Br. Med. J.,* 1:1049, 1979.

16. Cockcroft, D. W., and M. H. Gault: Prediction of creatinine clearance from serum creatinine, *Nephron,* 16:13, 1976.

17. Mitch, W. E., M. Walser, G. A. Buffington, and J. Lemann, Jr.: A simple method of estimating progression of chronic renal failure, *Lancet,* 2:1326, 1976.

18. Dubb, J. W., R. M. Stote, R. G. Familiar, K. Lee, and F. Alexander: Effect of cimetidine on renal function in normal man, *Clin. Pharmacol. Therap.,* 24:76, 1978.

19. Berglund, F., J. Killander, and R. Pompeius: Effect of trimethoprim-sulfamethoxazole on the renal excretion of creatinine in man, *J. Urol.,* 114:802, 1975.

20. Molitch, M. E., E. Rodman, C. A. Hirsch, and E. Dubinsky: Spurious serum creatinine elevations in ketoacidosis, *Ann. Intern. Med.,* 93:280, 1980.

21. Mascioli, S. R., J. P. Bantle, E. F. Freier, and B. J. Hoogwerf: Artifactual elevation of serum creatinine level due to fasting, *Arch. Intern. Med.,* 144: 1575, 1984.

22. Saah, A. J., T. R. Koch, and G. L. Drusano: Cefoxitin falsely elevates creatinine levels, *J. Am. Med. Assoc.,* 247:205, 1982.

23. Mitchell, E. K.: Flucytosine and false elevation of serum creatinine level (letter), *Ann. Intern. Med.,* 101:278, 1984.

24. Rocci, M. L., Jr., P. H. Vlasses, and R. K. Ferguson: Creatinine serum concentrations and H_2-receptor antagonists, *Clin. Nephrol.,* 22:214, 1984.

25. Dossetor, J. B.: Diagnosis and treatment, creatininemia versus uremia: The relative significance of blood urea nitrogen and serum creatinine concentrations in azotemia, *Ann. Intern. Med.,* 65:1287, 1966.

26. Smith, H. W., W. Goldring, and H. Chasis: The measurement of the tubular excretory mass, effective blood flow and filtration rate in the normal human kidney, *J. Clin. Invest.,* 17:263, 1938.

27. Lubowitz, H., E. Slatopolsky, S. Shankel, R. E. Rieselbach, and N. S. Bricker: Glomerular filtration rate: Determination in patients with chronic renal disease, *J. Am. Med. Assoc.,* 199:252, 1967.

28. Deen, W. M., D. A. Maddox, C. R. Robertson, and B. M. Brenner: Dynamics of glomerular ultrafiltration in the rat. VII. Response to reduced renal mass, *Am. J. Physiol.,* 227:556, 1974.

29. Hostetter, T. H., J. L. Olson, H. G. Rennke, M. A. Venkatachalam, and B. M. Brenner: Hyperfiltration in remnant nephrons: A potentially adverse response to renal ablation, *Am. J. Physiol.,* 241:F85, 1981.

30. Brenner, B. M., T. W. Meyer, and T. H. Hostetter:

Dietary protein intake and the progressive nature of kidney disease: The role of hemodynamically mediated glomerular injury in the pathogenesis of progressive glomerular sclerosis in aging, renal ablation, and intrinsic renal disease, *N. Engl. J. Med.,* 307:652, 1983.

31. Bosch, J. P., A. Lauer, and S. Glabman: Short-term protein loading in assessment of patients with renal disease, *Am. J. Med.,* 77:873, 1984.

32. Premen, A. J., J. E. Hall, and M. J. Smith, Jr.: Post-prandial regulation of renal hemodynamics: Role of pancreatic glucagon, *Am. J. Physiol.,* 248:F656, 1985.

33. Castellino, P., B. Coda, and R. A. DeFronzo: Effect of amino acid infusion on renal hemodynamics in humans, *Am. J. Physiol.,* 251:F132, 1986.

34. Brenner, B. M.: Nephron adaptation to renal injury or ablation, *Am. J. Physiol.,* 249:F324, 1985.

35. Maschio, G., L. Oldrizzi, N. Tessitore, A. D'Angelo, E. Valvo, A. Lupo, C. Loschiavo, A. Fabris, L. Gammaro, C. Rugiu, and G. Panzetta: Effects of dietary protein and phosphorus restriction on the progression of early renal failure, *Kidney Int.,* 22: 371, 1982.

36. Mogensen, C. E.: Long-term antihypertensive treatment inhibiting progression of diabetic nephropathy, *Br. Med. J.,* 285:685, 1982.

37. Baran, R. B., and E. Rowles: Factors affecting coloration of urine and feces, *J. Am. Pharm. Assoc.,* 13:139, 1973.

38. Cone, T. E.: Diagnosis and treatment: Some syndromes, diseases, and conditions associated with abnormal coloration of the urine or diaper, *Pediatrics,* 41:654, 1968.

39. Evans, B.: The greening of urine: Still another "Cloret sign" (letter), *N. Engl. J. Med.,* 300:202, 1979.

40. Pimstone, N. R.: Renal degradation of hemoglobin, *Semin. Hematol.,* 9:31, 1972.

41. Lathem, W.: The renal excretion of hemoglobin: Regulatory mechanisms and the differential excretion of free and protein-bound hemoglobin, *J. Clin. Invest.,* 38:652, 1959.

42. Lowenstein, J., D. A. Faulstick, M. J. Yiengst, and N. W. Shock: The glomerular clearance and renal transport of hemoglobin in adult males, *J. Clin. Invest.,* 40:1172, 1961.

43. Brenner, B. M., T. H. Hostetter, and H. D. Humes: Molecular basis of proteinuria of glomerular origin, *N. Engl. J. Med.,* 298:826, 1978.

44. Venkatachalam M. A., and H. G. Rennke: The structure and molecular basis of glomerular filtration, *Circ. Res.,* 43:337, 1978.

45. Kreisberg, J. I., and M. J. Karnovsky: Glomerular cells in culture, *Kidney Int.,* 23:439, 1983.

46. Kerjaschki, D., A. T. Vernillo, and M. G. Farquhar: Reduced sialation of podocalyxin—the major sialoprotein of rat kidney glomerulus—in aminonucleoside nephrosis, *Am. J. Pathol.,* 118:343, 1985.

47. Vehaskari, V. M., C. T.-C. Chang, J. K. Stevens, and A. M. Robson: The effects of polycations on vascular permeability in the rat, *J. Clin. Invest.,* 73:1053, 1984.

48. Bohrer, M. P., W. M. Deen, C. R. Robertson, and B. M. Brenner: Mechanisms of angiotensin II-induced proteinuria in the rat, *Am. J. Physiol.,* 233:F13, 1977.

49. Olivetti, G., K. Kithier, F. Giacomelli, and J. Wiener: Characterization of glomerular permeability and proteinuria in acute hypertension in the rat, *Kidney Int.,* 25:599, 1984.

50. Edwards, R. M.: Segmental effects of norepinephrine and angiotensin II on isolated renal microvessels, *Am. J. Physiol.,* 244:F526, 1983.

51. Myers, B. D., W. M. Deen, and B. M. Brenner: Effects of norepinephrine and angiotensin II on the determinants of glomerular ultrafiltration and proximal tubule fluid reabsorption in the rat, *Circ. Res.,* 37:101, 1975.

52. Vernier, R. L., D. J. Klein, S. P. Sisson, J. D. Mahan, T. R. Oegema, and D. M. Brown: Heparan sulfate-rich anionic sites in the human glomerular basement membrane. Decreased concentration in congenital nephrotic syndrome, *N. Engl. J. Med.,* 309: 1001, 1983.

53. Meyers, B. D., T. B. Okarma, S. Friedman, C. Bridges, J. Ross, S. Asseff, and W. M. Deen: Mechanisms of proteinuria in human glomerulonephritis, *J. Clin. Invest.,* 70:732, 1982.

54. Hunsicker, L. G., T. P. Shearer, and S. J. Shaffer: Acute reversible proteinuria induced by infusion of the polycation hexadimethrine, *Kidney Int.,* 20:7, 1981.

55. Carrie, B. J., M. Hilberman, J. S. Schroeder, and B. D. Myers: Albuminuria and the permselective properties of the glomerulus in cardiac failure, *Kidney Int.,* 17:507, 1980.

56. Peterson, A., E. Evrin, and I. Berggård: Differentiation of glomerular, tubular, and normal proteinuria: Determinations of urinary excretion of β_2-microglobulin, albumin, and total protein, *J. Clin. Invest.,* 48:1189, 1969.

57. Butler, E. A., and F. V. Flynn: The proteinuria of renal tubular disorders, *Lancet,* 2:978, 1958.

58. Perry, M. C., and R. A. Kyle: The clinical sign-

ificance of Bence-Jones proteinuria, *Mayo Clin. Proc.,* 50:234, 1975.

59. Muggia, F. M., H. O. Heinemann, M. Farhangi, and E. F. Osserman: Lysozymuria and renal tubular dysfunction in monocytic and myelomonocytic leukemia, *Am. J. Med.,* 47:351, 1969.

60. Carone, F. A., and D. R. Peterson: Hydrolysis and transport of small peptides by the proximal tubule, *Am. J. Physiol.,* 238:F151, 1980.

61. Viberti G. C., R. D. Hill, R. J. Jarrett, A. Argyropoulos, U. Mahmud, and H. Keen: Microalbuminuria as a predictor of clinical nephropathy in insulin-dependent diabetes mellitus, *Lancet,* 1:1430, 1982.

62. Mogensen, C. E., and C. K. Christensen: Predicting diabetic nephropathy in insulin-dependent patients, *N. Engl. J. Med.,* 311:89, 1984.

63. Thysell, H.: A comparison between albustix, hemacombistix, labstix, the sulphosalicylic-acid test, Heller's nitric-acid test, and a biuret method, *Acta Med. Scand.,* 185:401, 1969.

64. Abuelo, J. G.: Proteinuria: Diagnostic principles and procedures, *Ann. Intern. Med.,* 98:186, 1983.

65. Wellborne, F. R., R. G., Claypool, and J. B. Copley: Nephrotic range pseudoproteinuria in a tolmetin-treated patient, *Clin. Nephrol.,* 19:211, 1983.

66. Rennie, I. D. B., and H. Keen: Evaluation of clinical methods for detecting proteinuria, *Lancet,* 2:489, 1967.

67. Clugh, G., and T. G. Reak: A "protein error," *Lancet,* 1:1248, 1964.

68. Lippman, R. W.: *Urine and the Urinary Sediment,* 2d ed., Charles C Thomas, Springfield, Illinois, 1957.

69. Ginsberg, J. M., B. S. Chang, R. A. Matarese, and S. Garella: Use of single voided urine samples to estimate quantitative proteinuria, *N. Engl. J. Med.,* 309:1543, 1983.

70. Rose, B. D.: *Clinical Physiology of Acid-Base and Electrolyte Disorders,* 2d ed., McGraw-Hill, New York, 1984, chap. 14.

71. Rose, B. D.: *Clinical Physiology of Acid-Base and Electrolyte Disorders,* 2d ed., McGraw-Hill, New York, 1984, chap. 1.

72. Rose, B. D.: *Clinical Physiology of Acid-Base and Electrolyte Disorders,* 2d ed., McGraw-Hill, New York, 1984, chap. 8.

73. Schoen, E. J.: Minimum urine total solute concentration in response to water loading in normal men, *J. Appl. Physiol.,* 10:267, 1957.

74. Miles, B. E., A. Paton, and H. E. de Wardener: Maximum urine concentration, *Br. Med. J.,* 2:901, 1954.

75. Miller, M., T. Dalakos, A. M. Moses, H. Fellerman, and D. H. P. Streeten: Recognition of partial defects in antidiuretic hormone secretion, *Ann. Intern. Med.,* 73:721, 1970.

76. Lindeman, R. D., H. C. van Buren, and L. G. Raisz: Osmolar renal concentrating ability in healthy young men and hospitalized patients without renal disease, *N. Engl. J. Med.,* 262:1306, 1960.

77. Rose, B. D.: *Clinical Physiology of Acid Base and Electrolyte Disorders,* 2d ed., McGraw-Hill, New York, 1984, pp. 498–500, 528–535.

78. Miller, T. R., R. J. Anderson, S. L. Linas, W. L. Henrich, A. S. Berns, P. A. Gabow, and R. W. Schrier: Urinary diagnostic indices in acute renal failure: A prospective study, *Ann. Intern. Med.,* 89:47, 1978.

79. Espinel, C. H., and A. W. Gregory: Differential diagnosis of acute renal failure, *Clin. Nephrol.,* 13:73, 1980.

80. Dorhout Mees, E. J.: Relation between maximal urinary concentration, maximal water reabsorption capacity, and mannitol clearance in patients with renal disease, *Br. Med. J.,* 1:1159, 1959.

81. Zwelling, L. A., and J. E. Balow: Hypersthenuria in high-dose carbenicillin therapy, *Ann. Intern. Med.,* 89:225, 1978.

82. Rose, B. D.: *Clinical Physiology of Acid-Base and Electrolyte Disorders,* 2d ed., McGraw-Hill, New York, 1984, chap. 9.

83. Luft, F. C., R. S. Sloan, N. S. Fineberg, and A. H. Free: The utility of overnight urine collections in assessing compliance with a low sodium diet, *J. Am. Med. Assoc.,* 249:1764, 1983.

84. Hall, J. E., J. P. Granger, M. J. Smith, and A. J. Premen: Role of renal hemodynamics and arterial pressure in aldosterone "escape," *Hypertension Suppl.* 6:I-183, 1984.

85. Levinsky, N. G., E. A. Alexander, and M. A. Venkatachalam: Acute renal failure, in B. M. Brenner and F. C. Rector, Jr. (eds.), *The Kidney,* 2d ed., Saunders, Philadelphia, 1981.

86. Maronde, R. F., M. Milgrom, N. D. Vlachakis, and L. Chan: Response of thiazide-induced hypokalemia to amiloride, *J. Am. Med. Assoc.,* 249:237, 1983.

87. Besarab, A., R. S. Brown, N. T. Rubin, E. Salzman, L. Wirthlin, T. Steinman, R. R. Atlia, and J. J. Skillman: Reversible renal failure following bilateral renal artery occlusive disease: Clinical features, pathology, and the role of surgical revascularization, *J. Am. Med. Assoc.,* 235:2838, 1976.

88. Danovitch, G. M., J. J. Bourgoignie, and N. S. Bricker: Reversibility of the "salt-losing" tendency of chronic renal failure, *N. Engl. J. Med.,* 296:14, 1977.

89. Oken, D. E.: On the differential diagnosis of acute renal failure, *Am. J. Med.*, 71:916, 1981.

90. Steiner, R. W.: Interpreting the fractional excretion of sodium, *Am. J. Med.*, 77:699, 1984.

91. Kirchner, K. A., J. H. Galla, and R. G. Luke: Factors influencing chloride reabsorption in the collecting duct segment of the rat, *Am. J. Physiol.*, 239:F552, 1980.

92. Sherman, R. A., and R. P. Eisinger: The use (and misuse) of urinary sodium and chloride measurements, *J. Am. Med. Assoc.*, 247:3121, 1982.

93. Rose, B. D.: *Clinical Physiology of Acid-Base and Electrolyte Disorders*, 2d ed., McGraw-Hill, New York, 1984, pp. 384–385.

94. Addis, T.: The number of formed elements in the urinary sediment of normal individuals, *J. Clin. Invest.*, 2:409, 1926.

95. Mariani, A. J., S. Luangphinith, S. Loo, A. Scottolini, and C. V. Hodges: Dipstick chemical urinalysis: An accurate cost-effective screening test, *J. Urol.*, 132:64, 1984.

96. Fairley, K. F., and D. F. Birch: Hematuria: A simple method for identifying glomerular bleeding, *Kidney Int.*, 21:105, 1982.

97. Fassett, R. G., B. A. Horgan, and T. H. Mathew: Detection of glomerular bleeding by phase-contrast microscopy, *Lancet*, 1:1432, 1982.

98. Fassett, R. G., B. Horgan, D. Gove, and T. H. Mathew: Scanning electron microscopy of glomerular and nonglomerular red blood cells, *Clin. Nephrol.*, 20:11, 1983.

99. Van Iseghem, Ph., D. Hauglustaine, W. Bollens, and P. Michielsen: Urinary erythrocyte morphology in acute glomerulonephritis, *Br. Med. J.*, 287:1183, 1983.

100. Ditlove, J., P. Weidmann, M. Bernstein, and S. G. Massry: Methicillin nephritis, *Medicine*, 56:483, 1977.

101. Russell, P. S.: Kidney transplantation, *Am. J. Med.*, 44:776, 1968.

102. Curt, G. A., A. Kaldany, L. G. Whitley, A. W. Crosson, A. Rolla, M. J. Merino, and J. A. D'Elia: Reversible rapidly progressive renal failure with nephrotic syndrome due to fenoprofen calcium, *Ann. Intern. Med.*, 92:72, 1980.

103. Stachura, I., S. Jayakumar, and E. Bourke: T and B lymphocyte subsets in fenoprofen nephropathy, *Am. J. Med.*, 75:9, 1983.

104. Comings, D. E.: Anisotropic lipids and urinary cholesterol excretion, *J. Am. Med. Assoc.*, 183:128, 1963.

105. Zimmer, J. G., R. Dewey, C. Waterhouse, and R. Terry: The origin and nature of anisotropic urinary lipids in the nephrotic syndrome, *Ann. Intern. Med.*, 54:205, 1961.

106. McQueen, E. G.: The composition of the urinary casts, *Lancet*, 1:397, 1966.

107. Rutecki, G. J., C. Goldsmith, and G. E. Schreiner: Characterization of proteins in urinary casts: Fluorescent antibody identification of Tamm-Horsfall mucoprotein in matrix and serum proteins in granules, *N. Engl. J. Med.*, 284:1049, 1971.

108. McKenzie, J. K., and E. G. McQueen: Immunofluorescent localization of Tamm-Horsfall mucoprotein in human kidney, *J. Clin. Pathol.*, 22:334, 1969.

109. Hoyer, J. R., S. P. Sisson, and R. L. Vernier: Tamm-Horsfall glycoprotein, *Lab. Invest.*, 41:168, 1979.

110. Imhof, P. R., J. Hushak, G. Schumann, P. Dukor, J. Wagner, and H. M. Keller: Excretion of urinary casts after the administration of diuretics, *Br. Med. J.*, 2:199, 1972.

111. McQueen, E. G., and G. B. Engel: Factors determining the aggregation of urinary mucoprotein, *J. Clin. Pathol.*, 19:392, 1966.

112. Addis, T.: A clinical classification of Bright's diseases, *J. Am. Med. Assoc.*, 85:163, 1925.

113. Schreiner, G. E.: The identification and clinical significance of casts, *Arch. Intern. Med.*, 99:356, 1957.

114. Brody, L., M. C. Webster, and R. M. Kark: Identification of urinary sediment with phase-contrast microscopy, *J. Am. Med. Assoc.*, 206:1777, 1968.

115. Clinicopathological Conference: Progressive renal failure with hematuria in a 62-year-old man, *Am. J. Med.*, 71:468, 1981.

116. Sigala, J. F., C. G. Biava, and H. N. Hulter: Red blood cell casts in acute interstitial nephritis, *Arch. Intern. Med.*, 138:1419, 1978.

117. Orita, Y., N. Imai, N. Ueda, K. Aoki, K. Sugimoto, A. Ando, Y. Fujiwara, S. Hirano, and H. Abe: Immunofluorescent studies of urinary casts, *Nephron*, 19:19, 1977.

118. Addis, T.: Renal failure casts, *J. Am. Med. Assoc.*, 84:1013, 1925.

119. Fairley, K. F., D. F. Birch, and I. Haines: Abnormal urinary sediment in patients on triamterene, *Lancet*, 1:421, 1983.

120. Segal, S., and S. O. Thier: Cystinuria., in J. B. Stanbury, J. B. Wyngaarden, D. S. Fredrickson, J. L. Goldstein, and M. S. Brown (eds.), *The Metabolic Basis of Inherited Disease*, McGraw-Hill, New York, 1983.

121. Parry, M. F., and R. Wallach: Ethylene glycol poisoning, *Am. J. Med.*, 57:143, 1974.

122. Kjellstrand, C. M., D. Campbell, II, B. von Hartitzsch, and T. J. Buselmeier: Hyperuricemic acute renal failure, *Arch. Intern. Med.,* 133:349, 1974.

123. Wright W. T.: Cell counts in urine, *Arch. Intern. Med.,* 103:76, 1959.

124. Larcom, R. C., Jr., and G. H. Carter: Erythrocytes in urinary sediment: Identification and normal limits, *J. Lab. Clin. Med.,* 33:875, 1948.

125. Barach, J.: Physiological and pathological effects of severe exertion (marathon race) on circulatory and renal systems, *Arch. Intern. Med.,* 5:382, 1910.

126. Alyea, E. P., and H. H. Parish: Renal response to exercise—urinary findings, *J. Am. Med. Assoc.,* 167:807, 1958.

127. Stewart, H. J., and N. S. Moore: The number of formed elements in the urinary sediment of patients suffering from heart disease, with particular reference to the state of heart failure, *J. Clin. Invest.,* 9:409, 1931.

128. Race, G. A., C. H. Scheifley, and J. E. Edwards: Albuminuria in congestive heart failure, *Circulation,* 13:329, 1956.

129. Reuben, D. B., T. J. Wachtel, P. C. Brown, and J. L. Driscoll: Transient proteinuria in emergency medical admissions, *N. Engl. J. Med.,* 306:1031, 1982.

130. Goldring, W.: Studies of the kidney in acute infection, III. Observations with the urine sediment count (Addis) and the urea clearance test in lobar pneumonia, *J. Clin. Invest.,* 10:355, 1931.

131. Marks, M. I., P. N. McLaine, and K. N. Drummond: Proteinuria in children with febrile illnesses, *Arch. Dis. Child.,* 45:250, 1970.

132. Richmond, J. M., W. J. Sibbald, A. M. Linton, and A. L. Linton: Patterns of urinary protein excretion in patients with sepsis, *Nephron,* 31:219, 1982.

133. King, S. E., and D. S. Baldwin: Production of renal ischemia and proteinuria in man by the adrenal medullary hormone, *Am. J. Med.,* 20:217, 1956.

134. Fassett, R. G., J. E. Owen, J. Fairley, D. F. Birch, and K. F. Fairley: Urinary red-cell morphology during exercise, *Br. Med. J.,* 285:1455, 1982.

135. Poortmans, J. R.: Postexercise proteinuria in humans. Facts and mechanisms, *J. Am. Med. Assoc.,* 253:236, 1985.

136. Elsom, K. A.: Renal function in obstructive jaundice, *Arch. Intern. Med.,* 60:1028, 1937.

137. Green, J., R. Beyar, L. Bomzon, J. P. M. Finberg, and O. S. Better: Jaundice, the circulation and the kidney, *Nephron,* 37:145, 1984.

138. Bolton, W. K., R. J. Tully, E. J. Lewis, and K. Ranniger: Localization of the kidney for percutaneous biopsy: A comparative study of methods, *Ann. Intern. Med.,* 81:159, 1974.

139. Rosenbaum, R., P. E. Hoffsten, R. J. Stanley, and S. Klahr: Use of computerized tomography to diagnose complications of percutaneous renal biopsy, *Kidney Int.,* 14:87, 1978.

140. Messing, E., R. Kessler, and P. B. Kavaney: Renal arteriovenous fistulas, *Urology,* 8:101, 1976.

2

DIAGNOSTIC APPROACH TO THE PATIENT WITH RENAL DISEASE

Burton D. Rose

The preceding chapter described the common laboratory tests that are useful in the evaluation of renal function. This chapter describes how and when to use these tests in the clinical setting. As will be seen, the tests usually provide information that allows the diagnostic possibilities to be narrowed to one or only a few disorders. The approach presented here is a general one, with the individual diseases being discussed in detail in the following chapters.

CLASSIFICATION

A simple classification of disorders impairing renal function can be derived from an understanding of normal renal physiology. Urine formation involves four basic steps:

1. Blood is delivered to the glomeruli by branches of the renal arteries.
2. An ultrafiltrate of plasma is then formed across the glomeruli.
3. The filtrate is altered by tubular reabsorp-

tion and, to a lesser degree, secretion.
4. The urine then leaves the kidney and drains sequentially into the renal pelvis, ureter, and bladder before being excreted through the urethra.

As a result, intrinsic renal disease can be produced by disorders involving the blood vessels, glomeruli, tubules, or the interstitium which separates the individual nephrons. In addition, kidney function can be impaired by two extrarenal (and possibly easily reversible) processes: a reduction in renal perfusion or obstruction to the flow of urine at any site in the urinary tract. Table 2–1 is a partial list of the major causes of kidney disease according to these potential mechanisms.

CLINICAL PRESENTATION

The patient with renal disease may present to the physician in a variety of ways, some of

TABLE 2-1. Major Causes of Kidney Disease

Prerenal disease
  True volume depletion
    Gastrointestinal, renal, or sweat losses or bleeding
  Heart failure
  Hepatic cirrhosis (including the hepatorenal
    syndrome)
  Nephrotic syndrome (particularly after diuretic
    therapy for edema)
  Hypotension
  Nonsteroidal anti-inflammatory drugs
  Bilateral renal artery stenosis (particularly after
    therapy with a converting enzyme inhibitor)
Obstructive uropathy
  Prostatic disease
  Malignancy
  Calculi
  Congenital abnormalities
Vascular disease
  Acute
    Vasculitis
    Malignant hypertension
    Scleroderma
    Thromboembolic disease
  Chronic
    Nephrosclerosis
Glomerular disease
  Glomerulonephritis
  Nephrotic syndrome
Tubular disease
  Acute
    Acute tubular necrosis
    Multiple myeloma
    Hypercalcemia
    Uric acid nephropathy
  Chronic
    Polycystic kidney disease
    Medullary sponge kidney
Interstitial disease
  Acute
    Pyelonephritis
    Interstitial nephritis (usually drug-induced)
  Chronic
    Pyelonephritis (due primarily to vesicoureteral
      reflux)
    Analgesic abuse

which may directly suggest a specific diagnosis. These modes of presentation include:

1. The presence of signs or symptoms directly referable to the kidney such as a decrease in urine output, red or brown urine (most often due to hematuria; see Fig. 1–4), or unilateral or bilateral flank pain. Unilateral pain is suggestive of obstruction, infection, or, rarely, infarction; bilateral pain, however, is much less specific since a variety of acute renal disorders can induce pain by stretching the renal capsule.

2. The presence of extrarenal signs or symptoms such as edema or hypertension. Edema is generally due to hypoalbuminemia in the nephrotic syndrome or to primary sodium and water retention resulting from a low GFR.[1,2] Hypertension is most often related to volume expansion, but enhanced renin release and increased sympathetic tone may also be important (see p. 159).[3-5]

3. The presence of a concurrent systemic disease, such as diabetes mellitus or systemic lupus erythematosus, that can affect the kidney.

4. The presence of signs or symptoms of severe renal failure such as marked anemia, lethargy, weakness, and anorexia. In this setting, the plasma creatinine concentration (P_{cr}) will be substantially elevated.

5. The incidental discovery of an abnormal urinalysis or an elevated P_{cr}.

DURATION OF DISEASE

As depicted in Table 2–1, knowing the duration of the renal disease (acute versus chronic) frequently narrows the differential diagnosis. This can be done most accurately if the patient has had a urinalysis or P_{cr} in the past. If, for example, the P_{cr} were 2.1 mg/dL 3 years ago, 3.2 mg/dL 1 year ago, and 4.0 mg/dL now, it is most likely that the patient has a chronic slowly progressive disease. In comparison, a P_{cr} that begins to rise in the hospital is probably related to something that has happened in the hospital, such as the administration of a nephrotoxic drug.

If previous data are not available, there are several clues that may be helpful in determining the course of the renal disease. First, the history may provide valuable information. A complaint of gross hematuria and edema following an upper respiratory infection suggests a postinfectious glomerulonephritis. The presence of a low urine output also points toward an acute component since prolonged oliguria (output less than 500 mL/day) rapidly leads to advanced renal failure and the symptoms of uremia.

Second, serial measurements of the P_{cr} should be made on successive days. A rising value shows that some acute process is present. A stable P_{cr} is more consistent with chronic disease.

Third, anemia is more common in advanced chronic renal disease (P_{cr} greater than 5 mg/dL) than it is in acute disease of similar severity. The anemia of renal failure is primarily due to reductions in both production of and responsiveness to erythropoietin.[6,7] Since erythropoietin stimulates the production of red cells by the bone marrow, fewer new cells are made. However, fewer than 1 percent of the circulating red cells are normally destroyed each day. Therefore, in the absence of bleeding, hemolysis, or hemodilution secondary to fluid retention (all of which may occur in renal insufficiency), the hematocrit will fall at a maximal rate of only 1 percent per day if erythropoietin production is diminished. As a result, the hematocrit in acute renal failure may be normal or near normal because not enough time has elapsed for anemia to occur. However, a relatively normal hematocrit also may occur in some forms of chronic renal failure such as polycystic disease in which it is thought that regional ischemia due to pressure from the cysts stimulates erythropoietin production.[8,9]

EVALUATION

GLOMERULAR FILTRATION RATE

The initial evaluation of the patient suspected of having kidney disease should begin with estimation of the glomerular filtration rate (GFR) and examination of the urine (Table 2-2). As described in the preceding chapter, the GFR is measured clinically as the creatinine clearance (C_{cr}) and can be estimated simply in men from the P_{cr}[10]:

$$C_{cr} \cong \frac{(140 - \text{age}) \times \text{LBW}}{P_{cr} \times 72}$$

where LBW is the approximate lean body weight in kilograms. This value should be multiplied by 0.85 in women who, at a given weight, have less muscle mass (and therefore less creatinine production) than men.

This formula is accurate *only* in the steady state when the P_{cr} is relatively constant. In a patient with acute renal failure in whom the P_{cr} is rising daily, the GFR is typically quite low. Although knowledge of the exact GFR is usually not necessary in this setting, it can be estimated from the C_{cr} using a 24-h urine collection:

$$C_{cr} = \frac{U_{cr} \times V}{P_{cr}}$$

TABLE 2-2. Laboratory Evaluation of Renal Disease

Estimation of glomerular filtration rate
Plasma creatinine concentration
BUN/P_{cr} ratio*
Examination of the urine
Urinalysis
Urine volume
Urine osmolality and sodium excretion
Radiologic studies

*BUN = blood urea nitrogen.

where V is the urine flow rate in milliliters per minute or liters per day. The average of the P_{cr} on the 2 days of the urine collection should be used in this formula since the P_{cr} is not stable.

Measurement of the GFR is useful for two reasons. First, it generally reflects disease severity since the total GFR is equal to the sum of the filtration rates in each of the functioning nephrons. Second, it is the best way to follow the course of the disease. Since the GFR varies inversely with the P_{cr} (see Fig. 1–2), serial measurements of the P_{cr} are most often used—a rising P_{cr} reflects disease progression, whereas a falling P_{cr} generally indicates improvement. Although a stable P_{cr} usually indicates stable disease, this may not be true when the P_{cr} is below 1.5 mg/dL. In this setting, compensatory hyperfiltration by relatively uninvolved glomeruli may balance the effect of nephron loss due to disease progression (see p. 9).

BUN/P_{cr} RATIO

Although the BUN, like the P_{cr}, will rise as the GFR falls, it is a less reliable test because of potentially variable rates of urea production and excretion. In the absence of urea overproduction (most often due to bleeding, corticosteroids, or excess tissue breakdown), the BUN and P_{cr} rise in parallel in renal disease with a normal ratio of 10 to 15:1. The major exception to this rule occurs in prerenal disease in which enhanced sodium and water reabsorption result in increased passive urea reabsorption and a preferential rise in the BUN. In this setting, the BUN/P_{cr} ratio usually exceeds 20:1.[11] Thus, a high ratio is a diagnostic point in favor of prerenal disease. A normal ratio, however, does not exclude this diagnosis since decreased protein intake (as commonly occurs with vomiting, for example) can limit the rise in the BUN.

EXAMINATION OF THE URINE

URINALYSIS

Examination of the urine, particularly the urinalysis, is the major noninvasive diagnostic tool available to the clinician. As depicted in Table 2–3, different urinary findings are typically associated with different diseases. In some, the changes are so characteristic that one or just a few diagnoses are suggested. For example, the presence of red cell casts, heavy proteinuria, and/or lipiduria is virtually diagnostic of glomerular disease or vasculitis, although some exceptions may rarely occur.[12,13] The absence of these changes, however, does not exclude the presence of glomerular disease since some patients may have only hematuria (without casts) and/or mild proteinuria. (Use of the urinalysis to help distinguish between the different forms of glomerular disease is reviewed on p. 164.)

When hematuria is present, identification of the site of bleeding is important both to establish the diagnosis and to determine the extent of the evaluation that will ensue (see "Isolated Urinary Abnormalities: Hematuria," below). In this regard, there are certain characteristics that distinguish glomerular bleeding from extraglomerular bleeding (as may occur with calculi, tumors, or infection) (Table 2–4).[14,15] These include the presence of red cell casts or proteinuria, the absence of blood clots (perhaps because the glomeruli have a fibrinolytic system),[16] and abnormal red cell morphology. Glomerular bleeding presumably occurs when red cells enter the urine through rents in the damaged glomerular basement membrane.[17,18] This process seems to damage many of the red cells, resulting in a dysmorphic appearance with blebs, budding, and segmental loss of membrane (see Plate 1a and b).[15] In comparison, the red cells have a relatively uniform, circular shape with extraglomerular lesions.

TABLE 2–3. Correlation between Urinalysis and Causes of Renal Dysfunction

Urinary Findings	Etiology
Hematuria with red cell casts Heavy proteinuria (>3.5 g/day or 50 mg/kg per day) Lipiduria	Any of these findings, singly or in combination, is virtually diagnostic of glomerular disease or vasculitis. The absence of these findings, however, does not exclude these diagnoses.
Renal tubular epithelial cells with granular and epithelial cell casts	In acute renal failure, strongly suggestive of acute tubular necrosis although marked hyperbilirubinemia alone can produce similar changes.
Pyuria with white cell and granular or waxy casts and no or mild proteinuria (<1.5 g/day)	Suggestive of tubular or interstitial disease or obstruction.
Hematuria and pyuria with no or variable casts or proteinuria	May be seen with glomerular disease, vasculitis, infection, obstruction, renal infarction, or acute, usually drug-induced, interstitial nephritis. The presence of eosinophils in the urine usually indicates the last diagnosis.
Hematuria alone	In acute renal failure, suggestive of vasculitis or obstruction. The evaluation of isolated hematuria or proteinuria with relatively normal renal function is discussed separately later in the chapter.
Normal or near normal (few cells with little or no proteinuria or casts); hyaline casts *not considered* an abnormal finding (see p. 24)	Acute: may be seen with prerenal disease obstruction, hypercalcemia, multiple myeloma,* some cases of acute tubular necrosis, or vascular diseases in which glomerular ischemia but not necrosis occurs (including scleroderma, atheroemboli, and rare cases of polyarteritis nodosa). Chronic: may be seen with prerenal disease, obstruction, tubular or interstitial diseases, and nephrosclerosis.

*Although the dipstick is likely to be negative (detecting primarily albuminuria), the sulfosalicylic acid test will be very positive in multiple myeloma since it will detect the presence of immunoglobulin light chains.

Changes in the urine color also may be helpful (Table 2–4). The urine in patients with mild hematuria will retain its normal yellow color. However, as little as 1 mL of blood in 1 L of urine can produce a visible color change.[19] With glomerular disease, the combination of prolonged transit time through the nephron and an acid urine pH may result in the forma-

TABLE 2-4. Differentiation between Glomerular and Extraglomerular Bleeding

Urinary Finding	Glomerular	Extraglomerular
Red cell casts	May be present	Absent
Red cell morphology	Dysmorphic	Uniform
Proteinuria (>500 mg/day)	May be present	Absent
Clots	Absent	May be present
Color	May be red or brown	May be red

tion of methemoglobin, which has a smoky brown color.* Contact time with the urine is reduced with extraglomerular bleeding, and only a pink or red color will be seen.

URINE VOLUME

In contrast to the urinalysis, the urine volume is usually of little diagnostic value since it can range from anuria to more than several liters per day even in patients with marked reductions in GFR. The reason for this variability is that the urine output is determined not by the GFR alone but by the *difference* between the GFR and tubular reabsorption. In a normal subject, the GFR may be 180 L/day (or 125 mL/min) with 179 L being reabsorbed and 1 L excreted. In severe renal disease, the GFR may be diminished to 10 L/day or less. If 9.5 L is reabsorbed, 500 mL will be excreted and the patient will be said to be oliguric. However, the daily urine volume will be 2 L if only 8 L is reabsorbed, even though the patient still has advanced renal insufficiency. Among the factors that may decrease tubular reabsorption and therefore increase the urine output in renal failure are sodium retention (which may act by reducing the secretion of aldosterone and by enhancing that of a natriuretic hormone),[20,21] an osmotic diuresis due to increased urea excretion per functioning nephron,[21] and damage to the tubular cells.[22]

*Red to brown urine also may be seen with other disorders such as myoglobinuria or hemoglobinuria (see Fig. 1-4).

As a result of the variable rate of tubular reabsorption, the urine output may be low (<500 mL/day), normal, or high (>2 L/day) in most forms of renal disease. One general exception is prerenal disease, in which the appropriate retention of sodium and water usually keeps the urine output well below 1 L/day. Even this is not absolute, however, as patients with impaired concentrating ability can maintain a urine output above 1 L/day despite the presence of volume depletion and a low U_{Na}.[23]

The one setting in which the urine volume may be of diagnostic importance is the presence of anuria (urine output less than 50 mL/day), which occurs in relatively few conditions. Common causes of acute renal failure such as acute tubular necrosis and prerenal disease are often accompanied by oliguria but rarely anuria. The primary disorders associated with anuria are shock (accompanied by severe renal vasoconstriction and usually marked hypotension) and complete urinary tract obstruction. Less commonly, renal cortical necrosis, bilateral vascular occlusion, e.g., that due to a dissecting aneurysm, or severe glomerulonephritis, hemolytic-uremic syndrome, or vasculitis is responsible.*

*Anuria can also be induced in some patients with advanced renal failure by the institution of dialysis. Since volume expansion and the high BUN tend to decrease tubular reabsorption and maintain the urine output in renal failure, their partial correction by dialysis can markedly lower the urine volume.[21]

URINE OSMOLALITY AND SODIUM EXCRETION

Measurement of the urine osmolality and sodium excretion is primarily useful in the distinction between prerenal disease and acute tubular necrosis as the cause of acute renal failure. The use of these parameters is discussed in detail on p. 67. Summarized briefly, the kidney appropriately retains water [via enhanced antidiuretic hormone (ADH) secretion] and sodium in hypovolemic states: these effects are usually characterized by U_{osm} greater than 500 mosmol/kg, a U_{Na} below 20 meq/L, and a fractional excretion of sodium (FE_{Na}) below 1 percent.[24] In comparison, tubular damage in acute tubular necrosis impairs water and sodium conservation. As a result, typical results show a relatively isosmotic urine (U_{osm} below 350 mosmol/kg), a U_{Na} above 40 meq/L, and an FE_{Na} above 2 percent.[22,24,25]

In addition to prerenal disease, the U_{Na} and FE_{Na} may also be low in other states in which the GFR is reduced but tubular function is initially normal, including acute glomerulonephritis or vasculitis and acute urinary tract obstruction.[24,26] However, measurement of urinary sodium excretion is usually not necessary in these settings since the correct diagnosis is suggested from the urinalysis (glomerulonephritis) or ultrasound examination (urinary tract obstruction).

One other point concerning the diagnosis of prerenal disease deserves emphasis: when this disorder is superimposed on underlying chronic renal disease, none of the characteristic laboratory features of hypovolemia may be present, since the primary renal disease can impair maximum sodium and water conservation and can produce an abnormal urinalysis.[20,27] In this setting, the presence of true volume depletion may be suggested from the history (vomiting or diuretic use) or physical examination (decreased skin turgor or postural tachycardia and hypotension). If there is reason to suspect hypovolemia, a careful trial of fluid repletion can improve renal function as manifested by a fall in the BUN and P_{cr}. This is an important diagnosis to make in a patient with recent worsening of renal function, since prerenal disease is reversible, whereas progression of the underlying disease may not be.

RADIOLOGIC STUDIES

Although different radiologic studies can provide a great deal of useful information (see Table 1-5), a plain film of the abdomen and ultrasonography are the major tests used in the initial evaluation of the patient with renal disease. The former can show renal size and shape and detect radiopaque calculi, whereas the latter can reliably detect the presence of hydronephrosis due to obstruction (see Fig. 9-3).[28,29]

OBSTRUCTION

Urinary tract obstruction is a particularly important diagnosis to make since it is frequently readily reversible. This disorder should be *suspected in any patient who presents with unexplained renal insufficiency.* If the process is acute, as with prostatic disease or ureteral calculi, suprapubic or flank pain may be present. However, many patients with gradual obstruction (most often due to malignancy or prostatic disease in adults) will have no symptoms referable to the urinary tract. Furthermore, the urinary findings are variable, ranging from relatively normal to hematuria (with calculi), pyuria (with infection or chronic obstruction), or mild proteinuria (usually less than 1 g/day). A common error is to assume that obstruction is excluded by the finding of a normal urine output. Although complete obstruction will result in anuria, the urine output (equal to the GFR minus tubular reabsorption) is as variable with partial obstruction as it is with intrinsic renal disease (see "Urine Volume," above).

The workup for obstruction should proceed in the following manner. First, a catheter should be inserted into the bladder to rule out urethral or prostatic obstruction. This diagnosis should be suspected if a large bladder can be palpated on physical examination or if suprapubic pain or tenderness is present. If catheterization of the bladder does not yield a large output, then obstruction, if present, must be at the level of the ureters or above. This can usually be detected by ultrasonography or CT scanning.[28,29] Since calculi in the renal pelvis can lead to a false-negative result on ultrasonography, a plain film of the abdomen should be included in the initial evaluation.[28,29]

CLINICAL EXAMPLES

The diagnostic approach outlined in this chapter can be illustrated by the following case histories. As will be seen, the urinalysis or the time course may point toward a particular diagnosis in some patients. In other patients, however, the initial findings are

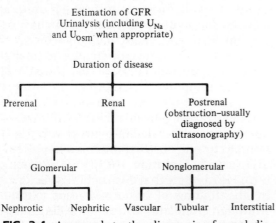

FIG. 2–1. Approach to the diagnosis of renal disease.

relatively nonspecific, and each of the major categories of disease must be considered separately (Fig. 2–1): prerenal; postrenal (obstruction); and intrinsic renal disorders involving the glomeruli, blood vessels, tubules, or interstitium.

Case History 2–1. A 47-year-old woman presents with a 3-month history of mild weakness. Prior to this, she has been essentially well and takes no prescribed medications. Physical examination reveals a blood pressure of 190/105, grade 2 hypertensive retinopathy, and mild cardiomegaly. Left ventricular hypertrophy with a strain pattern is noted on the electrocardiogram. The BUN is 52 mg/dL, P_{cr} is 4.1 mg/dL, and hematocrit is 30 percent. A P_{cr} 2 years ago was 1.9 mg/dL. The urinalysis reveals 1^+ proteinuria, 10 to 15 white cells per HPF (high power field), and an occasional white cell or granular cast. Urine culture is negative.

Comment. The history, previous P_{cr}, and anemia suggest that the renal disease reflects a chronic process. The retinal and electrocardiographic changes indicate that the hypertension also has been present for a relatively long time. There is no evidence in the history or physical examination for prerenal diseases. The urinalysis tends to exclude glomerular disease and vasculitis but is compatible with many of the chronic nonglomerular diseases (Table 2–1). Thus, the initial differential diagnosis includes obstruction, nephrosclerosis due to prolonged hypertension, and some form of chronic tubular or interstitial disease.

With these disorders in mind, ultrasonography was performed and revealed symmetric, slightly small kidneys with no evidence of obstruction or cystic disease. Thus, the differential diagnosis narrows further to nephrosclerosis and a chronic interstitial disease such as analgesic abuse nephropathy. Upon closer questioning, the patient admitted to a long history of headaches for which she had taken analgesic compounds containing aspirin and phenacetin. An intravenous pyelogram was performed and showed bilateral papillary necrosis consistent with this diagnosis (see Fig. 8–2).

Case History 2–2. A 53-year-old man is admitted to the hospital with anorexia and a 10-kg weight loss. He has a history of non-insulin-dependent diabetes mellitus with mild retinopathy, a P_{cr} of 2 mg/dL, 24-h urine protein excretion of 3.7 g, and an otherwise normal urinalysis. An intravenous pyelogram (IVP) is performed on the fourth hospital day as part of the evaluation for malignancy. Shortly thereafter, the urine output falls and the BUN and P_{cr} begin to rise. The urinalysis is unchanged. The patient is on no other medications except for insulin.

Comment. This patient has acute superimposed upon chronic renal disease. The history of diabetes and the presence of retinopathy and heavy proteinuria makes glomerular disease due to diabetes the most likely diagnosis of his primary renal problem.

When acute renal failure develops in the hospital, it is frequently possible, as in this case, to identify the date of onset. In this setting, either some nephrotoxic event occurred on that day or the cumulative effect of some nephrotoxin first became apparent as with the continued administration of an aminoglycoside antibiotic. In this patient, there is a strong temporal relationship to the IVP and no other obvious cause of renal dysfunction. Acute renal failure following radiocontrast media is a relatively common disorder, particularly in diabetics with underlying renal insufficiency (see Chap. 3).[30] Spontaneous recovery typically occurs within 4 to 10 days.

Case History 2–3. A 71-year-old man with a recent anterior myocardial infarction complains of the acute onset of left flank pain. He denies fever or chills. The P_{cr} is 2.1 mg/dL, increased from the baseline value of 1.4 mg/dL. The urinalysis shows 20 to 30 white and red cells per HPF, findings which had not been present in the past.

Comment. The unilateral nature of the symptoms, recent rise in the P_{cr}, and abnormal urinalysis point toward an acute process in the left kidney. The differential diagnosis includes acute pyelonephritis (which is somewhat unlikely since this disorder does not usually impair renal function), ureteral obstruction, and renal infarction. A renal ultrasound showed no evidence of obstruction, but a renal flow scan showed markedly reduced flow to the left kidney, probably due to an embolus from a mural thrombus in the heart. Rapid diagnosis is particularly important in this setting since local fibrinolytic therapy or perhaps heparin may cause clot lysis and preserve renal function (see Chap. 7).

Case History 2–4. A 67-year-old woman is admitted for nonspecific complaints of weakness and fatigue. She has a past history of mild hypertension but is currently on no medications. Physical examination shows a blood pressure of 105/80 with slightly cool extremities but no signs of peripheral or pulmonary edema; skin turgor is normal. During the first 48 h, it is noted that the patient is oliguric and the BUN and P_{cr} have risen from 15/1.0 mg/dL to 48/1.6 mg/dL. The urinalysis is normal, the U_{Na} is <10 meq/L, the FE_{Na} is 0.3 percent, and the U_{osm} is 511 mosmol/kg.

Comment. This patient clearly has acute renal failure. The high BUN/P_{cr} ratio and the normal urinalysis suggested prerenal disease, a diagnosis that was then confirmed by the low U_{Na} and FE_{Na} and the high U_{osm}. It is not, however, clear *why* the patient is effectively volume-depleted. There is no history of vomiting, diarrhea, or diuretic use, and there is no history or signs of heart failure, hepatic cirrhosis, or the nephrotic syndrome. In this setting, an *occult cardiopulmonary event* must be excluded as the cause of the reduced tissue perfusion. As a result, an electrocardiogram was obtained which demonstrated an acute anterior myocardial infarction. In retrospect, the apparently "normal" blood pressure of 105/80 was probably low for this patient, considering the history of mild hypertension. In addition, the presence of cool extremities on physical examination was another sign suggesting hypoperfusion.

ISOLATED URINARY ABNORMALITIES

When an abnormal urinalysis is found in conjunction with a reduced GFR, it is clear that some form of renal disease is present and the evaluation should proceed as described above. However, it is not uncommon to see patients with normal renal function who have an isolated abnormality on the urinalysis such as proteinuria, hematuria, or pyuria. In these patients, kidney disease may or may not be present since hematuria or pyuria can arise from any site in the urinary tract. Even when the abnormality is of renal origin, the disease is frequently benign, particularly in children.[31] In patients over the age of 25, however, the prognosis may not be as good since proteinuria or hematuria is frequently associated with potentially serious disease in the urinary tract.

PROTEINURIA

The initial approach to the patient with isolated proteinuria (Table 2–5) involves asking three questions:

1. What type of protein is excreted?
2. How much protein is excreted?
3. Under what conditions is protein excreted?

WHAT TYPE OF PROTEIN IS EXCRETED?

In proteinuric states, the primary urinary protein may be either albumin or low-molecular-weight proteins (MW less than 50,000) (see p. 14). Albuminuria, which is more common, is due to an increase in the permeability of the glomerular capillary wall. The result is enhanced filtration and subsequent excretion of albumin and other plasma proteins (called *glomerular* proteinuria). In comparison, low-molecular-weight proteins are normally filtered and then almost entirely reabsorbed in the proximal tubule. Increased excretion of these proteins (called *tubular* proteinuria) can occur in two settings: (1) when production is increased as with immunoglobulin light chains in multiple myeloma or lysozyme in acute (usually myelomonocytic) leukemia[32,33] or (2) when proximal tubular function is impaired as in the Fanconi syndrome or in disorders that cause tubular damage such as acute tubular necrosis due to aminoglycoside toxicity or chronic interstitial nephritis.[34,35,35a]

Differentiating between glomerular and tubular proteinuria is extremely important since the evaluation, therapy, and prognosis

TABLE 2-5. Etiology of Isolated Proteinuria

Glomerular proteinuria
   Transient or intermittent proteinuria
   Orthostatic or postural proteinuria
   Benign persistent proteinuria
   Early or mild glomerular disease
Tubular proteinuria
   Decreased proximal tubular reabsorption
      Fanconi syndrome
      Tubulointerstitial diseases
      Sepsis
   Increased production
      Multiple myeloma
      Leukemia (particularly acute myelomonocytic leukemia)

of patients with multiple myeloma, for example, differs from that of patients with increased glomerular permeability. The presence of low-molecular-weight proteins in the urine can be easily detected by testing the urine with both the dipstick, which senses primarily albumin, and sulfosalicylic acid, which senses all proteins (see Table 1–2).[36,37] A more positive response with sulfosalicylic acid indicates the presence of nonalbumin proteins. This can be confirmed by immunoelectrophoresis of the urine.

HOW MUCH PROTEIN IS EXCRETED?

In patients whose only urinary abnormality is glomerular proteinuria, the quantity of protein excreted may indicate whether benign or serious renal disease is present. Since the dipstick and sulfosalicylic acid measure only the urine protein concentration, which is a function of urine volume as well as the quantity of protein excreted, a quantitative assessment of the degree of proteinuria is best obtained with a 24-h urine collection for protein and creatinine. (The latter is measured to assess the completeness of the collection; see p. 5.)

A simpler alternative, which may be particularly useful in monitoring for changes in protein excretion, is to measure the protein/creatinine ratio (milligram/milligram) in a random daytime urine specimen. In adults, this ratio correlates closely with total protein excretion, i.e., a ratio of 2 represents protein excretion of approximately 2 g/day per 1.73 m^2 body surface area.[38] A similar relationship exists in children.[39]

Patients with the benign forms of isolated proteinuria (which occur primarily in children) usually excrete less than 1 g/day (upper limit of normal less than 150 mg),[40–42] although values as high as 2 g may be seen.[43,44] If more than 2 g is excreted, serious renal disease usually is present.[45,46] Values greater than 3.5 g (or 50 mg/kg) per day represent nephrotic range proteinuria and are

usually accompanied by hypoalbuminemia, edema, and hyperlipidemia (see Chap. 5).

Since the degree of proteinuria is of prognostic significance, it is important to be aware that the quantity of protein excreted is influenced by the GFR and the plasma albumin concentration as well as glomerular permeability.[47,48] If either of the first two factors is reduced, less albumin will be filtered and protein excretion will diminish. Patients excreting less than 2 g of protein per day usually do not develop hypoalbuminemia since hepatic albumin production can be increased to maintain a normal plasma albumin concentration.[49] In contrast, hypoalbuminemia is commonly seen in patients with the nephrotic syndrome who excrete more than 3.5 g/day. In some of these patients, however, the fall in the plasma albumin concentration can result in a decrease in daily protein excretion to less than nephrotic levels. Thus, the finding of otherwise unexplained hypoalbuminemia in a patient with moderate proteinuria (1.5 to 3.5 g/day) is strongly suggestive of the nephrotic syndrome. This suspicion can be confirmed by an intravenous infusion of albumin which will raise the plasma albumin concentration and markedly increase urinary albumin excretion.[47,48]

UNDER WHAT CONDITIONS IS PROTEIN EXCRETED?

Mild proteinuria can be divided into three categories[50]:

1. Transient, or intermittent
2. Orthostatic, or postural
3. Persistent

Transient, or intermittent, proteinuria is by far the most common. Up to 4 percent of men and 7 percent of women have proteinuria on a single examination with resolution in almost all on repeated examinations.[50,51] Stresses such as exercise and fever may be responsible in at least some cases (see p. 32).[52,53] Transient proteinuria is also found in about 10 percent of acutely ill patients admitted to the hospital (primarily with heart failure or infection).[54]

The mechanism by which these conditions induce proteinuria is not known. Glomerular and tubular components appear to be present as both albumin and low-molecular-weight protein excretion may be increased.[55] It is possible that stress hormones (norepinephrine and angiotensin II) may be involved in this response. These hormones can increase albumin excretion, perhaps by a hemodynamic effect or by enhancing glomerular pore size.[56,57] They might also cause tubular proteinuria by inducing mild ischemic tubular damage.[52] Regardless of the mechanism, transient proteinuria is a benign disorder.

Orthostatic, or postural, proteinuria is characterized by protein excretion that is increased in the upright position but is *normal during recumbency*.[50,58] Total protein excretion is generally under 1 g/day, but values in excess of 3 g/day may occasionally be seen.[59] Orthostatic proteinuria occurs in 2 to 5 percent of adolescents but is rarely seen over the age of 30. The assumption of the upright posture is associated with venous pooling in the legs, resulting sequentially in a reduction in the effective circulating volume[60] and increases in sympathetic tone and the activity of the renin-angiotensin system.[61] These neurohumoral changes could then be responsible for the proteinuria.[56,57] Consistent with this theory is the observation that the inhibition of venous pooling with an antigravity suit prevents orthostatic proteinuria.[62]

Although mild glomerular abnormalities are present on histologic examination in more than 50 percent of patients with orthostatic proteinuria, the long-term (up to 40 to 50 years) prognosis is excellent.[50,58] Renal function remains normal, the incidence of hypertension is not increased, and there is a gradual disappearance of proteinuria—49 percent positive at 10 years, but only 17 percent positive at 20 years.[58]

Patients with *persistent* proteinuria have a fixed disorder in which total protein excretion is usually below 1 to 2 g/day.[42-46,63] These patients are much more likely to have definite renal disease than those with transient or orthostatic proteinuria.[42,45,46,63] In addition to intrinsic renal diseases, hemodynamic disturbances such as heart failure can also be associated with persistent, mild proteinuria.[64]

The prognosis of persistent proteinuria in which there is no apparent cause appears to vary with age. Patients younger than 25 frequently follow a benign course.[40,42-44] However, the prognosis is likely to be worse in older patients, since a variety of renal diseases can present with mild isolated proteinuria, including diabetic nephropathy, nephrosclerosis, and membranous nephropathy.[45,46,65] In the Framingham study, for example, cardiovascular mortality was enhanced threefold in men with mild, persistent proteinuria. This increased risk appeared to be limited to those patients with hypertension, diabetes mellitus, or left ventricular hypertrophy, suggesting that underlying diabetic nephropathy or nephrosclerosis was responsible for the proteinuria.[51]

DIAGNOSIS

The diagnostic approach to the patient with isolated proteinuria should begin with the exclusion of potentially contributing systemic disorders such as diabetes mellitus, hypertension, systemic lupus erythematosus, heart failure, and acute infections. In addition, the personal (previous episode of poststreptococcal glomerulonephritis) and family history (positive for polycystic kidney disease or hereditary nephritis) may provide important information. Poststreptococcal glomerulonephritis, for example, may be associated with mild isolated proteinuria for several years after recovery from the acute episode.[66]

In the patient who has no evidence of an

underlying disease, at least three urinalyses (using both the dipstick and sulfosalicylic acid) should be performed to document that the proteinuria is persistent. To quantitate the amount of protein excreted and, in patients under the age of 25, to test for orthostatic proteinuria, a 24-h urine collection for protein and creatinine should then be obtained as outlined in Table 2-6. An orthostatic increase in protein excretion commonly occurs in a variety of benign as well as potentially serious renal diseases.[67] The specific diagnosis of benign orthostatic proteinuria requires that *protein excretion be normal in recumbency*—less than 50 mg per 8 h (that is, a rate less than 150 mg per day). In the absence of orthostatic proteinuria, a renal ultrasound or intravenous pyelogram (IVP) should be performed to rule out disorders such as chronic pyelonephritis, obstruction, or polycystic kidney disease, all of which can induce mild proteinuria.

The finding of lipiduria, as manifested by free fat droplets, oval fat bodies, or fatty casts (see Plates 1 and 2), also may be helpful. This lipid is assumed to enter the urine as a lipoprotein, which is filtered across an abnormally permeable glomerulus. Thus, lipiduria points strongly toward a primary glomerular disease. Occasional exceptions do occur, however, particularly in polycystic kidney disease.[68] It is not clear if the lipiduria in this setting originates from secondary glomerular damage or protein leakage from the tubular cells lining the cysts.

Since many patients with persistent proteinuria follow a benign course, a renal biopsy is not part of the routine evaluation. In the absence of a known cause for the proteinuria, a biopsy should be done when there is evidence of serious renal disease such as a reduced GFR, protein excretion in excess of 2 g/day, concurrent hematuria, or unexplained hypoalbuminemia (in which case infusing albumin to raise the plasma albumin concentration will markedly raise protein excretion if glomerular disease is present).*,[47,48] Patients who have no indications for biopsy on initial evaluation may develop evidence of progressive disease in the future. Therefore, a urinalysis, a random daytime urine protein/creatinine ratio (if the proteinuria persists),[38,39] and a P_{cr} should be obtained at regular intervals (every 6 months initially).

HEMATURIA

In contrast to proteinuria, which originates in the kidney, hematuria (defined as more than 2 red cells per HPF; see p. 32) can arise from any site in the urinary tract (Table 2-7). It is a relatively common and frequently transient problem. In one study of 1000 young men who had yearly urinalyses for 15 years (between the ages of 18 and 33), hematuria was found in 39 percent on at least one occasion and in 16 percent on two or more examinations.[69] In the great majority, no cause for this typically transient hematuria could be demonstrated.

TABLE 2-6. Procedure for 24-h Urine Collection in Evaluation of Isolated Proteinuria

1. At 7 a.m., the first morning void is discarded.
2. With the patient performing normal activities, a 16-h collection should be completed at 11 p.m.
3. To prevent contamination of the recumbent collection with urine formed in the upright position, the patient should remain recumbent after 9 p.m.
4. An 8-h recumbent collection should start at 11 p.m. (with the patient urinating just before the collection is begun) and be completed with the first morning void at 7 a.m.

*The glomerular diseases that can cause proteinuria are discussed in Chap. 6. Heavy proteinuria alone is not an indication for biopsy in *children* because minimal change disease, which usually is corticosteroid-responsive, accounts for the great majority of cases. Therefore, children with heavy proteinuria are first treated with steroids and biopsied only if they are steroid-resistant. Since minimal change disease is less common in adults, steroids are less effective and a biopsy should be performed before therapy is started.

TABLE 2-7. Major Causes of Isolated Hematuria

Extrarenal bleeding
  Ureters: calculi, carcinoma
  Bladder: hemorrhagic cystitis due to infection
    (including *Schistosoma haematobium* in endemic areas) or cyclophosphamide, carcinoma, catheterization, calculi
  Prostate: hypertrophy, carcinoma, or prostatitis
  Urethra: urethritis, trauma
Extraglomerular renal bleeding
  Carcinoma of the kidney or renal pelvis
  Trauma
  Crystalluria: hypercalciuria, rarely sulfonamides, mercaptopurine
  Vascular malformations: hemangiomas, arteriovenous fistulas, varices
  Sickle cell trait or disease
  Coagulation disorders (anticoagulant therapy, hemophilia)
  Cystic disease: polycystic kidney disease, medullary sponge kidney
  Renal tuberculosis
  Renal infarction
  Vasculitis
  Interstitial nephritis
Glomerular bleeding
  Mild forms of glomerulonephritis
  Benign hematuria
  Malignant hypertension
  Long-distance running

The major *identifiable* causes of isolated hematuria in adults* are prostatic disease, renal or ureteral calculi, malignancy (of the prostate, kidney, or bladder), and trauma.[71-73] Glomerular disease generally accounts for less than 5 percent of cases. Other renal diseases such as vasculitis and interstitial nephritis also can cause hematuria. However, they usually present with other urinary abnormalities or a reduced GFR and therefore are not examples of isolated hematuria.

In children, the etiologic distribution is somewhat different, as glomerular disease, hypercalciuria (with or without identifiable calculi), and perineal irritation or trauma are most common.[40,70,74] The importance of hypercalciuria (defined as calcium excretion exceeding 4 mg/kg per day) has only recently been appreciated.[74-76] In one study of 83 chil-

*In both adults and children, urinary tract infection may account for more than 25 percent of cases with hematuria.[70,71] However, this diagnosis is usually suspected by the concurrent findings of dysuria, frequency, pyuria, and bacteriuria.

dren with isolated hematuria, 23 had hypercalciuria (17 had glomerular disease and 38 of the remainder were of uncertain etiology).[74] Of the 23 with hypercalciuria, 77 percent had a positive family history of kidney stones (versus only 15 percent in the normocalciuric group), and 2 subsequently developed stones. It has been postulated that microcalculi or tubular damage from crystalluria is responsible for the hematuria. Regardless of the mechanism, lowering urinary calcium excretion with a calcium-restricted diet or a thiazide diuretic usually leads to cessation of hematuria.[74-76]

DIAGNOSIS

The initial aim in the evaluation of hematuria with little or no proteinuria is to identify the source of the bleeding. The magnitude of bleeding is not helpful since gross or microscopic hematuria can occur with most of the disorders in Table 2-7. Furthermore, the presence of red or brown urine does not necessarily indicate heavy bleeding, since as little as 1 mL of blood in 1 L of urine can produce a visible color change.[77]

As described previously (Table 2–4), examination of the urine frequently allows glomerular and extraglomerular bleeding to be distinguished. In particular, the finding of dysmorphic red cells (see Plate 1*b*) or red cell casts is virtually diagnostic of glomerular disease (or vasculitis). An interesting application of these principles can be seen with hematuria due to *long-distance running*. Although it had been assumed that bladder trauma was responsible, almost all patients have dysmorphic red cells and up to 30 percent have red cell casts and mild proteinuria, strongly suggesting a glomerular origin.[78]

In addition to the urinalysis, the history and physical examination may provide important clues to the diagnosis.

1. If the patient complains of gross hematuria, he or she should be asked if it is more prominent in the initial or terminal parts of the urinary stream. Initial hematuria points toward a urethral lesion, whereas terminal hematuria is suggestive of a localized bladder abnormality in the region of the trigone.[77,79] This history, if present, can be confirmed by examining split urine specimens—first few drops, midstream, and last few drops—and comparing the degree of hematuria. In contrast, renal, ureteric, and diffuse bladder bleeding all result in hematuria throughout the stream.

2. The history of a recent upper respiratory infection, particularly in the presence of gross hematuria, is suggestive of some form of acute postinfectious glomerulonephritis. In some patients, particularly those with IgA nephropathy or benign hematuria, there may be a history of recurrent episodes following viral infections.

3. Dysuria, urinary frequency, and suprapubic tenderness suggest hemorrhagic cystitis due to bacterial infection. Pyuria also is present, and the diagnosis can be confirmed by a urine culture. Dysuria, hematuria, and pyuria also may be the mode of presentation of urinary tuberculosis.[80] This diagnosis should be suspected if, in this setting, the urine culture is negative for bacteria. It can be confirmed by culture of the urine for *Mycobacterium tuberculosis.*

4. Unilateral flank pain suggests a unilateral process and may be due to the underlying disease (ureteric calculus, polycystic kidney disease, renal infarction) or to an obstructing blood clot in the ureter. Bilateral flank pain, however, is less specific and occurs with many forms of glomerulonephritis due to stretching of the renal capsule.

5. The patient should be questioned for signs of a systemic disease such as systemic lupus erythematosus, vasculitis, or a bleeding disorder, e.g., hemophilia or anticoagulant therapy,[81] particularly if there are signs of bleeding elsewhere.

6. Black patients should be tested for sickle cell trait or a combined hemoglobinopathy such as hemoglobin SC disease. These disorders may be associated with repeated episodes of hematuria, presumably due to sickling of erythrocytes in the hypertonic, hypoxemic medulla, resulting in local papillary infarcts.[82,83]

7. A positive family history of renal disease raises the possibility of hereditary nephritis or polycystic kidney disease.

8. A drug history should be obtained, since some drugs can lead to hematuria, including cyclophosphamide, which produces a sterile hemorrhagic cystitis,[84] or sulfonamides or mercaptopurine, which can induce crystalluria.[85]

9. The presence of hypertension is of little diagnostic benefit unless it is severe or known to be of recent onset. Malignant hypertension frequently is associated with hematuria. The findings of a very high diastolic pressure, hematuria, and

papilledema usually make this diagnosis apparent (see Chap. 11). If the onset of hypertension is temporally associated with the hematuria, acute glomerulonephritis may be present. However, other causes of isolated hematuria such as ureteral obstruction and polycystic disease also can produce an increase in blood pressure.[86,87]

10. Older men should be asked about symptoms of prostatic disease, such as hesitancy, dribbling, and frequency. Rectal examination may reveal prostatic enlargement or a prostatic mass.

In many patients, the initial evaluation does not suggest a definite diagnosis. In this setting, a plain film of the abdomen and an IVP should be performed. Renal masses, stones, hydronephrosis, and polycystic kidney disease all may be detected by these procedures. In addition, unilateral non-visualization suggests obstruction or severe ischemia due, for example, to a renal artery embolus.

If the IVP is normal, a cystoscopic examination of the bladder is usually the next step, looking primarily for tumor, prostatic disease, or cystitis. Although cystoscopy is warranted in patients over the age of 40, it is probably not necessary in most younger patients, since the incidence of malignancy or prostatic disease and, therefore, the diagnostic yield would be very low.[40,69] One exception occurs in patients with recurrent or persistent gross hematuria in whom cystoscopic examination during an episode may localize the bleeding to one kidney (in which case some anatomic abnormality is probably present)[88] or to both kidneys (making glomerulonephritis most likely).

Renal arteriography (and in some instances, venography), also has a role, particularly in patients with a solid renal mass (see p. 414), proven unilateral bleeding by cystoscopy, or persistent gross hematuria. As many as one-half of patients in the last two groups will, on arteriography or venography, be found to have a vascular abnormality such as an arteriovenous fistula, hemangioma, or varices.[89,90] If these tests are negative in patients with proven unilateral gross hematuria, operative nephroscopy may be very effective in localizing the site and source of the bleeding (frequently due to small submucosal hemangiomas).[88]

GLOMERULAR DISEASE

Some form of glomerulonephritis should be suspected if there are characteristic urinary changes (such as dysmorphic red cells or red cell casts), bilateral bleeding is identified on cystoscopy, or the above work-up is negative. This does not mean that a renal biopsy should be performed, however, since "benign hematuria" is a common cause of hematuria in children and may also occur in adults (see Chap. 6).[40,63,91-96] This disorder is typically characterized by episodes of gross hematuria that occur within 1 to 3 days after a viral upper respiratory infection. (Poststreptococcal glomerulonephritis can also lead to gross hematuria, but the latent period is generally longer at 7 to 21 days and recurrent episodes are unusual.)

Benign hematuria has an excellent long-term prognosis and requires no therapy. Renal biopsy is not helpful in this disorder since it usually reveals only nonspecific, focal proliferative changes in the mesangium.[63,94,96] In some patients, particularly those with a positive family history, electron microscopy will demonstrate marked thinning of the glomerular basement membrane.[97,98]

A renal biopsy *is* indicated when there are reasons to believe that a more serious type of glomerulonephritis may be present, including IgA nephropathy, membranoproliferative glomerulonephritis, and hereditary nephritis. Clues to the presence of potentially progressive disease include persistent proteinuria (particularly if more than 1 g/day), a reduced GFR, the concurrent development of hypertension, persistent hypocomplementemia (suggestive of membranoproliferative glomerulonephritis), and a positive family history of renal disease.[63,95,97,99] On the other hand, the absence of cellular or granular casts seems to be a strong predictor of minimal histologic changes.[100]

Isolated hematuria due to focal glomerulonephritis also may occur with systemic diseases such as poststreptococcal glomerulonephritis, systemic lupus erythematosus, Henoch-Schönlein purpura (and other forms of vasculitis), and subacute bacterial endocarditis (see Chaps. 6 and 7). Symptoms and findings consistent with these disorders, such as fever, sore throat, skin rash, arthralgias, or a heart murmur, usually are present. Although these diseases can progress to renal failure, the focal forms tend to follow a more benign course.

In approximately 10 percent of patients, no cause for hematuria will be found nor will there be criteria for performing a renal biopsy.[71-73] In this setting, urine cytology may uncover an occult malignancy.[77] It might also be worthwhile to obtain a 24-h urine collection for calcium and creatinine. As described above, hypercalciuria with presumed crystalluria is responsible for many cases of unexplained hematuria in children.[74-76] It is not known whether these results also apply to adults, but a trial of hydrochlorothiazide seems reasonable if hypercalciuria is found. If these tests are negative, the patient should be carefully followed and reevaluated at periodic intervals.

CLINICAL EXAMPLE

The approach to the patient with isolated hematuria can be illustrated by the following case history.

Case History 2-5. A 32-year-old man presented with moderate right flank pain and, on urinalysis, 5 to 10 red cells per HPF. Since the pain suggested a process in the right kidney, an IVP was performed, revealing a right renal mass. Renal arteriography confirmed the diagnosis of a renal carcinoma, and a right nephrectomy was performed. Histologic examination showed a renal cell carcinoma with the remainder of the kidney appearing normal.

Postoperatively, there was persistent microscopic hematuria without casts, proteinuria, or any symptoms. Residual tumor seemed to be the most likely diagnosis, so cystoscopy and renal arteriography were repeated and were negative. The hematuria continued over the next 8 years (without deterioration in renal function) with consistently negative results on cystoscopy and arteriography that were performed at 1- to 2-year intervals. Finally, the urine was examined again after the importance of dysmorphic red cells had become appreciated. More than 80 percent of the red cells had a dysmorphic appearance, suggesting a glomerular rather than a neoplastic origin. Light microscopic examination of the "normal" tissue in the nephrectomy specimen again appeared normal. This tissue was then looked at under electron microscopy, which revealed diffuse marked thinning of the glomerular basement membranes, the presumed cause of the benign microscopic hematuria.[97,98]

Comment. The presence of dysmorphic red cells in this patient both pointed toward the correct diagnosis (after 8 years of fruitless searching) and also obviated the need for repeated diagnostic procedures.

PYURIA

Pyuria is defined as more than 4 white blood cells per HPF on a clean-voided specimen. In patients with symptoms of dysuria and frequency, the concurrent presence of pyuria generally indicates infection due to bacteria or, less commonly, organisms that are not recovered on routine culture such as *Chlamydia* or *M. tuberculosis.*[80,101]

In asymptomatic subjects, the finding of isolated pyuria is frequently transient and not representative of underlying urinary tract disease.[102] Persistent pyuria should be evalu-

ated, however, beginning with a urine culture. If this is negative, a tubulointerstitial disease may be present, such as chronic pyelonephritis or analgesic abuse nephropathy.[103] An IVP may be helpful in this setting, possibly revealing papillary necrosis in the latter and calyceal blunting and cortical scarring in the former (see Chap. 8).

REFERENCES

1. Meltzer, J. I., H. J. Keim, J. H. Laragh, J. E. Sealey, K. M. Jan, and S. Chien: Nephrotic syndrome: Vasoconstriction and hypervolemic types indicated by renin-sodium profiling, *Ann. Intern. Med.,* 91:688, 1979.
2. Geers, A. B., H. A. Koomans, J. C. Roos, P. Boer, and E. J. Dorhout Mees: Functional relationships in the nephrotic syndrome, *Kidney Int.,* 26:324, 1984.
3. Acosta, J. H.: Hypertension in chronic renal disease, *Kidney Int.,* 22:702, 1982.
4. Vertes, V., J. L. Cangiano, L. B. Berman, and A. Gould: Hypertension in end-stage renal disease, *N. Engl. J. Med.,* 280:978, 1969.
5. Beretta-Piccoli, C., P. Weidmann, H. Schiffl, C. Cottier, and F. C. Reubi: Enhanced cardiovascular pressor activity to norepinephrine in mild renal parenchymal disease, *Kidney Int.,* 22:297, 1982.
6. McGonigle, R. J. S., F. Husserl, J. D. Wallin, and J. W. Fisher: Hemodialysis and continuous ambulatory peritoneal dialysis effects on erythropoiesis in renal failure, *Kidney Int.,* 25:430, 1984.
7. McGonigle, R. J. S., J. D. Wallin, R. K. Shadduck, and J. W. Fisher: Erythropoietin deficiency and inhibition of erythropoiesis in renal insufficiency, *Kidney Int.,* 25:437, 1984.
8. Basu, T. K., and R. M. Stein: Erythrocytosis associated with chronic renal disease, *Arch. Intern. Med.,* 133:422, 1974.
9. Friend, D. G., R. G. Haskins, and M. W. Kirkin: Relative erythrocytemia (polycythemia) and polycystic kidney disease with uremia: Report of a case with comments on frequency of occurrence, *N. Engl. J. Med.,* 264:17, 1961.
10. Cockcroft, D. W., and M. H. Gault: Prediction of creatinine clearance from serum creatinine, *Nephron,* 16:13, 1976.
11. Dossetor, J. B.: Creatininemia versus uremia. The relative significance of blood urea nitrogen and serum creatinine concentrations in azotemia, *Ann. Intern. Med.,* 65:1287, 1966.
12. Clinicopathological Conference: Progressive renal failure with hematuria in a 62 year-old man, *Am. J. Med.,* 71:468, 1981.
13. Sigala, J. F., C. G. Biava, and H. N. Hulter: Red blood cell casts in acute interstitial nephritis, *Arch. Intern. Med.,* 138:1419, 1978.
14. Northway, J. D.: Hematuria in children, *J. Pediatr.,* 78:381, 1971.
15. Fairley, K. F., and D. F. Birch: Hematuria: A simple method for identifying glomerular bleeding, *Kidney Int.,* 21:105, 1982.
16. Sanchez-Ibarrola, A., S. Qazzaz, and P. Naish: Clearance of fibrin from glomeruli. Renal cortical fibrinolytic response after thromboplastin infusion in the rat., *Clin. Sci.,* 60:47, 1981.
17. Min, K. W., F. Gjorkey, P. Gjorkey, J. J. Yium, and G. Eknoyan: The morphogenesis of glomerular crescents in rapidly progressive glomerulonephritis, *Kidney Int.,* 5:47, 1974.
18. Burkholder, P. M.: Ultrastructural demonstration of injury and perforation of glomerular capillary basement membrane in acute proliferative glomerulonephritis, *Am. J. Pathol.,* 56:251, 1969.
19. Boyd, P. J. R.: Hematuria, *Br. Med. J.,* 2:445, 1977.
20. Danovitch, G. M., J. J. Bourgoignie, and N. S. Bricker: Reversibility of the "salt-losing" tendency of chronic renal failure, *N. Engl. J. Med.,* 296:14, 1977.
21. Yeh, B. P. Y., D. J. Tomki, W. K. Stacy, E. S. Bear, H. T. Haden, and W. F. Falls, Jr.: Factors influencing sodium and water excretion in uremic man, *Kidney Int.,* 7:103, 1975.
22. Levinsky, N. G., E. A. Alexander, and M. A. Ven-

katachalam: Acute renal failure, in B. M. Brenner and F. C. Rector, Jr. (eds), *The Kidney*, 2d ed., Saunders, Philadelphia, 1981.

23. Miller, P. D., R. A. Krebs, B. J. Neal, and D. O. McIntyre: Polyuric prerenal failure, *Arch. Intern. Med.*, 140:907, 1980.

24. Miller, T. R., R. J. Anderson, S. L. Linas, W. L. Henrich, A. S. Berns, P. A. Gabow, and R. W. Schrier: Urinary diagnostic indices in acute renal failure: A prospective study, *Ann. Intern. Med.*, 89:47, 1978.

25. Steiner, R. W.: Interpreting the fractional excretion of sodium, *Am. J. Med.*, 77:699, 1984.

26. Hoffman, L. M., and W. N. Suki: Obstructive uropathy mimicking volume depletion, *J. Am. Med. Assoc.*, 236:2096, 1976.

27. Dorhout Mees, E. J.: Relation between maximal urine concentration, maximal water reabsorption capacity, and mannitol clearance in patients with renal disease, *Br. Med. J.*, 1:1159, 1959.

28. Editorial, Diagnosing obstruction in renal failure, *Lancet*, 2:848, 1984.

29. Webb, J. A. W., R. H. Reznek, F. E. White, W. R. Cattell, I. Kelsey Fry, and L. R. I. Baker: Can ultrasound and computed tomography replace high-dose urography in patients with impaired renal function?, *Q. J. Med.*, 53:411, 1984.

30. L. S.-T. Fang: Contrast medium-induced acute renal failure, *Med. Grand Rounds*, 2:263, 1983.

31. Dodge, W. F., E. F. West, E. H. Smith, and H. Bunce: Proteinuria and hematuria in school children: Epidemiology and early natural history, *J. Pediatr.*, 88:327, 1976.

32. Perry, M. C., and R. A. Kyle: The clinical significance of Bence Jones proteinuria, *Mayo Clin. Proc.*, 50:234, 1975.

33. Muggia, F. M., H. O. Heinemann, M. Farhangi, and E. F. Osserman: Lysozymuria and renal tubular dysfunction in monocytic and myelomonocytic leukemia, *Am. J. Med.*, 47:351, 1969.

34. Peterson, A., E. Evrin, and I. Berggård: Differentiation of glomerular, tubular, and normal proteinuria: Determinations of urinary excretion of β_2-microglobulin, albumin, and total protein, *J. Clin. Invest.*, 48:1189, 1969.

35. Schentag, J. J., and M. E. Plaut: Patterns of urinary β_2-microglobulin excretion by patients treated with aminoglycosides. *Kidnet Int.*, 17:654, 1980.

35a. Portman, R. J., J. M. Kissane, and A. M. Robson: Use of β_2-microglobulin to diagnose tubulointerstitial renal lesions in children, *Kidney Int.*, 30:91, 1986.

36. Thysell, H.: A comparison between albustix, hemacombistix, labstix, the sulphosalicylic-acid test, Heller's nitric acid test, and a biuret method, *Acta Med. Scand.*, 185:401, 1969.

37. Clugh, G., and T. G. Reak: A "protein error," *Lancet*, 1:1248, 1964.

38. Ginsberg, J. M., B. S. Chang, R. A. Matarese, and S. Garella: Use of single voided urine samples to estimate quantitative proteinuria, *N. Engl. J. Med.*, 309:1543, 1983.

39. Houser, M.: Assessment of proteinuria using random urine samples, *J. Pediatr.*, 104:845, 1984.

40. West, C. D.: Asymptomatic hematuria and proteinuria in children: Causes and appropriate diagnostic studies, *J. Pediatr.*, 89:173, 1976.

41. Muth, R. G.: Asymptomatic mild intermittent proteinuria: A percutaneous renal biopsy study, *Arch. Intern. Med.*, 115:569, 1965.

42. Chen, B. T. M., B. S. Ooi, K. K. Tan, and C. H. Lim: Comparative studies of asymptomatic proteinuria and hematuria, *Arch. Intern. Med.*, 134:901, 1974.

43. McLaine, P. N., and K. N. Drummond: Benign persistent asymptomatic proteinuria in childhood, *Pediatrics*, 46:548, 1970.

44. Urizar, R. D., B. O. Tinglof, F. G. Smith, Jr., and R. M. McIntosh: Persistent asymptomatic proteinuria in children: Functional and ultrastructural evaluation with special reference to glomerular basement membrane thickness, *Am. J. Clin. Pathol.*, 62:461, 1974.

45. Phillippi, P. J., J. Reynolds, H. Yamauchi, and S. C. Beering: Persistent proteinuria in asymptomatic individuals: Renal biopsy studies on 50 patients, *Mil. Med.*, 131:1311, 1966.

46. Pollak, V. E., C. L. Pirani, R. C. Muehrcke, and R. M. Kark: Asymptomatic persistent proteinuria: Studies by renal biopsies, *Guy's Hosp. Rep.*, 10:353, 1958.

47. Hardwicke, J., and J. R. Squire: The relationship between plasma albumin concentration and protein excretion in patients with proteinuria, *Clin. Sci.*, 14:509, 1955.

48. Shemesh, O., W. M. Deen, B. M. Brenner, E. McNeely, and B. D. Myers: Effect of colloid volume expansion on glomerular barrier size-selectivity in humans, *Kidney Int.*, 29:916, 1986.

49. Rothschild, M. A., M. Oratz, and S. S. Schreiber: Albumin synthesis, *N. Engl. J. Med.*, 286:748, 816, 1972.

50. Robinson, R. R.: Isolated proteinuria in asymptomatic patients, *Kidney Int.*, 18:395, 1980.

51. Kannel, W. B., M. J. Stampfer, W. P. Castelli, and J. Verter: The prognostic significance of proteinuria: The Framingham study, *Am. Ht. J.*, 108:1347, 1984.

52. Poortmans, J. R.: Postexercise proteinuria in humans. Facts and mechanisms, *J. Am. Med. Assoc.,* 253:236, 1985.

53. Marks, M. I., P. N. McLaine, and K. N. Drummond: Proteinuria in children with febrile illnesses, *Arch. Dis. Child.,* 45:250, 1970.

54. Reuben, D. B., T. J. Wachtel, P. C. Brown, and J. L. Driscoll: Transient proteinuria in emergency medical admissions, *N. Engl. J. Med.,* 306:1031, 1982.

55. Richmond, J. M., W. J. Sibbald, A. M. Linton, and A. L. Linton: Patterns of urinary protein excretion in patients with sepsis, *Nephron,* 31:219, 1982.

56. Bohrer, M. P., W. M. Deen, C. R. Robertson, and B. M. Brenner: Mechanisms of angiotensin II-induced proteinuria in the rat, *Am. J. Physiol.,* 233: F13, 1977.

57. Olivetti, G., K. Kithier, F. Giacomelli, and J. Wiener: Characterization of glomerular permeability and proteinuria in acute hypertension in the rat, *Kidney Int.,* 25:599, 1984.

58. Springberg, P. D., L. E. Garrett, Jr., A. L. Thompson, N. F. Collins, R. E. Lordon, and R. R. Thompson: Fixed and reproducible orthostatic proteinuria: Results of a 20-year follow-up study, *Ann. Intern. Med.,* 97:516, 1982.

59. Rytand, D. A., and S. Spreiter: Prognosis in postural (orthostatic) proteinuria. Forty to fifty-year follow-up of six patients after diagnosis by Thomas Addis, *N. Engl. J. Med.,* 305:618, 1981.

60. Epstein, F. H., A. N. Goddyer, F. D. Laurason, and A. S. Relman: Studies of the antidiuresis of quiet standing: The importance of changes in plasma volume and glomerular filtration rate, *J. Clin. Invest.,* 30:62, 1951.

61. Gordon, R. D., O. Kuchel, G. W. Liddle, and D. P. Island: Role of the sympathetic nervous system in regulating renin and aldosterone production in man, *J. Clin. Invest.,* 46:599, 1967.

62. Grenier, T., and J. P. Henry: Mechanism of postural proteinuria, *J. Am. Med. Assoc.,* 157:1373, 1955.

63. Brown, E. A., K. Upadhyaya, J. P. Hayslett, M. Kashgarian, and N. J. Siegel: The clinical course of mesangial proliferative glomerulonephritis, *Medicine,* 58:295, 1979.

64. Carrie, B. J., M. Hilberman, J. S. Schroeder, and B. D. Myers: Albuminuria and the permselective properties of the glomerulus in cardiac failure, *Kidney Int.,* 17:507, 1980.

65. Levinsky, N. G.: Interpretation of proteinuria and the urinary sediment, *Dis. Mon.,* 1967.

66. Potter, E. V., S. A. Lipschultz, S. Abidh, T. Poon-King, and D. P. Earle: Twelve to seventeen-year follow-up of patients with poststreptococcal acute glomerulonephritis in Trinidad, *N. Engl. J. Med.,* 307:725, 1982.

67. King, S. E.: Postural adjustments and protein excretion by the kidney in renal disease, *Ann. Intern. Med.,* 46:360, 1957.

68. Duncan, K. A., F. E. Cuppage, and J. J. Grantham: Urinary lipid bodies in polycystic kidney disease, *Am. J. Kid. Dis.,* 5:49, 1985.

69. Froom, P., J. Ribak, and J. Benbassat: Significance of microhaematuria in young adults, *Br. Med. J.,* 288:20, 1984.

70. Inglefinger, J. R., A. E. Davis, and W. E. Grupe: Frequency and etiology of gross hematuria in a general pediatric setting, *Pediatrics,* 59:557, 1977.

71. Carter, W. C., and S. N. Rous: Gross hematuria in 110 adult urologic hospital patients, *Urology,* 18: 342, 1981.

71a. Mohr, D. N., K. P. Offord, R. A. Owen, and L. J. Melton, III: Asymptomatic hematuria and urologic disease. A population-based study, *J. Am. Med. Assoc.,* 256:224, 1986.

72. Burkholder, G. V., N. Dotin, W. B. Thomason, and O. D. Beach: Unexplained hematuria: How extensive should the evaluation be?, *J. Am. Med. Assoc.,* 210:1729, 1969.

73. Carson, C. C., J. W. Segura, and L. F. Greene: Clinical importance of microscopic hematuria, *J. Am. Med. Assoc.,* 241:149, 1979.

74. Stapleton, F. B., S. Roy, III, H. N. Noe, and G. Jenkins: Hypercalciuria in children with hematuria, *N. Engl. J. Med.,* 310:1345, 1984.

75. Roy, S., III, F. B. Stapleton, H. N. Noe, and G. Jenkins: Hematuria preceding renal calculus formation in children with hypercalciuria, *J. Pediatr.,* 99: 712, 1981.

76. Kalia, A., L. B. Travis, and B. H. Brouhard: The association of idiopathic hypercalciuria and asymptomatic gross hematuria in children, *J. Pediatr.,* 99: 716, 1981.

77. Boyd, P. J. R.: Hematuria, *Br. Med. J.,* 2:445, 1977.

78. Fassett, R. G., J. E. Owen, J. Fairley, D. F. Birch, and K. F. Fairley: Urinary red-cell morphology during exercise, *Br. Med. J.,* 285:1455, 1982.

79. Northway, J. D.: Hematuria in children, *J. Pediatr.,* 78:381, 1971.

80. Simon, H. B., A. J. Weinstein, M. S. Pasternak, M. N. Swartz, and L. J. Kunz: Genitourinary tuberculosis: Clinical features in a general hospital population, *Am. J. Med.,* 63:410, 1977.

81. Small, M., P. E. Rose, N. McMillan, J. J. F. Belch, E. B. Rolfe, C. D. Forbes, and J. Stuart: Haemophilia and the kidney: Assessment after 11-year follow-up, *Br. Med. J.,* 285:1609, 1982.

82. De Jong, P. E., and L. W. Statius van Eps: Sickle cell nephropathy: New insights into its pathophysiology, *Kidney Int.,* 27:711, 1985.

83. Chapman, A. Z., R. S. Reeder, I. A. Friedman, and Y. A. Baker: Gross hematuria in sickle-cell trait and sickle cell hemoglobin-C disease, *Am. J. Med.,* 19:773, 1955.

84. Wall, R. L., and K. P. Clausen: Carcinoma of the urinary bladder in patients receiving cyclophosphamide, *N. Engl. J. Med.,* 293:271, 1975.

85. Duttera, M. J., R. L. Carolla, J. F. Gallelli, D. S. Gullion, D. E. Keim, and E. S. Henderson: Hematuria and crystalluria after high-dose 6-mercaptopurine administration, *N. Engl. J. Med.,* 287:292, 1972.

86. Weidmann, P., C. Beretta-Picoli, D. Hirsh, F. C. Reubin, and S. G. Massry: Curable hypertension with unilateral hydronephrosis, *Ann. Intern. Med.,* 87:437, 1977.

87. Nash, D. A., Jr.: Hypertension in polycystic kidney disease without renal failure, *Arch. Intern. Med.,* 137:1571, 1977.

88. Gittes, R. F., and S. Varady: Nephroscopy in chronic unilateral hematuria, *J. Urol.,* 126:297, 1981.

89. Hayashi, M., T. Kume, and H. Nihira: Abnormalities of renal venous system and unexplained renal hematuria, *J. Urol.,* 124:12, 1980.

90. Jonsson, K.: Renal angiography in patients with hematuria, *Am. J. Roentgenol. Rad. Therap. Nucl. Med.,* 116:758, 1972.

91. Johnston, C., and S. Shuler: Recurrent haematuria in childhood: A five-year follow-up, *Arch. Dis. Child.,* 44:483, 1969.

92. McConville, J. M., C. D. West, and A. J. McAdams: Familial and non-familial benign haematuria, *J. Pediatr.,* 69:207, 1966.

93. Glasgow, E. F., M. W. Moncrieff, and R. H. R. White: Symptomless haematuria in childhood, *Br. Med. J.,* 2:687, 1970.

94. Labovitz, E. D., S. R. Steinmuller, L. W. Henderson, D. K. McCurdy, and M. Goldberg: "Benign" hematuria with focal glomerulonephritis in adults, *Ann. Intern. Med.,* 77:723, 1972.

95. Hendler, E. D., M. Kashgarian, and J. P. Hayslett: Clinicopathological correlations of primary haematuria, *Lancet,* 1:458, 1972.

96. Pardo, V., M. G. Berian, D. F. Levi, and J. Strauss: Benign primary hematuria. Clinicopathologic study of 65 patients, *Am. J. Med.,* 67:817, 1979.

97. Trachtman, H., R. A. Weiss, B. Bennett, and I. Greifer: Isolated hematuria in children: Indications for a renal biopsy, *Kidney Int.,* 25:94, 1984.

98. Rogers, P. W., N. A. Kurtzman, S. M. Bunn, and M. G. White: Familial benign essential hematuria, *Arch. Intern. Med.,* 131:257, 1973.

99. Nicholls, K. M., K. F. Fairley, J. P. Dowling, and P. Kincaid-Smith: The clinical course of mesangial IgA associated nephropathy in adults, *Q. J. Med.,* 53:227, 1984.

100. Györy, A. Z., C. Hadfield, and C. S. Lauer: Value of urine microscopy in predicting histological changes in the kidney: Double blind comparison, *Br. Med. J.,* 288:819, 1984.

101. Stamm, W. E., K. F. Wagner, R. Amsel, E. R. Alexander, M. Turck, G. W. Counts, and K. K. Holmes: Causes of the acute urethral syndrome in women, *N. Engl. J. Med.,* 303:409, 1980.

102. Benbassat, J., P. Froom, M. Feldman, and S. Margaliot: The importance of leukocyturia in young adults, *Arch. Intern. Med.,* 145:79, 1985.

103. Gault, M. G., T. C. Rudwal, W. D. Engles, and J. B. Dossetor: Syndrome associated with the abuse of analgesics, *Ann. Intern. Med.,* 68:906, 1968.

3

ACUTE RENAL FAILURE—PRERENAL DISEASE VERSUS ACUTE TUBULAR NECROSIS

Burton D. Rose

Acute renal failure, a common clinical problem, is characterized by an abrupt decrease in renal function. Since this is associated with a fall in glomerular filtration rate (GFR), the initial clinical manifestations are elevations in the blood urea nitrogen (BUN) and plasma creatinine concentration (P_{cr}) and frequently a reduction in urine output. Even when renal function has previously been normal, a patient with acute renal failure may within 1 week develop the symptoms of uremia and require dialysis. In other patients, the course is more benign, and only a mild reduction in renal function is seen. Regardless of severity, most forms of acute renal failure are reversible. Thus, a proper approach to diagnosis and management is essential to allow time for renal function to improve.

The definition of what constitutes *acute,* as opposed to *subacute,* or *chronic,* renal failure is somewhat arbitrary. The simplest definition of *acute renal failure* is a recent increase in the P_{cr} of at least 0.5 mg/dL if the baseline P_{cr} is less than 3.0 mg/dL and at least 1.0 mg/dL if the baseline P_{cr} is higher. Although these changes in the P_{cr} are numerically small, they usually represent a large reduction in GFR if the baseline P_{cr} is under 2.0 mg/dL (see p. 6). In contrast, a 1.0-mg/dL elevation in the P_{cr} may reflect a drop of 5 mL/min or less in patients with advanced chronic renal disease (P_{cr} greater than 4 mg/dL). Even this small decrement may be clinically significant, however, since a fall in GFR from 10 to 15 mL/min may require the institution of dialysis to maintain life.

The major causes of acute renal failure are depicted in Table 2-1 (Chap. 2). Although the table lists a variety of disorders, this chapter reviews in detail only the two conditions that account for approximately 70 to 75 percent of cases: prerenal disease, in which decreased renal perfusion is responsible for the renal dysfunction; and acute tubular necrosis (ATN).[1,2] These disorders are particularly common when acute renal failure develops *in the hospital* since the other causes (such as glomerulonephritis, vasculitis, or obstruction) most often begin prior to hospitalization.

Both prerenal disease and ATN can occur in a variety of settings (Tables 3-1 and 3-2). In some cases, distinguishing between these disorders may be difficult, particularly since prerenal factors are the primary cause of ATN. This distinction is extremely important clinically since volume repletion will restore

TABLE 3-1. Causes of Prerenal Disease

True volume depletion
    Gastrointestinal losses: vomiting, diarrhea, bleeding, tube drainage
    Renal losses: diuretics, glucose osmotic diuresis, hypoaldosteronism, salt-wasting nephropathy, diabetes insipidus
        (only if abnormal thirst prevents replacement of water losses)
    Skin or respiratory losses: insensible losses, sweat, burns
    Third-space sequestration: intestinal obstruction, crush injury or skeletal fracture, acute pancreatitis
Hypotension
    Shock
    Posttreatment of severe hypertension
Edematous states
    Heart failure
    Hepatic cirrhosis
    Nephrotic syndrome
Selective renal ischemia
    Hepatorenal syndrome
    Nonsteroidal anti-inflammatory drugs
    Bilateral renal artery stenosis (frequently made worse by converting enzyme inhibition)
    Calcium channel blockers

TABLE 3-2. Causes of Acute Tubular Necrosis

Postischemia
    All causes of severe prerenal disease, particularly hypotension
Nephrotoxins
    Drugs and exogenous toxins
        Common: Aminoglycoside antibiotics, radiocontrast media, cisplatin
        Rare: Cephalosporins, rifampin, amphotericin B, polymixins, methoxyflurane, acetaminophen overdose, heavy
            metals (mercury, arsenic, uranium), carbon tetrachloride, EDTA, tetracyclines
    Heme pigments
        Rhabdomyolysis → myoglobinuria
        Intravascular hemolysis → hemoglobinuria

renal function in prerenal disease but will be ineffective (and may actually induce pulmonary or peripheral edema) in ATN.

DIAGNOSIS

The general diagnostic approach to the patient with renal failure has been presented in detail in Chap. 2. However, the distinction of prerenal disease from ATN deserves particular emphasis. To begin with, the history may identify potential causes of either of these disorders. Timing the onset of renal failure also may be helpful. In hospitalized patients, for example, it is frequently possible to determine the day on which the BUN and P_{cr} begin to rise. In this setting, either some renal insult occurred on that day (such as an episode of hypotension or the administration of radiocontrast media) or the cumulative effect of some prior insult became clinically apparent, as with the administration of an aminoglycoside antibiotic. With respect to drug toxicity, the duration of usage is another important facet of the history. Aminoglycosides, for example, accumulate in the renal cortex and usually do not produce clinical nephrotoxicity for at

least 7 to 10 days.[3] Thus, renal failure developing after just a few days of therapy is not likely to be due to the aminoglycoside.

The physical examination also may provide important information. Decreased skin turgor, a low jugular venous pressure, and postural tachycardia and hypotension are signs of true volume depletion. In contrast, the presence of peripheral or pulmonary edema or ascites most often points toward heart failure, hepatic cirrhosis, or the nephrotic syndrome.

In most patients, however, laboratory tests are required to establish the correct diagnosis (Table 3-3). When evaluating the accuracy of the different tests, it is important to define the "gold standard": the return of renal function to normal within 24 to 72 h of increasing the effective circulating volume (for example, by administering fluids or treating heart failure or hypotension) is considered diagnostic of prerenal disease; continued renal failure despite adequate fluid repletion is called ATN.[4]

It is also important to note that the laboratory tests are most useful in *oliguric* patients (urine output ≤500 mL/day). Patients with *nonoliguric* ATN appear to have less severe tubular damage (see "Acute Tubular Necro-

TABLE 3-3. Laboratory Tests Useful in the Diagnosis of Acute Renal Failure

Test	Favors Prerenal Disease	Favors ATN
BUN/P_{cr} ratio	>20:1	10–15:1
Rise in P_{cr}	Variable rate of rise with downward fluctuations in some patients	Progressive increase of ≥0.5 mg/dL per day, particularly in oliguric patients
Urinalysis	Normal or near normal; hyaline casts may be seen but are not an abnormal finding	Many granular casts with renal tubular epithelial cells and epithelial cell casts
U_{osm}	>500 mosmol/kg	<350 mosmol/kg
U_{Na}	<20 meq/L	>40 meq/L
FE_{Na}	<1 percent	>2 percent

sis,'' below),[5,6] and there may be a greater overlap with the results found in prerenal disease. As will be seen, this overlap is sufficiently common that *many of the tests are useful only at the extremes* when the values are clearly high or low.

BUN/P_{cr} RATIO

A reduction in the GFR, regardless of cause, will raise the BUN and the P_{cr}, maintaining the normal BUN/P_{cr} ratio of 10 to 15:1. However, an additional factor is operative in prerenal disease. The concomitant increase in proximal tubular sodium and water reabsorption enhances passive urea reabsorption, thereby raising the BUN out of proportion to the fall in GFR. As a result, the BUN/P_{cr} ratio frequently exceeds 20 to 30:1.[7] Thus, a high ratio is strongly suggestive of prerenal disease, unless there is some cause of increased urea production such as gastrointestinal bleeding, increased tissue breakdown, or high-dose corticosteroid therapy. A normal ratio is less useful diagnostically. It is characteristic of ATN but also may be seen in prerenal disease if protein intake is reduced (as with vomiting) or marked liver disease is present (the liver being the site of urea synthesis).

The *rate of rise* in the P_{cr} also may be helpful. Once renal failure begins in oliguric ATN, the P_{cr} typically increases by 0.5 mg/dL or more per day in a progressive fashion until a plateau is reached or dialysis is required.[8] A lesser daily increment, particularly if associated with occasional downward fluctuations in the P_{cr}, favors the diagnosis of prerenal disease.[9] The transient reductions in the P_{cr} in this setting are presumably due to transient improvements in renal perfusion. The rate of rise in the P_{cr} is not as useful in nonoliguric ATN in which lesser daily increments in the P_{cr} may be present.

URINALYSIS

The urinalysis in ATN typically reveals many dark brown granular casts and renal tubular epithelial cells and epithelial cell casts (see Plates 1 and 2, in Chap. 1). However, 20 to 30 percent of patients may lack these characteristic changes.[10]

In comparison, the urinalysis is relatively normal in prerenal disease since there is no structural damage present. Hyaline casts may be present but are not an abnormal finding.

In some patients with persistent hypovolemia, there may be a slow evolution from reversible prerenal disease to ATN. During this *interphase*, granular casts indicative of some tubular damage may be seen in the urine sediment. Although this finding suggests incipient ATN, the presence of a relatively high urine osmolality (U_{osm}), low urine sodium concentration (U_{Na}), or low fractional excretion of sodium (FE_{Na}) may indicate that fluid repletion or therapy with mannitol or furosemide (see "Acute Tubular Necrosis: Treatment," below) can still restore renal function.[11] If the course is not reversed, however, there will usually be a reduction in the U_{osm} and an increase in the U_{Na} and FE_{Na} to values that are typical of ATN.[12]

The urinalysis may be helpful in one other respect. Drug-induced acute renal failure may represent an allergic reaction (usually manifested as interstitial nephritis or vasculitis) as well as nephrotoxic ATN. In the former condition, the most commonly involved drugs are the penicillins (particularly methicillin) or sulfa drugs, not the aminoglycosides (see Chap. 8). The urine sediment in this disorder typically reveals findings very different from those in ATN: red cells, white cells (including eosinophils in some patients), white cell casts, and, if vasculitis is present, red cell casts.[13,14] Peripheral allergic manifestations also may present, including rash and eosinophilia. Establishing the correct diagnosis is extremely important since treatment with corticosteroids may hasten the recovery of renal function in allergic interstitial nephritis[13] but is without effect in ATN. If the diagnosis remains in doubt, a renal biopsy may have to be performed.[15]

URINE OSMOLALITY

The U_{osm} may distinguish between prerenal disease and ATN. Hypovolemia is a potent stimulus to the release of antidiuretic hormone (ADH),[16] which will result in a highly concentrated urine if tubular function is intact. In contrast, the U_{osm} in ATN is generally below 350 mosmol/kg (U_{osm} less than 1.2 times the P_{osm}).[4,12,17]

The almost uniform and early reduction in concentrating ability in ATN is due to several factors. Renal ischemia predominantly affects the medulla, which has a much lower rate of blood flow and oxygenation than the cortex (see "Acute Tubular Necrosis: Pathogenesis of Renal Failure," below). This can lead to preferential necrosis of the cells of the thick ascending limb of the loop of Henle, the segment that is responsible for the creation of the countercurrent gradient that is essential for urinary concentration.[18] Furthermore, marked medullary ischemia also affects the collecting tubules, resulting in reduced responsiveness to ADH.[19] Similar changes may occur with nephrotoxins. Aminoglycosides, for example, also impair the collecting tubule response to ADH, an effect that may be secondary to binding of the cationic drug to anionic phospholipids in the luminal membrane.[20]

Unfortunately, there is a wide overlap in the U_{osm} in patients with acute renal failure (Fig. 3–1). *A value above 500 mosmol/kg is strongly suggestive of prerenal disease, but lower values are*

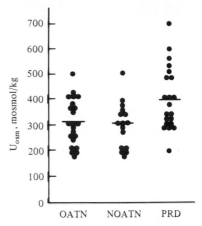

FIG. 3–1. Urine osmolality in 61 patients with oliguric or nonoliguric ATN (OATN and NOATN) or prerenal disease (PRD). Horizontal bars represent mean values. (*Adapted from C. H. Espinel and A. W. Gregory, Clin. Nephrol., 13:73, 1980.*)

not helpful.[4,17] This overlap is primarily due to an inappropriately low U_{osm} in certain patients with prerenal disease. This problem can occur in elderly patients or those with chronic renal disease in whom concentrating ability is impaired.[21,22] In addition, renal ischemia may diminish loop of Henle function in some patients without producing overt tubular necrosis.[23]

URINE SODIUM CONCENTRATION

The U_{Na} is another test that, in theory, should be very important diagnostically. Sodium retention is an appropriate response to prerenal disease, whereas tubular damage limits sodium reabsorption in ATN. However, there is again considerable overlap with only clearly high or low values being helpful: a U_{Na} above 40 meq/L is usually due to ATN; a U_{Na} below 20 meq/L generally, but not always, represents prerenal disease (Fig. 3–2).[4,17]

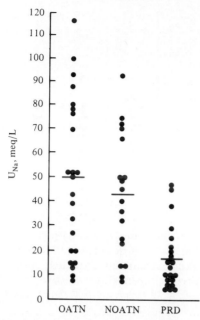

FIG. 3–2. Urine sodium concentration in 61 patients with oliguric or nonoliguric ATN or prenal disease *(Adapted from C. H. Espinel and A. W. Gregory, Clin. Nephrol., 13:73, 1980.)*

FRACTIONAL EXCRETION OF SODIUM

One of the major problems with the U_{Na} is that it is affected by the degree of *water* as well as sodium reabsorption. If the former is relatively low in ATN, the U_{Na} will be reduced by dilution. On the other hand, increased water reabsorption in prenal disease can raise the U_{Na} above 20 meq/L, even when there is avid sodium retention. These effects of water transport can be overcome by measuring the FE_{Na} which is a *direct* measure of sodium excretion* (see p. 19):

$$FE_{Na} \, (\%) = \frac{U_{Na} \times P_{cr}}{P_{Na} \times U_{cr}} \times 100$$

*Another way to estimate the degree of water reabsorption is to measure the urine-to-plasma creatinine ratio (U/P_{cr}). This ratio is 1 in the glomerular filtrate and increases progressively as water is reabsorbed but fil-

A variety of studies have confirmed that the FE_{Na} more clearly differentiates (with above 90 percent accuracy) between prenal disease and ATN than any of the above tests: a value below 1 percent favoring the former and greater than 2 percent strongly favoring the latter (Fig. 3–3).[4,17,24,25] In other words, marked sodium retention in prenal disease is characterized by the reabsorption of more than 99 percent and the excretion of less than 1 percent of the filtered sodium load.

The utilization of the FE_{Na} can be illustrated by the following laboratory data from a patient with severe hepatic cirrhosis, slowly progressive renal failure, and a normal urinalysis:

$$P_{cr} = \quad 2.4 \text{ mg/dL}$$
$$P_{Na} = 132 \text{ meq/L}$$
$$U_{osm} = 428 \text{ mosmol/kg}$$
$$U_{Na} = \quad 31 \text{ meq/L}$$
$$U_{cr} = 312 \text{ mg/dL}$$

Comment. The clinical impression was that the patient had prenal disease due to the hepatorenal syndrome. However, neither the U_{osm} nor the U_{Na} was in the diagnostic range. The laboratory diagnosis of prenal disease could be confirmed only by calculation of the FE_{Na}:

$$FE_{Na} = \frac{31 \times 2.4}{132 \times 312} \times 100 = 0.18\%$$

The reason that the U_{Na} was relatively high despite the extremely low FE_{Na} was

tered creatinine (plus some secreted creatinine) remains in the tubular lumen. Thus the U/P_{cr} is a rough measure of the degree of water reabsorption; that is, the more water reabsorbed, the higher the U/P_{cr}. If, for example, creatinine secretion is ignored, then a U/P_{cr} of 40:1 indicates that 39/40 or almost 98 percent of the filtered water has been reabsorbed, a relatively high value. Although there is overlap between 20:1 and 40:1, a U/P_{cr} above 40:1 usually indicates prenal disease, whereas a value below 20:1 is suggestive of ATN.[4,17] However, the U/P_{cr} is infrequently used because it is less accurate than the FE_{Na}.[4,17]

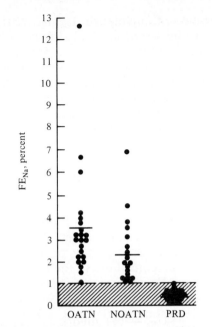

FIG. 3-3. FE_{Na} in 61 patients with oliguric or nonoliguric ATN or prerenal disease. Although this study shows essentially no overlap, other studies have shown that the FE_{Na} is below 1 percent in approximately 10 percent of patients with nonoliguric ATN and between 1 and 2 percent in about 10 percent of patients with prerenal disease.[4,25] (*Adapted from C. H. Espinel and A. W. Gregory, Clin. Nephrol., 13:73, 1980.*)

that the patient was also avidly reabsorbing water. This can be appreciated from the U/P_{cr} ratio of 130:1, indicating that as much as 129/130 or more than 99 percent of the filtered water also had been reabsorbed.

Although the FE_{Na} is the most accurate single test, an FE_{Na} below 1 percent has occasionally been reported in a variety of causes of acute renal failure other than prerenal disease (Table 3-4).[4,17,25-33] In these conditions, ATN is superimposed upon a chronic prerenal state, or net tubular function is assumed to be relatively intact, with renal

TABLE 3-4. Causes of Acute Renal Failure in Which FE_{Na} May Be below 1 Percent

Prerenal disease
ATN
10 percent of nonoliguric cases[4,25]
Superimposed upon chronic prerenal state
Hepatic cirrhosis[26]
Heart failure[27]
Severe burns[28]
Myoglobinuria or hemoglobinuria[29]
Radiocontrast media[30]
Sepsis[31]
Acute glomerulonephritis or vasculitis[4,17]
Acute obstructive uropathy[17,32]
Acute interstitial nephritis[33]

vasoconstriction, decreased glomerular permeability (particularly in acute glomerulonephritis), or tubular obstruction being responsible for the reduction in GFR (see "Acute Tubular Necrosis: Pathogenesis of Renal Failure," below).

It is important to note that use of the U_{Na} or FE_{Na} to diagnose prerenal disease is dependent on intact sodium reabsorptive capacity. When sodium reabsorption is impaired, the U_{Na} may be inappropriately high, despite the presence of volume depletion. This problem can occur with diuretic therapy, underlying chronic renal disease,[34] hypoaldosteronism, or metabolic alkalosis with bicarbonaturia. In the last setting, the excretion of excess plasma bicarbonate results in obligatory sodium losses to maintain electroneutrality. The presence of volume depletion in metabolic alkalosis can still be detected by measuring the U_{Cl} (or FE_{Cl}), which remains appropriately low.[35]

SUMMARY

Distinguishing between prerenal disease and ATN is clinically important because the former is reversible with appropriate therapy and generally produces less renal dysfunction. For example, dialysis is frequently required in patients with ATN but is rarely necessary with hypovolemia.[24] Unfortunately, there is no single test that can clearly differentiate between these disorders. Furthermore, the distinction is often blurred because prolonged renal hypoperfusion can ultimately progress into overt ATN.[11,12]

As a result, the history and multiple laboratory tests must all be taken into account (Table 3–3). Granular casts in the urine sediment, a U_{osm} below 350 mosmol/kg, and an FE_{Na} above 2 percent strongly favor the diagnosis of ATN. In contrast, prerenal disease is almost certainly present if the urinalysis is normal, the P_{cr} rises slowly with occasional downward fluctuations, the U_{osm} is greater than 500 mosmol/kg, and the FE_{Na} is less than 1 percent. The few patients with ATN (usually nonoliguric) who share one or more of these features generally have less severe tubular damage. This is also the setting in which early treatment with mannitol or furosemide is most likely to prevent progressive renal failure (see "Acute Tubular Necrosis: Treatment," below).[6,11]

PRERENAL DISEASE

Renal failure due to prerenal disease occurs in two basic settings: when renal ischemia is part of a generalized decrease in tissue perfusion or, less commonly, when there is selective renal ischemia as with bilateral renal artery stenosis or the hepatorenal syndrome (Table 3–1).

Systemic hypoperfusion is initially sensed by the cardiac and arterial baroreceptors (such as those in the carotid sinus and afferent glomerular arteriole), which respond to changes in pressure (or stretch).[36–38] When the mean arterial pressure is reduced, due to a reduction either in cardiac output or in systemic vascular resistance, activation of these receptors increases sympathetic neural tone and the release of both renin (leading to the generation of angiotensin II) and ADH.[16,36,37] The ensuing arteriolar and venular constriction and stimulation of cardiac function then returns the systemic blood pressure and cardiac output toward normal. Furthermore, the arteriolar vasoconstriction occurs primarily in the renal, splanchnic, and musculocutaneous circulations, resulting in the relative preservation of blood flow to the heart and brain.

Although these are appropriate systemic responses, the renal vasoconstriction diminishes renal blood flow and usually the GFR, which is flow-dependent.[39] If the compensatory responses are incomplete, persistent reductions in cardiac output or arterial pressure also can contribute to the decline in the GFR. A simple example of the sensitivity of this system is illustrated by the hemodynamic response to standing. Pooling of blood in the lower extremities leads sequentially to decreased venous return to the heart, a reduction in cardiac output, an increase in sympathetic tone, and a fall in GFR of 10 to 15 percent.[40,41] Sodium and water excretion also are reduced in an attempt to expand the effective circulating volume toward normal.[40]

It is important to note that effective volume depletion also occurs in edematous states such as heart failure or hepatic cirrhosis. The decrease in tissue perfusion is due to reduced cardiac function in the former and to splanchnic venous pooling, systemic vasodilatation, and ascites accumulation in the latter (see below). As a result, these disorders, when severe, are characterized by the same neurohumoral responses as true volume depletion: increased secretion of norepinephrine, renin, and ADH.[42–44]

TRUE VOLUME DEPLETION

Gastrointestinal, renal, skin, or respiratory losses or acute third-space sequestration can result in plasma volume depletion (Table 3–1).

DIAGNOSIS

The history, physical examination, and laboratory data all may be important in the diagnosis of true volume depletion. A history of vomiting, diarrhea, diuretic use, or polyuria may identify the source of fluid loss. Common physical findings which should be present when volume depletion is severe enough to cause renal failure include decreased skin turgor, estimated jugular venous pressure below 5 cmH$_2$O, and postural tachycardia with or without hypotension.[45]

The clinical syndrome of hypovolemic shock occurs with more pronounced volume loss and is most often due to bleeding or third-space sequestration. In this disorder, a marked increase in sympathetic tone and angiotensin II production leads to intense vasoconstriction. This decrease in peripheral perfusion is manifested by cold, clammy extremities, cyanosis, and agitation and confusion due to reduced cerebral blood flow. Although hypotension is generally present, it is not required for the diagnosis of shock since some patients vasoconstrict enough to maintain a relatively normal blood pressure.

Abnormalities in electrolyte and acid balance frequently occur with true volume depletion and, when the history is not helpful, can be of diagnostic importance.[45] For example, elderly patients with decreased mentation may become volume-depleted due to lack of replacement of insensible water losses. This sequence must produce hypernatremia because water is lost in excess of sodium. If the P$_{Na}$ is normal, however, then *sodium and water must have been lost in proportion* and some source of sodium loss must be identified. More often, hyponatremia accompanies volume depletion as the combination of a low GFR and increased ADH secretion promotes the retention of ingested or administered water.

Changes in acid-base balance also may be helpful. Metabolic alkalosis, usually associ-ated with hypokalemia, is suggestive of diuretic therapy or the loss of gastric secretions due to vomiting or tube drainage. Metabolic acidosis, on the other hand, is typically seen with diarrhea, the glucose-mediated osmotic diuresis in diabetic ketoacidosis, underlying chronic renal disease, and lactic acidosis due to shock. The anion gap is normal with diarrhea (or the loss of pancreaticobiliary secretions) but is elevated in the other disorders.[46]

TREATMENT

The aim of therapy in true volume depletion is fluid repletion. The major questions concern the type of fluid given and the rate of fluid administration.*[47] The tonicity of the fluid administered is usually determined by the P$_{Na}$, which almost always varies with the plasma osmolality. If the patient is hypernatremic, hypotonic fluids should be given. This may vary from dextrose in water to half-isotonic saline, depending on whether there has been concurrent sodium losses. Hyponatremia with hypoosmolality, on the other hand, should be treated with isotonic or, if the P$_{Na}$ is below 115 meq/L, hypertonic saline. Isotonic or half-isotonic saline can be used if the P$_{Na}$ is normal. In addition, blood may be required if the patient is actively bleeding or has marked anemia.

The ionic composition of the administered fluid is also determined by other electrolyte abnormalities that may be present. Consider the following laboratory tests in an elderly hypovolemic patient with diarrhea:

$$\begin{aligned} \text{Plasma Na} &= 150 \text{ meq/L} \\ \text{K} &= 3.4 \text{ meq/L} \\ \text{HCO}_3 &= 10 \text{ meq/L} \\ \text{Cl} &= 130 \text{ meq/L} \\ \text{pH} &= 7.25 \end{aligned}$$

*Treatment should also be directed at the underlying disease such as diarrhea or diabetic ketoacidosis.

Comment. The high P_{Na} means that water has been lost in excess of solute. In addition, there are also potassium and bicarbonate deficits. Thus, an appropriate *hypotonic* replacement fluid is 1 L of quarter-isotonic saline (Na concentration equals 37 meq/L) to which 22 meq of $NaHCO_3$ and 30 meq of KCl have been added.

In the absence of shock or symptomatic renal failure, there is no necessity to rapidly replace the fluid deficit. This is particularly true for patients with underlying cardiac disease in whom overzealous fluid therapy can lead to pulmonary edema. As a general rule, the administration of fluids at 75 to 100 mL/h to adults is adequate when no emergency exists. A more rapid rate is required in the presence of marked hypernatremia,[48] continued fluid loss, or shock.

The adequacy of fluid repletion will become apparent by improvement in skin turgor, jugular venous pressure, arterial pressure, and the urine output. The U_{Na} can be followed since it usually varies directly with effective renal perfusion.[36] For example, a rise in the U_{Na} from 5 to 55 meq/L indicates that normovolemia has probably been achieved.

HYPOVOLEMIC SHOCK

Early and aggressive therapy is required in hypovolemic shock to prevent tissue necrosis or the development of irreversible shock.[45] Blood should be given if bleeding is the primary problem. In general, the hematocrit should not be raised above 35 percent, since higher values are not necessary for adequate oxygen transport but can increase blood viscosity and lead to stasis in the already impaired capillary circulation.

Other than blood, isotonic electrolyte solutions (saline or Ringer's lactate) are the preferred replacement fluids. Albumin-containing solutions have been claimed both to expand the plasma volume more effectively and, by increasing the plasma oncotic pressure, to minimize the risk of pulmonary edema. However, controlled studies have failed to confirm either of these potential advantages in the absence of underlying hypoalbuminemia.[45,49-51]

Whichever fluid is chosen, as much as 1 to 2 L should be given in the first hour in an attempt to restore adequate tissue perfusion as rapidly as possible. It is not possible to predict in a given patient what the total fluid deficit will be, particularly if bleeding or third-space sequestration continues. If the patient does not improve quickly, further fluids should be administered while monitoring the central venous or preferably the pulmonary capillary wedge pressure. The development of peripheral edema does not necessarily indicate that fluids should be stopped since it may result from dilutional hypoalbuminemia, even though plasma volume depletion persists.[52]

Other therapeutic modalities also may be of use in hypovolemic shock. If available, military antishock trousers can raise the systemic blood pressure both by increasing vascular resistance (by mechanical compression of the legs) and by translocation of fluid from the legs into the central (cardiopulmonary) circulation.[52,53] Prolonged usage should be avoided, however, since it can lead to an ischemic compartment syndrome. There is also preliminary clinical and experimental evidence suggesting that endorphins may be responsible for some of the harmful consequences of shock and that the use of opiate antagonists (such as naloxone) may be beneficial in otherwise refractory patients.[54,55] In contrast, vasopressors such as dopamine or norepinephrine have little role in hypovolemic shock, since they will not correct the underlying fluid deficit and may, via vasoconstriction, intensify the tissue ischemia.

UNDERLYING RENAL DISEASE

True volume depletion may be superimposed upon underlying intrinsic renal disease. It is important to be aware of this complication since *hypovolemia is reversible in contrast to progression of the primary disease, which is frequently irreversible.* Furthermore, a small reduction in GFR can lead to a relatively large elevation in the P_{cr}. For example, a 10 mL/min reduction in the GFR from 20 to 10 mL/min can increase the P_{cr} from 6 to 12 mg/dL (see Fig. 1-2). In comparison, a similar change in a normal subject with a GFR of 120 mL/min would only raise the P_{cr} from 1.0 to 1.1 mg/dL.

The diagnosis of volume depletion may be difficult to establish in the patient with renal disease. Since a 10 mL/min reduction in GFR may be seen with a decrease in cardiac output of only 300 to 400 mL/min* (about a 10 percent fall), the physical findings of true volume depletion may be absent. In addition, the characteristic urinary findings of hypovolemia (normal urinalysis, high U_{osm}, low U_{Na}) may be missing since chronic renal disease impairs maximum water and sodium conservation.[22,34] Thus, the physician must be aware that *subclinical hypovolemia* may be responsible for an acute decline in renal function in a patient with chronic renal disease. This diagnosis can be confirmed by reductions in the BUN and P_{cr} after a fluid load. A similar sequence may be seen when there is a primary decrease in cardiac output, as with a myocardial infarction. In this setting, restoration of cardiac function rather than fluids is required for renal function to improve.

---

*Under normal conditions, approximately 20 percent of the cardiac output is delivered to the kidneys. Thus, a 350 mL/min fall in cardiac output should lower renal blood flow (RBF) by about 70 mL/min. If the hematocrit is 30 percent (anemia being a common finding in advanced renal disease), this decrease in RBF reduces renal plasma flow (RPF) by 50 mL/min. Since 20 percent of the RPF normally undergoes glomerular filtration, a 50 mL/min drop in RPF should diminish GFR by 10 mL/min. To the degree that hypovolemia results in enhanced sympathetic tone and renal vasoconstriction, RPF may fall by 50 mL/min with less than a 350 mL/min decrease in cardiac output.

HYPOTENSION

A fall in blood pressure can directly reduce the GFR by lowering the hydrostatic pressure in the glomerular capillary (P_{GC}). The P_{GC} is the major driving force for glomerular filtration.[39,56] It has a normal mean value of approximately 45 mmHg, much lower than the mean arterial pressure of 85 to 95 mmHg. Both the P_{GC} and the GFR (as well as renal blood flow) are regulated by the resistances at the afferent and efferent arterioles. Figure 3-4 illustrates the effects of arteriolar vasoconstriction. An increase in *afferent* tone (as might be produced by norepinephrine, which can constrict both arterioles)[57,58] lowers P_{GC} and the GFR by allowing less of the systemic pressure to be transmitted to the glomerulus. In comparison, an increase in *efferent* tone (as can be selectively produced by angiotensin II)[57,58] tends to raise these parameters.

Hypotension can affect renal hemodynamics in one of two ways. If only renal perfusion pressure is reduced, as with bilateral renal artery stenosis or aortic occlusion, the P_{GC}, GFR, and RBF are initially maintained at normal levels until there is marked intrarenal hypotension (Fig. 3-5). This phenomenon, which can also be demonstrated with muscle and cerebral flow, is called *autoregulation*.[39,59]

The autoregulation of P_{GC} and GFR in the presence of hypotension could occur in two ways, afferent dilation or efferent constriction. Both of these changes appear to occur: the former mediated by a local myogenic response and tubuloglomerular feedback, and the latter mediated by angiotensin II.*[39,60] If the autoregulatory response is impaired, then

---

*Angiotensin II has a dual effect on the GFR. The initial increase in efferent arteriolar resistance tends to maintain the GFR during the autoregulatory response. However, higher levels of angiotensin II can lead to reductions in both renal blood flow (by efferent constriction) and glomerular permeability (by mesangial contraction), ultimately leading to a fall in GFR. For example, increased angiotensin II plays an important role in the reduction of GFR with heart failure.[61]

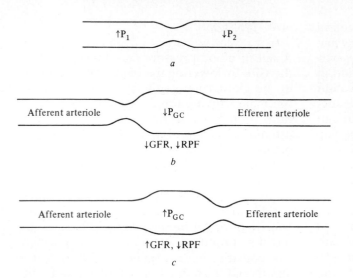

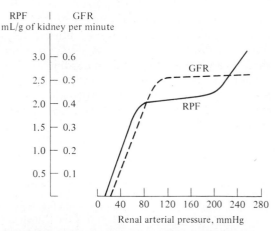

FIG. 3-4. Relationship between arteriolar resistance, GFR, and RPF. (*a*) If flow is contant, constriction of a vessel results in a rise in pressure proximally (P_1) and a fall distally (P_2). (*b*) Constriction of the afferent arteriole reduces P_{GC} and GFR. (*c*) Constriction of the efferent arteriole increases P_{GC} and GFR. Since constriction of either arteriole also increases renal vascular resistance, RPF will fall in both (*b*) and (*c*). Arteriolar vasodilatation has the opposite effects.

a fall in renal perfusion pressure will be more likely to reduce the GFR. This mechanism probably explains the acute renal failure that may occur when a converting enzyme inhibitor, which inhibits the production of angiotensin II, is given to a patient with bilateral renovascular disease (see "Bilateral Renal Artery Stenosis," below).[62-64]

Clinically, a reduction in renal perfusion is most often due to systemic hypotension, not selective renal ischemia as with renovascular disease. In this setting, the GFR may begin to fall with relatively minor reductions in blood pressure. This effect is mediated by marked increases in sympathetic tone and angiotensin II production, which lead to renal vasoconstriction (not afferent arteriolar dilation), a reduction in renal blood flow, and a lesser decrease in GFR (as efferent arteriolar constriction tends to maintain P_{GC} and GFR).[57,58,61] When hypotension is due to sepsis, the renal vasoconstrictive effects of endotoxin also contribute to the renal failure.[65]

To some degree, this renal ischemia is ameliorated by increased production of vasodilator prostaglandins and kinins.[57,65-68] As a result, blocking prostaglandin synthesis with nonsteroidal anti-inflammatory drugs, which

are widely used in the treatment of rheumatologic disorders, can exacerbate the renal vasoconstriction and increase the severity of renal failure (see "Nonsteroidal Anti-inflammatory Drugs," below).[69,70]

Acute renal failure due to hypotension is

FIG. 3-5. Autoregulation of GFR and RPF in the dog. Both parameters are maintained in the presence of hypotension until the mean renal arterial pressure falls below 80 mmHg. (*Adapted from R. E. Shipley and R. S. Study, Am. J. Physiol., 167:676, 1951.*)

seen in two basic situations: shock (due to hypovolemia, cardiac dysfunction, or sepsis) and the treatment of chronic, severe hypertension. In the latter disorder, a decrease in GFR may be seen with an acute reduction in systemic pressure, even if not to hypotensive levels. This response occurs when arteriolar intimal hyperplasia has developed because of prolonged hypertension. The increase in the thickness of these vessels impairs their ability to dilate when the blood pressure is

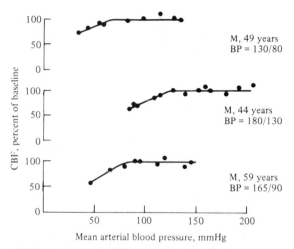

lowered toward normal, causing a decrease in tissue perfusion that is not limited to the kidney (Fig. 3–6).[59,71-73] Thus, elevations in the BUN and P_{cr} may be seen if the blood pressure is rapidly and appropriately lowered to 90 to 100 mmHg in a patient with severe hypertension (Fig. 3–7).[71,72] Fortunately, this effect is usually transient, since continued control of the blood pressure permits intimal hyperplasia to regress and renal perfusion to improve over a period of 1 to 3 months (Fig. 3–7). Antihypertensive medications do not need to be discontinued unless there has been an excessive fall in blood pressure or converting enzyme inhibitors have been given to a patient with possible bilateral renovascular disease (see below).[62,63]

This potential problem in hypertensive patients illustrates another important point: What level of blood pressure represents hypotension? As depicted in Fig. 3–6, both normal and hypertensive subjects autoregulate as the blood pressure falls, but they do so at different pressures. If hypotension is defined as the level at which tissue perfu-

FIG. 3–6. Autoregulation of the cerebral circulation in normotensive and hypertensive humans. In a normal subject (*upper panel*), cerebral blood flow (CBF) remains constant until the mean arterial pressure falls below 70 mmHg. In contrast, CBF begins to decrease at a much higher pressure (about 125 mmHg) in a patient with uncontrolled hypertension (*middle panel*). A curve similar to that in normal subjects may be seen with chronic control of severe hypertension (*lower panel*). In each case, CBF does not begin to fall until the blood pressure has been lowered more than 20 to 25 mmHg below the baseline value (arrow). A similar effect of hypertension and its control may be present in the renal circulation (*From S. Strandgaard, N. Engl. J. Med., 288:372, 1973. Reprinted by permission from the New England Journal of Medicine.*)

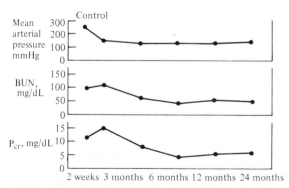

FIG. 3–7. Serial changes in mean arterial pressure, BUN, and P_{cr} following intensive antihypertensive treatment in a patient with severe hypertension. (*From W. R. Mroczek, M. Davidov, L. Gavrilovich, and F. A. Finnerty, Jr., Circulation, 40:893, 1969. By permission of the American Heart Association, Inc.*)

sion* begins to fall, then, from Fig. 3–6, this requires a drop in blood pressure of at least 20 to 25 mmHg *below the patient's previous baseline.*[59,74] Thus, a blood pressure of 120/80 is generally considered "normal" but actually represents hypotension in a previously hypertensive patient with a baseline blood pressure of 180/100.

HEART FAILURE

The hemodynamic changes that occur in heart failure can be appreciated from the Frank-Starling relationship between stroke volume and the left ventricular end-diastolic pressure (LVEDP) (Fig. 3–8). If a normal subject develops mild cardiac failure, there will initially be a reduction in stroke volume and cardiac output (line AB). The reduction in cardiac output appropriately induces sodium and water retention by the kidney, a response that is mediated in part by increased activity of the renin-angiotensin-aldosterone system.[75] The net result is an increase in plasma volume and cardiac filling pressure which will tend to normalize the stroke volume (line BC). (Other factors such as enhanced sympathetic tone and heart rate will also act to restore the cardiac output.) At this point, the patient is in a new steady state of *compensated* heart failure in which the cardiac output is normal (at least at rest), sodium excretion matches intake, and aldosterone secretion has returned to normal.[75] However, the restoration of tissue perfusion has occurred only after there has been an elevation in the LVEDP, perhaps to a level sufficient to produce pulmonary edema.

Although decreased contractility is most often responsible for the cardiac dysfunction,

---

*Neurohumorally mediated vasoconstriction may actually cause tissue perfusion to fall with a lesser reduction in blood pressure. This does not apply, however, to the cerebral circulation, which does not respond to norepinephrine or angiotensin II.

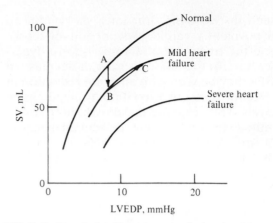

FIG. 3–8. Frank-Starling curves relating stroke volume (SV) to left ventricular end-diastolic pressure (LVEDP) in normal subjects and patients with heart failure. See text for details. (*Adapted from J. N. Cohn, Am. J. Med., 55:131, 1973.*)

as many as 35 to 40 percent of patients with heart failure have normal systolic function and a normal ejection fraction.[76,77] In this setting, abnormal *diastolic* function is of primary importance, as decreased compliance of the ventricular wall impairs ventricular filling. This distinction, which most often occurs in hypertensive or ischemic heart disease,[77,78] has important therapeutic implications (see below).

Renal ischemia in heart failure occurs primarily in two situations: when there is severe cardiac dysfunction (Fig. 3–8, lowest curve), or when cardiac filling pressures are reduced by diuretic therapy, e.g., by moving from point C to point B in Fig. 3–8.[79,80] In general, diuretics produce symptomatic relief by relieving pulmonary and peripheral edema with no, or only a clinically insignificant, decrease in tissue perfusion. However, in some patients with severe congestive heart failure, diuretic therapy leads to progressive and otherwise unexplained elevations in the BUN and P_{cr} (which indicate that flow is reduced to other organs as well). At this time, further diuresis should be avoided and vasodilator or inotropic therapy should be instituted.

Both the decrease in cardiac output and renal vasoconstriction (due to increased sympathetic activity and angiotensin II) contribute to the development of renal failure in this setting.[61,81] The enhanced secretion of these vasoconstrictors, which do increase the blood pressure, also has another deleterious effect: the rise in vascular resistance increases afterload, further diminishing cardiac performance.[42,79]

TREATMENT

The treatment of renal failure due to cardiac disease requires an improvement in cardiac function. In some patients, this occurs spontaneously, as with recovery from severe coronary ischemia. However, cell function may become sufficiently impaired during the period of ischemia (the "stunned" myocardium) that recovery may require 3 to 5 days after coronary flow has been restored.[82]

Increasing the cardiac output is usually attempted by combining digitalis[83,84] with vasodilators.[85,86] The latter agents act by lowering vascular (arteriolar) resistance, thereby reducing the impedance to cardiac contraction. Those agents that are also venous dilators (such as converting enzyme inhibitors, nitroprusside, and prazosin) have the added advantage of diminishing the pulmonary capillary pressure, thereby relieving pulmonary congestion. A converting enzyme inhibitor or hydralazine (primarily an arteriolar dilator) is preferable in patients with renal failure, since they augment renal blood flow and may increase the GFR.[61,87,88] In contrast, prazosin does not improve renal perfusion.[88] The reason for this difference is not known.

Inotropic agents other than digitalis also can improve cardiac function, particularly if given with vasodilators. Thus, the intravenous administration of dopamine or dobutamine with nitroprusside can substantially enhance the cardiac output and lower the pulmonary capillary pressure.[89] In some patients, the acute effects of dopamine or dobutamine persist for weeks to months after the infusion is discontinued.[90,91] The mechanism by which this occurs is uncertain. The role of newer *oral* inotropic agents such as milrinone is currently being evaluated.[92]

Therapy with inotropic agents and vasodilators is aimed at patients with impaired systolic contractility. This regimen, however, may be deleterious in patients with diastolic dysfunction since there may be a further limitation to diastolic filling.[78] These conditions can be differentiated by measuring the ejection fraction which is normal in the latter group. When diastolic dysfunction is the primary problem, use of a calcium channel blocker or β-adrenergic blocker may improve cardiac performance by enhancing ventricular compliance during diastole.[77,78]

HEPATIC CIRRHOSIS AND THE HEPATORENAL SYNDROME

Hepatic cirrhosis is one of the best illustrations of the concept of the *effective* circulating volume, i.e., the volume that is perfusing the tissues. The plasma volume is typically increased in this disorder because of slowly circulating blood in the dilated splanchnic venous system.[93] The cardiac output is also frequently elevated, probably due to the presence of multiple arteriovenous fistulas,* such as spider angiomas on the skin.[94] Despite these hemodynamic changes which suggest volume expansion, cirrhotic patients are *effectively volume depleted* as evidenced by a low rate of urinary sodium excretion and increased plasma levels of norepinephrine, angiotensin II, and ADH.[43,44,95]

---

*Blood flowing through these fistulas bypasses the capillary circulation and therefore is circulating ineffectively.

A variety of factors contribute to this decrease in effective tissue perfusion: increased hepatic sinusoidal pressure, which leads to fluid accumulation both in the peritoneum and in the dilated splanchnic venous system; peripheral vasodilatation (due to arteriovenous fistulas and enhanced production of prostaglandins), which augments vascular capacity; and hypoalbuminemia, which promotes fluid movement out of the vascular space into the interstitium.[96]

One proof of the presence of effective volume depletion has come from studies involving immersion to the neck in warm water. In this setting, the hydrostatic pressure of the water on the lower extremities results in the redistribution of intravascular fluid from the legs to the chest. In patients with cirrhosis, the ensuing increase in central blood volume and cardiac output results in enhanced urinary sodium and water excretion and a reduction in the secretion of the "hypovolemic" hormones, norepinephrine, renin, and ADH.[97,98] Similar results occur with ascites reinfusion via a peritoneovenous shunt (see "Treatment," below).[99,100]

In addition to these systemic changes, *active renal vasoconstriction* leads to selective renal ischemia in hepatic cirrhosis.[101] This is manifested by a marked decrease in the fraction of the cardiac output that is delivered to the kidney, particularly to the outer cortex, which contains 85 percent of the glomeruli.[101-103] These hemodynamic changes begin relatively early in the disease, as the increase in hepatic sinusoidal pressure appears to initiate an hepatorenal reflex, resulting in enhanced renal sympathetic nerve activity and renal vasoconstriction.[104,105] As more severe hepatic disease leads to effective volume depletion, this increase in renal vascular tone becomes more pronounced because of the production of angiotensin II and norepinephrine.[43,44,106] This tendency to renal ischemia is, at first, partially counteracted by enhanced

secretion of vasodilator prostaglandins and kinins.[44,68,107] However, these adaptive responses become impaired with more severe hepatic disease as both prostaglandin and kinin production are reduced.[44,106,107] These changes may occur because the liver is the site of both the production of prekallikrein (which, when activated to kallikrein, cleaves lysyl-bradykinin from kininogen) and of the conversion of linoleic acid to arachidonic acid (the latter being the precursor of the prostaglandins).[44,106,108] Thus, progressive hepatic disease results in

1. A progressive decrease in the effective circulating volume, leading to increased production of the vasoconstrictors angiotensin II, norepinephrine, and ADH.[43,44] The degree of effective hypovolemia becomes so severe that, in many patients, the cardiac output falls from an initially high level to one that is below normal.[103]
2. Increased renal sympathetic neural tone due to the rise in hepatic sinusoidal pressure.[105]
3. Reduced production of vasodilator prostaglandins and bradykinin with advanced disease.[44,106,107]

As a result of these changes, there is a progressive decrease in the GFR with increasingly severe hepatic disease (Fig. 3–9).[101,102,109] The hepatorenal syndrome, characterized by acute renal failure, is therefore not a separate disease but merely the end stage of a progressive process.

The continued decline in renal function is frequently masked in its early stages because a rise in the BUN and P_{cr} may be minimized by reductions in urea and creatinine synthesis. The latter is due to the associated malnutrition and consequent fall in muscle mass and perhaps to decreased hepatic production of creatine, the precursor of creatinine.[110] The net effect is that a seemingly normal P_{cr} of 1.0 to 1.3 mg/dL may be accompanied by

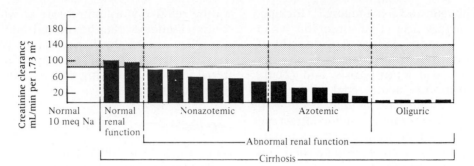

FIG. 3–9. The GFR, as estimated from the creatinine clearance (C_{cr}), in normal subjects on a 10 meq sodium diet and cirrhotic patients of increasing severity. (*Adapted from M. Epstein, D. P. Berk, N. K. Hollenberg, D. F. Adams, T. C. Chalmers, H. L. Abrams, and J. P. Merrill, Am. J. Med., 49:175, 1970.*)

a GFR as low as 15 to 40 mL/min (as illustrated by the nonazotemic patients in Fig. 3-9).[44,110] The GFR can be more accurately estimated from a 24-h urine collection for creatinine clearance:

$$C_{cr} = \frac{U_{cr} \times V}{P_{cr}}$$

However, this may still be an overestimate by as much as 50 percent or more because a progressively greater fraction of the excreted creatinine is derived from tubular secretion (see p. 4). A 24-h collection is also helpful in documenting a decrease in creatinine production, as reflected by a reduction in creatinine excretion ($U_{cr} \times$ urine flow rate: normal values are greater than 15 mg/kg per day in women and 20 mg/kg per day in men).

A variety of findings confirm that these changes in renal function are due to prerenal disease. The urinary criteria for prerenal disease (low U_{Na}, FE_{Na}, and high U_{osm}) are typically present.[10,109,111] Furthermore, the kidney itself is normal histologically[10,111,112] and has been used successfully for renal transplantation.[113] The one finding that may be absent is a normal urinalysis since marked hyperbilirubinemia alone can induce changes in the urine sediment more typical of ATN.[114]

CLINICAL CHARACTERISTICS

The hepatorenal syndrome most often occurs with advanced Laennec's cirrhosis but may also be seen with other disorders such as metastatic involvement of the liver or, rarely, viral hepatitis.[*,10,105,112,116] The onset of renal failure may be insidious or precipitated by an acute insult such as bleeding, paracentesis, or the use of diuretics. Once it begins, the hepatorenal syndrome is characterized by oliguria and slowly progressive increases in the BUN and P_{cr}. (The latter may change by as little as 0.1 mg/dL per day with occasional periods of stablization or even slight improvement.) Hepatic encephalopathy, ascites, and biochemical abnormalities such as hypoalbuminemia, hyperbilirubinemia, and hyponatremia commonly are present.

DIAGNOSIS

The diagnosis of the hepatorenal syndrome should be made only after excluding other

*It is of interest that sodium retention and ascites formation are late events and the hepatorenal syndrome is unusual in patients with primary biliary cirrhosis. The renal vasodilator and natriuretic effects of retained bile salts may be responsible for the relative preservation of renal function in this disorder.[115]

forms of hepatic and renal failure.[112] Included in this category are: (1) disorders in which both the liver and kidney are directly affected, such as collagen vascular diseases, amyloidosis, and leptospirosis; and (2) the superimposition of acute renal failure upon chronic hepatic disease as may occur with aminoglycoside therapy or radiocontrast media. The history and urinary findings usually allow these disorders to be distinguished from the hepatorenal syndrome.

The presence of hepatic cirrhosis as the cause of the ascites and peripheral edema is typically apparent from the history and physical examination (the latter showing spider angiomas and palmar erythema in many patients). On occasion, it may be difficult to differentiate primary hepatic disease from chronic right-sided heart failure which can also produce both hepatic cirrhosis (from chronic passive congestion) and renal failure. This distinction can usually be made on physical examination from estimation of the jugular venous pressure.[117] This pressure is elevated in heart failure but is normal or reduced (less than 7 cmH_2O) in hepatic cirrhosis since fluid accumulates below the hepatic sinusoids.[103,118] One exception to this general rule occurs with tense ascites in which the venous pressure may be elevated because upward pressure on the diaphragm raises the intrathoracic pressure.[118] However, the venous pressure rapidly falls when the tension is relieved by the removal of a small amount of ascitic fluid.[118]

One final disorder that can simulate the hepatorenal syndrome is the administration of diuretics to a patient with hepatic cirrhosis and ascites.[119,120] This is most likely to occur if there has been rapid fluid removal in a patient without peripheral edema; in this setting, the plasma volume can be protected from diuretic-induced losses only by mobilization of ascites. This is a relatively slow process (the safe *maximum* rate being only about 300 to 700 mL per day), in comparison to the relatively unlimited rate at which peripheral edema can be mobilized.[119] Thus the diagnosis of the hepatorenal syndrome requires that there be no improvement in renal function following an adequate trial of fluid repletion.

TREATMENT

The prognosis in the hepatorenal syndrome is extremely poor, since it generally occurs in patients with severe hepatic disease who frequently have hepatic encephalopathy or gastrointestinal bleeding. When recovery of renal function is seen, it is associated with improved hepatic function, occurring either spontaneously (usually in patients with less severe hepatic disease) or after a liver transplant.[116,121,122]

Initial therapy consists of general supportive measures and avoidance of situations which can further impair renal function, such as continued diuresis or the administration of nonsteroidal anti-inflammatory drugs (see below). Attempting to increase the effective circulating volume with saline or dextran has been at best only transiently effective.[103,123,124] Also unsuccessful have been attempts to reverse renal vasoconstriction with vasodilators such as acetylcholine, α-adrenergic blockers, or prostaglandins.[101,102] In theory, inhibiting angiotensin II might be more effective, since circulating levels are so high.[43,44,100] However, this modality is limited by its systemic effects. Patients with severe cirrhosis or the hepatorenal syndrome typically have a systolic blood pressure of 90 to 100 mmHg, as the high level of systemic vasoconstrictors is counterbalanced by the vasodilatation of hepatic desease.[103] In this setting, decreasing the effect of angiotensin II (with a converting enzyme inhibitor or the competitive antagonist saralasin) can lower the blood pressure by as much as 25 mmHg, leading to marked hypotension.[125]

The most effective therapy has been insertion of a peritoneovenous shunt, which reinfuses the ascitic fluid into the internal jugular vein. This procedure, initially accompanied by loop diuretics to begin the diuresis, increases the urine output and improves renal function in many patients with the hepatorenal syndrome.[99,100]

The mechanism by which the peritoneovenous shunt works is incompletely understood. Although ascites reinfusion substantially increases the intravascular volume, similar volume expansion with saline, dextran, or immersion in warm water does not produce the same beneficial effects.[98,103,123,124] These findings suggest that some other factor may be important. The peritoneovenous shunt has been shown to reduce hepatic sinusoidal pressure.[126] This could diminish renal sympathetic nerve activity (via a hepatorenal reflex),[104,105] which could then lead to increased renal perfusion. How intrahepatic pressure is reduced in this setting is uncertain. However, it is interesting to note that a side-to-side portasystemic shunt—which also diminishes ascites formation and lowers hepatic sinusoidal pressure—has effectively improved renal function in some patients.[100,127]

Despite the dramatic success that can occur with the peritoneovenous shunt, its use has been limited by a relatively high incidence of potentially fatal complications. These include infection of the shunt, which can lead to bacteremia; disseminated intravascular coagulation due to entry into the bloodstream of endotoxin or procoagulant material in the ascitic fluid; variceal bleeding; and small bowel obstruction.[99,128-130]

The net effect is that the perioperative mortality rate can reach 25 percent in patients with severe hepatic failure.[130] It has been suggested, although not proven, that the incidence of postoperative complications can be reduced by intraoperative drainage of the ascites.[130] This will minimize those problems that are directly related to ascites reinfusion: volume overload, increased portal pressure, and disseminated intravascular coagulation.

Considering these potential complications, the peritoneovenous shunt is best used in those patients with the hepatorenal syndrome who have relatively stable hepatic function, are not encephalopathic, and have not had a recent variceal bleed. In a patient who does not satisfy these criteria, peritoneal dialysis or hemodialysis can be used to treat uremic signs and symptoms. However, survival is poor in this setting.[131]

NEPHROTIC SYNDROME

Effective volume depletion also may occur in the nephrotic syndrome. In this disorder, urinary albumin losses lead to hypoalbuminemia, which favors the movement of fluid from the vascular space into the interstitium. The ensuing plasma volume depletion activates the renin-angiotensin-aldosterone system, thereby promoting renal sodium retention. Some of the excess sodium stays in the vascular space to replete the vascular volume, but most enters the interstitium where it becomes detectable as edema.

This "underfilling" sequence is most likely to occur in some patients with minimal change disease.[132] In comparison, patients with other glomerular lesions tend to have a low baseline GFR, leading directly to fluid retention, volume expansion, and relatively low plasma renin levels.[132] An intrarenal defect also appears to play a major role in many patients with minimal change disease.[133-135] As a result, most patients with this disorder have a relatively normal blood volume.[134] Thus, acute renal failure due to prerenal disease is uncommon in the nephrotic syndrome and occurs primarily in minimal change disease *after* diuretic therapy has been given to remove the edema fluid, thereby lowering the plasma volume to less than normal levels.[132,136,137] At this point, further diuretic therapy should be avoided, with correction of the underlying disease, if possible, being the most effective therapy (see Chap. 4).

Infrequently, acute renal failure with a low FE_{Na} occurs in patients with minimal change disease and marked hypoalbuminemia *prior* to therapy.[137,138] This problem may reflect marked interstitial edema or low filtration surface area due to foot process fusion (see p. 190). Renal function rapidly improves with corticosteroid-induced remission[137] or with diuretic therapy alone if interstitial edema is the primary abnormality.[138]

NONSTEROIDAL ANTI-INFLAMMATORY DRUGS

As described above, angiotensin II and norepinephrine increase renal vasodilator prostaglandin synthesis, resulting in amelioration of the arteriolar constriction[57] and consequently of the renal ischemia.[66,67] Since angiotensin II and norepinephrine production are increased in any of the prerenal states,[42-44] blocking prostaglandin synthesis in these settings with any of the nonsteroidal anti-inflammatory drugs (NSAID), including high-dose aspirin and sulfinpyrazone, would be expected to intensify the renal ischemia and lower the GFR.[69,70,139,140] Thus, acute renal failure, beginning soon after the institution of NSAID therapy, has been reported in true volume depletion,[66] heart failure,[*,141,142] hepatic cirrhosis (Fig. 3–10),[†,44,107,143] and the

---

*In addition to worsening renal function, NSAID can impair cardiac function in patients with severe heart disease.[141] The decrease in prostaglandin synthesis increases systemic vascular resistance and cardiac afterload, thereby diminishing cardiac contractility. This is opposite to the beneficial effect achieved with vasodilators.

†Renal prostaglandin production initially rises in hepatic cirrhosis because of the increases in circulating angiotensin II and norepinephrine levels.[44,107,143] Reduced prostaglandin synthesis, perhaps related to decreased conversion of linoleic acid to arachidonic acid, does not occur until the hepatic disease is far-advanced as in the hepatorenal syndrome.[44,107]

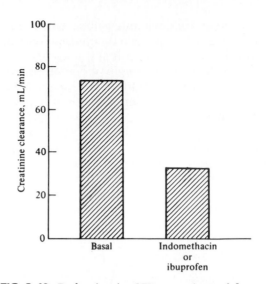

FIG. 3–10. Reduction in GFR, as estimated from the creatinine clearance, from a mean of 73 to 32 mL/min following the administration of indomethacin or ibuprofen to 12 patients with stable hepatic cirrhosis and ascites. Urinary PGE excretion in the patients in the basal state was substantially greater than in normal subjects. (*From R. D. Zipser, J. C. Hoefs, P. F. Speckhart, P. K. Zia, and R. Horton, J. Clin. Endocrinol. Metab., 48:895, 1979. Copyright by The Endocrine Society, 1979.*)

nephrotic syndrome.[144] Patients with glomerulonephritis, lupus nephritis, hypercalcemia, or who are concomitantly using triamterene also are at risk of developing this reversible complication.[139,145-147] In comparison, hemodynamically normal subjects are not at risk since basal renal prostaglandin production is relatively low and does not have an important effect on renal hemodynamics.[148]

One possible exception to the deleterious renal effects of NSAID* appears to be sulindac. In most[145,149-151] but not all[152] studies,

---

*An alteration in renal hemodynamics is not the only mechanism by which NSAID can produce acute renal failure. An acute interstitial nephritis typically associated with the nephrotic syndrome also may occur, particularly after the use of fenoprofen (see Chap. 8). This diagnosis is suggested by the abnormal urinalysis which shows red cells, white cells, and marked proteinuria.

sulindac produces either no or a relatively small reduction in renal prostaglandin synthesis. This effect may be related to the presence of oxidative enzymes in the kidney that rapidly convert the active drug into an inactive metabolite[153] or to sulindac being a somewhat weaker cyclooxygenase inhibitor, since platelet thromboxane release is reduced less than with other NSAIDs.[151,154] Regardless of the mechanism, sulindac can usually be used safely in most patients with one of the above disorders. This protection is not absolute, however, and careful monitoring is still required.

BILATERAL RENAL ARTERY STENOSIS

Renal artery stenosis can lower renal blood flow enough to result in renal insufficiency when both kidneys are involved or when one kidney is affected in a patient whose other kidney is absent or diseased.[155-157] This is most likely to occur in patients with atherosclerotic disease. Since the kidneys are anatomically normal (assuming that there is no underlying disease and that the ischemia is not so severe that infarction occurs), the urinary findings are similar to those in other forms of prerenal disease.[156]

Bilateral renovascular disease should be strongly considered in a patient with the triad of severe or refractory hypertension, renal insufficiency, and a relatively normal urinalysis. In one series of 21 such patients, 10 had bilateral renal artery stenosis.[157] Establishing this diagnosis is important clinically, since restoration of more normal renal perfusion with surgery or percutaneous transluminal angioplasty can both improve renal function and lower the blood pressure.*,[155-157]

*The diagnosis and treatment of renal artery stenosis is discussed in detail in Chap. 12.

EFFECT OF CONVERTING ENZYME INHIBITION

Patients with bilateral renovascular disease are prone to develop acute renal failure with the use of converting enzyme inhibitors (captopril or enalapril).[62,63,158-160] This unusual sensitivity is based upon the disparity between systemic and intrarenal pressures due to the stenotic lesion(s). Prior to treatment, the systemic pressure is elevated, but the intrarenal pressures are relatively normal. As antihypertensive agents are given to lower the systemic pressure, the intrarenal pressures fall below normal. In this setting, the GFR is initially maintained by autoregulation, a process that in part is due to angiotensin II–mediated constriction of the efferent arteriole (see Fig. 3–4).[39,60] However, the GFR may fall if angiotensin II formation is inhibited by converting enzyme inhibition (CEI).

Acute reversible renal failure has been described in CEI-treated patients with bilateral renal artery stenosis, stenosis of a solitary functioning kidney, and intrarenal vascular diseases such as chronic transplant rejection (see Fig. 12–7).[62,63,158-160] However, this is not a uniform complication in these conditions, occurring in 30 to up to 60 percent of patients, most of whom have only a mild decline in GFR.[158-160] Thus, the administration of a CEI (which is likely to effectively lower the blood pressure)[159] can be tried in patients with bilateral renovascular disease as long their renal function is carefully monitored.

One important risk factor for developing a decline in renal function with CEI therapy appears to be concurrent diuretic-induced volume depletion. Hypovolemia increases renin secretion and makes maintenance of the GFR more angiotensin II–dependent. As a result, the impairment in autoregulation by CEI is more marked in the presence of volume depletion.[161] This may explain the observation that almost all patients with CEI-induced acute renal failure were also taking a diuretic.[62,159] In some of these patients, stopping the diuretic and liberalizing sodium intake led to an improvement in GFR (as manifested by a fall in the plasma creatinine concentration) even though the CEI was continued.[162]

Similar hemodynamic changes following CEI therapy may occur in the stenotic kidney in patients with unilateral renal artery stenosis. In one study, for example, the administration of a CEI led to almost complete cessation of GFR (as estimated by radionuclide scanning) in 7 of 14 patients.[163] However, the presence of the normally perfused contralateral kidney generally prevents a decline in GFR,[158,163] unless secondary nephrosclerosis has developed in that kidney.[158,160] Despite the typical maintenance of total GFR, it is possible that prolonged loss of GFR can lead to irreversible atrophy of the stenotic kidney. As a result, patients with unilateral renal artery stenosis who are treated with a CEI should probably undergo a radionuclide scan to estimate GFR and different therapy instituted if function in the stenotic kidney has substantially declined (see p. 565).

Other antihypertensive agents that do not interfere with angiotensin II formation generally do not diminish renal function with renal artery stenosis[62-64] unless the intrarenal pressure falls below the level at which the GFR can be maintained by autoregulation (see Fig. 3-5). This can occur when there are severe bilateral stenoses or when there is a marked reduction in systemic pressure (see Fig. 12-8).[157,164] Patients with essential hypertension are not at risk of developing this complication since there is no pressure gradient across the renal arterial tree and therefore no need to autoregulate unless the systemic pressure is lowered excessively.[165]

CALCIUM CHANNEL BLOCKERS

Calcium channel blockers infrequently can produce an acute, rapidly reversible decline in renal function in patients with underlying chronic renal disease.[166] It is presumed that this change is mediated by an alteration in intrarenal hemodynamics, similar to that seen with an NSAID or a CEI. The mechanism by which this might occur is not known.

SUMMARY

Acute renal failure due to prerenal disease occurs in a variety of clinical settings. The underlying disorder can usually be ascertained from the history and physical examination, whereas the specific diagnosis of prerenal disease as the cause of renal failure is based upon the characteristic laboratory findings: elevated BUN/P_{cr} ratio, normal urinalysis, high U_{osm}, low U_{Na}, and FE_{Na} less than 1 percent.

An important diagnostic problem may arise when the laboratory tests point toward prerenal disease but no cause is readily apparent. In this setting, an occult cardiopulmonary event (such as an acute myocardial infarction) is frequently present (see Case history 2-4). Thus, an electrocardiogram should be obtained and the patient examined for signs of poor tissue perfusion such as cool, clammy extremities, obtundation, or a fall in blood pressure. Alternatively, bilateral renal artery stenosis should be suspected if the patient is markedly hypertensive. Establishing the correct diagnosis is extremely important since treatment varies with the underlying disease.

ACUTE TUBULAR NECROSIS

Tubular necrosis represents a nonspecific response to a variety of renal insults. Nevertheless, the clinical course of the disease usually follows a relatively uniform pattern. After the initial insult, there is an abrupt decline in renal function with the BUN and P_{cr} progressively rising, in many cases to levels requiring dialysis. This phase usually lasts 7 to 21 days and is typically followed by a gradual improvement in renal function back to baseline levels if the patient survives. Despite the ready reversibility of the renal disease, ATN frequently develops in patients with serious underlying diseases such as sepsis and shock. As a result, the mortality rate remains high, exceeding 50 percent in certain settings (see "Prognosis," below).

The causes of ATN can be divided into two broad categories: postischemic and nephrotoxic (Table 3–2). However, this distinction is frequently blurred because both factors are operative in many patients.[167] For example, a septic patient with hypotension may be treated with an aminoglycoside antibiotic. Furthermore, these problems may have synergistic nephrotoxicity. In one experimental model, neither mild volume depletion nor low doses of gentamicin impaired renal function, but the combination produced tubular necrosis.[168] How this synergism occurs can be best appreciated by a review of the factors that lead to tubular necrosis. An understanding of these mechanisms also has important implications for therapy and prevention.

POSTISCHEMIC ATN

ROLE OF MEDULLARY ISCHEMIA

An apparent paradox in ATN is that cell necrosis is generally limited to the kidneys, yet renal blood flow in the basal state is extremely high. When expressed in milliliters per minute per 100 g, renal blood flow is 5 times that of the heart and 8 times that of the liver and brain.[18] However, the unique anatomy of the renal medulla makes this segment particularly susceptible to ischemia. The vasa recta capillaries that perfuse the medulla do not course through the medulla but have a hairpin configuration with descending and ascending limbs (Fig. 3–11).

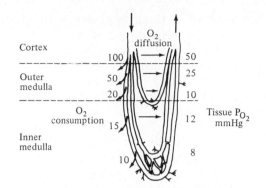

FIG. 3–11. Development of medullary hypoxia due to the exchange of oxygen between the descending and ascending limbs of the vasa recta capillaries (straight arrows) and to oxygen consumption by the medullary cells (curved arrows). (*From M. Brezis, S. Rosen, P. Silva, and F. H. Epstein, Kidney Int., 26:375, 1984. Reprinted by permission from Kidney International.*)

Blood entering the medulla has a high P_{O_2}, similar to that in the cortex. However, some of this oxygen diffuses into the relatively poorly oxygenated blood in the ascending limb. The combination of this diffusion plus oxygen utilization by the tubular cells lowers the P_{O_2} to 10 to 20 mmHg by the end of the outer medulla. This hypoxia is particularly important because of the high metabolic activity of the tubular cells in the proximal straight tubule (or pars recta which ends in the outer medulla) and in the thick ascending limb of the loop of Henle; the latter cells, for example, have the highest sodium-potassium-ATPase activity in the nephron.[169]

The net effect of relatively low oxygen delivery and relatively high metabolic rate is manifested by the outer medulla normally utilizing approximately 80 percent of the oxygen delivered to it, in comparison to 8 percent for the rest of the kidney.[18] Thus, the cells in the outer medulla are normally on the verge of hypoxia and are particularly susceptible to ischemic damage.

Although all nephron segments may be damaged during an ischemic episode,[19] the degree of cellular necrosis is frequently most severe in the outer medulla (where oxygen delivery is lowest)[170-173] and in the early proximal convoluted tubule (which has a limited capacity for anaerobic metabolism and is therefore highly sensitive to hypoxia).[173] Ischemic injury to these segments can result in sloughing of the brush border from the proximal convoluted and straight tubules and the release of Tamm-Horsfall mucoprotein (the major component of urinary casts; see p. 24) from the thick ascending limb.[18,170,171] These changes are pathogenetically important since the cellular debris and cast formation contribute to the intratubular obstruction that plays a major role in the development of renal failure (see "Pathogenesis of Renal Failure," below). The impairment in loop of Henle function may also explain the almost uniform loss of concentrating ability in this disorder.[18]

Preferential loop of Henle ischemia also has potential therapeutic implications. The likelihood that a thick ascending limb cell will develop ischemic damage is dependent on the relationship between energy delivery and energy consumption. If delivery is reduced, the cell still can be protected by diminishing energy requirements. This can be achieved by the use of loop diuretics, since almost one-half of thick limb energy utilization is involved in active sodium chloride transport.[174] In experimental forms of ischemic ATN, furosemide has been shown to preserve renal function, at least in part by minimizing the degree of cell necrosis (Fig. 3-12).[175-177] It is not yet proven that similar protection can be achieved in humans, in part because therapy must be begun early, before overt tubular necrosis has occurred (see "Treatment," below).

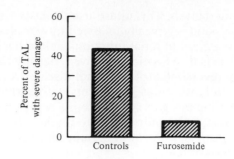

FIG. 3–12. Degree of necrosis in medullary thick ascending limbs (TAL) due to ischemia in the isolated perfused kidney. Furosemide has a marked protective effect. This is probably due to a reduction in cell work, i.e., active sodium chloride transport; similar protection is afforded if active transport is impaired by digitalis (which inhibits the sodium-potassium-ATPase pump) or by abolishing the GFR (which prevents sodium chloride from being delivered to the loop of Henle). (*Adapted from M. Brezis, S. Rosen, P. Silva, and F. H. Epstein, Kidney Int., 25:65, 1984. Reprinted by permission from Kidney International.*)

EVENTS DURING REFLOW

In addition to direct ischemic damage, events occurring during the reestablishment of tissue perfusion also appear to contribute to cell necrosis and the development of renal failure. Mitochondrial function initially increases with the return of flow but then has a secondary fall despite continued adequate oxygenation.[178] Mitochondrial accumulation of calcium may play an important role in this process.[178,179] During the period of ischemia, phospholipids in the tubular cell membrane may be altered, resulting in an increase in membrane permeability. When calcium is then delivered to the cell during reflow, there is increased calcium entry and subsequent accumulation in the mitochondria, producing mitochondrial dysfunction and decreased ATP synthesis. The last effect decreases the activity of the sodium-potassium-ATPase pump, which can lead to a vicious cycle characterized by cell swelling (since sodium is less efficiently pumped out of the cell), a further increase in membrane permeability, more calcium entry, and more mitochondrial damage. Mannitol, which has been effective in minimizing cell necrosis and renal failure in experimental animals[176,180] and may be beneficial in humans (see "Treatment," below),[11] appears to act primarily as an osmotic agent which prevents cell swelling and, therefore, continued calcium accumulation in the cell.[180]

It is highly probable that calcium is not the sole factor responsible for cell necrosis in this setting.[179] In particular, the local accumulation of oxygen-derived free radicals (O_2^-·) and fatty acids may play an important role.[181,182] During the ischemic phase, ATP is converted to AMP and ultimately hypoxanthine. Both calcium and oxygen are then delivered to the cell with reflow. The increase in cell calcium activates xanthine oxidase, allowing free radicals to be generated by the following simplified reaction[183]:

$$\text{Hypoxanthine} + O_2 \xrightarrow[\text{oxidase}]{\text{xanthine}} \text{uric acid} + O_2^-\cdot$$

ETIOLOGY

Although renal ischemia is the most common cause of ATN, the sensitivity of individual patients to a decrease in renal perfusion is variable. In some patients, a few minutes of hypotension is sufficient to induce ATN, whereas others are able to tolerate hours of renal ischemia without structural damage to the kidney, displaying the findings of only prerenal disease such as a normal urinalysis and a low FE_{Na}. Even these latter patients, however, can eventually develop ATN if renal perfusion is not improved. At this point, renal function can no longer be restored by volume repletion.

The importance of the *duration* of ischemia has been demonstrated in humans by studies of patients undergoing abdominal aortic aneurysm surgery.[184,185] Some patients require clamping of the aorta above the renal arteries, leading to a period of total renal ischemia lasting 15 to 90 min.*[185,186] After surgery, the GFR is reduced and the urinary findings are typical of ATN: high urine sodium concentration and urine osmolality similar to that of plasma. Within 3 days, however, renal function has essentially returned to normal.[185] This rapid recovery assumes that renal perfusion remains intact after the aortic clamp is removed. A more prolonged course is seen in the complicated patient in whom the cardiac output or systemic blood pressure is reduced in the postoperative period because of bleeding, infection, or myocardial dysfunction[184] or in the preoperative period because of aneurysmal rupture.[187]

Although any of the disorders associated with prerenal disease can result in ATN, renal damage most commonly occurs in patients with hypotension, particularly in the settings of *surgery, sepsis, or obstetrical complications.* The relationship to surgery is due in part to the associated hemodynamic changes. Preoperative fluid depletion, anesthesia, and intraoperative fluid losses can lead to volume depletion and enhanced ADH secretion.[188] The net effects are reductions in GFR (up to 30 to 45 percent), urine volume, and sodium excretion.[185,188] Most patients tolerate these changes well and do not develop renal failure. However, ATN may ensue if an additional insult is added, such as hypotension or hemolysis.

---

*The more common infrarenal clamping produces a relatively small reduction in GFR and, if the surgery is uncomplicated, little renal damage.[185,186]

The surgical procedures associated with the highest risk of ATN are abdominal aortic aneurysm repair,[185-187] open-heart surgery, and surgery in the presence of obstructive jaundice. With open-heart surgery, the underlying cardiac disease plus hypotension and hemolysis during cardiopulmonary bypass all may play a role in the development of renal failure.[12,24,189] Many patients remain prerenal in this setting, but progression to ATN is not uncommon.[24]

The mechanism by which obstructive jaundice predisposes toward ATN is incompletely understood. The reduction in GFR immediately following surgery is almost twice as great (60 versus 30 percent) in patients with obstructive jaundice than in those with other conditions.[190] This effect may be related to the systemic actions of endotoxin that has been absorbed from the gut.[191,192] Endotoxin induces renal ischemia both by lowering systemic blood pressure and by causing renal vasoconstriction.[65,193] Endotoxin absorption is normally limited, perhaps because bile salts have a detergent effect on the lipopolysaccharide endotoxin molecule. Patients with obstructive jaundice lose this protective effect since bile salt entry into the intestinal lumen is impaired. Although this hypothesis is unproven, the preoperative administration of oral bile salts appears to prevent both the endotoxinemia and the renal dysfunction.[191,192] Endotoxin also may be responsible for the development of ATN in the septic patient.

During pregnancy, ATN may be seen after a septic abortion or with severe bleeding at term, particularly due to abruptio placentae.[194,195] An amniotic fluid embolus or a retained dead fetus also can lead to acute renal failure in the pregnant patient. However, these disorders are typically associated with renal cortical necrosis and disseminated intravascular coagulation, rather than ATN.[194]

Finally, a low cardiac output due to heart failure represents one prerenal state in which the development of ATN is extremely unusual.[196] This protective effect may be related to a *cardiorenal reflex* in which an increase in left heart filling pressure reduces renal sympathetic tone, even though total sympathetic activity is enhanced because of the low flow state.[197,198] Heart failure is also associated with increased release of atrial natriuretic peptide, which can act as a renal vasodilator.[199] By either of these mechanisms, renal perfusion may be better maintained in heart failure than in other prerenal conditions in which intracardiac pressures are typically reduced.[198]

NEPHROTOXIC ATN

A variety of nephrotoxins can induce ATN*,[200] (Table 3-2), the most common being aminoglycoside antibiotics, radiocontrast media, cisplatin, and heme pigments.

AMINOGLYCOSIDE ANTIBIOTICS

Acute tubular necrosis is a relatively common complication of the prolonged administration of aminoglycoside antibiotics,[3,201,202] occurring in 5 to 15 percent of patients in most studies.[203,204] The nephrotoxicity of these agents is in part related to their preferential accumulation in the renal cortex. The aminoglycosides are freely filtered across the glomerulus and are then taken up by and stored in the proximal tubular cells. As long as 28 days after the drug is given, the concentration in the renal cortex may exceed that achieved in the plasma on the day of administration.[205] This distribution probably explains the observation that ATN may first

---

*Nephrotoxins also can induce acute renal failure by mechanisms other than tubular necrosis.[200] For example, the penicillins can cause an allergic vasculitis or interstitial nephritis (see Chaps. 7 and 8).

become clinically apparent several days after the drug has been discontinued.

The renal damage with aminoglycosides represents a cumulative effect that is initially manifested by increased excretion of low-molecular-weight proteins (such as β_2-microglobulin), due to decreased proximal reabsorption.[206] This is typically followed in 2 to 7 days by elevations in the BUN and P_{cr}.[206] Thus the development of renal insufficiency usually requires at least 7 days of drug administration.[3,203]

The number of cationic amino groups (NH_3^+) per molecule appears to correlate closely with nephrotoxicity.[201] Streptomycin (3 per molecule) produces the least renal damage and neomycin (6) the most. Gentamicin, tobramycin, netilmicin (5), amikacin and kanamycin (4) have intermediate toxicity.

The role of molecular charge seems to be related to the binding of the cationic aminoglycoside to anionic phospholipid receptors in the luminal and subcellular membranes.[3,201] At the luminal membrane, this interaction promotes drug movement from the tubular lumen into the cell. Within the cell, the aminoglycoside accumulates within lysosomes,[207] an effect that may be mediated by a similar charge interaction. The observation that other small cationic compounds (such as poly-L-lysine) can produce similar changes is further proof of the importance of molecular charge.[20,201]

Interference with lysosomal function may be responsible for the pathologic and functional changes induced by the aminoglycosides. These drugs inhibit phospholipase activity in the lysosome. The ensuing accumulation of phospholipids may lead to the formation of lamellar myeloid bodies within the lysosome, which are characteristic of aminoglycoside nephrotoxicity.[201,208] Either decreased lysosomal function or the release of lysosomal enzymes into the cytosol may then lead to cell necrosis.[3,201]

Toxic changes are not limited to the proximal tubule, although they are most prominent in this segment. Binding of the drug to anionic phospholipids in the collecting tubule cell membrane may interfere with the response to ADH.[20] The ensuing decrease in collecting tubule water reabsorption may account at least in part for the high frequency of *nonoliguric* ATN following aminoglycoside usage.[209] Hypomagnesemia due to urinary magnesium wasting also may be seen, although the mechanism by which it occurs is not known.[210]

Aminoglycoside toxicity in animals may also be associated with renal vasoconstriction and decreased glomerular capillary permeability, changes that can contribute to the fall in GFR. Angiotensin II appears to play an important role in this response; however the factors responsible for activation of the renin-angiotensin system in this setting are unclear.[211]

Although acute renal failure may develop when the plasma aminoglycoside level is kept within the therapeutic range,[212,213] many cases are associated with the administration of excessive amounts of the drug.[203,204] Drug dosage must be correlated with the GFR, since excretion occurs primarily by glomerular filtration. Three errors are commonly made in estimating the correct dose in relation to renal function.

1. A small elevation in the P_{cr} may be ignored. For example, a P_{cr} of 1.5 mg/dL may reflect a fall in GFR of more than 50 percent.
2. The effect of decreased muscle mass leading to decreased creatinine production also may be ignored. A P_{cr} of 1.0 mg/dL may indicate a normal GFR of 100 mL/min in a 40-year-old 70-kg man, but a GFR of only 40 mL/min in a 70-year-old 50-kg woman. The creatinine clearance can be estimated from the following for-

mula, which accounts for decreased muscle mass in older, smaller patients:

$$C_{cr} \cong \frac{(140 - age) \times LBW}{P_{cr} \times 72}$$

when LBW is the approximate lean body weight, in kilograms. This value should be multiplied by 0.85 in women who, at a given body weight, have a smaller muscle mass than men.

3. The P_{cr} can be used as an estimate of the GFR only in the steady state. In a patient with acute renal failure in whom the P_{cr} is rising each day, calculating the aminoglycoside dose on the basis of the P_{cr}[214] can lead to excessive drug administration.

Because of these potential problems, aminoglycosides are most safely given if serum levels are carefully monitored, particularly in high-risk patients.

In addition to increasing dose and duration of treatment, other risk factors for the development of aminoglycoside nephrotoxicity include advanced age, underlying renal disease, and concurrent volume depletion.[3,201,203] The first two factors are most likely related to a decline in GFR, which would favor excess drug accumulation. The effect of volume depletion may also reflect decreased perfusion to the tubular cells, making them more sensitive to the metabolic derangements induced by the aminoglycoside.[168]

Two other questions remain unresolved: the relative nephrotoxicity of gentamicin and tobramycin, and possible enhanced toxicity when an aminoglycoside is given with cephalothin. Initial studies appeared to show that tobramycin was less nephrotoxic than gentamicin,[212,213,215] suggesting some additional effect of gentamicin, since both drugs have the same number of cationic amino groups per molecule.[201] There were, however, methodologic problems with these studies, and more recent reports indicate that there is probably no clinically significant renal sparing effect of tobramycin.[203,204]

The potential risk of concurrent cephalosporin administration is uncertain. Early studies suggested than an aminoglycoside plus cephalothin was more nephrotoxic than an aminoglycoside plus a penicillin derivative.[213,216,217] Even if this effect is real (which has been questioned),[204] it is unclear if the added toxicity applies to cephalosporinlike drugs other than cephalothin. It appears, for example, that at least cefazolin and moxalactam can be safely administered with an aminoglycoside.[203,217,218]

RADIOCONTRAST MEDIA

Renal failure may follow the administration of radiocontrast media.[219,220] This complication most often occurs after intravenous pyelography, angiography, and contrast-enhanced CT scanning but also may rarely follow cholecystography or cholangiography. Two major risk factors have been identified, *renal insufficiency* and *diabetes mellitus*,[219-225] although the quantity of contrast administered and the adequacy of renal perfusion may also be important.[221] Patients with a P_{cr} below 1.5 mg/dL have less than a 1 to 2 percent incidence of renal failure which, when it occurs, is mild and transient.[222-224] Even patients with moderate renal insufficiency (P_{cr} 1.5 to 2.5 mg/dL) are at relatively low risk.[226] However, the incidence of renal failure increases substantially with more advanced renal disease, a risk that is dependent in part on the presence of other potentiating factors. For example, the likelihood of developing contrast-induced renal failure can reach as high as 90 percent when the P_{cr} exceeds 4.5 mg/dL in a patient with diabetic nephropathy.[222-225] In comparison, the risk is only about 2 percent in a patient with a P_{cr} above 2 mg/dL who has only one study, involving the administration of less than 125 mL of contrast, and who is nondiabetic and has a relatively normal cardiac output.[221]

Radiocontrast media also may potentiate the nephrotoxicity of excreted light chains in patients with multiple myeloma.[227] However, the development of acute renal failure in this setting is more likely related to prior dehydration promoting the precipitation of intratubular casts.[228]

The mechanism by which contrast media induce renal failure is not clear. The few biopsies that have been performed showed some tubular necrosis, suggesting a direct toxic effect.[229,230] However, the observation that the U_{Na} and FE_{Na} are usually typical of prerenal disease[30] argues against tubular necrosis as being the primary problem. Contrast media have been shown to reduce renal blood flow,[231] to induce aggregation of red cells in the glomerular capillaries,[232] to promote the intratubular precipitation of Tamm-Horsfall mucoprotein,[233] and to increase uric acid excretion,[234] all of which can lead to renal failure.

The course of contrast-induced renal failure also differs from typical ATN in that the duration is shorter. The P_{cr} typically begins to rise after the x-ray study, peaks at 3 to 7 days (versus 7 to 21 days in other forms of ATN), and then rapidly returns to baseline levels.[219] Many patients are asymptomatic, and the deterioration in renal function will be missed if the P_{cr} is not measured. Others, however, will have a more severe course, requiring dialysis with possibly irreversible changes. This uncommon result is most likely when the baseline P_{cr} exceeds 5 mg/dL, particularly in patients with type 1 diabetes mellitus.[223,225]

There is no specific treatment once renal failure has developed, but prevention is important. In high-risk patients, ultrasonography or unenhanced CT scanning can frequently provide the same information achieved with radiocontrast media. If contrast agents must be given, hydration during and after the study may ameliorate or prevent the renal failure. Although saline solutions may offer some protection,[224] 250 mL of 20 percent mannitol given over 1 h after the study is probably more effective.[235] The ensuing urinary losses must be replaced to avoid volume depletion.

CISPLATIN

Cisplatin is a very effective chemotherapeutic agent that also is a frequent nephrotoxin.[236,237] About 25 to 35 percent of patients will develop a mild and partially reversible decline in renal function after the first course of therapy.[237] The incidence and severity of renal failure increases with continued drug administration. The concurrent administration of an aminoglycoside appears to potentiate the nephrotoxicity.[236,238]

Cisplatin is a direct tubular toxin, preferentially affecting the proximal straight tubule (pars recta) and the distal and collecting tubules.[236] These changes are manifested by renal failure and, in many patients, hypomagnesemia due to urinary losses.[239]

Two disorders must be differentiated from cisplatin-induced ATN: prerenal disease due to drug-induced vomiting and thrombotic microangiopathy when cisplatin is given with bleomycin.[240] The former is associated with the signs of prerenal disease and is easily corrected with volume repletion. The latter may have a more acute course, but the diagnosis is suggested by the development of the characteristic hematologic changes of microangiopathic hemolytic anemia and thrombocytopenia (see Chap. 7).

Minimizing the renal toxicity of cisplatin is particularly important since it allows more drug to be given, thereby producing a greater antineoplastic effect. This can be achieved by vigorous intravenous hydration (250 mL/h of saline) and by administering the drug in a concentrated saline solution (preferentially 250 mL of 3% saline).[241] This regimen appears to change the chemical form of cisplatin in a manner that limits entry into the renal cells.

HEME PIGMENTS

ATN may result from the release of heme pigments as occurs with myoglobinuria due to rhabdomyolysis or hemoglobinuria due to intravascular hemolysis. These disorders are typically associated with red to brown urine (see p. 10) unless the GFR is very low or the plasma has been cleared of the pigment because of extrarenal metabolism.[242] The accumulation of unexcreted myoglobin or hemoglobin can produce similar, evanescent color changes in the plasma.

Rhabdomyolysis leading to acute renal failure occurs in a variety of conditions.[242,243] The most common are trauma (including ischemic tissue damage following a drug overdose), alcoholism, seizures, and exertional heat stroke, particularly in untrained subjects or those with sickle cell trait.[242-250] Hypokalemia is another rare cause, but it can potentiate any of these problems, both by interfering with cell metabolism and by limiting the release of potassium from exercising muscle cells, a normally important factor in the local vasodilatation that increases blood flow to these areas.[251,252] For example, heat stroke in young, untrained men typically occurs during the second week of exercise, the same time as the maximum potassium deficit (due to very high sweat losses) is achieved.[252,253]

A characteristic triad that is frequently present in patients with rhabdomyolysis consists of pigmented granular casts in the urine sediment, a positive orthotolidine (Hematest) reaction in the urine supernatant indicating the presence of heme, and a marked elevation in the plasma level of creatine phosphokinase due to the release of this enzyme from damaged muscle cells.[245] Other cellular constituents also may be released resulting

in hyperphosphatemia, hypocalcemia (due to precipitation of calcium phosphate in the injured muscle,* hyperkalemia, hyperuricemia, a high anion gap metabolic acidosis (due to the entry of cellular organic acids into the extracellular fluid), and an unusually rapid increase in the P_{cr} out of proportion to the duration of renal failure.[242,244,245,254-256] For example, the plasma potassium concentration increases at a maximum daily rate of less than 0.3 meq/L in patients with renal failure who are not hypercatabolic[257]; in comparison, the daily increment can exceed 1.0 meq/L with rhabdomyolysis.[244]

Intravascular hemolysis of any cause can lead to ATN[258-261] and is associated acutely with red plasma (see p. 11) and a drop in the hematocrit. The most common etiology is a transfusion reaction. In this setting, chills and hypotension also may be present.

The mechanism by which heme pigments lead to renal failure is incompletely understood. In general, neither hemoglobin nor myoglobin is directly nephrotoxic, as concurrent renal vasoconstriction or volume depletion is necessary for renal failure to occur.[262-265] These potentiating changes could result from fluid accumulation in the damaged muscle, sweat losses with exertion, hypotension due to a transfusion reaction, and renal vasoconstriction due to hemoglobin itself or the release of vasoactive substances in the red cell membrane or skeletal muscle.[264-266] It may be, for example, that decreased renal perfusion slows the rate of urine flow in the tubules, an effect that would promote the precipitation of the char-

---

*Approximately 20 to 30 percent of patients with rhabdomyolysis-induced acute renal failure become *hypercalcemic* during the recovery phase as the deposited calcium phosphate is mobilized and returned to the extracellular fluid.[254,255] Both correction of hyperphosphatemia (resulting from the rise in GFR) and a poorly understood increase in 1,25-dihydroxyvitamin D appear to contribute to this response.[254] Consequently, the administration of calcium should be avoided, if possible, during the period of hypocalcemia.

acteristic heme pigment casts. These casts, which cause intratubular obstruction,[262,263,267] plus the renal vasoconstriction are probably responsible for the renal failure.[29,268] True tubular necrosis is generally not a prominent finding,[263,267] an observation which is compatible with the low U_{Na} and FE_{Na} (less than 1 percent) that are frequently found in these patients.[29]

MISCELLANEOUS

A variety of other substances are infrequent causes of ATN (see Table 3–2). Included in this group are antimicrobials (cephalosporins, rifampin, amphotericin B, and polymixins),[269–273] heavy metals (mercury, arsine, arsinic, and uranium),[274,275] an acetaminophen overdose,[276,277] the anesthetic methoxyflurane,[278] carbon tetrachloride ingestion,[279,280] and ethylenediaminetetraacetic acid (EDTA) which is used in the treatment of lead poisoning.[281] Tetracyclines can also impair renal function, particularly in patients with underlying renal disease.[282] However, these changes are primarily due to the antianabolic effect of the tetracyclines (resulting in an elevation in the BUN)[283] and to prerenal disease produced by the side effects of vomiting and diarrhea.[282]

Acute renal failure due to ATN or, in some cases, interstitial nephritis may be associated with Legionnaires' disease.[284] It is possible that a toxin released by the microorganism is responsible for the renal damage in this setting.

PATHOLOGY

There are two major histologic changes in ATN: tubular necrosis with denuding of the epithelium and occlusion of the tubular lumina by casts and cell debris.[10,173,285] However the distribution of these lesions is somewhat different in the two forms of ATN. Tubular necrosis is typically patchy in ischemic ATN.

Although any nephron segment may be affected,[19] damage is generally most severe in the lesser oxygenated outer medulla (see Fig. 3–11), particularly the proximal straight tubule which also shows extensive loss of its brush border.[170,171,285] The brush border, other cellular debris, and pigmented casts all may occlude the tubular lumina, particularly in the distal and collecting tubules. Patients with prolonged ATN may have evidence of fresh necrotic lesions, indicating continued episodes of renal ischemia.[285] As healing occurs, nuclear mitoses indicative of tubular regeneration are frequently seen.

In contrast, the pathologic changes in nephrotoxic ATN are usually limited to the proximal convoluted and straight tubules, probably because this is the major site of reabsorption of potential nephrotoxins.[201] In addition, the tubular injury is relatively uniform in contrast to the focal distribution following ischemia. An exception to this general rule is cisplatin, which produces damage in both proximal and distal nephron segments.[236]

With either type of ATN in humans, the glomeruli and blood vessels usually are normal by light and electron microscopy.[286] Mild glomerular changes of uncertain significance have been described in animals.

PATHOGENESIS OF RENAL FAILURE

The mechanism by which ATN results in renal failure is incompletely understood. At least three factors have been thought to contribute to the decline in GFR:

1. Tubular obstruction
2. Backleak of the glomerular filtrate through the damaged tubular cells
3. A primary reduction in glomerular filtration

The data supporting these theories have been derived primarily from studies in experimental animals using both renal ischemia (renal artery occlusion, norepinephrine) and nephrotoxins (mercury, uranium). The applicability of these models to human disease is uncertain since they differ in some ways from human ATN.[10,285] Nevertheless, these models provide insight into the mechanisms that may be operative.

TUBULAR OBSTRUCTION

Tubular obstruction appears to be an important problem in many forms of ATN.[170,171,287-289] Cellular debris (particularly loss of the brush border in the proximal straight tubule), the release from damaged loop of Henle cells of Tamm-Horsfall mucoprotein (the primary matrix of tubular casts; see p. 24), and heme pigments all may contribute to this process.[10,18,170,171,267] The ensuing increase in intratubular pressure would then retard glomerular filtration.

Tubular occlusion may also have an important secondary mechanism in producing ATN. As the tubules dilate proximal to the obstruction, the ensuing elevation in the peritubular interstitial pressure can compress the adjacent peritubular capillaries.[289,290] This effect is most prominent in the outer medulla, particularly around the proximal straight tubules.[10,290] The net result is more medullary ischemia which can contribute to further cellular injury.

In some nephrons, the initially elevated intratubular pressure falls to or below normal.[287,288] This effect is due to a reduction in tubular flow resulting from either a primary decrease in glomerular filtration or increased reabsorption by tubular backleak (see below). Regardless of the mechanism, tubular obstruction may still be present, since enhancing tubular flow can once again elevate the intratubular pressure.[287]

The secondary decrease in tubular flow and pressure may also explain why the degree of tubular necrosis and dilatation is often relatively mild in humans with ATN.[18,291] Furthermore, the lack of evident necrosis does not mean that the tubules are unaffected, since markedly impaired function can occur in cells that appear histologically normal.[19,292]

BACKLEAK OF FILTRATE

If a substantial portion of the glomerular filtrate leaks back through damaged epithelial cells, urinary excretion will fall, resulting in elevations in the BUN and P_{cr}. This sequence has been demonstrated in both ischemic and nephrotoxic forms of ATN.[170,293] For example, the dye lissamine green normally is not reabsorbed by the tubules. Thus, if the dye is injected into Bowman's space, its green color normally can be seen as it moves down the nephron. In contrast, the green color disappears from the lumen in mercury-induced ATN, presumably owing to backleak.[293]

There is also indirect evidence suggesting that backleak occurs in humans, at least when ATN follows cardiac surgery.[12,24] Both freely filtered inulin (molecular radius 14 Å) and dextran molecules (molecular radius 22 to 30 Å) were infused into these patients. Neither compound is usually reabsorbed. In normals, the renal clearance of inulin exceeds that of dextran because the latter is larger and therefore less completely filtered. These results are reversed, however, in patients with ATN, presumably because filtered inulin leaks back through damaged tubular cells (and is thus not excreted) at a greater rate than the larger dextran molecules. By comparing their clearances, it was estimated that as much as 40 percent of the filtrate was reabsorbed by backleak. (In comparison, no backleak could be demonstrated in patients with prerenal disease.[24])

Although backleak does seem to occur, it

is not of primary importance in the renal failure. When the degree of backleak is accounted for, the total GFR still remains under 20 mL/min in many patients.[24]

REDUCTION IN GFR

The severe decrease in GFR that is characteristic of ATN may also be due in part to some primary change in glomerular function. Arteriolar vasoconstriction leading to renal and glomerular ischemia is frequently present in ATN, as evidenced by a 50 to 75 percent reduction in renal blood flow in humans with this disorder.[294,295] This increase in arteriolar resistance could represent a secondary response to tubular obstruction, a change that can be viewed as being somewhat appropriate in that perfusion is shunted away from obstructed nephrons toward those with better function.[296]

However, the role of renal ischemia in perpetuating the renal failure is uncertain. In both postischemic and nephrotoxic models, the normalization of renal blood flow by volume expansion or the use of vasodilators has been ineffective in increasing the GFR.[287,297,298] There data suggest that, although renal ischemia is important initially (both in postischemic ATN and by potentiating the toxicity of aminoglycosides, cisplatin, and heme pigments; see above), it is not necessary for the persistent reduction in GFR.

Another possibility, for which there is substantial experimental evidence, is that a decrease in glomerular capillary permeability contributes to the fall in GFR.[207,297-299] This change could be mediated by swelling of the endothelial cells, for which there is conflicting evidence,[299,300] or by contraction of the mesangium, thereby decreasing the surface area available for filtration. Mesangial contraction could be induced by a direct effect of angiotensin II[211,301] or by tubuloglomerular feedback.[302]

Tubuloglomerular feedback is a phenomenon in which flow to the distal nephron is regulated by receptors in the macula densa in the early distal tubule.[39,303] If distal flow were inappropriately increased, the reabsorptive capacity of the distal and collecting tubules could be overwhelmed, leading to severe volume depletion. This sequence is prevented by tubuloglomerular feedback, which reduces the GFR until distal flow is returned to normal. Viewed in terms of proximal and loop damage and decreased reabsorption in ATN, a marked reduction in GFR could be considered a successful adaptation to prevent progressive fluid depletion.[302] This decrease in filtration appears to be mediated by afferent arteriolar constriction and/or mesangial contraction, which lower glomerular capillary pressure and permeability, respectively.[303,304] The mechanism by which these changes occur is uncertain, but both intrarenally produced adenosine and angiotensin II may play a role.[39]

Although there is experimental evidence supporting a contribution of tubuloglomerular feedback in ATN, this phenomenon appears to decrease the GFR only by a maximum of about 50 percent[305] and therefore cannot alone explain the severe renal failure that frequently occurs.

SUMMARY

It does not seem likely that a single factor is responsible for the decline in GFR that accompanies ATN, as tubular obstruction, backleak, and a reduction in GFR all have been demonstrated. It may be that different factors are responsible for the initiation and perpetuation of the renal failure. For example, hypotension or a nephrotoxin may induce tubular necrosis, leading to tubular obstruction. This causes an increase in intratubular pressure, which then may fall to normal or below because of tubular backleak or a decrease in glomerular function. Tubular obstruction may still be present at this point, as the recovery of renal function seems to begin by the washout of obstructing debris and casts.[289,306]

CLINICAL COURSE

The course of ATN can be divided into three stages: (1) the renal failure phase, (2) the diuretic phase, and (3) the recovery phase.

RENAL FAILURE PHASE

The decrease in renal function seen in ATN may begin abruptly after a hypotensive episode or insidiously after the administration of a nephrotoxin such as gentamicin. In a typical patient, the daily increments in the BUN and P_{cr} are 10 to 25 mg/dL and 0.5 to 2.5 mg/dL, respectively.[8,257] These changes may be even more pronounced in patients who are hypercatabolic, as the BUN may rise by more than 50 mg/dL per day.[244] Hyperkalemia and hyperphosphatemia also are more common in this setting, owing to the release of potassium and phosphate from damaged cells.

The clinical problems occurring during this phase include fluid overload, electrolyte disorders (such as hyperkalemia, hyperphosphatemia, and hypocalcemia), and the signs and symptoms of uremia such as lethargy, vomiting, pericarditis, and bleeding.

Another frequent complication is infection, which is the most common cause of death.[187,307] Part of this problem is related to the underlying disorder such as abdominal surgery. In addition, renal failure can impair host defenses, especially when the BUN exceeds 80 to 100 mg/dL.[308-310] The primary sites of infection are in the lungs, abdomen, and urinary tract (particularly with prolonged indwelling bladder catheterization).[307] Wound infections with delayed healing also may be present in postoperative patients.

NONOLIGURIC VERSUS OLIGURIC ATN

The urine volume is variable in ATN, with many patients being nonoliguric (output greater than 500 mL/day) despite the marked reduction in GFR.[5,6] In general, a low or high urine output can be seen with any of the causes of ATN, although the aminoglycoside antibiotics, which inhibit ADH-induced water reabsorption in the collecting tubules,[20] most commonly induce the nonoliguric form.[5,209]

The presence of nonoliguric ATN is important because it frequently represents a less severe disease than the oliguric form.[5,6,167] This was manifested in one study by a lower FE_{Na}, lower peak P_{cr} (6 versus 9 mg/dL), less frequent requirement for dialysis (28 versus 84 percent), and lower mortality rate (26 versus 50 percent).[5] These findings are consistent with experimental data, which suggest that the difference in urine output is due to the presence of more functioning nephrons in nonoliguric as compared to oliguric animals.[289] This general rule, however, is not always applicable since many nonoliguric patients will have severe enough disease to require dialysis.[24]

It should also be noted that the relatively good prognosis of *spontaneous* nonoliguric ATN does not appear to apply to the conversion of oliguric into nonoliguric ATN by the administration of loop diuretics. In patients with established oliguric ATN, the administration of high doses of intravenous furosemide may increase the urine output but does not change the renal prognosis when compared to untreated patients.[311] This can be explained by the diuretic decreasing tubular reabsorption in those few nephrons that are still functioning; improved renal function would require the recruitment of new nephrons, and this does not seem to occur.

The average duration of the renal failure phase is approximately 7 to 21 days.[10,312] However, this does not apply to all patients, as a shorter period may occur following either the administration of radiocontrast media[219] or transient renal ischemia during abdominal aortic aneurysm surgery.[184,185] On the other hand, the period of renal failure is prolonged in some patients, lasting up to 3 to 6 months.[184,209,313] This is most likely to occur with persistent, severe infection, as with pneumonia or an intraabdominal abscess. In this setting, there is a persistent renal insult and a prolonged hypercatabolic state. The latter prevents the regeneration of new tubular cells that is required for complete recovery to occur.

DIURETIC AND RECOVERY PHASES

The renal failure phase is usually followed by gradual improvement in renal function characterized by an increase in GFR (and reduction in P_{cr}) most of or all the way to the previous baseline level.[312,314-316] This elevation in GFR is associated with a progressive increase in urine output (particularly in oliguric patients) that can initially average 50 to 100 percent per day. It is important to be aware, however, that an elevation in urine output can also be due to a decrease in tubular reabsorption. In this setting, the GFR will remain low, as detected by a continued elevation in the P_{cr}.

Experimental studies suggest that improvement in renal function begins with the relief of tubular obstruction by the washout of casts and cellular debris.[289,306] A similar course may occur in humans since persistent backleak (indicating tubular injury) has been demonstrated during the early recovery phase.[12] Thus, the initial improvement in GFR does not require the restoration of normal tubular function.

The increase in urine output that occurs during the diuretic phase may be non-physiologic because of this delay in the recovery of tubular function. If tubular reabsorption is unable to increase as rapidly as the GFR, the net result may be inappropriate sodium and water loss in the urine. True volume depletion will then ensue if these losses are not replaced.

CHANGES IN P_{cr}

The P_{cr}, which is determined by the relationship between creatinine production and excretion, follows a triphasic pattern in ATN (Fig. 3–13). When the GFR is reduced in the renal failure phase, there is a marked fall in creatinine excretion, resulting in the reten-

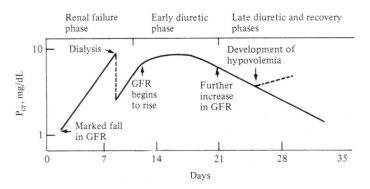

FIG. 3–13. Sequential changes in the P_{cr} in a typical case of ATN. See text for details.

tion of creatinine and a progressive elevation in the plasma level until the rates of production and excretion are again equal. In some oliguric patients who become volume-expanded owing to fluid retention, dilution of the extracellular fluid can initially minimize or even prevent the expected rise in the P_{cr}.[317] This effect, however, is transient, as continued creatinine retention must increase the P_{cr}.

During the early diuretic phase, the initial elevation in GFR toward normal enhances creatinine excretion. As the rate of excretion approaches that of production, the daily increments in the P_{cr} become smaller. Thus, the P_{cr} may continue to rise slowly for several days, even though the GFR has increased. When excretion equals production, there will be a plateau in the P_{cr}. With further improvement in the GFR, creatinine excretion exceeds production, resulting in a gradual reduction in the P_{cr} toward normal. If, however, inappropriate urinary losses are not replaced, the ensuing volume depletion may cause a secondary rise in the P_{cr} (Fig. 3–13). This problem can be reversed with fluid repletion.

DIAGNOSIS

The basic aspects of the diagnosis of ATN have been discussed above (see Table 3–3). Even when the diagnosis seems evident, it is still important to exclude other causes of renal failure that might be present. For example, acute renal failure following an arteriogram does not always represent a toxic reaction to radiocontrast media. In patients with erosive atherosclerosis, insertion of the arteriogram catheter into the aorta can result in atheroemboli to the kidney (and to other organs as well, possibly resulting in pancreatitis or gangrene of the toes) (see Chap 7). The distinction between these two causes of

renal failure is important because a reaction to contrast media is generally reversible, whereas atheroembolic changes tend to persist and cause chronic renal failure.

TREATMENT

The therapy of ATN includes attempts at prevention as well as treatment of established disease during the renal failure and diuretic phases.

PREVENTION

There are certain principles that may be generally effective in reducing the frequency of ATN.

1. Hypovolemia should be prevented or, if present, rapidly corrected. This includes avoiding the use of nonsteroidal anti-inflammatory drugs in volume-depleted states, since the inhibition of prostaglandin synthesis can intensify the renal ischemia and increase the risk of renal failure.[318] In addition to its direct effect, hypovolemia also enhances the toxicity of aminoglycosides.[168,201] and heme pigments.[262]

2. Fluid loading may prevent the development of ATN in certain settings. Saline has been effective with cisplatin,[241] and mannitol may reduce the risk of radiocontrast studies in high-risk patients (such as diabetics with a $P_{cr} > 1.5$ mg/dL).[235] In the latter group, it is also frequently possible to avoid the administration of radiocontrast media by using ultrasonography or unenhanced CT scanning.

3. The incidence of aminoglycoside-induced ATN can probably be diminished by carefully following plasma drug levels and by discontinuing the drug once the P_{cr} begins to rise without another apparent cause.

Attempts may also be made to prevent or minimize cell necrosis and subsequent tubular obstruction. In experimental animals with renal ischemia, the administration of magnesium ATP leads to more rapid recovery of ATP stores during reflow.[319] This results in the preservation of sublethally injured tubular cells and a lesser degree of renal failure.[320,321] Although these studies are not directly applicable to humans, they do indicate the possible efficacy of trying to prevent cell necrosis.

In an effort to achieve this goal, mannitol and loop diuretics (particularly furosemide) have been widely used during episodes of renal ischemia.* Both drugs appear to preserve cellular integrity in experimental animals,[176,177] mannitol by diminishing cell swelling[180] and furosemide by decreasing active transport and therefore energy requirements in the cells in the medullary thick ascending limb of the loop of Henle (see Fig. 3–12).[18,175]

These drugs also may have other beneficial effects. Both produce a diuresis which could minimize the degree of tubular obstruction by washing out cellular debris and casts.[322,323] Mannitol also is a renal vasodilator, thereby increasing glomerular capillary hydrostatic pressure.[324,325] This effect can maintain the GFR even in the presence of marked hypotension.[325,326]

Despite this extensive experimental literature, the proof that these agents are effective in humans is not yet conclusive. In such high-risk settings as open-heart surgery, surgery for an abdominal aortic aneurysm, prolonged renal ischemia, or rhabdomyolysis, mannitol has been reported to be effective in preserving renal function in at least some

*Mannitol and loop diuretics generally have little use in nephrotoxic ATN (except for mannitol following radiocontrast media). With aminoglycosides, for example, the duration of the toxic insult is much more prolonged because of drug accumulation in the proximal tubular cells.[205]

patients.[11,186,188,327–329] However, these studies were not controlled, and their results have not been confirmed by others.[189,330,331] Not surprisingly, mannitol is not effective in reversing established ATN (more than 48 h after onset) in which the tubular damage has already occurred.[332,333]

Unfortunately, most of the studies utilizing loop diuretics have been done in established oliguric ATN, not early in the ischemic phase when they would be most likely to be effective.[11] Although some oliguric patients can be made nonoliguric in this setting, no definite improvement in renal function could be demonstrated.[311,333–336] These results suggest that loop diuretics can increase the output in those nephrons that are still functioning but that there is little recruitment of previously nonfunctioning nephrons.

Two recent studies shed some light on therapy early in the ischemic phase. In one, oliguric patients who did not respond to mannitol or furosemide were treated with intravenous furosemide (30 to 50 mg/h) plus dopamine (3 μg/kg per min).[337] Nineteen of twenty-four patients responded to this regimen with a substantial increase in urine output. The responders had a shorter duration of oliguria (17 versus 33 h), a lower U_{Na} (perhaps indicating less severe tubular damage), and more rapid recovery of renal function (10 versus 41 days). All 5 nonresponders but only 5 of 19 responders required dialysis. These data, although limited and uncontrolled, suggest that early treatment (within 24 h) might provide at least partial protection against ischemic damage. It is not known if dopamine has an independent beneficial effect or merely acts by increasing furosemide delivery to the kidney via renal vasodilatation.[337]

In the second study, all patients undergoing open-heart surgery were treated prophylactically with mannitol, furosemide, and dopamine during and after the operation.[24]

Sixteen patients with ATN were identified, all of whom were nonoliguric rather than oliguric, as had been the previous experience. These findings indicate that treatment seems to be effective in converting oliguric into nonoliguric ATN. They do not, however, provide any information as to whether the *incidence* of ATN was reduced. Furthermore, the benefit of this conversion is unclear. Although spontaneous non-oliguric ATN is associated with a low requirement for dialysis (under 30 percent),[5,167] this modality was necessary in 14 of 16 patients (88 percent) in this study. These findings suggest that prophylactic therapy increased the urine output in functioning nephrons but offered no protection against net nephron loss.

In summary, the efficacy of mannitol or loop diuretics in preventing or ameliorating ischemic ATN has not been proven. Nevertheless, these drugs have little toxicity, and it seems reasonable to use mannitol (12.5 to 25 g intravenously over 10 to 30 min)[338] and a loop diuretic such as furosemide (working up to a maximum dose of 5 mg/kg) to maintain an adequate urine output in oliguric patients at high risk of developing postischemic ATN (postsurgery, rhabdomyolysis, sepsis). Therapy is most likely to be effective if begun within the first 24 h.[11,337] If the urine output does increase, urinary losses must be replaced to prevent further volume depletion and worsening renal ischemia. If, however, there is no response, dopamine (3 to 5 μg/kg per min) can be tried with a loop diuretic.[337]

If this regimen fails to produce a diuresis, multiple doses should not be given. The retention of hypertonic mannitol in the extracellular space can lead to hyperosmolality, hyponatremia (due to osmotic water movement out of the cells), extracellular volume expansion, and possibly pulmonary edema.[339] For these reasons, the use of mannitol should be avoided in patients with heart failure, as only a loop diuretic and dopamine should be tried. Repeated doses of a loop diuretic also may be toxic, producing deafness which may be permanent.[*,311,340]

RENAL FAILURE PHASE

The treatment of renal failure due to ATN is similar to that due to other diseases. The basic goals are the maintenance of fluid and electrolyte balance, adequate nutrition, and if present, the treatment of infection and uremia. Hyperkalemia and fluid overload are more likely to occur in oliguric patients. These problems can be minimized by restricting potassium intake and matching sodium and water intake to urinary and insensible losses. When estimating insensible losses, it is important to take into account endogenous water formation due to the metabolism of proteins, carbohydrates, and fats (to carbon dioxide and water) and to intracellular water released from cell catabolism.[344] Although insensible losses may be 1000 mL/day, endogenous water formation averages 450 mL/day. Thus, only 550 mL of water has to be replaced in the absence of fever or hyperventilation.

Early diagnosis and treatment of infection is also essential. In patients with renal failure, the usual findings of fever and leukocytosis may be minimal or absent,[345,346] with the only signs of infection being dyspnea or un-

---

*There is some preliminary evidence that, when given intravenously in high doses, bumetanide may be less ototoxic than either furosemide or ethacrynic acid.[341,342] This difference may be related to the relative potency of these drugs in inhibiting different transport systems. Within the kidney, for example, bumetanide is about 40 times more effective than a similar dose of furosemide in inhibiting the Na-K-2Cl carrier protein in the luminal membrane of the thick ascending limb of the loop of Henle.[342,343] In comparison, bumetanide may be *less potent* in impairing the activity of other transport proteins,[343] which may be important in the production of endolymph. As a result, when equally effective diuretic doses are used (furosemide 40 times that of bumetanide), inhibition of these other proteins and therefore ototoxicity may be substantially less with bumetanide.[341,342] This hypothesis, however, remains unproven.

explained tachycardia or hypotension. Consequently, a careful physical examination and, when indicated, chest x-ray and cultures may provide the first clues to the presence of infection. To minimize the frequency of infection in the urinary tract, indwelling bladder catheters should be used only when necessary. For example, the urine output in oliguric patients can be safely measured by intermittent (every 12 to 24 h) bladder catheterization. Continuous catheterization adds little additional information and carries a higher risk of infection.

Once an infecting organism is identified, antimicrobial dosage must be adjusted for those drugs that are excreted in the urine (see Chap. 13). For example, gentamicin (in a dose of 1 mg/kg) can be given every 36 to 72 h in patients with severe renal failure, depending on the plasma level. The dosage must also be changed when dialysis is begun, since gentamicin is dialyzable. In patients on hemodialysis, the above dose should be given after each dialysis. The regimen is different with peritoneal dialysis. After the initial loading dose, 10 mg of gentamicin can be added to every 2 L of dialysis fluid. This will maintain the plasma gentamicin concentration at a therapeutic level of approximately 5 μg/mL.

DIALYSIS

Many patients, particularly those with oliguric ATN, will eventually require dialysis. Definite indications for dialysis are an inability to control hyperkalemia with cation-exchange resins (particularly in hypercatabolic states in which severe hyperkalemia may develop rapidly), fluid overload, and the signs of uremia such as pericarditis, colitis, or confusion. Dialysis should also be performed in a patient with significant bleeding who has a prolonged bleeding time. The latter indicates uremia-induced platelet dysfunction,[347] an effect that becomes promi-

nent when the BUN exceeds 80 mg/dL.[348] Cryoprecipitate, transfusions to raise the hematocrit above 30 percent, estrogens, and dDAVP (the synthetic analog of antidiuretic hormone) have also been used to normalize platelet function in this setting.[349-351]

It has also been suggested that *prophylactic* dialysis to keep the BUN under 80 to 100 mg/dL (independent of fluid overload or uremic symptoms) may improve survival.[352-354] The rationale for early dialysis is that maintaining the BUN under this level will prevent the impairment in phagocytic and platelet function that can lead to infection, bleeding, and death. However, the above studies were largely uncontrolled, comparing patients from different time periods. A recent controlled study demonstrated no benefit from prophylactic dialysis.[355]

When dialysis is required, either peritoneal dialysis or hemodialysis can be used. In general, hemodialysis is preferred in hypercatabolic patients, since the increased solute clearance with this method removes more of the urea and potassium being released from damaged cells. On the other hand, peritoneal dialysis is preferred in the presence of hypotension,[356] since it avoids the potential problems of hemodynamic instability induced by hemodialysis. Recent abdominal surgery is *not* a contraindication to peritoneal dialysis, as this procedure has been safely used as soon as 4 days after the operation.[357]

HYPERALIMENTATION

Maintaining adequate nutrition is an important component of therapy since many patients with ATN are in a catabolic state. Furthermore, 10 to 20 g of amino acids may be lost per day in patients being dialyzed. In addition to this general rationale, a high-calorie, low-protein, high essential amino acid regimen has been advocated in an attempt to minimize protein breakdown and therefore the rate of rise in the BUN. Initial studies indicated that this regimen effectively slowed the increase in BUN and also reduced the frequency of dialysis, duration of renal failure, and mortality rate.[358,359] A proposed mechanism for this beneficial effect is that the increased energy supply enhances the rate of new membrane formation, thereby allowing tubular regeneration to occur more quickly.[360]

However, these early positive results have not been confirmed in other studies in animals or humans.[361,362] These contrasting data could be related to possible deleterious effects of the administration of amino acids. If more amino acids are given than can be utilized for anabolism, they will be converted to urea in the liver, further raising the BUN.[363] Amino acids also may potentiate the severity of ischemic tubular injury.[364] This effect could be related to the energy utilized for amino acid reabsorption and metabolism in the proximal tubular cells.[365] Thus, energy requirements are increased at a time when energy delivery is inadequate. In summary, the effectiveness of specific renal failure diets in hastening the recovery of renal function must be considered unproven. Hyperalimentation may, however, be of general benefit, increasing survival in severely ill patients with multisystem abnormalities.[359]

DIURETIC PHASE

As described earlier, the increased sodium and water excretion during the diuretic phase may be nonphysiologic. Thus, fluid balance must be carefully monitored and urinary losses replaced if the signs of volume depletion appear.

PROGNOSIS

Despite the availability of dialysis, the mortality rate of all patients with ATN has remained between 40 and 60 percent, with infection and the underlying disease (such as hypotension following open-heart surgery) being the major causes of death.[2,10,187,359,366] However, this statistic is somewhat misleading since the *mortality rate is largely dependent on the general health of the patient and the cause of the renal failure.* For example, when ATN follows surgery or trauma, the overall mortality is 40 to 80 percent.[2,27,187,244,367] In comparison, survival is much improved in those patients who do not develop other medical complications such as infection, bleeding, or respiratory failure.[359] The prognosis also is better with nonoliguric ATN (in part because the renal damage appears to be less severe)[5,6] and, since the patients tend to be otherwise healthy, with ATN due to a transfusion reaction, an obstetrical complication, or antibiotics (without continuing infection).[2,368] In these last settings, the mortality rate is under 10 percent. The importance of extrarenal disturbances in determining patient survival is not surprising, since dialysis should be able to correct most of the abnormalities directly associated with renal failure.

In those patients who survive, the GFR typically returns to or near the previous baseline level.[312,314-316] Recovery typically begins within 21 days but occasionally may be prolonged for 3 to 6 months.[184,209,213] Irreversible renal insufficiency is unusual but may occur, particularly following aortic aneurysm surgery.[187,369] In this setting, it is possible that atheroemboli released during aortic manipulation are responsible for the persistent renal dysfunction.[187]

When recovery is delayed, performing a radionuclide renogram (using a radioactively labeled compound such as iodohippurate) may be a useful guide to prognosis.[313] If both kidneys visualize normally, eventual return of renal function is highly likely. Recovery may also occur if there is faint or no visualization, but it is this group that is at risk for the development of chronic renal failure. Since hippurate is delivered to the kidneys by renal blood flow and then enters the tubules by tubular secretion, lack of visualization implies poor blood flow or poor tubular function, either of which could lead to persistent renal disease.

CLINICAL EXAMPLE

The problems in diagnosis and management that may occur in acute renal failure can be illustrated by the following case history.

Case History 3-1. A 74-year-old man complained of the acute onset of abdominal pain and weakness. On physical examination, the patient was pale and appeared acutely ill. The pertinent findings were: blood pressure 60/40 (recumbent); pulse 130 per minute and regular; cool extremities; moist skin; a large, tender, pulsatile mass in the abdomen; and intact peripheral pulses. The laboratory data revealed a hematocrit of 28 percent, BUN 15 mg/dL, P_{cr} 1.0 mg/dL, and a normal urinalysis.

The clinical impression was that the patient had a ruptured abdominal aortic aneurysm. This diagnosis was confirmed at surgery, and a Dacron graft was inserted. Postoperatively, the patient was hypotensive and oliguric for several hours. With fluid administration, his blood pressure rose only to 100/60, and urine output increased over several days to 60 mL/h (1500 mL/day).

Despite the maintenance of a good urine output, progressive elevations in the BUN (from 40 to 88 to 132 mg/dL) and P_{cr} (from 2.3 to 3.6 to 5.0 mg/dL) were noted over the next 3 days. The plasma potassium concentration, which had been normal, increased to 6.9 meq/L. Examination of the urine prior to and the day after surgery revealed a normal urine sediment and a U_{Na} of 6 meq/L. However, in the second and third postoperative days, the U_{Na} increased to 19 and then 69 meq/L with the

urine osmolality being 336 mosmol/kg. The urine sediment at this time showed many granular casts and occasional renal tubular cells. In addition to his renal problems, the patient also developed respiratory failure and gram-negative bacteremia.

In an attempt to treat the renal failure and hyperkalemia, hemodialysis was begun. The patient required 6 h of dialysis every day to keep his BUN under 100 mg/dL. During this time, his urine output fell to 250 to 400 mL/day. Gentamicin was administered after each dialysis to treat the septicemia. On the seventh postoperative day, the patient expired from septic shock.

Comment. Several common problems were encountered in this patient. First, the initial decrease in renal function was due to prerenal disease as evidenced by the normal urinalysis and low U_{Na}. However, the prolonged hypotension and persistent renal ischemia eventually led to the development of ATN and its characteristic urinary changes. It is possible that the use of mannitol and furosemide when the patient was first oliguric could have ameliorated the degree of tubular damage and renal failure.

Second, the increase in urine output produced by the administration of fluids in the immediate postoperative period initially suggested that the oliguria had been largely due to reduced renal perfusion. However, the progressive elevations in the BUN and P_{cr} indicated that the GFR had remained very low and that the augmented output was due to a decrease in tubular reabsorption.

Third, the patient was extremely hypercatabolic (presumably due to the effects of surgery and the absorption of blood from the abdomen), resulting in hyperkalemia and daily increments in the BUN of 45 to 50 mg/dL. As a result, the patient had to be dialyzed every day to maintain his BUN under 100 mg/dL. In comparison, patients who are not hypercatabolic usually require dialysis only 2 to 3 times per week.

Fourth, a marked fall in urine output commonly occurs after the institution of dialysis. This is due both to lowering of the BUN (since urea acts as an osmotic diuretic in renal failure) and to the removal of excess fluid (since volume expansion reduces sodium and water reabsorption).[370]

Fifth, since gentamicin is dialyzable, the drug dosage must be adjusted. One method to maintain adequate plasma gentamicin levels in the patient on hemodialysis is to give a normal dose (1 mg/kg) after each dialysis.

Sixth, postoperative ATN is associated with a high mortality rate. In spite of optimum therapy of his renal failure, this patient died from infection, the most common cause of death in patients with ATN.

REFERENCES

1. Hou, S. H., D. A. Bushinsky, J. B. Wish, J. J. Cohen, and J. T. Harrington: Hospital-acquired renal insufficiency: A prospective study, *Am. J. Med.,* 74:243, 1983.

2. Balslov, J. T., and H. E. Jorgensen: A survey of 499 patients with acute anuric renal insufficiency: Causes, treatment, complications and mortality, *Am. J. Med.,* 34:753, 1963.

3. Whelton, A., and K. Solez: Aminoglycoside nephrotoxicity—A tale of two transports, *J. Lab. Clin. Med.,* 99:148, 1982.

4. Miller, T. R., R. J. Anderson, S. L. Linas, W. L. Henrich, A. S. Berns, P. A. Gabow, and R. W. Schrier: Urinary diagnostic indices in acute renal failure: A prospective study, *Ann. Intern. Med.,* 89:47, 1978.

5. Anderson, R. J., S. L. Linas, A. S. Berns, W. L. Henrich, T. R. Miller, P. A. Gabow, and R. W. Schrier: Non-oliguric acute renal failure, *N. Engl. J. Med.,* 296:1134, 1977.

6. Dixon, B. S., and R. J. Anderson: Nonoliguric acute renal failure, *Am. J. Kid. Dis.,* 6:71, 1985.

7. Dossetor, J. B.: Creatininemia versus uremia. The relative significance of blood urea nitrogen and serum creatinine concentrations in azotemia, *Ann. Intern. Med.,* 65:1287, 1966.

8. Kilby, J. E., S. R. Powers, and R. T. Beebe: Acute renal failure: Eighty cases of acute tubular necrosis, *N. Engl. J. Med.,* 262:481, 1960.

9. Oken, D. E.: On the differential diagnosis of acute renal failure, *Am. J. Med.,* 71:916, 1981.

10. Levinsky, N. G., E. A. Alexander, and M. A. Venkatachalam: Acute renal failure, in B. M. Brenner and F. C. Rector, Jr. (eds.), *The Kidney,* 2d ed., Saunders, Philadelphia, 1981.

11. Luke, R. G., J. D. Briggs, M. E. M. Allison, and A. C. Kennedy: Factors determining response to mannitol in acute renal failure, *Am. J. Med. Sci.,* 259:168, 1970.

12. Myers, B. D., B. J. Carrie, R. R. Yee, M. Hilberman, and A. S. Michaels: Pathophysiology of hemodynamically mediated acute renal failure in man, *Kidney Int.,* 18:495, 1980.

13. Galpin, J. E., J. H. Shinaberger, T. M. Stanley, M. J. Blumenkrantz, A. S. Bayer, G. S. Friedman, J. Z. Montgomerie, L. B. Guze, J. W. Coburn, and R. J. Glassock: Acute interstitial nephritis due to methicillin, *Am. J. Med.,* 65:756, 1978.

14. Ditlove, J., P. Weidmann, M. Bernstein, and S. G. Massry: Methicillin nephritis, *Medicine,* 56:483, 1977.

15. Beaufils, M.: Glomerular disease complicating abdominal sepsis, *Kidney Int.,* 19:609, 1981.

16. Rose, B. D.: *Clinical Physiology of Acid-Base and Electrolyte Disorders,* 2d ed., McGraw-Hill, New York, 1984, chap. 8.

17. Espinel, C. H., and A. W. Gregory: Differential diagnosis of acute renal failure, *Clin. Nephrol.,* 13:73, 1980.

18. Brezis, M., S. Rosen, P. Silva, and F. H. Epstein: Renal ischemia. A new perspective, *Kidney Int.,* 26:375, 1984.

19. Hanley, M. J.: Isolated nephron segments in a rabbit model of ischemic acute renal failure, *Am. J. Physiol.,* 239:F17, 1980.

20. Humes, H. D., and J. M. Weinberg: The effect of gentamicin on antidiuretic hormone-stimulated osmotic water flow in the toad urinary bladder, *J. Lab. Clin. Med.,* 101:472, 1983.

21. Sporn, I. N., R. G. Lancestremere, and S. Papper: Differential diagnosis of oliguria in aged patients, *N. Engl. J. Med.,* 267:130, 1962.

22. Dorhout Mees, E. J.: Relation between maximal urine concentration, maximal water reabsorption capacity, and mannitol clearance in patients with renal disease, *Br. Med. J.,* 1:1159, 1959.

23. Miller, P. D., R. A. Krebs, B. J. Neal, and D. O. McIntyre: Polyuric prerenal failure, *Arch. Intern. Med.,* 140:907, 1980.

24. Myers, B. D., M. Hilberman, R. J. Spencer, and R. L. Jamison: Glomerular and tubular function in non-oliguric acute renal failure, *Am. J. Med.,* 72:642, 1982.

25. Steiner, R. W.: Interpreting the fractional excretion of sodium, *Am. J. Med.,* 77:699, 1984.

26. Diamond, J. R., and D. C. Yoburn: Nonoliguric acute renal failure associated with a low fractional excretion of sodium, *Ann. Intern. Med.,* 96:597, 1982.

27. Hilberman, M., B. D. Myers, B. J. Carrie, G. Derby, R. L. Jamison, and E. B. Stinson: Acute renal failure following cardiac surgery, *J. Thorac. Cardiovasc. Surg.,* 77:880, 1979.

28. Planas, M., T. Wachtel, H. Frank, and L. W. Henderson: Characterization of acute renal failure in the burned patient, *Arch. Intern. Med.,* 142:2087, 1982.

29. Corwin, H. L., M. J. Schreiber, and L. S.-T. Fang: Low fractional excretion of sodium. Occurrence with hemoglobinuric- and myoglobinuric-induced acute renal failure, *Arch. Intern. Med.,* 144:981, 1984.

30. Fang, L. S- T., R. A. Sirota, T. H. Ebert, and N. S. Lichtenstein: Low fractional excretion of sodium with contrast media-induced acute renal failure, *Arch. Intern. Med.,* 140:531, 1980.

31. Vaz, A. J.: Low fractional excretion of urine sodium in acute renal failure due to sepsis, *Arch. Intern. Med.,* 143:738, 1983.

32. Hoffman, L. M., and W. N. Suki: Obstructive uropathy mimicking volume depletion, *J. Am. Med. Assoc.,* 236:2096, 1976.

33. van Ypersele de Strihou, C.: Acute oliguric interstitial nephritis, *Kidney Int.,* 16:751, 1979.

34. Danovitch, G. M., J. J. Bourgoignie, and N. S. Bricker: Reversibility of the "salt-losing" tendency of chronic renal failure, *N. Engl. J. Med.,* 296:14, 1977.

35. Rose, B. D.: *Clinical Physiology of Acid-Base and Electrolyte Disorders,* 2d ed., McGraw-Hill, New York, 1984, pp. 384–385.

36. Rose, B. D.: *Clinical Physiology of Acid-Base and Electrolyte Disorders,* 2d ed., McGraw-Hill, New York, 1984, chap. 9.

37. Skorecki, K. L., and B. M. Brenner: Body fluid hoemostasis in man, *Am. J. Med.,* 70:77, 1981.

38. Scher, A.: Control of arterial blood pressure, in T. C. Ruch and H. D. Patton (eds.), *Physiology and Biophysics,* vol. 2, Saunders, Philadelphia, 1974.

39. Rose, B. D.: *Clinical Physiology of Acid-Base and Electrolyte Disorders,* 2d ed., McGraw-Hill, New York, 1984, chap. 3.

40. Epstein, F. H., A. N. Goddyer, F. D. Laurason, and A. S. Relman: Studies of the antidiuresis of quiet standing: The importance of changes in plasma volume and glomerular filtration rate, *J. Clin. Invest.,* 30:62, 1951.

41. Eisenberg, S., and P. Wolf: Plasma volume after posture changes in hypertensive subjects, *Arch. Intern. Med.,* 115:17, 1965.

42. Francis, G. S., S. R. Goldsmith, T. B. Levine, M. T. Olivari, and J. N. Cohn: The neurohumoral axis in congestive heart failure, *Ann. Intern. Med.,* 101:370, 1984.

43. Bichet, D. G., M. J. VanPutten, and R. W. Schrier: Potential role of increased sympathetic activity in impaired sodium and water excretion in cirrhosis, *N. Engl. J. Med.,* 307:1552, 1982.

44. Pérez-Ayuso, R. M., V. Arroyo, J. Campos, A. Rimola, J. Gaya, J. Costa, F. Rivera, and J. Rodés: Evidence that renal prostaglandins are involved in renal water metabolism in cirrhosis, *Kidney Int.,* 26:72, 1984.

45. Rose, B. D.: *Clinical Physiology of Acid-Base and Electrolyte Disorders,* 2d ed., McGraw-Hill, New York, 1984, chap. 15.

46. Rose, B. D.: *Clinical Physiology of Acid-Base and Electrolyte Disorders,* 2d ed., McGraw-Hill, New York, 1984, pp. 399–403.

47. Rose, B. D.: *Clinical Physiology of Acid-Base and Electrolyte Disorders,* 2d ed., McGraw-Hill, New York, 1984, pp. 294–306.

48. Rose, B. D.: *Clinical Physiology of Acid-Base and Electrolyte Disorders,* 2d ed., McGraw-Hill, New York, 1984, pp. 535–538.

49. Virgilio, R. W., C. L. Rice, D. E. Smith, D. R. James, C. K. Zarins, C. F. Hobelmann, and R. M.

Peters: Crystalloid vs. colloid resuscitation: Is one better?, *Surgery,* 85:129, 1979.

50. Moss, G. S., R. J. Lowe, J. Jilek, and H. D. Levine: Colloid or crystalloid in the resuscitation of hemorrhagic shock: A controlled clinical trial, *Surgery,* 89:434, 1981.

51. Monafo, W.: Expensive salt water, *Surgery,* 80:525, 1981.

52. Shine, K. I., M. Kuhn, L. S. Young, and J. H. Tillisch: Aspects of the management of shock, *Ann. Intern. Med.,* 93:723, 1980.

53. Kaback, K. R., A. B. Sanders, and H. W. Meslin: MAST suit update, *J. Am. Med. Assoc.,* 252:2598, 1984.

54. Higgins, T. L., E. D. Sivak, D. M. O'Neil, J. W. Graves, and D. G. Foutch: Reversal of hypotension by continuous naloxone infusion in a ventilator-dependent patient, *Ann. Intern. Med.,* 98:47, 1983.

55. Curtis, M. T., and A. M. Lefer: Protective actions of naloxone in hemorrhagic shock, *Am. J. Physiol.,* 239:H416, 1980.

56. Brenner, B. M., and H. D. Humes: Mechanics of glomerular ultrafiltration, *N. Engl. J. Med.,* 297:148, 1977.

57. Edwards, R. M.: Effects of prostaglandins on vasoconstrictor action in isolated renal arterioles, *Am. J. Physiol.,* 248:F779, 1985.

58. Myers, B. D., W. M. Deen, and B. M. Brenner: Effects of norepinephrine and angiotensin II on the determinants of glomerular ultrafiltration and proximal tubule fluid reabsorption in the rat, *Circ. Res.,* 37:101, 1975.

59. Strandgaard, S.: Treating hypertension, *N. Engl. J. Med.,* 288:372, 1973.

60. Schnermann, J., J. P. Briggs, and P. C. Weber: Tubuloglomerular feedback, prostaglandins, and angiotensin in the autoregulation of glomerular filtration rate, *Kidney Int.,* 25:53, 1984.

61. Ichikawa, I., J. M. Pfeffer, M. A. Pfeffer, T. H. Hostetter, and B. M. Brenner: Role of angiotensin II in the altered renal function of congestive heart failure, *Circ. Res.,* 55:669, 1984.

62. Hricik, D. E., P. J. Browning, R. Kopelman, W. E. Goorno, N. E. Madias, and V. J. Dzau: Captopril-induced functional renal insufficiency in patients with bilateral renal-artery stenoses or renal artery stenosis in a solitary kidney, *N. Engl. J. Med.,* 308:373, 1983.

63. Curtis, J. J., R. G. Luke, J. D. Whelchel, A. G. Diethelm, P. Jones, and H. P. Dustan: Inhibition of angiotensin-converting-enzyme in renal-transplant recipients with hypertension, *N. Engl. J. Med.,* 308:377, 1983.

64. Helmchen, U., H. J. Gröne, E. J. Kirchertz, H. Bader, R. M. Bohle, U. Kneissler, and M. C. Khosla: Contrasting renal effects of different antihypertensive agents in hypertensive rats with bilaterally constricted renal arteries, *Kidney Int.,* 22(suppl. 12):S-198, 1982.

65. Henrich, W. L., Y. Hamasaki, S. I. Said, W. P. Campbell, and R. E. Cronin: Dissociation of systemic and renal effects in endotoxemia, *J. Clin. Invest.,* 69:691, 1982.

66. Oliver, J. A., J. Pinto, R. R. Sciacca, and P. J. Cannon: Increased renal secretion of norepinephrine and prostaglandin E_2 during sodium depletion in the dog, *J. Clin. Invest.,* 66:748, 1980.

67. Henrich, W. L., T. Berl, K. M. McDonald, R. J. Anderson, and R. W. Schrier: Angiotensin II, renal nerves, and prostaglandins in renal hemodynamics, *Am. J. Physiol.,* 235:F46, 1978.

68. Johnston, P. A., N. S. Perrin, D. B. Bernard, and N. G. Levinsky: Control of rat renal vascular resistance at reduced perfusion pressure, *Circ. Res.,* 48:734, 1981.

69. Clive, D. M., and J. S. Stoff: Renal syndromes associated with nonsteroidal antiinflammatory drugs, *N. Engl. J. Med.,* 310:563, 1984.

70. Garella, S., and R. A. Matarese: Renal effects of prostaglandins and clinical adverse effects of nonsteroidal anti-inflammatory agents, *Medicine,* 63:165, 1984.

71. Woods, J. W., and W. Blythe: Management of malignant hypertension complicated by renal insufficiency, *N. Engl. J. Med.,* 277:57, 1967.

72. Mroczek, W. J., M. D. Davidov, L. Gavrilovich, and F. A. Finnerty, Jr.: The value of aggressive therapy in the hypertensive patient with azotemia, *Circulation,* 40:893, 1969.

73. Ledingham, J. G. G., and B. Rajagopalan: Cerebral complications in the treatment of accelerated hypertension, *Q. J. Med.,* 48:25, 1979.

74. Johansson, B., S. Strandgaard, and N. A. Lassen: On the pathogenesis of hypertensive encephalopathy: The hypertensive "breakthrough" of autoregulation of cerebral blood flow with forced vasodilation, flow increase, and blood-brain-barrier damage, *Circ. Res.,* 34(suppl. 1):167, 1974.

75. Watkins, L., Jr., J. A. Burton, E. Haber, J. R. Cant, F. W. Smith, and A. C. Barger: The renin-angiotensin-aldosterone system in congestive failure in conscious dogs, *J. Clin. Invest.,* 57:1606, 1976.

76. Dougherty, A. H., G. V. Maccarelli, E. L. Gray, C. H. Hicks, and R. A. Goldstein: Congestive heart failure with normal systolic function, *Am. J. Cardiol.,* 54:778, 1984.

77. Soufer, R., D. Wohlgelertner, N. A. Vita, M. Amuchestegui, H. D. Sostman, H. J. Berger, and B. L. Zaret: Intact systolic left ventricular function in clinical congestive heart failure, *Am. J. Cardiol.,* 55:1032, 1985.

78. Topol, E. J., T. A. Traill, and N. J. Fortuin: Hypertensive hypertrophic cardiomyopathy of the elderly, *N. Engl. J. Med.,* 312:277, 1985.

79. Cohn, J. N.: Blood pressure and cardiac performance, *Am. J. Med.,* 55:351, 1973.

80. Stampfer, M., S. E. Epstein, G. D. Beiser, and E. Braunwald: Hemodynamic effects of diuresis at rest and during intense exercise in patients with impaired cardiac function, *Circulation,* 37:900, 1968.

81. Millard, R. W., C. B. Higgins, D. Franklin, and S. F. Vatner: Regulation of the renal circulation during severe exercise in normal dogs and dogs with experimental heart failure, *Circ. Res.,* 31:881, 1972.

82. Braunwald, E., and R. A. Kloner: The stunned myocardium: Prolonged postischemic ventricular dysfunction, *Circulation,* 66:1146, 1982.

83. Arnold, S. B., R. C. Byrd, W. Meister, K. Melman, M. D. Cheitlin, D. J. Bristow, W. W. Parmley, and K. Chatterjee: Long-term digitalis therapy improves left ventricular function in heart failure, *N. Engl. J. Med.,* 303:1443, 1980.

84. Lee, D. C-S., R. A. Johnson, J. B. Bingham, M. Leahy, R. E. Dinsmore, A. H. Goroll, J. B. Newell, H. W. Strauss, and E. Haber: Heart failure in outpatients: A randomized trial of digoxin versus placebo, *N. Engl. J. Med.,* 306:699, 1982.

85. Mason, D. T.: Symposium on vasodilator and inotropic therapy, *Am. J. Med.,* 65:101, 1978.

86. Braunwald, E., and W. S. Colucci: Vasodilator therapy of heart failure. Has the promissory note been paid?, *N. Engl. J. Med.,* 310:459, 1984.

87. Creager, M. A., J. L. Halperin, D. B. Bernard, D. P. Faxon, C. D. Melidossian, H. Gavras, and T. J. Ryan: Acute regional circulatory and renal hemodynamic effects of converting-enzyme inhibition in patients with congestive heart failure, *Circulation,* 64:484, 1981.

88. Magorien, R. D., D. W. Triffon, C. E. Desch, W. H. Bay, D. V. Unverferth, and C. V. Leier: Prazosin and hydralazine in congestive heart failure, *Ann. Intern. Med.,* 95:5, 1981.

89. Cohn, J. N., and J. A. Franciosa: Selection of vasodilator, inotropic or combined therapy for the management of heart failure, *Am. J. Med.,* 65:181, 1978.

90. Liang, C-S., L. G. Sherman, J. U. Doherty, K. Wellington, V. W. Lee, and W. B. Hood: Sustained improvement of cardiac function in patients with congestive heart failure after short-term infusion of dobutamine, *Circulation,* 69:113, 1984.

91. Leier, C. V., P. Huss, R. P. Lewis, and D. V. Unverferth: Drug-induced conditioning in congestive heart failure, *Circulation,* 65:1382, 1982.

92. Colucci, W. S., R. F. Wright, and E. Braunwald: New positive inotropic agents in the treatment of congestive heart failure: Mechanisms of action and recent clinical developments, *N. Engl. J. Med.,* 314:290, 349, 1986.

93. Lieberman, F. L., and T. B. Reynolds: Plasma volume in cirrhosis of the liver: Its relation to portal hypertension, ascites, and renal failure, *J. Clin. Invest.,* 46:1297, 1967.

94. Lancestremere, R. G., P. L. Davidson, L. E. Earley, F. J. O'Brien, and S. Papper: Renal failure in Laennec's cirrhosis, II: Simultaneous determination of cardiac output and renal hemodynamics, *J. Clin. Invest.,* 41:531, 1965.

95. Arroyo, V., J. Bosch, J. Gaya-Beltran, D. Kravetz, L. Estrada, F. Rivera, and J. Rodés: Plasma renin activity and urinary sodium extretion as prognostic indicators in nonazotemic cirrhosis with ascites, *Ann. Intern. Med.,* 94:198, 1981.

96. Better, O. S., and R. W. Schrier: Disturbed volume homeostasis in patients with cirrhosis of the liver, *Kidney Int.,* 23:303, 1983.

97. Bichet, D. G., B. M. Groves, and R. W. Schrier: Mechanisms of improvement of water and sodium excretion by immersion in decompensated cirrhotic patients, *Kidney Int.,* 24:788, 1983.

98. Bichet, D. G., B. G. Groves, and R. W. Schrier: Effect of head-out water immersion on hepatorenal syndrome, *Am. J. Kid. Dis.,* 3:258, 1984.

99. Epstein, M.: Peritoneovenous shunt in the management of ascites and the hepatorenal syndrome, *Gastroenterology,* 82:790, 1982.

100. Schroeder, E. T., G. H. Anderson, and H. Smulyan: Effects of a portacaval or peritoneovenous shunt on renin in the hepatorenal syndrome, *Kidney Int.,* 15:54, 1979.

101. Epstein, M., D. P. Berk, N. K. Hollenberg, D. F. Adams, T. C. Chalmers, H. L. Abrams, and J. P. Merrill: Renal failure in patients with cirrhosis, *Am. J. Med.,* 49:175, 1970.

102. Arieff, A. I., and C. A. Chidsey: Renal function in cirrhosis and effects of prostaglandin A, *Am. J. Med.,* 56:695, 1974.

103. Tristani, R. E., and J. N. Cohn: Systemic and renal hemodynamics in oliguric hepatic failure: Effect of volume expansion, *J. Clin. Invest.,* 46:1894, 1967.

104. Kostreva, D. R., A. Castaner, and J. P. Kampine: Reflex effects of hepatic baroreceptors on renal and cardiac sympathetic nerve activity, *Am. J. Physiol.*, 238:R390, 1980.

105. DiBona, G. F.: Renal neural activity in hepatorenal syndrome, *Kidney Int.*, 25:841, 1984.

106. Wong, P. Y., R. C. Talamo, and G. H. Williams: Kallikrein-kinin and renin-angiotensin systems in functional renal failure of cirrhosis of the liver, *Gastroenterology*, 73:1114, 1977.

107. Laffi, G., G. La Villa, M. Pinzani, G. Ciabbatoni, P. Patrignani, M. Mannelli, F. Cominelli, and P. Gentilini: Altered renal and platelet arachidonic acid metabolism in cirrhosis, *Gastroenterology*, 90:274, 1986.

108. Bagdasarian, A., B. Lahiri, R. C. Talamo, P. Wong, and R. W. Colman: Immunochemical studies of plasma kallikrein, *J. Clin. Invest.*, 54:1444, 1974.

109. Baldus, W. P., R. N. Feichter, and W. H. J. Summerskill: The kidneys in cirrhosis, I: Clinical and biochemical features of azotemia in hepatic failure, *Ann. Intern. Med.*, 60:353, 1964.

110. Papadakis, M. A., and A. I. Arieff: Hepatorenal syndrome: An expanded definition (abstract), *Kidney Int.*, 25:173, 1984.

111. Papper, S., J. L. Belsky, and K. H. Bleifer: Renal failure in Laennec's cirrhosis of the liver, I: Description of clinical and laboratory features, *Ann. Intern. Med.*, 51:759, 1959.

112. Metz, R. J., and R. K. Thompkins: The hepatorenal syndrome, *Surg. Gynecol. Obstet.*, 143:297, 1976.

113. Koppel, M. H., J. W. Coburn, M. D. Mimes, H. Goldstein, J. D. Boyle, and M. E. Rubini: Transplantation of cadaveric kidneys from patients with hepatorenal syndrome: Evidence for the functional nature of renal failure in advanced liver disease, *N. Engl. J. Med.*, 280:1367, 1969.

114. Eknoyan, G.: Renal disorders in hepatic failure (letter), *Br. Med. J.*, 2:670, 1974.

115. Better, O. S.: Renal and cardiovascular dysfunction in liver disease. *Kidney Int.*, 29:598, 1986.

116. Wilkinson, S. P., M. H. Davies, B. Portmann, and R. Williams: Renal failure in otherwise uncomplicated acute viral hepatitis, *Br. Med. J.*, 2:338, 1978.

117. Rose, B. D.: *Clinical Physiology of Acid-Base and Electrolyte Disorders*, 2d ed., McGraw-Hill, New York, 1984, pp. 327–329.

118. Guazzi, M., A. Polese, F. Magrini, C. Fiorentini, and M. T. Olivar: Negative influences of ascites on the cardiac function of cirrhotic patients, *Am. J. Med.*, 59:165, 1975.

119. Pockros, P. J., and T. B. Reynolds: Rapid diuresis in patients with ascites from chronic liver disease: the importance of peripheral edema, *Gastroenterology*, 90:1827, 1986.

120. Sherlock, S., B. Sensiviratne, A. Scott, and J. G. Walker: Complications of diuretic therapy in hepatic cirrhosis, *Lancet*, 1:1049, 1966.

121. Goldstein, H., and J. D. Boyle: Spontaneous recovery from hepatorenal syndrome: Report of four cases, *N. Engl. J. Med.*, 272:895, 1965.

122. Iwatsuki, S., M. M. Popovtzer, J. L. Corman, M. Ishikawa, C. W. Putnam, F. H. Katz, and T. E. Starzl: Recovery from "hepatorenal syndrome" after orthotopic liver transplantation, *N. Engl. J. Med.*, 289:1155, 1973.

123. McCloy, R. M., W. P. Baldus, F. T. Maher, and W. H. J. Summerskill: Effects of changing plasma volume, serum albumin concentration and plasma osmolality on renal function in cirrhosis, *Gastroenterology*, 53:229, 1967.

124. Reynolds, T. B., F. L. Lieberman, and A. Redeker: Functional renal failure with cirrhosis: The effect of plasma expansion therapy, *Medicine*, 46:191, 1967.

125. Schroeder, E. T., G. H. Anderson, S. H. Goldman, and D. H. P. Streeten: Effect of blockade of angiotensin II on blood pressure, renin and aldosterone in cirrhosis, *Kidney Int.*, 9:511, 1976.

126. Greig, P. D., L. M. Blendis, B. Langer, B. R. Taylor, and R. F. Colapinto: Renal and hemodynamic effects of the peritoneovenous shunt, II. Long-term effects, *Gastroenterology*, 80:119, 1981.

127. Schroeder, E. T., P. J. Numann, and B. E. Chamberlain: Functional renal failure in cirrhosis: Recovery after portocaval shunt, *Ann. Intern. Med.*, 72:923, 1970.

128. Greig, P. D., B. Langer, L. M. Blendis, B. R. Taylor, and M. F. X. Glynn: Complications after peritoneovenous shunting for ascites, *Am. J. Surg.*, 139:125, 1980.

129. Harmon, D. C., Z. Demerjian, L. Ellman, and J. E. Fischer: Disseminated intravascular coagulation with the peritoneovenous shunt, *Ann. Intern. Med.*, 90:774, 1979.

130. Smadja, C., and D. Franco: The LeVeen shunt in the elective treatment of ascites in cirrhosis. A prospective study of 140 patients, *Ann. Surg.*, 201:488, 1985.

131. Wilkinson, S. P., M. J. Weston, and V. Parsons: Dialysis in the treatment of renal failure in patients with liver disease, *Clin. Nephrol.*, 8:287, 1977.

132. Meltzer, J. I., H. J. Keim, J. H. Laragh, J. E. Sealey, K-M. Jan, and S. Chien: Nephrotic syndrome: Vasoconstriction and hypervolemic types indicated by renin-sodium profiling, *Ann. Intern. Med.,* 91:688, 1979.

133. Ichikawa, I., H. G. Rennke, J. R. Hoyer, K. F. Badr, N. Schor, J. L. Troy, C. P. Lechene, and B. M. Brenner: Role for intrarenal mechanisms in the impaired salt excretion of experimental nephrotic syndrome, *J. Clin. Invest.,* 71:91, 1983.

134. Dorhout Mees, E. J., J. C. Roos, P. Boer, O. H. Yoe, and T. A. Simatupang: Observations on edema formation in the nephrotic syndrome in adults with minimal lesions, *Am. J. Med.,* 67:378, 1979.

135. Brown, E. A., N. Markandu, G. A. Sagnella, B. E. Jones, and G. A. MacGregor: Sodium retention in nephrotic syndrome is due to an intrarenal defect: Evidence from steroid-induced remission, *Nephron,* 39:290, 1985.

136. Garnet, E. S., and C. E. Webber: Changes in blood volume produced by treatment in the nephrotic syndrome, *Lancet,* 2:798, 1967.

137. Nolasco, F., J. S. Cameron, E. F. Heywood, J. Hicks, C. S. Ogg, and D. G. Williams: Adult-onset minimal change nephrotic syndrome: A long-term follow-up, *Kidney Int.,* 29:1215, 1986.

138. Lowenstein, J., R. G. Schacht, and D. S. Baldwin: Renal failure in minimal change nephrotic syndrome. *Am. J. Med.,* 70:227, 1981.

139. Kimberly, R. P., and P. H. Plotz: Aspirin-induced depression of renal function, *N. Engl. J. Med.,* 296:418, 1977.

140. Lijnen, P., J. Boelart, P. Van Eeghem, R. Daneels, M. Schurgers, P. DeJaeger, E. Van der Stichele, J. Vincke, R. Fagard, J. Verschuernen, and A. Amery: Decrease in renal function due to sulphinpyrazone treatment early after myocardial infarction, *Clin. Nephrol.,* 19:143, 1983.

141. Dzau, V. J., M. Packer, L. S. Lilly, S. L. Swartz, N. K. Hollenberg, and G. H. Williams: Prostaglandins in severe congestive heart failure, *N. Engl. J. Med.,* 310:347, 1984.

142. Walsh, J. J., and R. C. Venuto: Acute oliguric renal failure induced by indomethacin: Possible mechanism, *Ann. Intern. Med.,* 91:47, 1979.

143. Zipser, R. D., J. C. Hoefs, P. F. Speckhart, P. K. Zia, and R. Horton: Prostaglandins: Modulators of renal function and pressor resistance in chronic liver disease, *J. Clin. Endocrinol. Metab.,* 48:895, 1979.

144. Arisz, L., A. J. M. Donker, J. R. H. Brentjens, and G. K. van der Hem: The effect of indomethacin on proteinuria and kidney function in the nephrotic syndrome, *Acta Med. Scand.,* 199:121, 1976.

145. Ciabattoni, G., G. A. Cinotti, A. Pierucci, B. M. Simonetti, M. Manzi, F. Pugliese, P. Barsotti, G. Pecci, F. Taggi, and C. Patrono: Effects of sulindac and ibuprofen in patients with chronic glomerular disease, *N. Engl. J. Med.,* 310:279, 1984.

146. Levi, M., M. A. Ellis, and T. Berl: Control of renal hemodynamics and glomerular filtration rate in chronic hypercalcemia. Role of prostaglandins, renin-angiotensin system, and calcium, *J. Clin. Invest.,* 71:1624, 1983.

147. Weinberg, M. S., R. J. Quigg, D. J. Salant, and D. B. Bernard: Anuric renal failure precipitated by indomethacin and triamterene, *Nephron,* 40:216, 1985.

148. Dunn, M. J., and V. L. Hood: Prostaglandins and the kidney, *Am. J. Physiol.,* 233:F169, 1977.

149. Bunning, R. D., and W. F. Barth: Sulindac: A potentially renal-sparing nonsteroidal anti-inflammatory drug, *J. Am. Med. Assoc.,* 248:2864, 1982.

150. Sedor, J. R., S. L. Williams, A. N. Chremos, C. L. Johnson, and M. J. Dunn: Effects of sulindac and indomethacin on renal prostaglandin synthesis, *Clin. Pharmacol. Therap.,* 36:85, 1984.

151. Roberts, D. G., J. G. Gerber, J. S. Barnes, G. O. Zerbe, and A. S. Nies: Sulindac is not renal sparing in man, *Clin. Pharmacol. Therap.,* 38:258, 1985.

152. Henrich, W. L., D. C. Brater, and W. B. Campbell: Renal hemodynamic effects of therapeutic plasma levels of sulindac sulfide during hemorrhage, *Kidney Int.,* 29:484, 1986.

153. Zambraski, E. J., A. N. Chremos, and M. J. Dunn: Comparison of the effects of sulindac with other cyclooxygenase inhibitors on prostaglandin production and renal function in normals and chronic bile duct ligated dogs and swine, *J. Pharmacol. Exp. Therap.,* 228:560, 1984.

154. Laffi, G., G. Daskalopoulos, I. Kronborg, W. Hsueh, P. Gentilini, and R. D. Zipser: Effects of sulindac and ibuprofen in patients with cirrhosis and ascites. An explanation for the renal-sparing effect of sulindac, *Gastroenterology,* 90:182, 1986.

155. Morris, G. C., Jr., M. E. DeBakey, and D. A. Cooley: Surgical treatment of renal failure of renovascular origin, *J. Am. Med. Assoc.,* 182:609, 1962.

156. Besarab, A., R. S. Brown, N. T. Rubin, E. Salzman, L. Wirthlin, T. Steinman, R. R. Atlia, and J. J.

Skillman: Reversible renal failure following bilateral renal artery occlusive disease: Clinical features, pathology, and the role of surgical revascularization, *J. Am. Med. Assoc.,* 235:2838, 1976.

157. Ying, C. Y., C. P. Tifft, H. Gavras, and A. V. Chobanian: Renal revascularization in the azotemic hypertensive patient resistant to therapy, *N. Engl. J. Med.,* 311:1070, 1985.

158. Jackson, B., P. G. Matthews, B. P. McGrath, and C. I. Johnston: Angiotensin converting enzyme inhibition in renovascular hypertension: Frequency of reversible renal failure, *Lancet,* 1:225, 1984.

159. Franklin, S. S., and R. D. Smith: Comparison of effects of enalapril plus hydrochlorothiazide versus standard triple therapy on renal function in renovascular hypertension, *Am. J. Med.,* 79(suppl. 3c):14, 1985.

160. Hollifield, J. W., L. C. Moore, S. D. Winn, M. A. Marshall, C. McCombs, M. G. Frazer, and V. Goncharenko: Angiotensin converting enzyme inhibition in renovascular hypertension, *Cardiovasc. Rev. Rep.,* 3:673, 1982.

161. Hall, J. E., A. C. Guyton, T. E. Jackson, T. G. Coleman, T. E. Lohmeier, and N. C. Trippodo: Control of glomerular filtration rate by renin-angiotensin system, *Am. J. Physiol.,* 233:F366, 1977.

162. Hricik, D. E.: Captopril induced renal insufficiency and the role of sodium balance, *Ann. Intern. Med.,* 103:222, 1985.

163. Wenting, G. J., H. L. Tan-Tjiong, F. H. M. Derkx, J. H. B. deBruyn, and A. J. Man in't Veld: Split renal function after captopril in unilateral renal artery stenosis, *Br. Med. J.,* 288:886, 1984.

164. Textor, S. E., A. Novick, R. C. Tarazi, V. Klimas, D. G. Vidt, and M. Pohl: Critical renal perfusion pressure for renal function in patients with bilateral atherosclerotic renal vascular disease, *Ann. Intern. Med.,* 102:308, 1985. .

165. Hollenberg, N. K., L. G. Meggs, G. H. Williams, J. Katz, J. D. Garnic, and D. P. Harrington: Sodium intake and renal responses to captopril in normal man and in essential hypertension, *Kidney Int.,* 20: 240, 1981.

166. Diamond, J. R., J. Y. Cheung, and L. S.-T. Fang: Nifedipine-induced renal dysfunction. Alterations in renal hemodynamics, *Am. J. Med.,* 77:905, 1984.

167. Rasmussen, H. H., and L. S. Ibels: Acute renal failure. Multivariate analysis of causes and risk factors, *Am. J. Med.,* 73:211, 1982.

168. Zager, R. A., and H. M. Sharma: Gentamicin increases renal susceptibility to an acute ischemic insult, *J. Lab. Clin. Med.,* 101:670, 1983.

169. Garg, L. C., M. A. Knepper, and M. B. Burg: Mineralocorticoid effects on Na-K-ATPase in individual nephron segments, *Am. J. Physiol.,* 240:F536, 1981.

170. Donohue, J. F., M. A. Venkatachalam, D. B. Bernard, and N. G. Levinsky: Tubular leakage and obstruction after renal ischemia: Structural-functional correlations, *Kidney Int.,* 13:208, 1978.

171. Venkatachalam, M. A., D. B. Bernard, J. F. Donohue, and N. G. Levinsky: Ischemic damage and repair in the rat proximal tubule: Differences among the S_1, S_2, and S_3 segments, *Kidney Int.,* 14:31, 1978.

172. Oliver, J., M. MacDowell, and A. Tracy: The pathogenesis of acute renal failure associated with traumatic and toxic injury: Renal ischemia, nephrotoxic damage and the ischemuric episode, *J. Clin. Invest.,* 30:1307, 1951.

173. Shanley, P. F., M. D. Rosen, M. Brezis, P. Silva, F. H. Epstein, and S. Rosen: Topology of focal proximal tubular necrosis after ischemia with reflow in the rat kidney, *Am. J. Pathol.,* 122:462, 1986.

174. Chamberlin, M. E., A. LeFurgey, and L. J. Mandel: Suspension of medullary thick ascending limb tubules from the rabbit kidney, *Am. J. Physiol.,* 247: F955, 1984.

175. Brezis, M., S. Rosen, P. Silva, and F. H. Epstein: Transport activity modifies thick ascending limb damage in the isolated perfused kidney, *Kidney Int.,* 25:65, 1984.

176. Hanley, M. J., and K. Davidson: Prior mannitol and furosemide infusion in a model of ischemic acute renal failure, *Am. J. Physiol.,* 241:F556, 1981.

177. Kramer, H. J., J. Schüürmann, C. Wasserman, and R. Dusing: Prostaglandin-independent protection by furosemide from oliguric ischemic renal failure in conscious rats, *Kidney Int.,* 17:455, 1980.

178. Wilson, D. R., P. E. Arnold, T. J. Burke, and R. W. Schrier: Mitochondrial calcium accumulation and respiration in ischemic acute renal failure in the rat, *Kidney Int.,* 25:519, 1984.

179. Burke, T. J., P. E. Arnold, J. A. Gordon, R. E. Bulger, D. C. Dobyan, and R. W. Schrier: Protective effect of intrarenal calcium membrane blockers before or after renal ischemia, *J. Clin. Invest.,* 74: 1830, 1984.

180. Schrier, R. W., P. E. Arnold, J. A. Gordon, and T. J. Burke: Protection of mitochondrial function by mannitol in ischemic acute renal failure, *Am. J. Physiol.,* 247:F365, 1984.

181. Poller, M. S., J. R. Hoidal, and T. F. Ferris: Oxygen free radicals in ischemic acute renal failure in the rat, *J. Clin. Invest.,* 74:1156, 1984.

182. Matthys, E., Y. Patel, J. Kreisberg, J. H. Stewart, and M. Venkatachalam: Lipid alterations induced by renal ischemia: Pathogenic factor in membrane damage, *Kidney Int.,* 26:153, 1984.

183. McCord, J. M.: Oxygen-derived free radicals in postischemic tissue injury, *N. Engl. J. Med.,* 312: 159, 1985.

184. Myers, B. D., and S. M. Moran: Hemodynamically mediated acute renal failure, *N. Engl. J. Med.,* 314: 97, 1986.

185. Myers, B. D., C. Miller, J. T. Mehigan, C. Olcott IV, H. Golbetz, C. R. Robertson, R. Spencer, and S. Friedman: Nature of the renal injury following total renal ischemia in man, *J. Clin. Invest.,* 73:329, 1984.

186. Barry, K. G., A. Cohen, J. P. Knochel, T. J. Whelan, Jr., W. R. Beisel, C. A. Bargas, and P. C. Leblanc, Jr.: Mannitol infusion, II. The prevention of acute functional renal failure during resection of an aneurysm of the abdominal aorta, *N. Engl. J. Med.,* 264:967, 1961.

187. Gornick, C. C., and C. M. Kjellstrand: Acute renal failure complicating aortic aneurysm surgery, *Nephron,* 35:145, 1983.

188. Barry, K. G., R. I. Mazze, and F. D. Schwartz: Prevention of surgical oliguria and renal hemodynamic suppression by sustained hydration, *N. Engl. J. Med.,* 270:1373, 1964.

189. Yeboah, E. D., A. Petrie, and J. L. Pead: Acute renal failure and open heart surgery, *Br. Med. J.,* 1:415, 1972.

190. Dawson, J. L.: Post-operative renal function in obstructive jaundice: Effect of a mannitol diuresis, *Br. Med. J.,* 1:82, 1965.

191. Evans, H. J. R., V. Torrealba, C. Hudd, and M. Knight: The effect of preoperative bile salt administration on postoperative renal function in patients with obstructive jaundice, *Br. J. Surg.,* 69: 706, 1982.

192. Cahill, C. J.: Prevention of postoperative renal failure in patients with obstructive jaundice—The role of bile salts, *Br. J. Surg.,* 70:590, 1983.

193. Gillenwater, J. Y., E. S. Dooley, and E. D. Frolich: Effects of endotoxins on renal function and hemodynamics, *Am. J. Physiol.,* 205:293, 1963.

194. Ober, W. E., D. E. Reid, S. L. Romney, and J. P. Merrill: Renal lesions and acute renal failure in pregnancy, *Am. J. Med.,* 21:781, 1956.

195. Smith, K., J. C. M. Brown, R. Shackman, and O. M. Wrong: Acute renal failure of obstetric origin: An analysis of 70 patients, *Lancet,* 2:351, 1965.

196. Schrier, R. W.: Acute renal failure, *Kidney Int.,* 15: 205, 1979.

197. Thames, M. D., and F. M. Abboud: Reflex inhibition of renal sympathetic nerve activity during myocardial ischemia mediated by left ventricular receptors with vagal afferents in dogs, *J. Clin. Invest.,* 63:395, 1979.

198. Gorfinkel, H. J., J. P. Szidon, L. J. Hirsch, and A. P. Fishman: Renal performance in experimental cardiogenic shock, *Am. J. Physiol.,* 222:1260, 1972.

199. Tikkanen, I., F. Fyhrquist, K. Metsarinne, and R. Leidenius: Plasma atrial natriuretic peptide in cardiac disease and during infusion in healthy volunteers, *Lancet,* 2:66, 1985.

200. Appel, G. B., and H. C. Neu: Nephrotoxicity of antimicrobial agents, *N. Eng. J. Med.,* 296:663, 772, 784, 1977.

201. Humes, W. D., J. M. Weinberg, and T. C. Knauss: Clinical and pathophysiologic aspects of aminoglycoside nephrotoxicity, *Am. J. Kid. Dis.,* 2:5, 1982.

202. Kaloyanides, G. J., and E. Pastoriza-Munoz: Aminoglycoside nephrotoxicity, *Kidney Int.,* 18: 571, 1980.

203. Meyer, R. D.: Risk factors and comparisons of clinical nephrotoxicity of aminoglycosides, *Am. J. Med.,* 80 (suppl. 6B):119, 1986.

204. Moore, R. D., C. R. Smith, J. J. Lipsky, E. D. Mellits, and P. S. Lietman: Risk factors for nephrotoxicity in patients treated with aminoglycosides, *Ann. Intern. Med.,* 100:352, 1984.

205. Fabre, J., M. Rudhardt, P. Blanchard, and C. Regamey: Persistence of sisomicin and gentamicin in renal cortex and medulla compared with other organs and serum of rats, *Kidney Int.,* 10:444, 1976.

206. Schentag, J. J., and M. E. Plaut: Patterns of urinary β_2-microglobulin excretion by patients treated with aminoglycosides, *Kidney Int.,* 17:654, 1980.

207. De Broe, M. E., G. J. Paulus, G. A. Verpooten, F. Roels, N. Buyssens, R. Wedeen, F. Van Hoof, and P. M. Tulkens: Early effects of gentamicin, tobramycin, and amikacin on the human kidney, *Kidney Int.,* 25:643, 1984.

208. Giuliano, R. A., G. J. Paulus, G. A. Verpooten, V. M. Pattyn, D. E. Pollet, E. J. Nouwen, G. Laurent, M-B. Carlier, P. Maldague, P. M. Turkens, and M. E. De Broe: Recovery of cortical phospholipidosis and necrosis after acute gentamicin loading in rats, *Kidney Int.,* 26:838, 1984.

209. Gary, E. N., L. Buzzeo, J. Salaki, and R. P. Eisinger: Gentamicin-associated acute renal failure, *Arch. Intern. Med.,* 136:1101, 1976.

210. Patel, R., and A. Savage: Symptomatic hypomag-

nesemia associated with gentamicin therapy, *Nephron,* 23:50, 1979.

211. Schor, N., I. Ichikawa, H. G. Rennke, J. L. Troy, and B. M. Brenner: Pathophysiology of altered glomerular function in aminoglycoside-treated rats, *Kidney Int.,* 19:288, 1981.

212. Smith, C. R., J. J. Lipsky, O. L. Laskin, D. B. Hellman, E. D. Mellits, J. Longstreth, and P. S. Lietman: Double-blind comparison of the nephrotoxicity and auditory toxicity of gentamicin and tobramycin, *N. Engl. J. Med.,* 302:1106, 1980.

213. Wade, J. C., C. R. Smith, B. G. Petty, J. J. Lipsky, G. Conrad, J. Ellner, and P. S. Lietman: Cephalothin plus an aminoglycoside is more nephrotoxic than methicillin plus aminoglycoside, *Lancet,* 2: 604, 1978.

214. Cutler, R. E., A. M. Gyselynck, P. Fleet, and A. W. Forrey: Correlation of serum creatinine concentration and gentamicin half-life, *J. Am. Med. Assoc.,* 219:1037, 1972.

215. Plaut, M. E., J. J. Schentag, and W. J. Jusko: Nephrotoxicity with gentamicin or tobramycin, *Lancet,* 2:526, 1979.

216. Plager, J. E.: Association of renal injury with combined cephalothin-gentamicin therapy among patients severely ill with malignant disease, *Cancer,* 37:1037, 1976.

217. Wade, J. C., S. C. Schimpff, and P. H. Wiernik: Antibiotic combination-associated nephrotoxicity in granulocytopenic patients with cancer, *Arch. Intern. Med.,* 141:1789, 1981.

218. DeJongh, C. A., J. C. Wade, S. C. Schimpff, K. A. Newman, R. S. Finley, P. C. Salvatore, M. R. Moody, H. C. Standiford, C. L. Fortner, and P. H. Wiernik: Empiric antibiotic therapy for suspected infection in granulocytopenic cancer patients, *Am. J. Med.,* 73:89, 1982.

219. Fang, L. S-T.: Contrast medium-induced acute renal failure, *Med. Grand Rounds,* 2:263, 1983.

220. Mudge, G. G.: Nephrotoxicity of urographic radiocontrast drugs, *Kidney Int.,* 18:840, 1980.

221. Taliercio, C. P., R. E. Vlietstra, L. D. Fisher, and J. C. Burnett: Risk for renal function with cardiac angiography, *Ann. Intern. Med.,* 104:501, 1986.

222. VanZee, B. E., W. E. Hoy, T. E. Talley, and J. R. Jaenike: Renal injury associated with intravenous pyelography in nondiabetic and diabetic patients, *Ann. Intern. Med.,* 89:51, 1978.

223. D'Elia, J. A., R. E. Gleason, M. Alday, C. Malarick, K. Godley, J. Warram, A. Kaldany, and L. A. Weinrauch: Nephrotoxicity from angiographic

contrast material. A prospective study, *Am. J. Med.,* 72:719, 1982.

224. Shafi, T., S-Y. Chou, J. G. Porush, and W. B. Shapiro: Infusion intravenous pyelography and renal function. Effects in patients with chronic renal insufficiency, *Arch. Intern. Med.,* 138:1218, 1978.

225. Weinrauch, L. A., R. W. Healy, O. S. Leland, H. H. Goldstein, S. D. Kassissiek, J. A. Libertino, F. J. Takacs, and J. A. D'Elia: Coronary angiography and acute renal failure in diabetic nephropathy, *Ann. Intern. Med.,* 86:56, 1977.

226. Cramer, B. C., P. S. Parfrey, T. A. Hutchinson, D. Baran, D. M. Melanson, R. E. Ethier, and J. F. Seely: Renal failure following infusion of radiologic contrast material. A prospective controlled study, *Arch. Intern. Med.,* 145:87, 1985.

227. Holland, M. D., J. H. Galla, P. W. Sanders, and R. G. Luke: Effect of urinary pH and diatrizoate on Bence Jones protein nephrotoxicity in the rat, *Kidney Int.,* 27:46, 1985.

228. Morgan, C., Jr., and W. J. Hammack: Intravenous urography in multiple myeloma, *N. Engl. J. Med.,* 275:77, 1966.

229. Krumlovsky, F. A., N. Simon, S. Santhanam, F. del Greco, D. Roxe, and M. M. Pomaranc: Acute renal failure: Association with administration of radiographic contrast media, *J. Am. Med. Assoc.,* 239:125, 1978.

230. Light, J. A., and G. S. Hill: Acute tubular necrosis in a renal transplant recipient: Complication from drip-infusion excretory urography, *J. Am. Med. Assoc.,* 232:1267, 1975.

231. Larson, T. S., K. Hudson, J. E. Mertz, J. C. Romero, and F. G. Knox: Renal vasoconstrictive response to contrast medium. The role of sodium balance and the renin-angiotensin system, *J. Lab. Clin. Med.,* 101:385, 1983.

232. Dean, R. E., J. H. Andrew, and R. C. Reed: The red cell factor in renal damage from angiographic media, *J. Am. Med. Assoc.,* 187:27, 1964.

233. Berdon, W. E., R. H. Schwartz, J. Becker, and D. H. Baker: Tamm-Horsfall proteinuria: Its relationship to prolonged nephrogram in infants and children and to renal failure following intravenous urography in adults with multiple myeloma, *Radiology,* 92:714, 1969.

234. Postlethwaite, A. E., and W. N. Kelley: Uricosuric effect of radiocontrast agents: A study in man of four commonly used preparations, *Ann. Intern. Med.,* 74:845, 1971.

235. Anto, H. R., S-Y. Chou, J. G. Porush, and W. B. Shapiro: Infusion intravenous pyelography and renal function. Effects of hypertonic mannitol in patients with chronic renal insufficiency, *Arch. Intern. Med.,* 141:1652, 1981.

236. Loehrer, P. L., and L. H. Einhorn: Cisplatin, *Ann. Intern. Med.,* 100:704, 1984.

237. Madias, N. E., and J. T. Harrington: Platinum nephrotoxicity, *Am. J. Med.,* 65:307, 1978.

238. Gonzalez-Vitale, J. C., D. M. Hades, E. Cvitkovic, and S. S. Sternberg; Acute renal failure after *cis*-dichlorodiamineplatinum (2) and gentamicin-cephalothin therapies, *Cancer Tr. Rep.,* 62:693, 1978.

239. Schilsky, R. L., and T. Anderson: Hypomagnesemia and renal magnesium wasting in patients receiving cisplatin, *Ann. Intern. Med.,* 90:929, 1979.

240. Jackson, A. M., B. D. Rose, L. G. Graff, J. B. Jacobs, J. H. Schwartz, G. M. Strauss, J. P. S. Yang, M. R. Rudnick, I. B. Elfenbein, and R. G. Narins: Thrombotic microangiopathy and renal failure associated with antineoplastic chemotherapy, *Ann. Intern. Med.,* 101:41, 1984.

241. Ozols, R. F., B. J. Corden, J. Jacob, M. N. Wesley, Y. Ostchega, and R. C. Young: High-dose cisplatin in hypertonic saline, *Ann. Intern. Med.,* 100:19, 1984.

242. Gabow, P. A., W. D. Kaehny, and S. P. Kelleher: The spectrum of rhabdomyolysis, *Medicine,* 61:141, 1982.

243. Honda, N.: Acute renal failure and rhabdomyolysis, *Kidney Int.,* 23:888, 1983.

244. Lordon, R. E., and J. R. Burton: Post-traumatic renal failure in military personnel in southeast Asia, *Am. J. Med.,* 53:137, 1972.

245. Grossman, R. A., R. W. Hamilton, B. M. Morse, A. S. Penn, and M. Goldberg: Nontraumatic rhabdomyolysis and acute renal failure, *N. Engl. J. Med.,* 291:807, 1974.

246. Koffler, A., R. M. Friedler, and S. G. Massry: Acute renal failure due to non-traumatic rhabdomyolysis, *Ann. Intern. Med.,* 85:23, 1976.

247. Vertel, R. M., and J. P. Knochel: Acute renal failure due to heat injury: An analysis of ten cases associated with a high incidence of myoglobinuria, *Am. J. Med.,* 43:435, 1967.

248. Knochel, J. P., L. N. Dotin, and R. J. Hamburger: Heat stress, exercise, and muscle injury: Effects on urate metabolism and renal function, *Ann. Intern. Med.,* 81:321, 1974.

249. Hamilton, R. W., B. Gardner, A. S. Penn, and M. Goldberg: Acute tubular necrosis caused by exercise-induced myoglobinuria, *Ann. Intern. Med.,* 77: 77, 1972.

250. Koppes, G. M., J. J. Daly, C. A. Coltman, and D. E. Butkus: Exertion-induced rhabdomyolysis with acute renal failure and disseminated intravascular coagulation in sickle cell trait, *Am. J. Med.,* 63:314, 1977.

251. Knochel, J. P., and E. M. Schlein: On the mechanism of rhabdomyolysis in potassium depletion, *J. Clin. Invest.,* 51:1750, 1972.

252. Knochel, J. P.: Neuromuscular manifestations of electrolyte disorders, *Am. J. Med.,* 72:521, 1982.

253. Knochel, J. P., L. N. Dotin, and R. J. Hamburger: Pathophysiology of intense physical conditioning in a hot climate. I. Mechanisms of potassium depletion, *J. Clin. Invest.,* 51:242, 1972.

254. Akmal, M., J. E. Bishop, N. Telfer, A. W. Norman, and S. G. Massry: Hypocalcemia and hypercalcemia in patients with rhabdomyoloysis with and without acute renal failure, *J. Clin. Endocrinol. Metab.,* 63:137, 1986.

255. Llach, F., A. J. Felsenfeld, and M. R. Haussler: The pathophysiology of altered calcium metabolism in rhabdomyolysis-induced acute renal failure, *N. Engl. J. Med.,* 305:117, 1981.

256. McCarron, D. A., W. C. Elliott, J. S. Rose, and W. M. Bennett: Severe mixed metabolic acidosis secondary to rhabdomyolysis, *Am. J. Med.,* 67:905, 1979.

257. Strauss, M.: Acute renal insufficiency due to lower-nephron nephrosis, *N. Engl. J. Med.,* 239:693, 1948.

258. Bull, G. M., and A. M. Joekes: Acute renal failure following intravascular hemolysis, *Lancet,* 1:114, 1957.

259. Pechel, E., H. D. McIntosh, T. W. Brown, Jr., and H. V. Murdaugh: Acute tubular necrosis after transfusion reaction due to antibodies: Report of a case and discussion of management, *J. Am. Med. Assoc.,* 167:1736, 1958.

260. Whelton, A., J. V. Donadio, Jr., and B. L. Elisberg: Acute renal failure complicating rickettsial infections in glucose-6-phosphate dehydrogenase deficient individuals, *Ann. Intern. Med.,* 69:323, 1968.

261. Tungsanga, K., D. Boonwichit, A. Lekhakula, and V. Sitprija: Urine uric acid and urine creatinine ratio in acute renal failure, *Arch. Intern. Med.,* 144: 934, 1984.

262. Jaenike, J. R.: The renal lesion associated with hemoglobinemia. I. Its production and functional evolution in the rat, *J. Exp. Med.* 123:523, 1966.

263. Jaenike, J. R.: The renal lesion associated with hemoglobinemia: A study of the pathogenesis of the excretory defect in the rat, *J. Clin. Invest.,* 46:378, 1967.

264. Blackburn, C. R. B., W. J. Hensley, D. K. Grant, and F. B. Wright: Studies on intravascular hemolysis in man: The pathogenesis of the initial stages of acute renal failure, *J. Clin. Invest.,* 33:825, 1954.

265. Blachar, Y., J. S. C. Fong, J-P. de Chadarévian, and K. N. Drummond: Muscle extract infusion in rabbits. A new experimental model of the crush syndrome, *Circ. Res.,* 49:114, 1981.

266. Miller, J. H., and R. K. McDonald: The effect of hemoglobin on renal function in the human, *J. Clin. Invest.,* 30:1033, 1951.

267. Schrier, R. W., H. S. Henderson, C. C. Tisher, and R. L. Tannen: Nephropathy associated with heat stress and exercise, *Ann. Intern. Med.,* 67:356, 1967.

268. Venkatachalam, M. A., H. G. Rennke, and D. J. Sandstrom: The vascular basis for acute renal failure in the rat: Preglomerular and postglomerular vasoconstriction, *Circ. Res.,* 38:267, 1976.

269. Tune, B. M., and D. Fravert: Mechanisms of cephalosporin nephrotoxicity: A comparison of cephaloridine and cephaloglycin, *Kidney Int.,* 18:591, 1980.

270. Kleinknecht, D., J. C. Homberg, and G. DeCroix: Acute renal failure after rifampicin, *Lancet,* 1:1238, 1972.

271. Cochran, M., P. J. Moorhead, and M. Platts: Permanent renal damage with rifampicin, *Lancet,* 1: 1428, 1975.

272. Porter, G. A., and W. M. Bennett: Nephrotoxic acute renal failure due to common drugs, *Am. J. Physiol.,* 241:F1, 1981.

273. Wolinsky, E., and J. D. Hines: Neurotoxic and nephrotoxic effects of colistin in patients with renal disease, *N. Engl. J. Med.,* 266:759, 1962.

274. Humes H. D., and J. M. Weinberg: Toxic nephropathies, in B. M. Brenner and F. C. Rector, Jr. (eds), *The Kidney,* 3d ed., Saunders, Philadelphia, 1986.

275. Fowler, B. A., and J. B. Weissberg: Arsine poisoning, *N. Engl. J. Med.,* 291:1171, 1974.

276. Curry, R. W., J. D. Robinson, and M. J. Sughrue: Acute renal failure after acetaminophen ingestion, *J. Am. Med. Assoc.,* 247:1012, 1982.

277. Cobden, I., C. O. Record, M. K. Ward, and D. N. S. Kerr: Paracetamol-induced acute renal failure in the absence of fulminant liver damage, *Br. Med. J.,* 284:21, 1982.

278. Mazze, R. I., J. R. Trudell, and M. J. Cousins: Methoxyflurane metabolism and renal dysfunction: Clinical correlations in man, *Anesthesiology,* 35:247, 1971.

279. Sirota, J. H.: Carbon tetrachloride poisoning in man, I. The mechanisms of renal failure and recovery, *J. Clin. Invest.,* 28:1421, 1949.

280. Sinicrope, R. A., J. A. Gordon, J. R. Little, and A. C. Schoolwerth: Carbon tetrachloride nephrotoxicity: A reassessment of pathophysiology based upon the urinary diagnostic indices, *Am. J. Kid. Dis.,* 3:362, 1984.

281. Moel, D. I., and K. Kumar: Reversible nephrotoxic reactions to a combined 2,3-dimercapto-1-propanol and calcium disodium ethylenediaminetetraacetic acid regimen in asymptomatic children with elevated blood lead levels, *Pediatrics,* 70:259, 1982.

282. Phillips, M. E., J. B. Eastwood, J. R. Curtis, P. E. Gower, and H. E. de Wardener: Tetracycline poisoning in renal failure, *Br. Med. J.,* 2:149, 1974.

283. Edwards, O. M., E. C. Huskisson, and R. T. Taylor: Azotemia aggravated by tetracycline, *Br. Med. J.,* 1:26, 1970.

284. Fenves, A. Z.: Legionnaire's disease associated with acute renal failure: A report of 2 cases and review of the literature, *Clin. Nephrol.,* 23:96, 1985.

285. Solez, K., L. Morel-Maroger, and J-D. Straer: The morphology of "acute tubular necrosis" in man: Analysis of 57 renal biopsies and a comparison with the glycerol model, *Medicine,* 58:362, 1979.

286. Dalgaard, O. Z.: An electron microscopic study of glomeruli in renal biopsies taken from human shock kidney, *Lab. Invest.,* 9:364, 1960.

287. Finn, W. F., W. J. Arendshorst, and C. W. Gottschalk: Pathogenesis of oliguria in acute renal failure, *Circ. Res.,* 36:675, 1975.

288. Flanigan, W. J., and D. E. Oken: Renal micropuncture study of the development of anuria in the rat with mercury-induced acute renal failure, *J. Clin. Invest.,* 44:449, 1965.

289. Finn, W. F.: Nephron heterogeneity in polyuric acute renal failure, *J. Lab. Clin. Med.,* 98:21, 1981.

290. Yamamoto, K., D. R. Wilson, and R. Baumal: Outer medullary circulatory defect in ischemic acute renal failure, *Am. J. Pathol.,* 116:253, 1984.

291. Finckh, E., S. D. Jeremy, and H. M. Whyte: Structural renal damage and its relation to clinical features in acute oliguric renal failure, *Q. J. Med.,* 31:429, 1962.

292. Johnston, P. A., H. G. Rennke, and N. G. Levinsky:

Recovery of proximal tubular function from ischemic injury, *Am. J. Physiol.,* 246:F159, 1984.

293. Bank, N., B. F. Mutz, and H. S. Aynedjian: The role of "leakage" of tubular fluid in anuria due to mercury poisoning, *J. Clin. Invest.,* 46:695, 1967.

294. Hollenberg, N. K., M. Epstein, S. M. Rosen, R. T. Basch, D. E. Oken, and J. P. Merrill: Acute oliguric renal failure in man: Evidence for preferential renal cortical ischemia, *Medicine,* 47:455, 1968.

295. Hollenberg, N. K., D. F. Adams, D. E. Oken, H. L. Abrams, and J. P. Merrill: Acute renal failure due to nephrotoxins: Renal hemodynamic and angiographic studies in man, *N. Engl. J. Med.,* 282:1329, 1970.

296. Tanner, G. A.: Effects of kidney tubule obstruction on glomerular function in rats, *Am. J. Physiol.,* 239: F379, 1979.

297. Cox, J. W., R. W. Baehler, H. Sharma, T. O'Dorisio, R. W. Osgood, J. H. Stein, and T. F. Ferris: Studies on the mechanism of oliguria in a model of unilateral acute renal failure, *J. Clin. Invest.,* 53:1547, 1974.

298. Stein, J. H.: The glomerulus in acute renal failure, *J. Lab. Clin. Med.,* 90:227, 1977.

299. Savin, V. J., R. V. Patak, G. Marr, A. S. Hermreck, S. M. Ridge, and K. Lake: Glomerular ultrafiltration coefficient after ischemic renal injury in dogs, *Circ. Res.,* 53:439, 1983.

300. Bulger, R. E., G. Eknoyan, D. J. Purcell, II, and D. C. Dobyan: Endothelial characteristics of glomerular capillaries in normal, mercuric chloride-induced, and gentamicin-induced acute renal failure in the rat, *J. Clin. Invest.,* 72:128, 1983.

301. Blantz, R. C., K. S. Konnen, and B. J. Tucker: Angiotensin II: Effects upon the glomerular microcirculation and ultrafiltration coefficient of the rat, *J. Clin. Invest.,* 57:419, 1976.

302. Thurau, K., and J. W. Boylan: Acute renal success: The unexpected logic of oliguria in acute renal failure, *Am. J. Med.,* 61:308, 1976.

303. Wright, F. S., and J. P. Briggs: Feedback regulation of glomerular filtration rate, *Am. J. Physiol.,* 233:F1, 1977.

304. Ichikawa, I.: Direct analysis of the effector mechanism of the tubuloglomerular feedback system, *Am. J. Physiol.,* 243:F447, 1982.

305. Wunderlich, P. F., F. P. Brunner, J. M. Davis, D. A. Häberle, H. Thölen, and G. Thiel: Feedback activation in rat nephrons by sera from patients with acute renal failure, *Kidney Int.,* 17:497, 1980.

306. Finn, W. F., and R. L. Chevalier: Recovery from postischemic acute renal failure in the rat, *Kidney Int.,* 16:113, 1979.

307. Montgomerie, J. Z., G. M. Kalmanson, and L. B. Guze: Renal failure and infection, *Medicine,* 47:1, 1968.

308. Goldstein, E., and G. M. Green: The effect of acute renal failure on the bacterial clearance mechanisms of the lung, *J. Lab. Clin. Med.,* 68:531, 1966.

309. Goldblum, S. E., and W. P. Reed: Host defenses and immunologic alterations associated with chronic hemodialysis, *Ann. Intern. Med.,* 93:597, 1980.

310. Newbery, W. M., and J. P. Sanford: Defective cellular immunity in renal failure: Depression of reactivity of lymphocytes to phytohemagglutinin by renal failure, *J. Clin. Invest.,* 50:1262, 1971.

311. Brown, C. B., C. S. Ogg, and J. S. Cameron: High dose frusemide in acute renal failure: A controlled trial, *Clin. Nephrol.,* 15:90, 1981.

312. Franklin, S. S., and J. P. Merrill: Acute renal failure, *N. Engl. J. Med.,* 262:711, 1960.

313. Harwood, T. H., D. R. Hierstermann, R. G. Robinson, D. E. Cross, F. C. Whittier, D. A. Dierderich, and J. J. Grantham: Prognosis for recovery of function in acute renal failure: value of renal image obtained using iodohippurate sodium I[131], *Arch. Intern. Med.,* 136:916, 1976.

314. Briggs, J. G., A. C. Kennedy, L. N. Young, R. G. Lukes, and M. Gray: Renal function after acute tubular necrosis, *Br. Med. J.,* 3:513, 1970.

315. Hall, J. W., W. J. Johnson, F. T. Maher, and J. C. Hunt: Immediate and long-term prognosis in acute renal failure, *Ann. Intern. Med.,* 73:515, 1970.

316. Lewers, D. T., T. H. Mathew, J. F. Maher, and G. E. Schreiner: Long-term follow-up of renal function and histology after acute tubular necrosis, *Ann. Intern. Med.,* 73:523, 1970.

317. Moran, S. M., and B. D. Myers: Course of acute renal failure studied by a model of creatinine kinetics, *Kidney Int.,* 27:928, 1985.

318. Torres, V. E., C. G. Strong, J. C. Romero, and D. M. Wilson: Indomethacin enhancement of glycerol-induced acute renal failure in rabbits, *Kidney Int.,* 7:170, 1975.

319. Siegel, N. J., M. J. Avison, H. F. Reilly, J. R. Alger, and R. G. Shulman: Enhanced recovery of renal ATP with post-ischemic infusion of ATP-MgCl$_2$ determined by ^{31}P-NMR, *Am. J. Physiol.,* 245:F530, 1983.

320. Gaudio, K. M., T. A. Ardito, H. F. Reilly, M. Kash-

garian, and N. J. Siegel: Accelerated cellular recovery after an ischemic renal injury, *Am. J. Pathol.,* 112:338, 1983.

321. Sumpio, B. E., I. H. Chaudry, M. G. Clemens, and A. E. Baue: Accelerated functional recovery of isolated rat kidney with ATP-MgCl$_2$ after warm ischemia, *Am. J. Physiol.,* 247:R1047, 1984.

322. Zageri, R. A.: Glomerular filtration rate and brush border debris excretion after mercuric chloride and ischemic acute renal failure: Mannitol versus furosemide diuresis, *Nephron,* 33:196, 1983.

323. Cronin, R. E., A. deTorrente, P. D. Miller, R. E. Bulger, T. J. Burke, and R. W. Schrier: Pathogenic mechanisms in early norepinephrine-induced acute renal failure: Functional and histological correlates of protection, *Kidney Int.,* 14:115, 1978.

324. Burke, T. J., R. E. Cronin, K. L. Duchin, L. N. Peterson, and R. W. Schrier: Ischemia and tubule obstruction during acute renal failure in dogs: Mannitol in protection, *Am. J. Physiol.,* 238:F305, 1980.

325. Johnston, P. A., D. B. Bernard, J. F. Donohue, N. S. Perrin, and N. G. Levinsky: Effect of volume expansion on hemodynamics of the hypoperfused rat kidney, *J. Clin. Invest.,* 64:550, 1979.

326. Johnston, P. A., D. B. Bernard, N. S. Perrin, and N. G. Levinsky: Prostaglandins mediate the vasodilatory effect of mannitol in the hypoperfused rat kidney, *J. Clin. Invest.,* 68:126, 1981.

327. Powers, S. R., Jr.: Prevention of postoperative acute renal failure with mannitol in 100 cases, *Surgery,* 55:15, 1964.

328. Barry, K. G., and J. P. Malloy: Oliguric renal failure: Evaluation and therapy by the intravenous infusion of mannitol, *J. Am. Med. Assoc.,* 179:510, 1962.

329. Eneas, J. F., P. Y. Schoenfeld, and M. H. Humphreys: The effect of infusion of mannitol-sodium bicarbonate on the clinical course of myoglobinuria, *Arch. Intern. Med.,* 139:801, 1979.

330. Beals, A. C., M. R. Holman, G. C. Morris Jr., and M. E. DeBakey: Mannitol-induced osmotic diuresis during vascular surgery, *Arch. Surg.,* 86:34, 1963.

331. Berman, L. B., L. L. Smith, G. D. Chisholm, and R. E. Weston: Mannitol and renal function in cardiovascular surgery, *Arch. Surg.,* 88:239, 1964.

332. Eliahou, H. E.: Mannitol therapy in oliguria of acute onset, *Br. Med. J.,* 1:807, 1964.

333. Auger, R. G., D. A. Dayton, C. E. Harrison, R. M. Tucker, and C. R. Anderson: Use of ethacrynic acid in mannitol resistant oliguric renal failure, *J. Am. Med. Assoc.,* 206:891, 1968.

334. Stott, R. B., C. S. Ogg, J. S. Cameron, and M. Bewick: Why the persistently high mortality in acute renal failure?, *Lancet,* 2:75,1972.

335. Epstein, M., N. S. Schneider, and B. Befeler: Effect of intrarenal furosemide on renal function and intrarenal hemodynamics in acute renal failure, *Am. J. Med.,* 58:510, 1975.

336. Kleinknecht, D., D. Ganeval, L. A. Gonzalez-Duque, and J. Fermanian: Furosemide in acute oliguric renal failure: A controlled trial, *Nephron,* 17:51, 1976.

337. Graziani, G., A. Cantaluppi, S. Casati, A. Citterio, A. Scalamogna, A. Aroldi, R. Silenzio, D. Branacaccio, and C. Ponticelli: Dopamine and frusemide in oliguric acute renal failure, *Nephron,* 37:39, 1984.

338. Warren, S. E., and R. C. Blantz: Mannitol, *Arch. Intern. Med.,* 141:493, 1981.

339. Aviram, A., A. Pfau, J. W. Czaczkes, and T. D. Ullman: Hyperosmolality with hyponatremia caused by inappropriate administration of mannitol, *Am. J. Med.,* 42:648, 1967.

340. Gallagher, K. L., and J. K. Jones: Furosemide-induced ototoxicity, *Ann. Intern. Med.,* 91:744, 1979.

341. Brown, R. D.: Comparative acute cochlear toxicity of intravenous bumetanide and furosemide in the purebred beagle, *J. Clin. Pharmacol.,* 21:620, 1981.

342. Feig, P. U.: Cellular mechanism of action of loop diuretics: Implications for drug effectiveness and adverse effects, *Am. J. Cardiol.,* 57:14A, 1986.

343. Aronson, P. S., and J. Seifter: Cl$^-$ transport via anion exchange, *Fed. Proc.,* 43:2483, 1984.

344. Bluemle, L. W., Jr., H. P. Potter, and J. R. Elkinton: Changes in body composition in acute renal failure, *J. Clin. Invest.,* 35:1094, 1956.

345. Walk, P. J., and M. A. Apicella: The effect of renal function on the febrile response to bacteremia, *Arch. Intern. Med.,* 138:1084, 1978.

346. Peresecenschi, G., M. Blum, A. Aviram, and Z. H. Spirer: Impaired neutrophil response to acute bacterial infection in dialyzed patients, *Arch. Intern. Med.,* 141:1301, 1981.

347. Deykin, D.: Uremic bleeding, *Kidney Int.,* 24:698, 1983.

348. Eknoyan, G., S. J. Wacksman, H. I. Glueck, and J. J. Will: Platelet function in renal failure, *N. Engl. J. Med.,* 280:677, 1969.

349. Janson, P. A., S. J. Jubelier, M. S. Weinstein, and D. Deykin: Treatment of bleeding tendency in uremia with cryoprecipitate, *N. Engl. J. Med.,* 303: 1318, 1980.

350. Livio, M., D. Marchesi, G. Remuzzi, E. Gotti, G.

Mecca, and G. de Gaetano: Uraemic bleeding: Role of anemia and beneficial effect of red cell transfusions, *Lancet,* 2:1013, 1982.

350a. Livio, M., P. M. Mannucci, G. Vigano, G. Mingardi, R. Lombardi, G. Mecca, and G. Remuzzi: Conjugated estrogens for the management of bleeding associated with renal failure, *N. Engl. J. Med.,* 315:731, 1986.

351. Mannucci, P., G. Remuzzi, F. Pusineri, R. Lombardi, C. Valsecchi, G. Mecca, and T. S. Zimmerman: Deamino-8-D-AVP shortens the bleeding time in uremia, *N. Engl. J. Med.,* 308:8, 1983.

352. Teschan, P. E., C. R. Baxter, T. F. O'Brien, J. N. Freyhof, and W. H. Hall: Prophylactic hemodialysis in the treatment of acute renal failure, *Ann. Intern. Med.,* 53:992, 1960.

353. Kleinknecht, C., P. Jungers, J. Chanard, C. Barbanel, and D. Ganeval: Uremic and nonuremic complications in acute renal failure: Evaluation of early and frequent dialysis on prognosis, *Kidney Int.,* 1:190, 1972.

354. Conger, J. D.: A controlled evaluation of prophylactic dialysis in posttraumatic acute renal failure, *J. Trauma,* 15:1056, 1975.

355. Gillum, D. M., and J. D. Conger: Intensive dialysis is of no value in acute renal failure (abstract), *Kidney Int.,* 27:162, 1985.

356. Erbe, R. W., J. A. Green, Jr., and J. M. Weller: Peritoneal dialysis during hemorrhagic shock, *J. Appl. Physiol.,* 22: 131, 1967.

357. Tzamaloukas, A. H., S. Garella, and J. A. Chazan: Peritonal dialysis for acute renal failure after major abdominal surgery, *Arch. Surg.,* 106:639, 1973.

358. Abel, R. M., C. H. Beck, W. M. Abbott, J. A. Ryan, G. O. Barnett, and J. E. Fischer: Improved survival from acute renal failure after treatment with intravenous essential L-amino acids and glucose, *N. Engl. J. Med.,* 288:695, 1973.

359. McMurray, S. D., F. C. Luft, D. R. Maxwell, R. J. Hamburger, D. Futty, J. J. Szwed, K. H. Lavalle, and S. A. Kleit: Prevailing patterns and predictor variables in patients with acute tubular necrosis, *Arch. Intern. Med.,* 138:950, 1978.

360. Toback, F. G., D. E. Teegarden, and L. J. Havener: Amino acid-mediated stimulation of renal phospholipid biosynthesis after acute tubular necrosis, *Kidney Int.,* 15:542, 1979.

361. Oken, D. E., F. M. Sprinkel, B. B. Kirschbaum, and D. M. Landwehr: Amino acid therapy in the treatment of experimental acute renal failure in the rat, *Kidney Int.,* 17:14, 1980.

362. Feinstein, E. I., M. J. Blumenkrantz, M. Healy, A. Koffler, H. Silberman, S. G. Massry, and J. D. Kopple: Clinical and metabolic responses to parenteral nutrition in acute renal failure, *Medicine,* 60: 124, 1981.

363. Smith, J. L., C. Arteaga, and S. B. Heymsfield: Increased ureagenesis and impaired nitrogen use during infusion of a synthetic amino acid formula. A controlled trial, *N. Engl. J. Med.,* 306:1013, 1982.

364. Zager, R. A., and M. A. Venkatachalam: Potentiation of ischemic renal injury by amino acid infusion, *Kidney Int.,* 24:620, 1983.

365. Brezis, M., P. Silva, and F. H. Epstein: Amino acids induce renal vasodilatation in isolated perfused kidney: Coupling to oxidative metabolism, *Am. J. Physiol.,* 247: H999, 1984.

366. Kennedy, A. C., J. A. Burton, R. G. Luke, J. D. Briggs, R. M. Lindsay, M. E. Allison, N. Edwards, and H. J. Dargie: Factors affecting the prognosis in acute renal failure: A survey of 251 cases, *Q. J. Med.,* 42:73, 1973.

367. Casali, R., R. L. Simmons, J. S. Najarian, B. von Hartitzsch, T. J. Buselmeier, and C. M. Kjellstrand: Acute renal insufficiency complicating major cardiovascular surgery, *Ann. Surg.,* 181:370, 1975.

368. Kilby, J. E., S. R. Powers, and R. T. Beebe: Acute renal failure: Eighty cases of acute tubular necrosis, *N. Engl. J. Med.,* 262:481, 1960.

369. Merino, G. E., T. J. Buselmeier, and C. M. Kjellstrand: Postoperative chronic renal failure: A new syndrome?, *Ann. Surg.,* 182:37, 1975.

370. Yeh, B. P. Y., D. J. Tomko, W. K. Stacy, E. S. Bear, H. T. Haden, and W. F. Falls, Jr.: Factors influencing sodium and water excretion in uremic man, *Kidney Int.,* 7:103, 1975.

iii

4

MECHANISMS OF PROGRESSION OF RENAL DISEASE

Burton D. Rose
Barry M. Brenner

Progression to end-stage renal failure is a common event in chronic renal disease once the P_{cr} exceeds 1.5 to 2.0 mg/dL. Furthermore, the rate of progression is relatively uniform in many patients, with the glomerular filtration rate (GFR) declining in a linear fashion with time.[1,2] As depicted in Fig. 4–1, the GFR in this setting can be simply estimated from the reciprocal of the P_{cr} ($1/P_{cr}$). The use of this parameter can be understood if we consider the formula for the creatinine clearance (C_{cr}), the most common clinical method for evaluating the GFR (see p. 4):

$$C_{cr} = \frac{U_{cr} \times \text{urine flow rate}}{P_{cr}}$$

The numerator of this equation ($U_{cr} \times$ urine flow rate) represents urinary creatinine excretion. This value in the steady state is equal to creatinine production, which remains relatively constant if muscle mass is unchanged. Thus, the C_{cr} (and therefore the GFR) varies with the reciprocal of the P_{cr}.

The factors responsible for progressive renal failure have been incompletely understood. Increasing severity of the primary disease and complicating problems such as poorly controlled hypertension, urinary tract infection or obstruction, or the intrarenal deposition of calcium phosphate all may play a role (see p. 131). However, many disorders associated with moderate but permanent nephron injury progress even when these risk factors are absent. Chronic pyelonephritis due to vesicoureteral reflux (see Chap. 8) is one example of this phenomenon. Once renal insufficiency and proteinuria are present, surgical correction of the reflux and maintenance of a sterile urine with antimicrobials do not prevent the ultimate development of renal failure.[3]

These observations suggest that, after a certain point, a reduction in functioning nephron number eventually leads to failure of the more normal nephron units. This sequence appears to be a *predictable result* of the glomerular hemodynamic response to widespread renal injury. Furthermore, reversal of these hemodynamic changes by restricting dietary protein intake or by lowering the systemic blood pressure may delay or prevent progressive renal failure in many patients. Before discussing the findings in humans, it is useful to first review the experimental data upon which this hemodynamic theory is based.

GLOMERULAR HYPERPERFUSION AND PROGRESSION OF EXPERIMENTAL RENAL DISEASE

The simplest experimental model to study the hemodynamic response to reduced nephron number is provided by surgical nephrectomy. In this setting, there is an increase in the single nephron GFR in the remaining (or remnant) nephrons.[4] Dilatation of the afferent and to a lesser degree efferent glomerular arterioles is responsible for this hyperfiltration by allowing an increase in both glomerular plasma flow and hydrostatic pressure.[5] The magnitude of the elevation in remnant nephron GFR (and of the associated reductions in arteriolar resistance) correlates closely with the amount of renal mass which has been removed. Thus, the remnant nephron GFR in rats increases by about 40 to 50 percent with uninephrectomy and to more than twice normal with 80 percent surgical ablation.[5]

Enhanced filtration by remnant nephrons has generally been regarded as "adaptive" since it partially offsets the loss of function that would otherwise occur. However, a growing body of evidence suggests that the hemodynamic changes that cause remnant nephron hyperfiltration eventually prove injurious to the glomeruli.[6] Although the remnant nephrons are initially normal, they undergo a series of histologic changes that include glomerular hypertrophy, fusion of the epithelial cell foot

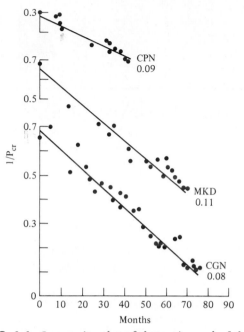

FIG. 4–1. Composite plot of the reciprocal of the P_{cr} (an estimate of the GFR) versus months of observation in three patients with chronic renal failure due to chronic pyelonephritis (CPN), medullary cystic kidney disease (MKD), and chronic glomerulonephritis (CGN). (*Adapted from W. E. Mitch, M. Walser, G. A. Buffington, and J. Lemann, Jr., Lancet, 2:1326, 1976.*)

processes, and expansion of the mesangium.[7] Progressive mesangial expansion then leads to collapse of capillary lumens and the appearance of areas of glomerular sclerosis.[7-9] These sclerosing lesions in the remnant glomeruli are, in their early phase, typically segmental (involving only parts of some glomeruli). With time, however, glomerular sclerosis becomes more widespread, ultimately producing renal failure.

The pace of injury to the remnant glomeruli, like the hemodynamic changes, increases in proportion to the loss of renal mass.[7,10,11] For example, uninephrectomy is associated with moderate acceleration of the glomerular sclerosis normally seen in aging rats with two kidneys.[12] In comparison, glomerular morphologic changes can be detected within 2 weeks after 90 to 95 percent nephrectomy.[11]

Evidence that increased glomerular capillary pressure and/or flow initiates this glomerular injury has been obtained from studies of nephrectomized rats. Severe restriction of dietary protein intake, which lowers the GFR in intact animals (see below),[13,14] was used to blunt the adaptive hyperfiltration following more than 90 percent ablation.[11] In animals fed a 6 percent protein diet (standard laboratory chow contains 24 percent protein), the elevations in nephron GFR, capillary pressure, and capillary flow were attenuated or prevented (Table 4-1). This was accompanied by much less extensive glomerular damage and a lower rate of protein excretion. Similar beneficial results with dietary protein restriction have also been obtained in rats subjected to lesser degrees of renal ablation[15-17] and in rats in which treatment was delayed until some glomerular injury had already occurred.[18]

The importance of these hemodynamic changes is not limited to models using surgical nephrectomy. A similar response has also been found when the number of functioning nephrons is reduced by advancing disease, a situation more analogous to that which occurs in humans. In experimental glomerulonephritis, for example, increased intraglomerular pressure and filtration rate may occur in relatively unaffected glomeruli.[19] These glomeruli are presumably at risk for future hemodynamic injury. Further evidence in support of the importance of hemodynamic factors in glomerular disease comes from the observation that enhancing the intraglomerular pressure and flow by uninephrectomy increases the severity of the glomerular lesions.[20,21]

Limitation of protein intake may again be beneficial, as it can retard the progression of immunologic and diabetic glomerular disease in rats and the lupuslike nephropathy of the NZB/NZW mouse.[22-26] This effect appears to be due primarily to alterations in intrarenal hemodynamics, since similar protection is attained when the intraglomerular pressure is reduced by antihypertensive agents (see "Role of Systemic Hypertension," below). However, other factors are also likely to play a contributory role. For example, recent experiments suggest an intriguing mechanism that may be responsible for at least part of the tubulointerstitial damage that accompanies any form of chronic renal disease.[27] Nephron loss leads to an increase in a variety of tubular functions as well as in the filtration rate in the remaining, less affected nephrons. One such adaptive change is a rise in ammonia production in an attempt to excrete the daily acid load. The ensuing local accumulation of ammonia can then activate

TABLE 4-1. Renal Hemodynamics in Normal and Nephrectomized Rats*

Condition	Single Nephron GFR, nL/min	Glomerular Plasma Flow, nL/min	Glomerular Hydrostatic Pressure, mmHg
Normal	28	74	49
90 percent nephrectomy	63	187	63
90 percent nephrectomy plus protein restriction	38	92	46

*Data from T. H. Hostetter, J. L. Olson, H. G. Rennke, H. A. Venkatachalam, and B. M. Brenner, *Am. J. Physiol.,* 241:F85, 1981.

the alternate complement pathway, leading to tubulointerstitial damage and worsening renal function. Lowering the acid load (and therefore the need to produce ammonia) by the administration of sodium bicarbonate appears to minimize the extent of tubulointerstitial injury. Since the daily acid load is generated largely from protein metabolism, the beneficial effect of dietary protein restriction could be mediated in part by a reduction in ammoniagenesis. Limiting protein intake could also be protective in immunologically mediated renal diseases by diminishing immune responsiveness.[28]

ROLE OF SYSTEMIC HYPERTENSION

Systemic hypertension, either primary or superimposed upon underlying renal disease, can cause glomerular injury. The degree to which this occurs depends on the magnitude of increase in pressure transmitted to the glomeruli. In animal models of primary hypertension associated with renal vasoconstriction (such as the spontaneously hypertensive rat), there is little change in glomerular hemodynamics and relatively little glomerular damage.[29,30] Those lesions that do occur are initially confined to the juxtamedullary glomeruli, which have higher filtration rates and presumably higher pressures than those in the outer cortex.[31,32]

In comparison, when hypertension is associated with a normal or reduced renal vascular resistance, intraglomerular pressure and flow will rise, directly promoting the development of glomerular sclerosis.[30,33,34] This is most often found in salt-sensitive forms of hypertension, including the administration of a mineralocorticoid and salt, the experimental equivalent of primary hyperaldosteronism.[33-35] In this setting in the rat, a low protein diet can prevent or minimize both the hemodynamic and morphologic changes.[35]

These findings may also be applicable to essential hypertension in humans. Most patients with this disorder have renal vasoconstriction and reduced renal blood flow demonstrable early in the course of the disease.[36] This may explain why mild to moderate hypertension is usually associated with at most only slowly progressive renal insufficiency.[30] However, some patients with essential hypertension have renal vasodilatation and increases in renal blood flow and GFR.[36,37] These patients are presumably at higher risk for the development of glomerular sclerosis.

Systemic hypertension may be even more deleterious when superimposed upon underlying renal disease, since the latter's compensatory hemodynamic changes noted above are associated with pronounced renal vasodilatation.[5] In addition, some *glomerular* diseases may be associated with early renal vasodilatation produced by two other mechanisms:

1. Although the glomerular permeability to water is reduced by the immunologic injury, the GFR may initially remain normal. This "adaptation" is mediated by a rise in glomerular capillary hydrostatic pressure that is induced by an unknown mechanism involving afferent arteriolar dilation.[38]
2. Insulin-dependent diabetes mellitus is characterized by vasodilatation and a high GFR soon after the development of hyperglycemia (see p. 203).[39-41]

These changes, which promote glomerular hypertension and hyperperfusion, probably explain why an elevation in systemic blood pressure seems to have a particularly adverse effect in primary glomerular diseases. Thus, the induction of hypertension has been shown to intensify the glomerular damage due to immune complex deposition, antiglomerular basement membrane antibody disease, or diabetic nephropathy.[42-45] If, for example, hypertension is induced by partially occluding one renal artery, the glomerular injury is asymmetric, being much more severe in the nonstenotic, contralateral kidney that is perfused at a higher pressure.[44,45] This deleterious effect of systemic hypertension, however, is apparent only if the increase in pressure is transmitted to the glomerulus. Thus, the course of immune-mediated glomerulonephritis is *not exacerbated* in the vasoconstricted, spontaneously hypertensive rat, which has a relatively normal intraglomerular pressure.[42,46]

The dependence of intrarenal pressure and flow on the systemic blood pressure also has important therapeutic implications. In animals with subtotal nephrectomy, diabetes mellitus, or glomerulonephritis, reducing the systemic blood pressure returns intrarenal hemodynamics toward normal and minimizes the degree of glomerular injury.[47-50] It is important to note in this regard that angiotensin converting enzyme inhibitors (such as enalapril or captopril) may be *particularly effective.* These agents directly lower the glomerular capillary pressure by reversing the angiotensin II–mediated constriction of the efferent (postglomerular) arteriole (Fig. 4–2). The net effect is that proteinuria and glomerular sclerosis are markedly diminished.[47,48,50] In contrast, antihypertensive agents which act in the kidney by dilating the afferent arteriole (such as the triad of hydrochlorothiazide-reserpine-hydralazine) may be less beneficial.[50-52] Although the systemic pressure is reduced with this regimen, the decrease in preglomerular resistance means that more of the systemic pressure is transmitted to the glomerulus (Fig. 4–2). As a result, the glomerular capillary pressure may be relatively unchanged with less protection against glomerular injury.[50,51] (The arteriolar sites of action of β-blockers and calcium channel blockers are at present unclear.[53])

Drugs other than antihypertensive agents also can affect intrarenal hemodynamics and, therefore, the rate of progression of renal disease. In particular, corticosteroids can produce renal vasodilatation and raise the intraglomerular pressure. In animals with subtotal nephrectomy, the concurrent administration of the equivalent of 60 mg of prednisone per day accelerates the development of proteinuria and glomerulosclerosis.[54] This deleterious effect of chronic, high-dose corticosteroid therapy could contribute to the apparently diminished effectiveness of this regimen (in comparison to cyclophosphamide therapy) in patients with diffuse proliferative lupus nephritis (see Fig. 6–24).

MECHANISM OF HEMODYNAMIC INJURY

The experiments with converting enzyme inhibitors also shed some light on the relative importance of the different hemodynamic changes that occur. These drugs decrease renal vascular resistance by dilating the efferent arteriole and can increase glomerular capillary permeability, reversing a direct effect of angiotensin II.[55] As a result, the glomerular capillary pressure is reduced to near normal, but there are persistent elevations in glomerular plasma flow (due to renal vasodilation) and filtration rate (due to increased water permeability).[47,48,50] Preferential lowering of intraglomerular pressure also occurs with dietary protein restriction (Table 4–1), although this response is mediated by afferent arteriolar constriction rather than efferent dilatation.[56] These findings suggest that the *elevation in glomerular capillary pressure* (not hyperfiltration itself) is of primary importance in hemodynamically mediated glomerular injury.[47,48,50] Increased glomerular plasma flow alone does not appear to be deleterious, but it may exacerbate the effect of intraglomerular hypertension.

Glomerular hypertension presumably acts by causing mechanical disruption of normal

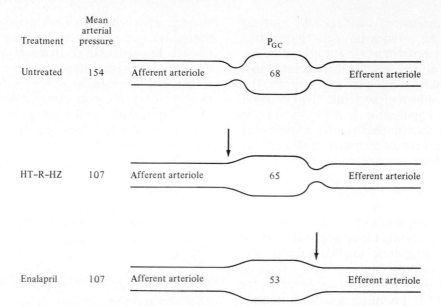

FIG. 4–2. Relationship between mean arterial pressure, arteriolar resistance, and glomerular capillary hydrostatic pressure (P_{GC}) in three groups of five-sixths nephrectomized rats. Untreated rats (*top panel*) are hypertensive and have an elevated P_{GC} (normal about 45 mmHg) that is largely responsible for the associated compensatory hyperfiltration. When the mean arterial pressure is reduced with hydrochlorothiazide-reserpine-hydralazine (HT-R-HZ; *middle panel*), the predominant dilation of the afferent arteriole (arrow) prevents a fall in P_{GC}. As a result, the percentage of glomeruli showing sclerotic lesions at 3 months is the same as in untreated rats (22 to 24 percent). In comparison, the converting enzyme inhibitor enalapril lowers both the arterial and, due to efferent arteriolar dilation, the intraglomerular pressures (*bottom panel*). The afferent arteriole also dilates in this setting, probably due to an autoregulatory response to maintain the GFR. In these rats in whom the intraglomerular hypertension is largely corrected, sclerotic lesions are seen in only 1.5 percent of the glomeruli. (*Adapted from S. Anderson, H. G. Rennke, and B. M. Brenner, J. Clin. Invest., 77:1993, 1986.*)

vascular integrity. For example, the proteinuria associated with the development of hemodynamically mediated glomerular sclerosis is due to impairment in both the size- and charge-selective properties of the glomerular basement membrane.[57] As a result, the combined effects of increased pressure and flow, which elevate the GFR, also enhance the transglomerular movement of macromolecules such as albumin. Studies using ferritin or carbon colloid have demonstrated increased mesangial deposition of these compounds after contralateral uninephrectomy, an effect that begins before glomerular sclerosis has developed.[57,58] It is possible, therefore, that overloading of the mesangium is the general mechanism for mesangial expansion, the forerunner of glomerular sclerosis.[57,58] The resulting loss of glomerular units leads to a further hemodynamic burden on less affected glomeruli, setting the stage for their eventual destruction as well.

MECHANISM OF HEMODYNAMIC CHANGES

The mechanism by which reduction in renal mass leads to structural and functional hypertrophy of the remaining nephrons is incompletely understood.[59,60] In the rat subjected to unilateral nephrectomy, increased renal ribonucleic acid and protein synthesis are seen within hours,[61] and kidney size and weight begin to increase within 1 to 2 days.[62] This structural hypertrophy involves both the glomeruli and the tubules and is accompanied by an increase in the single nephron GFR[63] due, as described above, to arteriolar dilation. By 2 weeks, whole kidney GFR and kidney weight rise in proportion by about 40 percent.[64]

Similar changes have been documented in humans in studies of renal transplant donors. Within the first weeks, glomerular filtration and renal plasma flow rates in the remaining kidney increase by about 40 percent.[65-67] The net effect is that the total GFR is about 70 percent of the prenephrectomy value.

Multiple factors that can influence this compensatory hypertrophy have been identified, including age (growth being greatest in the young), androgens, pituitary hormones (particularly growth hormone), sensitization of the tubular cells to nonspecific growth factors as a result of the rise in nephron GFR, and possibly specific, as yet unidentified "renotropins".[68,69] The retention of compounds normally excreted in the urine also may be an important stimulus to growth. If, for example, half the urine volume of rats is reinfused continuously (thus halving excretory function while maintaining renal mass), bilateral renal hypertrophy may be seen.[69]

It is likely that the need to excrete protein metabolites also plays a role in the compensatory elevation in GFR.[14] In the setting of reduced nephron number, an increase in GFR in the remaining nephrons maximizes the filtration and subsequent excretion of these compounds. If, however, protein intake is diminished, nephron GFR falls toward normal (see Table 4–1).

This effect of protein intake can also be demonstrated in normal experimental animals and humans.[14] For example, chronically changing from a low to a normal protein diet in humans can raise the GFR by 15 to 20 mL/min or more.[70,71] The effect of an acute protein load is even more prominent, as the increment in GFR can transiently exceed 35 to 40 mL/min.[71] It is interesting to note that this response is progressively attenuated as renal function declines, there being little rise in GFR with protein loading once the creatinine clearance is below 40 to 70 mL/min.[71-73] It is probable, in this setting, that the underlying renal disease has already produced a near maximal compensatory increase in nephron GFR.

The mechanism by which protein intake affects the GFR is uncertain. Amino acids, but not urea or the associated acid load, appear to be responsible.[14] Pituitary ablation or the administration or somatostatin can abolish the protein effect on GFR in both animals and humans.[74-76] These findings suggest at least a permissive role for a circulating hormone, although neither growth hormone nor glucagon appears to be responsible.[75-77] It is also possible that intrarenal factors can contribute. The filtration and reabsorption of the extra amino acids may increase renal oxygen consumption, an effect that could promote renal vasodilatation in an attempt to enhance oxygen delivery.[78,79]

Regardless of the mechanism, it seems reasonable to assume that the renal hemodynamic response to protein loading reflects an evolutionary adaptation to the excretory needs of animals whose protein intake was not constant because of intermittent feeding.[14] The increase in GFR with meals facilitates the excretion of protein metabolites as well as that of other solutes and water.

PROGRESSION OF HUMAN RENAL DISEASE

Studies in humans, although generally less direct, also support the view that hyperperfused nephrons ultimately fail. Morphologic studies in human renal disease have demonstrated hypertrophy (presumably reflecting hyperperfusion and hyperfiltration) of those nephrons least damaged by disease (Fig. 4–3).[80] Furthermore, sclerotic lesions (similar to those in animals with hemodynamically mediated injury) are most likely to develop in these enlarged glomeruli.[81]

Progressive loss of renal function, proteinuria, and segmental or widespread glomerular sclerosis has been demonstrated in a variety of disorders in which damage has occurred, but the underlying process has remitted spontaneously or been controlled therapeutically (Table 4–2). To give some examples:

1. Patients with poststreptococcal glomerulonephritis who apparently recover from the initial episode may develop proteinuria, hypertension, glomerular sclerosis, and renal failure decades later.[82,83]
2. Patients with chronic pyelonephritis (due to vesicoureteral reflux) and proteinuria inevitably develop renal failure with increasing glomerular sclerosis, despite surgical correction of the reflux and prevention of infection with antimicrobials.[3,84–86] Moreover, glomerular sclerosis has been found in the contralateral unscarred kidney in patients with unilateral disease.[87]
3. Patients with analgesic nephropathy often progress to renal failure despite discontinuation of analgesic use.[88] This is as-

sociated with focal areas of glomerular sclerosis.[89]
4. Patients with bilateral renal cortical necrosis who require dialysis during the acute phase frequently recover stable, although reduced, renal function before eventually proceeding to end-stage renal failure.[90]

Similar findings occur when there is a primary reduction in the number of functioning nephrons, a situation analogous to the animal experiments with subtotal nephrectomy described above. Oligomeganephronia is a rare congenital disease characterized by a markedly reduced (up to 80 percent) nephron number and compensatory hypertrophy in the remaining nephrons. Hyperfiltration in these nephrons initially maintains the total GFR at an acceptable level,[91] but progressive proteinuria, glomerular sclerosis, and renal failure typically are seen by adolescence.[91,92] The same changes may be found with unilateral renal agenesis, a more common disorder which occurs in approximately 1 in 1000 people.[81,93,94] However, the development of

TABLE 4–2. Possible Hemodynamic Glomerulopathies in Humans

Decreased number of functioning nephrons
  Oligomeganephronia
  Unilateral renal agenesis
  Unilateral nephrectomy
Parenchymal disease causing loss of functioning renal
  mass
  Examples: Poststreptococcal glomerulonephritis
           Chronic pyelonephritis
           Analgesic nephropathy
           Renal cortical necrosis
Primary renal vasodilatation
  Diabetes mellitus
  Sickle cell disease
  Familial dysautonomia
Poorly controlled hypertension
  Especially if underlying renal disease is present
Relative intraglomerular hypertension
  Aging
  Hereditary nephritis

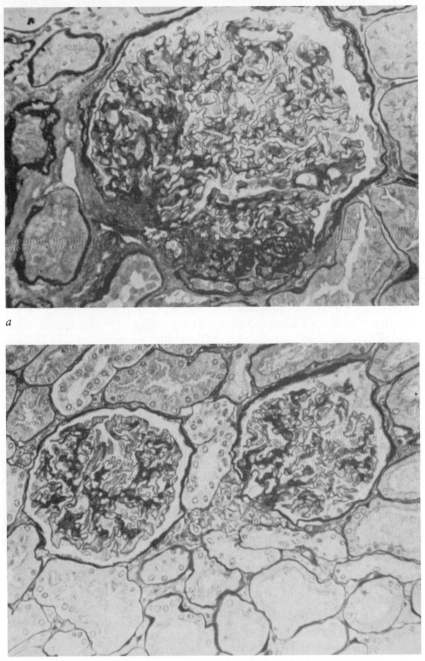

a

b

FIG. 4–3. Renal tissue from (*a*) a 27-year-old man with unilateral renal agenesis and (*b*) a 27-year-old normal control at identical magnification (390×). Both the glomeruli and tubules are markedly enlarged in *a*, with the glomerular volume being more than 4× normal. The lower segment of this glomerulus also shows consolidation and early sclerosis. (*From D. B. Bhathena, B. A. Julian, R. G. McMorrow, and R. W. Baehler, Am. J. Kid. Dis., 5:226, 1985.*)

glomerular sclerosis is less predictable than in oligomeganephronia, presumably because there are more functioning nephrons with unilateral agencies and therefore less pronounced intraglomerular hemodynamic changes.

The risk of hemodynamically mediated glomerular injury is greater in males[95,96] and in young children. Thus, glomerular sclerosis can occur following unilateral nephrectomy[95,96] but is probably less common than with unilateral agenesis. This can be appreciated from studies of renal transplant donors. After more than 10 to 15 years of follow-up, the GFR tends to remain unchanged although there is a somewhat increased incidence of proteinuria and hypertension.[97,98] However, isolated cases of focal glomerular sclerosis have been reported in previously healthy transplant donors and in recipients of grafts from identical twins (in whom chronic rejection can be excluded).[99-101] Taken together, these findings suggest that removal of one-half of the renal mass can be deleterious in the long-run but that the risk is enhanced with a more marked reduction in nephron number (as in oligomeganephronia).

The glomerular changes in diseases associated with primary renal vasodilatation or poorly controlled hypertension also support the importance of intraglomerular hypertension. With renal vasodilatation, more of the systemic pressure is transmitted to the glomeruli. This could explain the development of glomerular sclerosis in diabetes mellitus (see p. 203),[39] sickle cell disease,[102,103] and familial dysautonomia,[104] in which hyperglycemia, medullary ischemia leading to increased prostaglandin production, and decreased sympathetic neural tone, respectively, are responsible for the fall in renal vascular resistance. Furthermore, glomerular sclerosis is most likely to occur in those patients with an initially elevated GFR.[103,105]

Systemic hypertension can also cause glomerular damage, in both patients with primary hypertension and those with underlying renal disease.[30] As in experimental animals,[44,45] unilateral renal artery stenosis in humans can lead to unilateral glomerulonephritis or diabetic nephropathy with the ischemic kidney being relatively protected.[106-108] In addition, those diabetics with higher blood pressure are at greater risk of developing renal disease.[105]

Finally, it is possible that "normal" glomerular pressure and flow can, in the long run, produce glomerular disease. Otherwise healthy adults show a progressive decline in GFR and renal blood flow after the age of 30 to 40; values in octogenarians are only one-half to two-thirds those of young adults.[109,110] This loss of renal function is associated with increasing glomerular sclerosis.[111] Similar glomerular changes can be demonstrated in aging animals.[112] The observations in animals that the severity of these lesions can be increased by uninephrectomy[113] and diminished by protein restriction,[114,115] suggest that they may be mediated by hemodynamic factors. Thus, the decline in renal function with age in humans may be due in part to chronic glomerular hyperperfusion induced by the protein-rich diet of modern society. Not surprisingly, the rate of decline also varies directly with the systemic blood pressure, being most rapid in hypertensive subjects.[116]

Relative intraglomerular hypertension also may be important in hereditary nephritis. This disorder is characterized by abnormal glomerular basement membranes which may be unable to tolerate even normal pressures and flows (see Chap. 6).

IMPLICATIONS FOR THERAPY

The experimental and human studies cited above suggest that reversing intraglomerular hypertension and hyperperfusion may delay or prevent progressive renal disease. One such intervention is dietary protein restriction; sample daily diets consist of 0.6 g/kg of high biologic value protein and 700 mg of phosphorus or 20 to 30 g of protein supplemented with amino acids and their keto analogues.[117-119] Plotting the $1/P_{cr}$ versus time and using the patients as their own controls, multiple studies have demonstrated marked slowing (more than 75 to 90 percent) or even cessation of the decline in GFR in many patients (Fig. 4–4).[72,118-123] This effect occurs in a wide variety of chronic renal diseases, including chronic glomerulonephritis, chronic pyelonephritis, and polycystic kidney disease.[72,120-122] However, limiting protein intake is less likely to be beneficial when the P_{cr} is greater than 8 mg/dL,[119] if the patient is hypertensive,[120] or with nephrosclerosis in which the vascular disease may prevent nephron hyperperfusion.[72]

Patient compliance is clearly important if this dietary regimen is to be effective. Assuming that daily intake does not vary widely and that the patient is in a steady state, then nitrogen excretion will be roughly equal to nitrogen intake. The former can be estimated from a 24-h urine collection[124]:

Urine nitrogen excretion
= urine urea nitrogen + nonurea nitrogen

Nonurea nitrogen excretion is relatively constant at about 30 mg/kg of body weight per day. Thus

Urine nitrogen excretion
= urine urea nitrogen + 30 mg/kg

Since each gram of nitrogen is derived from 6.25 g of protein,

Estimated protein intake
= 6.25(urine urea nitrogen + 30 mg/kg)

If, for example, 24-h urine urea nitrogen excretion is 9 g in a 70-kg man, then

Estimated protein intake
= 6.25(9 + 2.1) = 79.4 g

The safety of dietary protein restriction in the presence of marked proteinuria is uncertain. In three studies of patients with the nephrotic syndrome, dietary protein restriction resulted in decreased proteinuria and no change in either the plasma albumin concentration or total albumin pool.[125-127] Al-

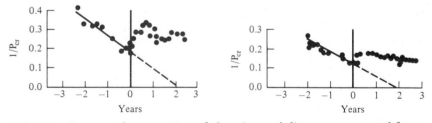

FIG. 4–4. The rate of progression of chronic renal disease as assessed from the reciprocal of the P_{cr} in two patients before and after (vertical bar) the institution of dietary protein restriction. The regression line for pretherapy values is shown as a solid line; the dashed line represents the expected change if treatment were not successful. Both patients had stabilization of their GFR. Stabilization or a slower rate of decline occurred in six of seven patients in this study with an initial P_{cr} below 8 mg/dL. (*Adapted from W. E. Mitch, M. Walser, T. I. Steinman, S. Hill, S. Zeger, and K. Tungsanga, N. Engl. J. Med., 311:623, 1984. Reprinted by permission from the New England Journal of Medicine.*)

though the mechanism by which protein excretion fell is not clear, these findings suggest that protein restriction may be well tolerated in nephrotic patients with no significant change in nitrogen balance. However, these results need to be confirmed in a larger number of patients before a definite conclusion can be made.

Another potentially important therapeutic modality is rigorous control of the systemic blood pressure. In experimental and human glomerular disease, hypertension can intensify the degree of glomerular injury.[42-45,106-108] In comparison, lowering the blood pressure in animals with surgical ablation, diabetic nephropathy, or glomerulonephritis can decrease the *intrarenal hypertension* and preserve renal function.[47-51] This beneficial effect can be demonstrated even in normotensive animals in whom the systemic pressure is reduced by about 15 mmHg.[48]

Clinical studies are currently underway in humans to evaluate the efficacy of blood pressure reduction (in both hypertensive and normotensive subjects) in slowing the progression of chronic renal disease. Antihypertensive therapy has already been shown to be effective in patients with marked primary hypertension[128-131] and those with diabetes mellitus.[132-134] Once the glomerular disease is established in diabetic nephropathy, correction of hypertension appears to minimize the further loss of renal function and to diminish the degree of proteinuria (Fig. 4–5).[132-134] In comparison, control of the plasma glucose concentration is ineffective at this relatively late stage.[135,136]

It is important to reemphasize that preliminary experimental data suggest that converting enzyme inhibitors may be particularly beneficial in this setting. In addition to lowering the systemic blood pressure, these agents directly lower the intraglomerular pressure by selectively dilating the efferent arteriole (see Fig. 4–2).[47,48,50] Other agents which dilate the afferent arteriole (such as

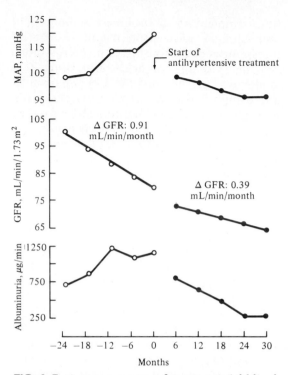

FIG. 4–5. Average course of mean arterial blood pressure (MAP), GFR, and the rate of albumin excretion before and after the institution of effective antihypertensive therapy in 10 patients with diabetic nephropathy. A reduction in blood pressure from 144/97 to 128/84 was associated with a much slower fall in GFR and less albuminuria. (*From H.-H. Parving, U. Smidt, A. R. Andersen, and P. A. Svendsen, Lancet, 1:1175, 1983.*)

the triad of hydrochlorothiazide-reserpine-hydralazine) may not reduce intraglomerular pressure and therefore may be less protective.[50-52]

SUMMARY

A large and increasing body of experimental and clinical data suggest that dietary protein restriction and lowering the systemic blood pressure delay or prevent the progression of many renal diseases, presumably by reversing the associated intraglomerular hypertension and hyperperfusion. One weakness in the human studies reported thus far is that efficacy has been determined by comparing the patient's course before and after the institution of therapy (Figs. 4–4 and 4–5). Such studies, however, can lead to potentially erroneous conclusions due in part to the "clinic effect" in which more comprehensive care, not the therapeutic intervention, is responsible for the observed benefit.[137] Appropriately controlled studies currently being performed should more accurately assess the effectiveness of dietary and antihypertensive therapy. If these studies confirm the experimental evidence, then the treatment of early renal insufficiency will be radically altered. In diabetic nephropathy, for example, control of intrarenal hemodynamics may be more important than strict regulation of the plasma glucose concentration.[39,48,138]

If protein restriction and more aggressive lowering of the systemic blood pressure become more widely used, patients will have to be carefully followed for possible unsuspected adverse effects. For example, reducing dietary protein intake diminishes the excretion of allopurinol and its active metabolite oxypurinol.[139] Both a fall in GFR and enhanced tubular reabsorption may contribute to this response. As a result, the dose of allopurinol should be reduced to minimize the likelihood of drug toxicity. It is at present unknown if limiting protein intake has an important effect on the renal excretion of other drugs.

ALTERNATIVE EXPLANATIONS OF PROGRESSIVE NATURE OF RENAL DISEASE

Several factors other than glomerular capillary hypertension and hyperperfusion also have been proposed to account for the progressive course of many renal diseases. It

has been suggested, for example, that the deposition of calcium phosphate in the renal interstitium (due to a rise in the circulating calcium phosphate product) contributes to the loss of renal function.[140,141] The observation that dietary phosphorus restriction (sufficient to induce hypophosphatemia) offers partial protection against the degree of renal injury and the decline in GFR is also compatible with this hypothesis.[140-142]

However, the morphological and functional deterioration in these studies *preceded* calcium phosphate deposition, indicating that the latter is a relatively late occurrence.[143,144] Thus, the protective effect of phosphate restriction must have been mediated by another mechanism.[142] Phosphate depletion can blunt tissue hypertrophy[144,145] and can lower the GFR,[146] effects that could minimize glomerular hyperperfusion in animals with renal disease.

The presence of immunoglobulins (particularly IgM) in diseased glomeruli in remnant kidneys and in humans with end-stage kidney disease[147] has raised the possibility that an immune response directed against renal antigens may contribute to the associated functional deterioration. However, immune complexes have not been found in the damaged remnant glomeruli,[11] making it likely that the IgM is nonspecifically absorbed onto the abnormal glomerular tissue. The primary importance of hemodynamic rather than immunologic factors in this setting is also suggested by the observation that accelerated glomerular sclerosis does not occur with the loss of less than one-half of functioning renal tissue.[11]

Another recent hypothesis proposed that progressive chronic renal disease may be mediated in part by abnormalities in lipid metabolism.[148] According to this view, the initial renal injury is followed by an elevation in plasma lipid levels, which then cause further damage to the glomeruli. However, the correlation between renal functional deterioration and hyperlipidemia is poor, and familial hyperlipidemias have not been shown to cause kidney disease.

Vascular coagulation with eventual thrombosis of the glomerular capillaries also may play a role in glomerular injury following renal ablation. Heparin, warfarin, and aspirin in combination with dipyridamole all have been shown to minimize glomerular damage in this model,[10,149-151] but the mechanism of the protective effect is unclear. Each of these therapies is associated with a significant fall in the systemic blood pressure as well as anticoagulation. It is uncertain, therefore, whether the observed benefit is due to pre-vention of thrombosis or to an effect on glomerular hemodynamics.

Finally, renal prostanoids also may play a role. Inhibiting prostaglandin synthesis with indomethacin has been reported to preserve renal function in different animal models.[152] In humans with the nephrotic syndrome, prostaglandin synthesis inhibitors can markedly reduce proteinuria with a modest fall in GFR.[153,154] These changes could reflect renal vasoconstriction and a decrease in intraglomerular pressure; the latter effect could be beneficial in the long term.

REFERENCES

1. Mitch, W. E., M. Walser, G. A. Buffington, and J. Lemann, Jr.: A simple method for estimating progression of chronic renal failure, *Lancet,* 2:1326, 1976.
2. Rutherford, W. E., J. Blondin, J. P. Miller, A. S. Greenwalt, and J. D. Vavra: Chronic progressive renal disease: Rate of change of serum creatinine, *Kidney Int.,* 11:62, 1977.
3. Torres, V. E., J. A. Velosa, K. E. Holley, P. P. Kelalis, G. B. Stickler, and S. B. Kurtz: The progression of vesicoureteral reflux, *Ann. Intern. Med.,* 92:776, 1980.
4. Hayslett, J. P.: Functional adaptation to reduction in renal mass, *Physiol. Rev.,* 59:137, 1979.
5. Deen, W. M., D. A. Maddox, C. R. Robertson, and B. M. Brenner: Dynamics of glomerular ultrafiltration in the rat. VII. Response to reduced renal mass, *Am. J. Physiol.,* 227:556, 1974.
6. Brenner, B. M.: Nephron adaptation to renal injury or ablation, *Am. J. Physiol.,* 249:F324, 1985.
7. Shimamura, T., and A. B. Morrison: A progressive glomerulosclerosis occurring in partial five-sixths nephrectomized rats, *Am. J. Pathol.,* 79:95, 1975.
8. Chanutin A., and E. B. Ferris: Experimental renal insufficiency produced by partial nephrectomy. I. Control diet, *Arch. Intern. Med.,* 49:767, 1932.
9. Kenner, C. H., A. P. Evan, P. Blomgren, G. R. Aronoff, and F. C. Luft: Effect of protein intake on renal function and structure in partially nephrectomized rats, *Kidney Int.,* 27:739, 1985.
10. Purkerson, M. L., P. E. Hoffsten, and S. Klahr: Pathogenesis of the glomerulopathy associated with renal infarction in rats, *Kidney Int.,* 9:407, 1976.
11. Hostetter, T. H., J. L. Olson, H. G. Rennke, M. A. Venkatachalam, and B. M. Brenner: Hyperfiltration in remnant nephrons: A potentially adverse response to renal ablation, *Am. J. Physiol.,* 241:F85, 1981.
12. Striker, G. E., R. B. Nagle, P. W. Kohnen, and E. A. Smuckler: Response to unilateral nephrectomy in old rats, *Arch. Pathol.,* 87:439, 1969.
13. Ichikawa, I., M. L. Purkerson, S. Klahr, J. L. Troy, M. Martinez-Maldonado, and B. M. Brenner: Mechanism of reduced glomerular filtration rate in chronic malnutrition, *J. Clin. Invest.,* 65:982, 1980.
14. Brenner, B. M., T. W. Meyer, and T. H. Hostetter: Dietary protein intake and the progressive nature of kidney disease: The role of hemodynamically mediated glomerular injury in the pathogenesis of progressive glomerular sclerosis in aging, renal ablation, and intrinsic renal disease, *N. Engl. J. Med.,* 307:652, 1982.
15. Hostetter, T. H., T. W. Meyer, H. G. Rennke, and B. M. Brenner: Chronic effects of dietary protein in the rat with intact and reduced renal mass, *Kidney Int.,* 30:509, 1986.
16. Madden, M. A., and S. W. Zimmerman: Protein restriction and renal function in the uremic rat (abstract), *Kidney Int.,* 23:217, 1983.
17. El Nahas, A. M., H. Paraskevakou, S. Zoob, A. J. Rees, and D. J. Evans: Effect of dietary protein

restriction on the development of renal failure after subtotal nephrectomy in rats, *Clin. Sci.,* 65:399, 1983.

18. Nath, K. A., D. Kaufman, and T. H. Hostetter: Effect of low protein diet after renal injury is established, abstract, *Kidney Int.,* 27:248, 1985.

19. Allison, M. E. M., C. B. Wilson, and C. W. Gottschalk: Pathophysiology of experimental glomerulonephritis in rats, *J. Clin. Invest.,* 53:1402, 1974.

20. Teoduru, C. V., A. Saifer, and H. Frankel: Conditioning factors influencing evolution of experimental glomerulonephritis in rabbits, *Am. J. Physiol.,* 196:457, 1959.

21. Beyer, M. M., A. D. Steinberg, A. D. Nicastri, and E. A. Friedman: Unilateral nephrectomy: Effect on survival in NZB/NZW mice, *Science,* 198:511, 1977.

22. Farr, L. E., and J. E. Smadel: The effect of dietary protein on the course of nephrotoxic nephritis in rats, *J. Exp. Med.,* 70:615, 1939.

23. Neugarten, J., H. D. Feiner, R. G. Schacht, and D. S. Baldwin: Amelioration of experimental glomerulonephritis by dietary protein restriction, *Kidney Int.,* 24:595, 1983.

24. Zatz, R., T. W. Meyer, H. G. Rennke, and B. M. Brenner: Predominance of hemodynamic rather than metabolic factors in the pathogenesis of diabetic nephropathy, *Proc. Natl. Acad. Sci. (U.S.A.),* 82: 5963, 1985.

25. El Nahas, A. M., S. Zoob, D. J. Evans, and A. J. Rees: Modification of the course of nephrotoxic nephritis by diet (abstract), *Kidney Int.,* 22:219, 1982.

26. Friend, P. S., G. Fernandes, R. A. Good, A. F. Michael, and E. J. Yunis: Dietary restrictions early and late: Effects on the nephropathy of the NZB/NZW mouse, *Lab. Invest.,* 38:629, 1978.

27. Nath, K. A., M. K. Hostetter, and T. H. Hostetter: Pathophysiology of chronic tubulo-interstitial disease in rats. Interactions of dietary acid load, ammonia, and complement component C3, *J. Clin. Invest.,* 76:667, 1985.

28. Agus, D., R. Mann, D. Cohn, L. Michaud, C. Kelly, M. Clayman, and E. G. Neilson: Inhibitory role of dietary protein restriction on the development and expression of immune-mediated antitubular basement membrane-induced tubulointerstitial nephritis in rats, *J. Clin Invest.,* 76:930, 1985.

29. Arendshorst, W. J., and W. H. Beierwaltes: Renal and nephron hemodynamics in spontaneously hypertensive rats, *Am. J. Physiol.,* 236:F246, 1979.

30. Baldwin, D. S., and J. Neugarten: Treatment of hypertension in renal disease, *Hypertension,* 5:A57, 1985.

31. Feld, L. G., J. B. vanLiew, R. G. Galaske, and J. W.

Boylan: Selectivity of renal injury and progression in the spontaneously hypertensive rat, *Kidney Int.,* 12:332, 1977.

32. Bank, N., L. Allerman, and H. S. Aynedjian: Selective JM nephron hyperfiltration in SHR rats with reduced renal mass (abstract), *Kidney Int.,* 23:211, 1983.

33. Azar, S., M. A. Johnson, B. Hertel, and L. Tobian: Single-nephron pressures, flows and resistances in hypertensive kidneys with nephrosclerosis, *Kidney Int.,* 12:28, 1977.

34. Azar, S., M. A. Johnson, J. Iwai, L. Bruno, and L. Tobian: Single-nephron dynamics in "post-salt" rats with chronic hypertension, *J. Lab. Clin. Med.,* 91:156, 1978.

35. Dworkin, L. D., T. H. Hostetter, H. G. Rennke, and B. M. Brenner: Hemodynamic basis for glomerular injury in rats with desoxycorticosterone-salt hypertension, *J. Clin. Invest.,* 73:1448, 1984.

36. Hollenberg, N. K., L. J. Borucki, and D. F. Adams: The renal vasculature in early essential hypertension, *Medicine,* 57:167, 1978.

37. Bianchi, G., D. Cusi, C. Barlassina, G. P. Lupi, P. Ferrari, G. B. Picotti, M. Gatti, and T. Polli: Renal dysfunction as a possible cause of essential hypertension in predisposed subjects, *Kidney Int.,* 23:870, 1983.

38. Sakai, T., F. H. Harris, D. J. Marsh, C. M. Bennett, and R. J. Glassock: Extracellular fluid expansion and autoregulation in nephrotoxic serum nephritis in rats, *Kidney Int.,* 25:619, 1984.

39. Hostetter, T. H., H. G. Rennke, and B. M. Brenner: The case for intrarenal hypertension in the initiation and progression of diabetic and other glomerulopathies, *Am. J. Med.,* 72:375, 1982.

40. Mogensen, C. E.: Diabetes mellitus and the kidney, *Kidney Int.,* 21:673, 1982.

41. Hostetter, T. H., J. L. Troy, and B. M. Brenner: Glomerular hemodynamics in experimental diabetes mellitus, *Kidney Int.,* 19:410, 1981.

42. Raij, L., S. Azar, and W. Keane: Role of hypertension in progressive glomerular immune injury, *Hypertension,* 7:398, 1985.

43. Tikkanen, I., F. Fyhrquist, A. Miettinen, and T. Tornroth: Autologous immune complex nephritis and DOCA-NaCl load: A new model of hypertension, *Acta Path. Microbiol. Scand.,* 88:241, 1980.

44. Neugarten, J., H. D. Feiner, R. G. Schacht, G. R. Gallo, and D. S. Baldwin: Aggravation of experimental glomerulonephritis by superimposed clip hypertension, *Kidney Int.,* 22:257, 1982.

45. Mauer, S. M., M. W. Steffes, S. Azar, S. K. Sandberg, and D. M. Brown: The effects of Goldblatt

hypertension on development of diabetic mellitus in the rat, *Diabetes,* 27:738, 1978.

46. Stein, H. D., R. B. Sterzel, J. D. Hunt, R. Pabst, and M. Kashgarian: No aggravation of the course of experimental glomerulonephritis in spontaneously hypertensive rats, *Am. J. Pathol.,* 122:520, 1986.

47. Anderson, S., T. W. Meyer, H. G. Rennke, and B. M. Brenner: Control of glomerular hypertension limits glomerular injury in rats with reduced renal mass, *J. Clin. Invest.,* 76:612, 1985.

48. Zatz, R., B. R. Dunn, S. Anderson, H. G. Rennke, and B. M. Brenner: Prevention of diabetic glomerulopathy by pharmacological amelioration of glomerular capillary hypertension, *J. Clin. Invest.,* 77:1925, 1986.

49. Neugarten, J., B. Kaminetsky, H. Feiner, R. G. Schacht, D. T. Liu, and D. S. Baldwin: Nephrotoxic serum nephritis with hypertension: Amelioration by antihypertensive therapy, *Kidney Int.,* 28:135, 1985.

50. Anderson, S., H. G. Rennke, and B. M. Brenner: Therapeutic advantage of converting enzyme inhibitors in arresting progressive renal disease associated with systemic hypertension in the rat, *J. Clin. Invest.,* 77:1993, 1986.

51. Dworkin, L. D., H. D. Feiner, and J. Randazzo: Evidence for hemodynamically mediated glomerular injury despite antihypertensive therapy in rats with desoxycorticosterone-salt hypertension (abstract), *Kidney Int.,* 27:189, 1985.

52. Azar, S., W. Keane, and L. Raij: Antihypertensive therapy in nephritic spontaneously hypertensive rats: Effects on nephron dynamics and morphology (abstract), *Kidney Int.,* 27:187, 1985.

53. Loutzenheiser, R., and M. Epstein: Effects of calcium antagonists on renal hemodynamics, *Am. J. Physiol.,* 249:F619, 1985.

54. Garcia, D. L., S. Anderson, H. G. Rennke, and B. M. Brenner: Chronic steroid therapy amplifies glomerular injury in rats with reduced renal mass (abstract), *Clin. Res.,* 34(2):697a, 1986.

55. Dworkin, L. D., I. Ichikawa, and B. M. Brenner: Hormonal modulation of glomerular function, *Am. J. Physiol.,* 244:F95, 1983.

56. Dworkin, L. D., and H. D. Feiner: Glomerular injury in uninephrectomized spontaneously hypertensive rats. A consequence of glomerular capillary hypertension, *J. Clin. Invest.,* 77:797, 1986.

57. Olson, J. L., T. H. Hostetter, H. G. Rennke, B. M. Brenner, and M. A. Venkatachalam: Altered glomerular permselectivity and progressive sclerosis following extreme ablation of renal mass, *Kidney Int.,* 22:112, 1982.

58. Grond, J., M. S. Schilthuis, J. Koudstaal, and J. D. Elema: Mesangial function and glomerular sclerosis in rats after unilateral nephrectomy, *Kidney Int.,* 22:338, 1982.

59. Preuss, H. G.: Compensatory renal growth symposium: An introduction, *Kidney Int.* 23:571, 1983.

60. Fine, L.: The biology of renal hypertrophy, *Kidney Int.,* 29:619, 1986.

61. Johnson, H. A., and J. M. Vera Roman: Compensatory renal enlargement: Hypertrophy versus hyperplasia, *Am. J. Pathol.,* 49:1, 1966.

62. Phillips, T. L., and G. F. Leong: Kidney cell proliferation after unilateral nephrectomy as related to age, *Cancer Res.,* 27:286, 1967.

63. Diezi, J., P. Michoud, A. Grandchamp, and G. Giebisch: Effects of nephrectomy on renal salt and water transport in the remaining kidney, *Kidney Int.,* 10:450, 1976.

64. Deen, W. M., D. A. Maddox, C. R. Robertson, and B. M. Brenner: Dynamics of glomerular ultrafiltration in the rat. VII. Response to reduced renal mass, *Am. J. Physiol.,* 227:556, 1974.

65. Boner, G., W. D. Shelp, M. Newton, and R. E. Rieselbach: Factors influencing the increase in glomerular filtration rate in the remaining kidney of transplant donors, *Am. J. Med.,* 55:169, 1973.

66. Pabico, R. C., B. A. McKenna, and R. B. Freeman: Renal function before and after unilateral nephrectomy in renal donors, *Kidney Int.,* 8:166, 1975.

67. Vincenti, F., W. J. Amend, Jr., G. Kaysen, N. Feduska, J. Birnbaum, R. Duca, and O. Salvatierra: Long-term renal function in kidney donors. Sustained compensatory hyperfiltration with no adverse effects, *Transplantation,* 36:626, 1983.

68. Yamamoto, N., H. Kanetake, and J. Yamada: In vitro evidence from tissue cultures to prove existence of rabbit and human renotropic growth factor, *Kidney Int.,* 23:624, 1983.

69. Harris, R. H., M. K. Hise, and C. F. Best: Renotrophic factors in urine, *Kidney Int.,* 23:616, 1983.

70. Pullman, T. N., A. S. Alving, R. J. Dern, and M. Landowne: The influence of dietary protein on specific renal functions in normal man, *J. Lab. Clin. Med.,* 44:320, 1954.

71. Bosch, J. P., A. Lauer, and S. Glabman: Short-term protein loading in assessment of patients with renal disease, *Am. J. Med.,* 77:873, 1984.

72. El Nahas, A. M., A. Masters-Thomas, S. A. Brady, K. Farrington, V. Wilkinson, A. J. W. Hilson, Z. Varghese, and J. F. Moorhead: Selective effect of low protein diets in chronic renal disease, *Br. Med. J.,* 289:1337, 1984.

73. ter Wee, P. M., J. B. Rosman, S. van der Geest,

W. J. Sluiter, and Ab. J. Donker: Renal hemodynamics during separation and combined infusions of amino acid and dopamine, *Kidney Int.,* 29:870, 1986.

74. Meyer, T. W., J. L. Troy, H. G. Rennke, and B. M. Brenner: Prevention of glomerular injury by pituitary ablation in rats with reduced nephron number (abstract), *Kidney Int.,* 25:250, 1984.

75. Castellino, P., B. Coda, and R. A. DeFronzo: Effect of amino acid infusion on renal hemodynamics in humans, *Am. J. Physiol.,* 251:F132, 1986.

76. Premen, A. J., J. E. Hall, and M. J. Smith, Jr.: Postprandial regulation of renal hemodynamics: Role of pancreatic glucagon, *Am. J. Physiol.,* 248:F656, 1985.

77. Hirschberg, R., K. Kleinman, R. J. Glassock, and J. D. Kopple: Effect of arginine infusion on renal plasma flow and GFR in normal and growth hormone deficient man (abstract), *Kidney Int.,* 29:190, 1986.

78. Brezis, M., P. Silva, and F. H. Epstein: Amino acids induce renal vasodilation in isolated perfused kidney: Coupling to oxidative metabolism, *Am. J. Physiol.,* 247:H999, 1984.

79. Baines, A. D., P. Ho, and H. James: Metabolic control of renal vascular resistance and glomerulotubular balance, *Kidney Int.,* 27:848, 1985.

80. Gottschalk, C. W.: Function of the chronically diseased kidney: The adaptive nephron, *Circ. Res.,* 28(suppl. I): I-1, 1971.

81. Bhathena, D. B., B. A. Julian, R. G. McMorrow, and R. W. Baehler: Focal sclerosis of hypertrophied glomeruli in solitary functioning kidneys of humans, *Am. J. Kid. Dis.,* 5:226, 1985.

82. Baldwin, D. S.: Chronic glomerulonephritis: Nonimmunologic mechanisms of progressive glomerular damage, *Kidney Int.,* 21:109, 1982.

83. Baldwin, D. S.: Poststreptococcal glomerulonephritis: A progressive disease?, *Am. J. Med.,* 62:1, 1977.

84. Senkkjian, H. O., B. J. Stinebaugh, C. A. Mattioli, and W. N. Suki: Irreversible renal failure following vesicoureteral reflux, *J. Am. Med. Assoc.,* 241:160, 1979.

85. Cotran, R. S.: Glomerulosclerosis in reflux nephropathy, *Kidney Int.,* 21:528, 1982.

86. Bhathena, D. B., J. H. Weiss, N. H. Holland, R. G. McMorrow, J. J. Curtis, B. A. Lucas, and R. G. Luke: Focal and segmental glomerulosclerosis in reflux nephropathy, *Am. J. Med.,* 68:886, 1980.

87. Kincaid-Smith, P.: Glomerular and vascular lesions in chronic atrophic pyelonephritis and reflux nephropathy, *Adv. Nephrol.,* 5:3, 1975.

88. Kincaid-Smith, P.: Analgesic abuse and the kidney, *Kidney Int.,* 17:250, 1980.

89. Bürgin, M., M. Schmidt, and F. Gloor: Focal segmental glomerulosclerosis in analgesic nephropathy (abstract), *Kidney Int.,* 23:900, 1983.

90. Kleinknecht, D., J. P. Grünfeld, P. C. Gomez, J. F. Moreau, and R. Garcia-Torres: Diagnostic procedures and long-term prognosis in bilateral cortical necrosis. *Kidney Int.,* 4:390, 1973.

91. Bernstein, J.: Renal hypoplasia and dysplasia, in C. M. Edelmann, Jr., J. Bernstein, A. F. Michael, and A. Spitzer (eds.), *Pediatric Kidney Disease.,* Little, Brown, Boston, 1978, p. 541.

92. McGraw, M., S. Poucell, J. Sweet, and R. Baumal: The significance of focal segmental glomerulosclerosis in oligomeganephronia. *Int. J. Ped. Nephrol.,* 5:67, 1984.

93. Kiprov, D. D., R. B. Colvin, and R. T. McCluskey: Focal and segmental glomerulosclerosis and proteinuria associated with unilateral renal agenesis, *Lab. Invest.,* 46:275, 1982.

94. Thorner, P. S., G. S. Arbus, D. S. Celermajer, and R. Baumal: Focal segmental glomerulosclerosis and progressive renal failure associated with a unilateral kidney, *Pediatrics,* 73:806, 1984.

95. Zucchelli, P., L. Cagnoli, S. Lasanova, U. Donini, and S. Pasquali: Focal glomerulosclerosis in patients with unilateral nephrectomy, *Kidney Int.,* 24:649, 1983.

96. Case Records of the Massachusetts General Hospital (Case 17-1985), *N. Engl. J. Med.,* 312:1111, 1985.

97. Hakim, R. M., R. C. Goldzer, and B. M. Brenner: Hypertension and proteinuria: Long-term sequelae of uninephrectomy in humans, *Kidney Int.,* 25:930, 1984.

98. Vincenti, F., W. J. C. Amend, Jr., G. Kaysen, N. Feduska, J. Birnbaum, R. Duca, and O. Salvatierra: Long-term renal function in kidney donors. Sustained compensatory hyperfiltration with no adverse effects, *Transplantation,* 36:626, 1983.

99. Chocair, P. R., L. B. Saldanha, A. M. Lucon, G. M. Goes, and E. Sabbaga: Long term follow up of related kidney donors. Incidence of hypertension and proteinuria, Abstracts, IXth Int. Congr. Nephrol., Los Angeles, 1984, p. 471A.

100. Parfey, P. S., D. J. Hollomby, N. J. Gilmore, J. Knaack, P. H. Schur, and R. D. Guttmann: Glomerular sclerosis in a renal isograft and identical twin donor: A family study, *Transplantation,* 38:343, 1984.

101. Rivolta, E., C. Ponticelli, E. Imbasciati, and A. Vegeto: De novo focal glomerular sclerosis in an identical twin renal transplant recipient, *Transplantation,* 35:328, 1983.

102. De Jong, P. E., and L. W. Statius van Eps: Sickle

cell nephropathy: New insights into its pathophysiology, *Kidney Int.,* 27:711, 1985.

103. Tejani, A., K. Phadke, O. Adamson, A. Nicastri, D. K. Chen, and D. Sen: Renal lesions in sickle cell nephropathy in children, *Nephron,* 39:352, 1985.

104. Pearson, J., G. Gallo, M. Gluck, and F. Axelrod: Renal disease in familial dysautonomia, *Kidney Int.,* 17:102, 1980.

105. Mogensen, C. E., and C. K. Christiansen: Predicting diabetic nephropathy in insulin-dependent patients, *N. Engl. J. Med.,* 311:89, 1984.

106. Palmer, J. H., S. L. Eversole, and T. A. Stamey: Unilateral glomerulonephritis, *Am. J. Med.,* 40:816, 1966.

107. Dikman, S. H., L. Strauss, L. J. Berman, N. S. Taylor, and J. Churg: Unilateral glomerulonephritis, *Arch. Pathol. Lab. Med.,* 100:480, 1976.

108. Berkman, J., and H. Rifkin: Unilateral nodular diabetic glomerulosclerosis (Kimmelstiel-Wilson): Report of a case, *Metabolism,* 22:715, 1973.

109. Anderson, S., and B. M. Brenner: Effects of aging on the renal glomerulus, *Am. J. Med.,* 80:435, 1986.

110. Rowe, J. W., R. Andres, J. D. Tobin, A. H. Norris, and N. W. Shock: The effect of age on creatinine clearance in man: A cross sectional and longitudinal study, *J. Gerontol.,* 31:155, 1976.

111. Kaplan, C., B. Pasternack, H. Shah, and G. Gallo: Age-related incidence of sclerotic glomeruli in human kidneys, *Am. J. Pathol.,* 80:227, 1975.

112. Couser, W. G., and M. M. Stilmant: Mesangial lesions and focal glomerular sclerosis in the aging rat, *Lab. Invest.,* 33:491, 1975.

113. Striker, G. E., R. B. Nagle, P. W. Kohnen, and E. A. Smuckler: Response to unilateral nephrectomy in old rats, *Arch. Pathol.,* 87:439, 1969.

114. Feldman, D. B., E. E. McConnell, and J. J. Knapka: Growth, kidney disease, and longevity of Syrian hamsters (Mesocricetus auratus) fed varying levels of protein, *Lab. Animal Sci.,* 32:613, 1982.

115. Spector, D., G. Hill, N. Diciani, D. Teller, and B. Sacktor: Low protein but not low phosphate diet inhibits proteinuria in aging rats (abstract), *Kidney Int.,* 27:251, 1985.

116. Lindeman, R. D., J. D. Tobin, and N. W. Shock: Association between blood pressure and rate of decline in renal function with age, *Kidney Int.,* 26:861, 1984.

117. Giordano, C.: Protein restriction in chronic renal failure, *Kidney Int.,* 22:401, 1982.

118. Maschio, G., L. Oldrizzi, N. D'Angelo, A. Valvo, E. Lupo, C. Loschiavo, A. Fabris, L. Gammaro, C. Rugiu, and G. Panzetta: Effects of dietary protein and phosphorus restriction on the progression of early renal failure, *Kidney Int.,* 22:371, 1982.

119. Mitch, W. E., M. Walser, T. I. Steinman, S. Hill, S. Zeger, and K. Tungsanga: The effects of a keto acid-amino acid supplement to a restricted diet on the progression of chronic renal failure, *N. Engl. J. Med.,* 311:623, 1984.

120. Oldrizzi, L., C. Rugiu, E. Valvo, A. Lupo, C. Loschiavo, L. Gammaro, N. Tessitore, A. Fabris, G. Panzetta, and G. Maschio: Progression of renal failure in patients with renal disease of diverse etiology on protein-restricted diet, *Kidney Int.,* 27: 553, 1985.

121. Gretz, N., E. Korb, and M. Strauch: Low-protein diet supplemented by ketoacids in chronic renal failure: A prospective controlled study, *Kidney Int.,* 24(suppl. 16):S-263, 1983.

122. Rosman, J. B., P. M. ter Wee, S. Meiser, T. Ph. M. Piers-Brecht, W. J. Sluiter, and Ab. J. M. Donker: Prospective randomized trial of early dietary protein restriction in chronic renal failure, *Lancet,* 2: 1291, 1984.

123. Bennett, S. E., G. I. Russell, and J. Walls: Low protein diets in uraemia, *Br. Med. J.,* 287:1344, 1983.

124. Maroni, B. J., T. I. Steinman, and W. E. Mitch: A method for estimating nitrogen intake of patients with chronic renal failure, *Kidney Int.,* 27:58, 1985.

125. Kaysen, G. A., J. Gambertoglio, I. Jimenez, H. Jones, and F. N. Hutchison: Effect of dietary protein intake on albumin homeostasis in nephrotic patients, *Kidney Int.,* 29:572, 1986.

126. van der Meulen, J., L. Gooren, and P. L. Oe: Low-protein diet increases serum albumin by decreasing proteinuria in some nephrotic patients (abstract), *Kidney Int.,* 28:299, 1985.

127. Zeller, K. R., P. Raskin, J. Rosenstock, and H. Jacobson: The effect of dietary protein restriction in diabetic nephropathy: Reduction in proteinuria (abstract), *Kidney Int.,* 29:209, 1986.

128. Moyer, J. H., C. Heider, K. Pevey, and R. V. Ford: The effect of treatment on the vascular deterioration associated with hypertension, with particular emphasis on renal function, *Am. J. Med.,* 24:177, 1958.

129. Mroczek, W. J., M. Davidov, L. Gavrilovich, and F. A. Finnerty, Jr.: The value of aggressive therapy in the hypertensive patient with azotemia, *Circulation,* 40:893, 1969.

130. Nabel, E. G., A. Kugelmass, G. Zins, E. Phipps, and V. J. Dzau: Does blood pressure control alter renal function in refractory hypertension, *Circulation,* 70 (suppl. II):II-213, 1984.

131. Woods, J. W., and W. B. Blythe: Management of malignant hypertension complicated by renal insufficiency, *N. Engl. J. Med.,* 277:57, 1967.

132. Mogensen, C. E.: Long-term antihypertensive treatment inhibiting progression of diabetic nephropathy, *Br. Med. J.,* 285:685, 1982.

133. Parving, H-H., U. M. Smidt, A. R. Andersen, and P. A. Svendsen: Early aggressive antihypertensive treatment reduces rate of decline in kidney function in diabetic nephropathy, *Lancet,* 1:1175, 1983.

134. Parving, H-H., A. R. Andersen, E. Hommel, and U. Smidt: Effects of long-term antihypertensive treatment on kidney function in diabetic nephropathy, *Hypertension,* 7(suppl. II):II-114, 1985.

135. Steno Study Group: Effect of 6 months of strict metabolic control on eye and kidney function in insulin-dependent diabetics with background retinopathy, *Lancet,* 1:121, 1982.

136. Viberti, G. C., R. W. Bilous, D. Mackintosh, J. J. Bending, and H. Keen: Long term correction of hyperglycaemia and progression of renal failure in insulin dependent diabetes, *Br. Med. J.,* 286:598, 1983.

137. Churchill, D. N., and D. W. Taylor: Thiazides for patients with recurrent calcium stones: Still an open question, *J. Urol.,* 133:749, 1985.

138. Zatz, R., T. W. Meyer, J. L. Noddin, A. W. Nunn, J. L. Troy, and B. M. Brenner: Dietary protein restriction limits glomerular hyperfiltration in experimental diabetes (abstract), *Kidney Int.,* 25:255, 1984.

139. Berlinger, W. G., G. D. Park, and R. Spector: The effect of dietary protein on the clearance of allopurinol and oxypurinol, *N. Engl. J. Med.,* 313:771, 1985.

140. Ibels, L. S., A. C. Alfrey, L. Haut, and W. E. Huffer: Preservation of function in experimental renal disease by dietary restriction of phosphate, *N. Engl. J. Med.,* 298:122, 1978.

141. Karlansky, M. L., L. Haut, B. Buddington, N. A. Schrier, and A. C. Alfrey: Preservation of renal function in experimental glomerulonephritis, *Kidney Int.,* 17:293, 1980.

142. Lumbertgul, D., T. J. Burke, D. M. Gillum, A. C. Alfrey, D. C. Harris, W. S. Hammond, and R. W. Schrier: Phosphate depletion arrests progression of chronic renal failure independent of protein intake, *Kidney Int.,* 29:658, 1986.

143. Alfrey, A. C.: Prevention of renal failure in experimental renal disease, *Am. J. Kid. Dis.,* 1:315, 1982.

144. Laouari, D., C. Kleinknecht, G. Cournot-Witmer, R. Habib, F. Mounier, and M. Broyer: Beneficial effect of a low phosphorus diet in uremic rats: A reappraisal, *Clin. Sci.,* 63:539, 1982.

145. Klahr, S., J. Buerkert, and M. L. Purkerson: Role of dietary factors in the progression of chronic renal disease, *Kidney Int.,* 24:579, 1983.

146. Harter, H. R., A. Mercado, W. E. Rutherford, H. Rodriguez, E. Slatopolsky, and S. Klahr: Effects of phosphate depletion and parathyroid hormone on renal glucose reabsorption, *Am. J. Physiol.,* 227:1422, 1974.

147. Velosa, J., K. Miller, and A. F. Michael: Immunopathology of the end-stage kidney: Immunoglobulin and complement component deposition in nonimmune disease, *Am. J. Pathol.,* 84:149, 1976.

148. Moorhead, J. F., M. K. Chan, A. M. El Nahas, and Z. Varghese: Lipid nephrotoxicity in chronic progressive glomerular and tubulo-interstitial disease. *Lancet,* 2:1309, 1982.

149. Olson, J. L.: Role of heparin as a protective agent following reduction of renal mass, *Kidney Int.,* 25:376, 1984.

150. Purkerson, M. L., J. H. Joist, J. M. Greenberg, D. Day, P. E. Hoffsten, and S. Klahr: Inhibition by anticoagulant drugs of the progressive hypertension and uremia associated with renal infarction in rats, *Thromb. Res.,* 26:227, 1982.

151. Purkerson, M. L., J. H. Joist, J. Yates, and S. Klahr: Role of hypertension and coagulation in the glomerulopathy of rats with subtotal renal ablation, Abstracts, IXth Int. Congr. Nephrol., Los Angeles, 1984, p. 359A.

152. Vanrenterghem, Y., L. Roels, B. Van Damme, and P. Michielsen: Influence of indomethacin treatment on the spontaneous glomerulosclerosis of the rat (abstract), *Kidney Int.,* 16:659, 1979.

153. Shemesh, O., J. C. Ross, W. M. Deen, G. W. Grant, and B. D. Myers: Nature of the glomerular capillary injury in human membranous nephropathy, *J. Clin. Invest.,* 77:868, 1986.

154. Velosa, J. A., V. E. Torres, J. V. Donadio, Jr., R. D. Wagoner, K. E. Holley, and K. P. Offord: Treatment of severe nephrotic syndrome with meclofenamate: An uncontrolled pilot study, *Mayo Clinic Proc.,* 60:586, 1985.

5

PATHOGENESIS, CLINICAL MANIFESTATIONS, AND DIAGNOSIS OF GLOMERULAR DISEASE

Burton D. Rose

Glomerular disease is the most common cause of chronic end-stage renal failure. It is not, however, a uniform problem since the different glomerular diseases have varying prognoses and responses to therapy. As a result, establishment of the correct diagnosis is extremely important. This is usually achieved by percutaneous renal biopsy. Examination of the renal tissue by light, immunofluorescent, and electron microscopy then allows disorders previously grouped under the general heading of "glomerulonephritis" to be separated into specific entities.

The different glomerular diseases are defined primarily by their morphologic changes. Thus, this chapter will first review normal glomerular anatomy, the types of histologic changes that can occur, and the pathophysiologic mechanisms responsible for glomerular damage. This will be followed by an approach to the clinical presentation, classification, and diagnosis of glomerular disease. The individual disorders will then be discussed in the next chapter.

GENERAL CONSIDERATIONS

NORMAL GLOMERULAR ANATOMY AND FUNCTION

The *glomerulus* is a tuft of branching capillaries interposed between two arterioles—the afferent and efferent arterioles. The capillary tufts are arranged in lobules and supported by a stalk consisting of mesangial cells and their basement membrane-like extracellular matrix (Fig. 5-1). In general, there are 2 to 3 mesangial cells in the central region of each lobule, separated from one another by the mesangial matrix.

The capillary wall, through which the filtrate must pass, is composed of three layers (Fig. 5-2): the inner, fenestrated endothelial cell; the glomerular basement membrane (GBM); and the outer epithelial cell, which is attached to the basement membrane by discrete cytoplasmic extensions, the foot processes. The foot processes are separated by narrow slit pores closed by a thin membrane, the slit diaphragm.

The major function of the glomerulus is to allow the filtration of small solutes (such as sodium and urea) and water. The combination of the high rate of renal blood flow and the relatively high permeability of the glomerular capillary wall results in an ultrafiltrate of plasma entering Bowman's space and then the proximal tubule at a rate of approximately 100 to 125 mL/min in normal adults.[1]

Small solutes cross the glomerulus easily, passing through the GBM and then the slit pores between the epithelial cell foot processes.[2] In comparison, there is a progressive restriction on the passage of larger molecules, such as albumin (Fig. 5-3). This is physiologically important in that it prevents the loss of these macromolecules in the urine. When glomerular permeability is abnormally increased in the nephrotic syndrome, for example, the loss of albumin can lead to hypoalbuminemia, edema, and hy-

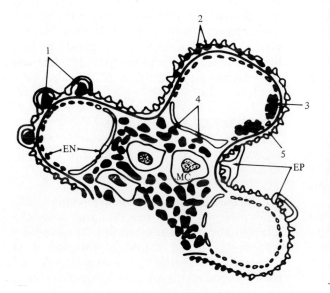

FIG. 5-1. Schematic depiction of the anatomy of the glomerulus and possible intraglomerular sites of immune complex deposition. A glomerular lobule is shown with three capillary loops on the periphery and the mesangium containing both mesangial matrix and mesangial cells (MC) in the center. Basement membrane surrounds both the loops and part of the mesangium, while some parts of the mesangium are separated from the capillary lumen only by the fenestrated endothelial cells (EN). The epithelial cells (EP) with their foot processes are on the outer aspect of the capillary loop.

Immune complexes can deposit in the subepithelial space between the epithelial cell and the basement membrane) in postinfectious glomerulonephritis (1) or membranous nephropathy (2), in the subendothelial space (between the endothelial cell and the basement membrane) (3), or in the mesangium (4). Anti-GBM antibodies also can deposit on the glomerular basement membrane itself (5) (see Fig. 5-5). (*Adapted from W. G. Couser, Kidney Int., 28:569, 1985. Reprinted by permission from Kidney International.*)

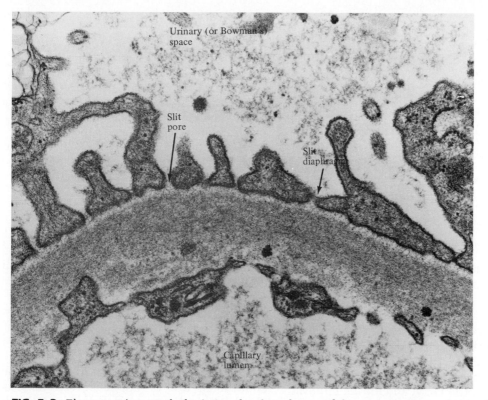

FIG. 5–2. Electron micrograph depicting the three layers of the normal glomerular capillary wall: fenestrated endothelial cell, basement membrane, and epithelial cell with foot processes. The foot processes are separated by slit pores, which are closed by a thin membrane, the slit diaphragm.

perlipidemia (see "Clinical Characteristics," below).

The basement membrane appears to be the primary barrier to the filtration of larger molecules, although the slit diaphragms between the epithelial cell foot processes may play a contributory role.[3,4] The size limitation to filtration depicted in Fig. 5–3 suggests that functional pores (perhaps reflecting the molecular organization of proteins) exist within the GBM.

Molecular *charge* is also an important determinant of filtration across the GBM.[4] As illustrated in Fig. 5–3, cationic and neutral dextrans are filtered to a greater degree than anionic dextrans of similar

molecular sizes. This effect of charge is mediated by negatively charged sialoproteins and proteoglycans (such as heparan sulfate) in the GBM[4,5]; these compounds interfere with the filtration of anions (such as albumin) but facilitate the filtration of cations. For example, the filtration of anions is very limited above a molecular weight of 70,000, whereas cations may continue to be filtered at a molecular weight as high as 480,000.[6]

Both experimental and clinical observations suggest that the loss of these anionic sites is responsible for the increased filtration of albumin seen in certain glomerular diseases.[7-9] The charge properties of the GBM also may determine where immune

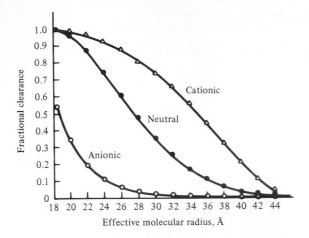

FIG. 5–3. Fractional clearances (the ratio of the filtration of a substance to that of inulin, which is freely filtered) of anionic, neutral, and cationic dextrans as a function of effective molecular radius. Both molecular size and charge are important as smaller or cationic molecules are more easily filtered. As a reference, the effective molecular radius of albumin is about 36 Å. (*From M. P. Bohrer, C. Baylis, H. D. Humes, R. J. Glassock, C. R. Robertson, and B. M. Brenner, J. Clin. Invest., 61:72, 1978, by copyright permission of the American Society for Clinical Investigation.*)

reactants are deposited, as cationic antigens or antibodies are best able to cross the GBM and accumulate in the subepithelial space (see "Pathophysiology: Immune Complex Deposition," below).

The glomerular cells also have synthetic, phagocytic, and endocrine functions. The epithelial cells are thought to be responsible for synthesis of the GBM and for the removal of macromolecules that pass through it.[10] Macromolecules (including immune complexes) that enter the capillary wall but are unable to cross the GBM localize in the mesangium. They are then phagocytosed by circulating macrophages that move in and out of the mesangium.[11,12] The resident mesangial cells, on the other hand, produce prostaglandins, a possible immunoregulatory factor, and respond to vasoactive hormones (such as angiotensin II), resulting in changes in glomerular capillary permeability and GFR.[13-15] In addition, the extraglomerular cells of the afferent arteriole produce renin.[1]

TERMINOLOGY

The terminology used to describe the different glomerular diseases is derived from the histologic changes that are found on light, electron, and immunofluorescent microscopy.

LIGHT MICROSCOPY

The light microscopy of a normal glomerulus is shown in Fig. 5–4. The capillary loops are open, the basement membrane is thin, an endothelial and/or epithelial cell may be seen with each loop, and the mesangial cells and matrix are located in the central part of the tuft. Within this framework, the following terms are used to describe the changes that may occur:

Diffuse. All glomeruli are involved to at least some degree by the pathologic process.

Focal. Only some glomeruli are affected, with others being completely or essentially normal.

Local or segmental. Only part of a glomerulus is affected by the disease process, with other segments being normal.

Global. Lesions that affect the entire capillary tuft of the involved glomeruli.

Proliferative. An increase in glomerular cellularity (excluding the infiltration of neutrophils, which is referred to as an *exudative change*). The cells that proliferate may be endocapillary (mesangial and/or

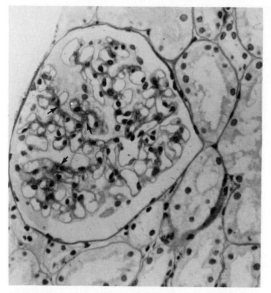

FIG. 5-4. Light microscopy of a normal glomerulus. Arrows indicate mesangial areas which are in the center of the lobules.

endothelial), extracapillary (epithelial cells of the glomerulus and Bowman's capsule), or infiltrating macrophages. Extracapillary proliferation characteristically leads to the formation of a crescentic cell mass within Bowman's space, which may ultimately compress the capillary tuft.

Membranous. An increase in the thickness of the glomerular capillary wall, frequently due to immune complex (antigen-antibody) deposition. This may be the only histologic abnormality (as in membranous nephropathy) or may be accompanied by cell proliferation (as in membranoproliferative glomerulonephritis).

Necrotizing. Death of tissue which is generally associated with the deposition of fibrinoid material (fibrinoid necrosis).

Sclerotic. A hypocellular fibrotic process that reflects scarring from previous glomerular injury.

ELECTRON MICROSCOPY

Electron microscopy is most useful in defining changes in the glomerular capillary wall. Thus, amyloid deposition, fusion of the foot processes in minimal change disease, and the location and morphology of immune complex deposits are some of the abnormalities that can be detected by this procedure. The normal appearance of the glomerular capillary wall on electron microscopy is shown in Fig. 5-2. When immune complexes are present, electron-dense deposits (which represent a large lattice of antigen and antibody molecules) may be localized at the following sites in the glomerulus (Fig. 5-5):

Subepithelial. Deposits are found between the epithelial cells and the GBM. These may be amorphous, dense deposits (also called epimembranous deposits) or semilunar humps. The latter are characteristic of postinfectious glomerulonephritis.

Subendothelial. Deposits are seen between the endothelial cell and the GBM.

Intramembranous. Deposits are located within the GBM.

Mesangial. Deposits are seen in the mesangial matrix.

The findings on electron microscopy are frequently diagnostically important since the different immunologically mediated glomerular diseases are associated with characteristic patterns of immune complex deposition (Table 5-1).

IMMUNOFLUORESCENT MICROSCOPY

That the electron-dense deposits found on electron microscopy represent aggregated immune (antigen-antibody) deposits has been confirmed by *immunofluorescence* studies.[16] By incubating the kidney tissue with fluorescein-labeled antibodies to the different immunoglobulins (IgG, IgA, IgM), components of the complement cascade (C3, C4), or

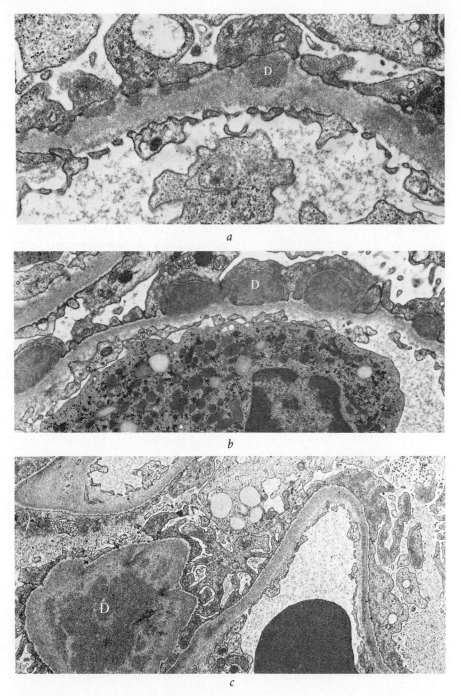

FIG. 5–5. Location of electron-dense deposits (D) on electron microscopy in different glomerular diseases. In each picture, the epithelial cell is on top and the endothelial cell on the bottom.

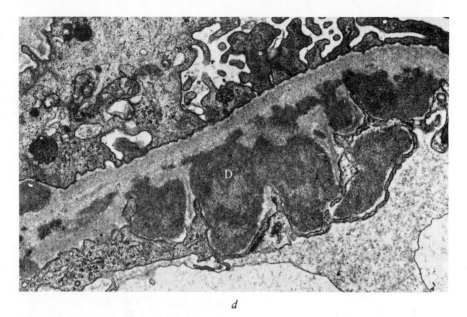

d

FIG. 5-5 (Continued). (*a*) Amorphous, subepithelial deposits in membranous nephropathy (stage I). (*b*) Subepithelial humps characteristic of postinfectious glomerulonephritis. (*c*) Mesangial, but not capillary loop, deposits in IgA nephropathy. (*d*) Subendothelial and, on the left side of the diagram, subepithelial deposits in diffuse proliferative lupus nephritis.

fibrin, the presence of these compounds in the glomerulus can be detected when the biopsy is viewed under ultraviolet light.

In patients with antigen-antibody deposition, discrete, granular ("lumpy-bumpy") deposits can be detected in the capillary wall or mesangium (Fig. 5-6*b* and *c*). Immunofluorescent microscopy has the advantage of identifying which immunoglobulins are present, a finding that may be of diagnostic importance. For example, IgA nephropathy is characterized histologically by focal or diffuse mesangial proliferation with IgA deposition in the mesangium. Although a variety of disorders have similar findings on light microscopy, only Henoch-Schönlein purpura (which is accompanied by signs of multisystem disease; see Chap. 7) also has predominant mesangial IgA deposition.[17,18]

In addition to demonstrating antibodies deposited in immune complexes, immunofluorescent microscopy can detect antibodies directed against antigens in the GBM. These antibodies tend to attach to the GBM in a diffuse, uniform manner, resulting in the deposition of IgG (and frequently C3) in a linear pattern (Fig. 5-6*a*). This is in contrast to the granular pattern observed with disorders mediated by immune complexes.

Immunofluorescence techniques have also been used in selected patients to detect the antigenic component of the deposited complexes. Included in this group are DNA (in lupus), hepatitis B virus, and bacterial antigens.

TABLE 5-1. Location of Electron-Dense Deposits in Glomerular Disease

Subepithelial
  Amorphous (epimembranous) deposits
    Membranous nephropathy
    Systemic lupus erythematosus
  Humps
    Acute postinfectious glomerulonephritis, e.g., poststreptococcal, bacterial endocarditis
Intramembranous
  Membranous nephropathy
  Membranoproliferative glomerulonephritis, type II
Subendothelial
  Systemic lupus erythematosus
  Membranoproliferative glomerulonephritis, type I
  Less commonly, bacterial endocarditis, IgA nephropathy, Henoch-Schönlein purpura, mixed cryoglobulinemia
Mesangial
  Focal glomerulonephritis
  IgA nephropathy
  Henoch-Schönlein purpura
  Systemic lupus erythematosus
  Mild or resolving acute postinfectious glomerulonephritis
Subepithelial and subendothelial
  Systemic lupus erythematosus
  Membranoproliferative glomerulonephritis, type III
  Postinfectious glomerulonephritis

PATHOPHYSIOLOGY

Although nonimmune factors are important in certain disorders (diabetes mellitus, hereditary nephritis, amyloidosis), antibody-mediated mechanisms are responsible for most glomerular diseases.[19] In the vast majority, antigen-antibody lattices form in the mesangium or the glomerular capillary wall. This may occur by the deposition of circulating immune complexes or the combination of circulating antibody with previously deposited antigen (called *in situ complex formation*).[19-21] A variety of antigens, both endogenous (DNA, tumor antigens, thyroglobulin) and exogenous (hepatitis B virus, drugs, bacteria), have been implicated in human glomerular diseases.

Less commonly (in fewer than 5 percent of cases), glomerular damage is due to the deposition of circulating antibodies directed against GBM antigens. It is also possible that cell-mediated immunity plays a role in some patients.

Much of the information concerning the manner in which immune mechanisms lead to glomerular disease has been derived from studies in experimental animals. Although it is frequently difficult to extrapolate from animal models to humans, each of the histologic patterns found in human disease has been duplicated in animals, suggesting that similar mechanisms may be involved.

IMMUNE COMPLEX DEPOSITION

The classic model of immune complex glomerulonephritis is serum sickness. If a large dose of a foreign antigen such as bovine serum albumin (BSA) is administered to a rabbit, antibodies begin to be produced in 6 to 8 days. These antibodies combine with antigen, resulting in the formation of antigen-antibody complexes in the glomerulus (and other capillaries) (Fig. 5–7). The net effect in the kidney is a diffuse proliferative glomerulonephritis, the severity of which is in part dependent on the number of complexes formed. If no further antigen is administered, the antigen is gradually removed from the circulation by antibody and the disease resolves. This sequence of an *acute,* self-limited disease is similar to that seen in humans with poststreptococcal glomerulonephritis.

However, different renal changes are seen with daily low-dose antigen administration over several weeks. In this setting of continued formation of immune complexes, a variety of *chronic* glomerular lesions may be seen, including focal or diffuse proliferation and basement membrane thickening without proliferative changes.[22,23] A human counterpart to these findings is systemic lupus erythematosus (SLE). In this disorder, circulating immune complexes (in which DNA

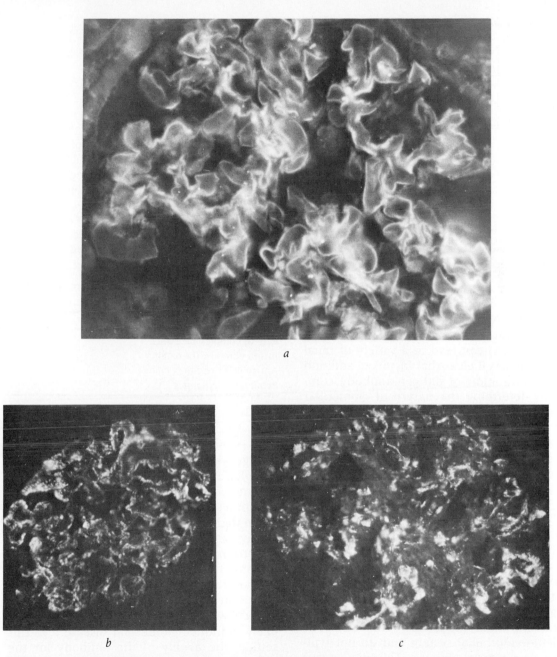

FIG. 5-6. Immunofluorescence patterns in immunologic glomerular diseases. (*a*) Linear deposition of IgG due to the presence of circulating antibodies directed against the glomerular basement membrane in Goodpasture's syndrome. (*b*) Discrete, granular deposition of IgG throughout the capillary loops in membranous nephropathy. (*c*) Granular deposition of IgA essentially limited to the mesangial areas in IgA nephropathy. Capillary loops are not outlined as in (*b*).

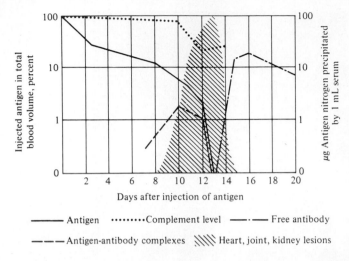

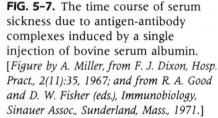

FIG. 5–7. The time course of serum sickness due to antigen-antibody complexes induced by a single injection of bovine serum albumin. [*Figure by A. Miller, from F. J. Dixon, Hosp. Pract., 2(11):35, 1967; and from R. A. Good and D. W. Fisher (eds.), Immunobiology, Sinauer Assoc., Sunderland, Mass., 1971.*]

is the primary antigen) can usually be demonstrated with focal, diffuse, or membranous changes in the glomeruli (see Chap. 6).[24]

The observation that one antigen (such as BSA or DNA) can lead to a variety of renal lesions makes it clear that factors in addition to the formation of antigen-antibody complexes determine the nature of glomerular injury. These include the characteristics of the host immune response, the rate of complex clearance, in situ complex formation, antigenic or complex charge, and renal hemodynamics (Table 5–2).[25]

HOST RESPONSE

Antigen and antibody must be delivered to the kidney to produce disease. The degree to which this occurs is in part dependent upon the host response and the ensuing size of the complexes that are formed.[26-28] Very large complexes (molecular weight greater than 1.5 million) are usually removed by the reticuloendothelial system and do not typically cause renal disease. This may occur when the primary antibody is IgM* or when

*IgM is both larger than IgG (970,000 versus 150,000) and has more binding sites per molecule (10 versus 2).

TABLE 5–2. Factors Affecting Glomerular Immune Complex Deposition

Host immune response
Rate of complex clearance
In situ complex formation
Antigenic or complex charge
Renal hemodynamics

a large amount of antibody is formed to a complex antigen with multiple antigenic sites per molecule. Small complexes (molecular weight less than 400,000), which are formed when there is a weak antibody response or a relatively simple antigen, also are infrequently nephrotoxic, perhaps because they are unable to form the large antigen-antibody lattices that are required to activate complement.[28,29] Thus, an intermediate immune response, usually with mild antibody excess, is most likely to induce glomerular disease.[20] In this setting, the avidity of the antibody for the antigen is another potential determinant of the type of lesion that is produced.[30]

It is also possible that autoantibodies contribute to the development of the antigen-antibody lattice. The antibodies that are initially produced contain unique determinants within the antigen-binding region that are called *idiotypes*. As more antibodies are produced, the idiotype itself is perceived as a new antigen since it has not previously been seen by the immune system. This leads to the formation of *anti-idiotypic antibodies* that usually serve to suppress the initial immune response.[31] In animal models,[32,33] and perhaps in humans,[34] idiotype-anti-idiotype complexes can be demonstrated in the glomeruli and may contribute to further tissue damage.

Genetic and perhaps environmental factors contribute to the variability in the immune response and therefore the likelihood of developing glomerular disease.[35-37] These factors can influence multiple steps in the immunoregulatory system, including the degree to which antigens are recognized as being foreign and the magnitude of the antibody response.

Complex Clearance. The rate of complex clearance by C3b and Fc receptors on macrophages in the liver and spleen[26,35] also can affect the susceptibility to glomerular disease. Decreased complex clearance, which results in greater delivery to the kidney, has been demonstrated in a variety of disorders including SLE, vasculitis, and IgA nephropathy.[38-40] This defect may result from (1) saturation of the receptors by previously circulating complexes,[39,41] (2) *not* from an inherited abnormality in Fc or C3b receptor-mediated clearance,[42,43] or (3) *not* from a congenital deficiency in one of the complement components.[44-46] C3b, derived from activation of the classic complement pathway, normally plays an important role in *preventing* immune complex disease, both by limiting growth of the antigen-antibody lattice (thereby minimizing the formation of large precipitating complexes that are more likely to produce renal damage) and by facilitating delivery of immune complexes (in part via attachment

to C3b receptors on erythrocytes) to their site of elimination in the reticuloendothelial system.[44] As a possible example of the importance of an intact complement system, a majority of patients with C2 deficiency have an immune complex disease, most often SLE.*,[44]

Although most studies have evaluated the effect of decreased complement removal, increasing the rate of complex elimination also can influence the course of immune-mediated glomerular disease. For example, stimulation of the reticuloendothelial system with *Corynebacterium parvum* protects against BSA-induced glomerulonephritis by enhancing the removal of circulating BSA-containing immune complexes.[47]

In Situ Complex Formation. The traditional theory of immune complex glomerulonephritis presumes that complex size is an important determinant of its site of deposition within the glomeruli. Larger circulating complexes are thought to be trapped initially in the mesangium, which is separated from the capillary lumen only by the fenestrated endothelial cell (see Fig. 5-1). If a large number of complexes are deposited, the absorptive capacity of the mesangium is overwhelmed and complexes begin to accumulate in the subendothelial space (see Fig. 5-5d). According to this hypothesis, subepithelial deposits (see Fig. 5-5a and b) are likely to occur only with smaller complexes (molecular weight 400,000 to 700,000) which can pass through the GBM.[22,23]

However, this model may not be correct, particularly with regard to subepithelial

---

*It is important to recognize that the complement system has a dual role in immune-mediated glomerular diseases: it *protects* against disease by promoting the elimination of immune complexes; but, if precipitating complexes have already deposited in the kidney, it *promotes* the development of tissue injury, in part by formation of the membrane attack complex (C5b-C9) (see "Mechanisms of Glomerular Damage: Complement," below).

deposits. Although circulating immune complexes can be demonstrated in many patients with glomerular disease, these complexes are in equilibrium with free antigen and antibody:

$$\text{Antigen} + \text{antibody} \rightleftharpoons \text{antigen-antibody complex}$$

Thus, it is possible that the separate deposition in the glomeruli of antigen and antibody, rather than intact complexes, is of primary importance. In animals, for example, the injection of preformed immune complexes can lead to mesangial and subendothelial deposits but only rarely to accumulation in the subepithelial space.[21] In comparison, the separate injection of antigen (primarily if cationic; see "Antigenic Charge," below) and then antibody can readily produce subepithelial deposits.[21,48] Furthermore, the degree of glomerular damage is generally greater than that achieved by the administration of intact complexes.[21]

These findings suggest the potential importance of *in situ complex formation:* antigen either exists in or is deposited in the capillary wall and then reacts with free circulating antibody. For example, an intrinsic renal antigen (called *renal tubular epithelial antigen*) is present in the brush border of the proximal tubule and in the cell membrane of the glomerular epithelial cells along the subepithelial aspect of the GBM.[49] If antibody to this antigen is infused directly into the renal artery, subepithelial deposits can be detected within seconds in a pattern similar to membranous nephropathy in humans (Fig. 5–5a).[50] It is likely that the epithelial cell slit diaphragms prevent passage of these complexes into the urinary space.[51]

The available evidence strongly suggests that subepithelial deposits, as occur in membranous nephropathy, result primarily from in situ immune complex formation.[21] This could explain why circulating intact complexes cannot be found in most patients with this disorder.[52,53]

The same in situ mechanism can also contribute to mesangial and subendothelial deposits. This can be illustrated by the following experiment.[54] Human IgG is administered to a rabbit, some of which accumulates in the mesangium. One kidney is then transplanted into another rabbit (to make certain that no circulating antigen is present), and antibodies to human IgG are given intravenously. The result is a marked mesangioproliferative glomerulonephritis, changes that are more prominent than those induced by the infusion of intact complexes.[21] Similarly, the administration of concanavalin A (con A) a plant lectin that binds to the GBM, followed by anti-con A antibodies can lead directly to the formation of subendothelial deposits.[55]

A human equivalent to these experiments may be found in SLE. Both free DNA and free anti-DNA antibodies can be detected in the circulation in patients with this disorder.[56] Furthermore, DNA (but not the antigen-antibody complex) has a high affinity for binding to basement membranes.[57] Thus, circulating DNA could be deposited along the GBM (as well as epidermal[58] and renal tubular[59] basement membranes) and later combine with circulating antibody to produce tissue damage.

Although in situ complex formation may be the initial step in immune-mediated disease, tissue damage is produced not by single complexes but by the growth of large antigen-antibody lattices which persist in the glomerulus and active effectors such as the complement system.[29,60] The incorporation of new antigen, antibody, or anti-idiotypic antibody all contribute to expansion of the lattice.

ANTIGENIC CHARGE

As described above, the ability of a macromolecule to cross the GBM is in part related to its charge (Fig. 5–3). Charge also appears to be an important determinant of the site of immune complex deposition. In the model of BSA-induced glomerulonephritis, for example, the administration of native anionic BSA leads to immune deposits in the mesangium but generally not in the glomerular capillary wall (Fig. 5–8). Only cationic BSA, which should more easily bind to and pass through the GBM, results in the formation of subepithelial deposits (Fig. 5–8).[61-63] Sequential electron microscopic studies have shown that the combination of this antigen with circulating antibody initially occurs in the *subendothelial* space.[6,64] This complex then dissociates, with both free antigen and antibody crossing the GBM and reforming an immune complex in the *subepithelial* space. Intact complexes that are cationic can also cross the GBM,[65] but this is probably a less important mechanism.

The relevance of these findings to human disease is unproven. Membranous nephropathy and poststreptococcal glomerulonephritis are the primary human diseases associated with subepithelial deposits (Fig. 5–5*a* and *b*). In some patients with the latter disorder, a cationic streptococcal antigen has been eluted from the glomeruli and could be responsible for the development of subepithelial deposits and glomerular disease.[66] The possible role of cationic antigens in membranous nephropathy remains to be demonstrated.

RENAL HEMODYNAMICS

The predisposition of antigen and antibody to localize in the glomerulus is probably related to its high blood flow and capillary hydrostatic pressure (45 mmHg versus 17 mmHg in muscle capillaries).[1] Changes in pressure can also influence the course of the glomerular disease. In particular, hypertension exacerbates the severity of experimental immune complex glomerulonephritis,[67,68] apparently by increasing the intraglomerular pressure.[67] A probable human counterpart has been described in patients with unilateral renal artery stenosis who developed glomerulonephritis only in the nonstenotic kidney which was perfused at a higher pressure.[69] It is not known if the elevation in pressure acts by increasing immune complex deposition in the glomeruli or by potentiating the severity of tissue damage. Regardless of the mechanism, these findings have important clinical implications, since lowering the blood pressure may minimize the extent of renal injury.[70]

In addition to systemic hypertension, a primary rise in *intraglomerular* pressure also can contribute to the development of progressive renal failure in patients with glomerular disease. At the single nephron level,

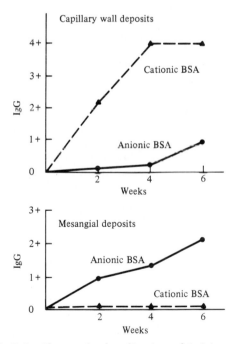

FIG. 5–8. Glomerular localization of IgG in animals receiving either anionic or cationic BSA. Capillary wall deposits, most of which were in the subepithelial space, were almost only seen with cationic BSA. (*From W. A. Border, H. J. Ward, E. S. Kamil, and A. H. Cohen, J. Clin. Invest., 69:451, 1982, by copyright permission of The American Society for Clinical Investigation.*)

the GFR may initially remain normal, even though glomerular permeability (K_f) has been reduced by the immunologic injury. This response is mediated by an increase in glomerular capillary hydrostatic pressure (the main driving force for filtration) that is induced by an unknown mechanism by afferent arteriolar dilation.[71] Similar hemodynamic changes (arteriolar dilation increasing glomerular pressure) can be induced by nephron loss (see Chap. 4). As some nephrons are damaged, other more normal nephrons hypertrophy, increasing their GFR in an attempt to maintain the total GFR. The elevation in glomerular pressure seen with reduced K_f or nephron loss is adaptive from the viewpoint of GFR but could intensify the glomerular damage. As a result, it is possible that reversing this intraglomerular hypertension by reducing the systemic blood pressure with a converting enzyme inhibitor could retard the development of progressive disease (see p. 123).

SUMMARY

The development of immune complex-mediated glomerular injury is dependent upon multiple factors. To begin with, the type and quantity of antibody produced (which is in part under genetic control) is an important determinant: glomerular disease is most likely to occur when there is an intermediate response with approximate antigen-antibody equivalence or mild antibody excess.[20] In this setting, immune complex lattices may develop by the deposition of circulating complexes or, more probably, by in situ complex formation.[21] The site of deposition within the glomerulus appears to be primarily determined by the charge on the antigen or possibly the intact complex: cationic antigen is more likely to cross the GBM, leading to subepithelial deposits; anionic antigens, on the other hand, tend to be restricted to the mesangium or subendothelial space (Fig. 5–8).[63]

The duration of antigen exposure is also important. Persistently active disease requires the continued presence of antigen and antibody. On the other hand, transient antigenemia leads to acute but short-lived glomerular injury in which the complexes are ultimately removed from viable glomeruli during the recovery phase. At least two factors appear to contribute to complex removal in this setting: activation of complement, which releases small soluble complexes from the lattice, and subsequent phagocytosis of these small complexes by infiltrating macrophages and neutrophils.[12,44,45]

ANTIBODY AGAINST GBM

Glomerular damage due to circulating antibodies to GBM antigens (another form of in situ complex formation) has been demonstrated in both experimental animals and humans.[72,73] This disorder is usually characterized by rapidly progressive renal failure, epithelial crescent formation on light microscopy, linear deposition of IgG and C3 on immunofluorescent microscopy* (Fig. 5–6a), and circulating antibodies to the GBM.[73]

Antibody charge also may be important in this setting. Cationic antibodies bind more avidly to the negatively charged GBM antigens and produce more severe disease.[76]

CELL-MEDIATED GLOMERULAR DISEASE

Although experimental models of cell-mediated (delayed hypersensitivity) glomerular

---

*Diffuse linear deposition of IgG is not specific for anti-GBM disease since it has been demonstrated in several other renal disorders, particularly diabetes mellitus.[74,75] In these settings, however, circulating anti-GBM antibodies are absent, IgG eluted from the glomeruli does not bind to the GBM when incubated with normal renal tissue, and albumin is also frequently deposited in a linear fashion. These findings suggest that the linear deposition of IgG in these disorders merely represents nonspecific protein absorption onto an abnormally permeable GBM.

disease have been described,[77,78] the clinical applicability of these findings is unclear since lymphocytic infiltration in the glomerulus is an unusual finding in humans. It is possible, however, that activated T cells against glomerular-bound antigen are present very early in the disease, a time at which renal biopsy is not performed.[79] These T cells could release lymphokines that promote the accumulation of macrophages, which then produce further glomerular damage.[79,80] Minimizing T-cell activation with cyclosporine in this setting can attenuate macrophage infiltration and glomerular injury without affecting the degree of immune complex deposition.[79,80] These experiments suggest that cell-mediated immunity may be substantially more important than previously considered.

Lymphokines can also contribute to glomerular disease by other mechanisms. In minimal change disease, for example, a lymphokine-mediated increase in glomerular permeability may be responsible for the proteinuria.[81]

MECHANISMS OF GLOMERULAR DAMAGE

Although immune complexes alone may be sufficient to cause damage in some forms of glomerular disease,[82,83] animal models generally indicate that mediators activated by antigen-antibody complexes or perhaps T cells are of primary importance in the associated glomerular damage (Table 5–3). Their role has been proven experimentally

TABLE 5–3. Mediators of Glomerular Damage

Complement
Neutrophils
Macrophages
Platelets
Vasoactive amines
Fibrin
Lymphokines

by beneficial therapeutic results obtained from antagonizing the specific mediator. The correlation with human disease is less certain, but the same therapeutic modalities (corticosteroids, cyclophosphamide, anticoagulants) have been effective in some diseases.

COMPLEMENT

In both immune complex and anti-GBM disease, complement tends to be deposited along with immunoglobulins. This can occur by activation via either the classic or alternate pathway (Fig. 5–9). The complement components can contribute to glomerular damage in several ways:[84]

1. The formation of C5b-C9, the membrane attack complex, is probably most important.[84] This complex can produce damage in part by causing mesangial cells and perhaps infiltrating macrophages to release toxic oxygen radicals and interleukin 1.[84,87] The membrane attack complex has been identified in proliferative disorders such as SLE[88] and in membranous nephropathy, where it may be responsible for the proteinuria since there is little if any cell proliferation or neutrophilic infiltration.[89,90]
2. C3a and C5a have chemotactic activity, promoting the local accumulation of neutrophils and macrophages.
3. C3a and C5a also increase vascular permeability (anaphylatoxin activity), which can facilitate further immune complex deposition and possibly contribute to the development of proteinuria.

Although complement seems to play an important role in almost all immunologically mediated glomerular diseases, the contribution of the other mediators in Table 5–3 is variable. This may in large part reflect the *site of formation* of the antigen-antibody complex.[91] Complexes in the mesangium or subendothelial space (due, for example, to anionic or large antigens that cannot cross

CLASSIC PATHWAY

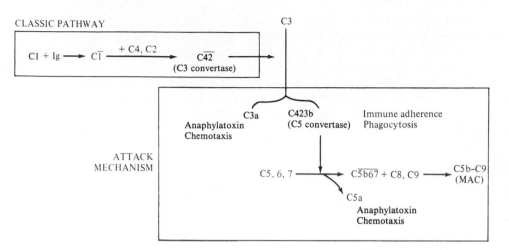

ATTACK
MECHANISM

ALTERNATE PATHWAY

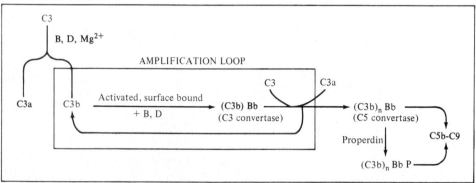

FIG. 5–9. Sequence of complement activation and effects of the activated complement components in the classic and alternate pathways. Activated products are indicated by an overbar, while fragments from enzymatic cleavage are indicated by small letters (C3 is cleaved to C3a + C3b). In the classic pathway, C1 is bound to the Fc receptor on the immunoglobulin (IgG) and reacts with C4 and then C2.[84] These components are cleaved, resulting in the formation of C42, a *C3 convertase* which cleaves C3 into two components, C3a and C3b. The latter combines with the C3 convertase to form C423b, a *C5 convertase* which activates the remaining components of the complement cascade, leading to the production of C5b-C9, the membrane attack complex (MAC).

In the alternate pathway, C3 is cleaved by factors B, D, and magnesium, independent of C1, C4, and C2.[84–86] The C3b that is formed is rapidly inactivated unless it is bound by, for example, the cell surface of a microorganism, damaged renal tissue, or IgA. The bound C3b combines with factor B, which is then cleaved by factor D to form C3bBb, the *C3 convertase* of the alternate pathway. This convertase produces further breakdown of C3, leading to a self-perpetuating cycle known as the amplification loop. As more C3b is generated, $(C3b)_nBb$ is produced, a *C5 convertase* that activates C5 to C9. Properdin contributes to this process by binding to the C3 and C5 convertases, thereby minimizing their inactivation.[84]

the GBM) are in relatively close contact with the circulation. Thus, activation of complement can lead to infiltration of neutrophils and macrophages, resulting in potentially severe glomerular damage. In comparison, subepithelial deposits (as in membranous nephropathy) are separated from the circulation by the GBM. In this setting, complement-mediated injury produces proteinuria,[89,90] but there is little cellular proliferation or involvement of other mediators.

The one apparent exception to this model occurs in postinfectious glomerulonephritis in which there is marked cellular proliferation and neutrophilic infiltration but usually only subepithelial deposits on electron microscopy (see Fig. 5–5b). There is evidence, however, that complexes in this disorder initially form in the sub*endo*thelial space before dissociating and crossing the GBM.[92]

NEUTROPHILS

Complement-mediated neutrophil accumulation can cause glomerular damage by the release of proteolytic enzymes and the formation of highly reactive hydroxyl radicals (OH).[93] The ensuing tissue injury can then activate other mediators such as macrophages and platelets which are responsible for perpetuating the glomerular disease. Neutrophils appear to be particularly important in experimental anti-GBM antibody disease[94–96] and in poststreptococcal glomerulonephritis in which prominent neutrophilic accumulation is commonly present. In the latter setting, occlusion of the capillary loops by the white cells can also contribute to the fall in GFR.[95]

MACROPHAGES

Infiltration of circulating macrophages occurs in a variety of experimental and human renal diseases.[96–101] Complement-mediated chemotaxis, attachment to the Fc receptor on immunoglobulins, or chemotaxis by thrombin or tissue breakdown products all

may contribute to this process. In experimental anti-GBM disease, for example, neutrophils are responsible for the initial glomerular damage, followed by the influx of macrophages at a time when neutrophils can no longer be found.[102] These macrophages can then release damaging proteolytic enzymes or soluble factors that can promote cellular proliferation or the formation of fibrin.[100,103,104]

PLATELETS AND VASOACTIVE AMINES

Increased platelet consumption has been demonstrated in a variety of glomerular diseases.[*,105–107] The local adherence and aggregation of platelets can be initiated by several mechanisms, including basement membrane damage induced by one of the above mediators or the release of soluble factors from infiltrating basophils.[108] These platelets can then contribute to the disease process by releasing vasoactive amines (such as serotonin and histamine) which enhance glomerular permeability, by releasing growth factors that promote cellular proliferation, or by activating the clotting system.[105] In addition, platelets secrete cationic proteins which can bind avidly to the anionic GBM.[109] The ensuing partial neutralization of the membrane's charge barrier could then facilitate immune complex deposition in the capillary wall.[110]

FIBRIN

Fibrin deposition also occurs in a variety of glomerular disorders.[111–113] It can contribute to the disease process either by forming thrombi[114] or by promoting the development of crescents (see p. 256).

Although the pathogenetic contribution of fibrin is well defined in certain disorders,

---

*Glomerular platelet and/or fibrin deposition also occurs in coagulopathies such as thrombotic thrombocytopenic purpura and in primary vascular diseases such as scleroderma or malignant nephrosclerosis. These disorders are discussed in Chaps. 7 and 11.

the mechanism of fibrin formation is less clear. Immunofluorescence studies in patients with crescentic glomerulonephritis have revealed glomerular deposition of fibrin but not factor VIII,[113] suggesting that fibrin may be formed without activation of the intrinsic clotting pathway. Also consistent with this possibility is the observation in experimental immune complex or anti-GBM disease that the administration of heparin does not prevent glomerular fibrin deposition.[115] One potential mechanism for this atypical fibrin formation is the release of procoagulant material from activated macrophages. Both a thromboplastin and a prothrombinase have been described, either of which could result in fibrin formation independent of factor VIII.[103,104]

THERAPEUTIC IMPLICATIONS

Knowledge of the factors which produce glomerular damage is clinically important since they can be affected to varying degrees by the drugs used to treat human glomerulopathies (see individual diseases in the next chapter). Corticosteroids, for instance, have multiple actions which could account for their beneficial effects in certain glomerular disorders. These include: (1) decreased release by macrophages of interleukin 1, the substance which activates helper T cells; (2) decreased accumulation of neutrophils at inflammatory sites because of reduced adherence to the vascular wall; and (3) decreased number of circulating monocytes/macrophages and lymphocytes due to redistribution into the bone marrow and lymph nodes.[116,117] The immunosuppressive agent cyclophosphamide also reduces the number of circulating lymphocytes, although by direct cellular toxicity not redistribution.[118,119]

Exactly how these drugs act in human disease is uncertain. The corticosteroid-induced reduction in circulating macrophages may be very important in those proliferative disorders in which macrophage accumulation is primarily responsible for glomerular damage.[96,120] Corticosteroids and cyclophosphamide are also very effective in minimal change disease, a disorder in which there is little or no cellular proliferation but in which abnormal T-cell function may be the major abnormality.[81] In this setting, the ability of these drugs to decrease T-cell number and function may account for the beneficial therapeutic result.

Atypical fibrin formation independent of the intrinsic clotting pathway may explain the variable and generally disappointing results with heparin or warfarin in both experimental and human forms of glomerular disease.[112,115,121-125] In comparison, directly preventing fibrin deposition by defibrination with pit-viper venom is much more effective than heparin in animals[125,126] and, in preliminary studies, may be beneficial in humans.[127] Antiplatelet agents have been used less extensively but may be effective in membranoproliferative glomerulonephritis, a disorder in which platelet consumption is enhanced.[107]

CLINICAL CHARACTERISTICS

The presence of a glomerular disease is frequently discovered incidentally by the finding of an abnormal urinalysis or an elevated plasma creatinine concentration (P_{cr}). In addition, patients may present with one or more of the following: edema, hypertension, gross hematuria, diminished urine output, or symptoms resulting from severe hypertension, uremia, or an associated underlying disease such as SLE, diabetes mellitus, or amyloidosis.

URINALYSIS

The urinary findings in glomerular diseases are variable, ranging from normal (seen primarily in subclinical disease)[128] to isolated hematuria or proteinuria (see Chap. 2) to a urinalysis in which proteinuria, hematuria, pyuria, lipiduria, and red cell and other casts all may be observed. The severity of these changes is also variable since hematuria can be either microscopic or grossly visible and the degree of proteinuria can range from just above normal (more than 150 mg/day) to greater than 20 g/day. The only changes that are generally diagnostic of glomerular disease (or vasculitis) are dysmorphic red cells (see Plates 1*a* and 1*b*),[129,130] red cell casts, daily protein excretion exceeding 3.5 g (or 50 mg/kg), and lipiduria (see Chap. 1).

Increased glomerular permeability is largely responsible for these urinary abnormalities. Focal disruptions in the capillary wall induced by the underlying disease process can allow the passage of normally nonfiltered red cells and white cells.[131] This form of damage also creates larger "pores" that permit the filtration of albumin and larger proteins such as IgG.[7,132] In addition, loss of the anionic charge barrier in the GBM (see Fig. 5–3) can also contribute to the development of proteinuria, particularly in minimal change disease.[7-9] These defects in glomerular function may be associated with the filtration of lipoproteins as well, leading to the appearance of free fat droplets, oval fat bodies, and fatty casts in the urine sediment (see p. 23).[133]

GLOMERULAR FILTRATION RATE

The glomerular filtration rate is variable in patients with glomerular disease. The initial glomerular injury primarily lowers the permeability coefficient (K_f) of the glomerular basement membrane, by reducing the surface area available for filtration and/or the unit permeability of the membrane.[*,134-137]

---

*It may seem contradictory to say that a low K_f is responsible for a decrease in GFR at the same time that an increase in glomerular permeability accounts for the

Despite this abnormality, the total GFR may, in the early stages, remain within or near the normal range because the low K_f is counteracted by an elevation in the glomerular capillary hydrostatic pressure (the main driving force for filtration).[135] Both afferent arteriolar dilation (which allows more of the systemic pressure to be transmitted to the glomerulus) and efferent arteriolar constriction (which raises the glomerular pressure by impairing flow into the efferent arteriole) appear to contribute to this response. These changes in resistance are mediated in part by angiotensin II and prostaglandins, although it is unclear how these humoral mechanisms are activated.[138] In addition, increased filtration in relatively unaffected glomeruli[136] also can maintain the GFR (see Chap. 4). The net effect is that *substantial glomerular damage can occur before the total GFR falls.* In this setting in which the P_{cr} will be unchanged, more prominent urinary abnormalities (such as increasing proteinuria) or the development of hypertension may be the only clues to the presence of progressive disease. With more severe disease, cell swelling or proliferation, fibrin deposition, and fibrosis during the healing phase all may contribute to a decrease in total GFR by further reducing the K_f and ultimately glomerular perfusion.

It should be remembered that an elevation in the P_{cr} may be due to some superimposed, potentially reversible process rather than progression of the glomerular disease. One common setting in which this may occur is with the use of diuretics to treat nephrotic edema. The combination of fluid removal plus hypoalbuminemia can lead to

---

presence of proteinuria. However, glomerular damage leading to a *reduction in the surface area available for filtration* will diminish the filtration of small solutes and water. At the same time, the *loss of negative charges in the capillary wall or the creation of abnormally large pores in the basement membrane* will allow the passage of normally poorly filtered macromolecules such as albumin.

plasma volume depletion and prerenal disease.[139,140]

EDEMA

Renal sodium and water retention leading to edema is a common occurrence in glomerular disease and may be produced by three different mechanisms. First, acute glomerular disease is characterized by a variable reduction in GFR but initially normal tubular function. As a result, these patients behave as if they have prerenal disease with enhanced tubular sodium and water reabsorption.[141-143] The ensuing decrease in sodium excretion will lead to edema if sodium intake is not restricted. However, edema is not a part of mild to moderate *chronic* glomerulonephritis (in the absence of the nephrotic syndrome or another edematous state such as heart failure). The maintenance of sodium balance in this setting is due to the presence of factors leading to decreased tubular sodium reabsorption such as tubular damage[142] and perhaps a natriuretic hormone.[144]

Second, fluid retention may be directly due to the low GFR in patients with end-stage renal failure. In this setting, the factors that reduce tubular reabsorption are unable to counteract the effect of the markedly reduced GFR.

Third, edema can be induced by hypoalbuminemia. In this setting, it has been presumed that hypoalbuminemia causes fluid to move from the vascular space into the interstitium, leading to plasma volume depletion which then promotes renal sodium and water retention.[139] However, this explanation is incomplete as some concurrent intrarenal defect such as a low GFR appears to be required for maximum fluid retention to occur.[143,145-148] This can be illustrated by serial studies in patients with minimal change disease undergoing corticosteroid-induced correction of the glomerular le-

sion.[146] In this setting, sodium retention *can be dissociated from hypoalbuminemia* as a diuresis, leading to partial resolution of the edema, occurs before any elevation in the plasma albumin concentration.

The clinical consequences of the edema formation are variable. With the first two mechanisms (increased tubular reabsorption and low GFR), the excess fluid expands the plasma volume and can produce both peripheral and pulmonary edema. As a result, removal of sodium and water with diuretics lowers the plasma volume toward normal, leading to symptomatic improvement without further reducing renal function.

In contrast, the plasma volume is usually normal (due in part to the compensatory sodium and water retention) when hypoalbuminemia is the primary problem.[147-149] Although gradual fluid removal is generally well tolerated,[148] the use of diuretics to remove all the edema fluid can occasionally produce plasma volume depletion and a reduction in GFR, particularly in patients with minimal change disease who have a plasma albumin concentration under 2.0 g/dL.[139,140,150] Thus, the blood urea nitrogen (BUN) and P_{cr} should be monitored as fluid is removed and diuretics discontinued if renal function deteriorates.

Although hypoalbuminemia alone can cause peripheral edema, pulmonary edema is rare.[151] This difference is due to the relatively high permeability of the pulmonary capillary wall, which allows some plasma proteins to enter the pulmonary interstitium. As a result, the importance of the plasma oncotic pressure (26 mmHg) in keeping fluid in the vascular space is diminished because it is partially counterbalanced by the pulmonary interstitial oncotic pressure (approximately 16 mmHg versus only 5 to 6 mmHg in the skeletal muscle capillary which is less permeable to macromolecules).[152] As hypoalbuminemia develops, the plasma and pulmonary interstitial oncotic pressures fall in parallel, producing little tendency toward edema.[151]

HYPERTENSION

Both volume and vasoconstrictor factors may participate in the hypertension that frequently accompanies glomerular disease. In acute disease, the elevation in blood pressure is primarily due to volume expansion as the level of vasoconstrictors (such as the renin-angiotensin system) is relatively low.[153,154] As a result, removal of the excess fluid with diuretics or dialysis usually lowers the blood pressure, frequently into the normal range.

The role of volume expansion (usually manifested by edema) may be of diagnostic importance. In a patient with apparent acute glomerulonephritis (by history and urinalysis), marked hypertension without edema suggests a different diagnosis: renin-mediated hypertension due to a vascular disease such as systemic vasculitis or the hemolytic-uremic syndrome.[154,155]

With chronic glomerular disease, factors in addition to hypervolemia may contribute. In particular, the activity of the renin-angiotensin system is frequently elevated, probably due to regional ischemia induced by scarring.[156] Increased activity of the sympathetic nervous system also may be important.[157] How this might occur is not known.

NEPHROTIC SYNDROME

The *nephrotic syndrome* is simply defined as the urinary excretion of more than 3.5 g or 50 mg/kg of protein per day* (excluding low-molecular-weight proteins such as immunoglobulin light chains). Although this may seem like an arbitrary dividing line, this

degree of proteinuria is virtually diagnostic of primary glomerular disease (or, less commonly, vasculitis), whereas a lower rate of protein excretion may be seen with many nonglomerular diseases and is therefore of lesser diagnostic importance. In addition, the other findings characteristic of the nephrotic syndrome (hypoalbuminemia, edema, hyperlipidemia, and a hypercoagulable state) are usually not seen with milder degrees of proteinuria.

The quantity of protein excreted varies directly with the GFR and plasma albumin concentration as well as glomerular permeability. Thus, protein excretion may fall below the nephrotic range if hypoalbuminemia or renal failure occurs. For example, the combination of hypoalbuminemia and mild proteinuria (1.5 to 3.5 g/day) suggests that a glomerular lesion may be present if no other cause of hypoalbuminemia such as liver disease or malnutrition is apparent. In the unusual patient in whom other signs of glomerular disease (lipiduria, dysmorphic red cells, red cell casts) are absent, the diagnosis of a glomerular lesion can be established in this setting by an intravenous infusion of albumin which will increase urinary protein excretion into the nephrotic range.[159] In addition to enhancing the load of albumin presented to the kidney (by raising the plasma albumin concentration), an albumin infusion also promotes proteinuria by exacerbating the glomerular defect in size selectivity, allowing more macromolecules to be filtered.[160] This change may be hemodynamically mediated, since the associated intravascular volume expansion raises both the glomerular capillary flow and hydrostatic pressure.

The dependence of proteinuria on the plasma albumin concentration also means

---

*Protein excretion can be quantified by a 24-h urine collection or estimated simply by measuring the protein/creatinine ratio (milligrams per milligram) in a random daytime urine specimen. This ratio correlates

closely with total protein excretion.[158] For example, a ratio of 2:1 represents protein excretion of approximately 2 g/day per 1.73 m^2 body surface area.

that patients with the same level of protein excretion do not necessarily have glomerular lesions of the same severity. Consider, for example, two patients with 5 g of proteinuria per day, one with a plasma albumin concentration of 2.5 g/dL and one with a near normal value of 3.7 g/dL. The former patient is hypoalbuminemic in part because he or she has a *much greater increase* in glomerular permeability. This could be demonstrated by the marked rise in protein excretion that would occur if the plasma albumin concentration were raised toward normal by an albumin infusion.[159]

The degree of proteinuria also varies directly with dietary protein intake. In particular, lowering protein intake in one study from 1.6 to 0.8 g/kg per day resulted in decreased proteinuria with no change in the plasma albumin concentration or total body albumin stores.[161] Although the mechanism by which this occurred is not known, it is clinically relevant since it implies that protein intake can be safely restricted in nephrotic patients in an attempt to prevent hemodynamically mediated injury and progressive renal failure (see Chap. 4).

HYPOALBUMINEMIA

The mechanism by which hypoalbuminemia develops is incompletely understood. Urinary albumin loss of as little as 3.5 g/day cannot be the whole explanation because normal subjects can increase hepatic albumin synthesis by as much as 30 g/day in the presence of a low plasma oncotic pressure.[162] As an example, patients on continuous ambulatory peritoneal dialysis lose between 4 and 5 g of albumin per day but do not become hypoalbuminemic, since hepatic albumin production is enhanced.[163] However, the plasma albumin concentration does fall in the nephrotic syndrome because the adaptive hepatic response usually does not occur as albumin synthesis is generally unchanged or only moderately elevated.[163,164] The reason for this abnormality in hepatic function is not known.[163]

In addition to the hepatic defect, it has also been proposed that the true renal albumin loss is underestimated because some of the filtered albumin is reabsorbed by and then catabolized in the proximal tubular cells, not excreted in the urine. However, this process is not likely to play a major role in most patients.[165] Nevertheless, the variability in the hepatic and renal responses to a glomerular protein leak accounts in part for the observation that there is no definite correlation between the degree of proteinuria and the fall in the plasma albumin concentration.[166]

EDEMA

The mechanism of edema formation with hypoalbuminemia is discussed above. The edema in this setting is soft, pits easily, and accumulates in dependent areas and where tissue pressure is low as in the periorbital region. Thus, the patient frequently complains of swelling of the face upon awakening and of the legs during the day. Ascites and pleural effusions also may be seen with severe hypoalbuminemia, but, as described above, pulmonary edema does not occur in the absence of heart failure or renal failure.

The degree of edema resulting from hypoalbuminemia is dependent upon two factors: the level of sodium intake and the plasma albumin concentration. Although augmented fluid movement out of the vascular space begins with the first reduction in the plasma albumin concentration, edema does not initially occur because of protective factors such as enhanced lymphatic flow, which returns the excess interstitial fluid to the circulation.[167] In general, edema does not become apparent until the plasma albumin concentration falls below 2.5 to 3.0 g/dL. Above this level, other causes of edema such as heart failure, renal failure, or inferior vena caval thrombosis (see below) should be excluded.

HYPERLIPIDEMIA

Elevations in the plasma concentrations of cholesterol, phospholipids, and triglycerides are common in nephrotic patients and are most often associated with a type IIa, IIb, or V pattern on lipoprotein electrophoresis.[166,168] (This is in contrast to chronic renal failure in which a type IV pattern is most common.)

Increased hepatic synthesis of very low density lipoproteins, some of which are then converted to low density lipoproteins (the major carrier of plasma cholesterol), appears to be the primary abnormality.[169,170] The mechanism by which this occurs is not well understood. It has been suggested that the low plasma oncotic pressure stimulates lipoprotein synthesis by the hepatocyte.[171] It is of interest in this regard that patients with the rare syndrome of congenital analbuminemia have similar disturbances in lipid metabolism.[172] In both the nephrotic syndrome and analbuminemia, raising the plasma oncotic pressure toward normal with albumin or dextran infusions rapidly lowers the plasma cholesterol concentration toward normal.[172-174]

An additional abnormality, decreased chylomicron removal, appears to be present in those patients with type V hyperlipoproteinemia.[166,170] This defect is probably related to deficient lipoprotein lipase activity. The mechanism by which this occurs is not understood although reduced activity of heparan sulfate, an important cofactor for lipoprotein lipase, may be involved.[175]

The consequences of these changes is uncertain. It might be expected that those patients with persistent nephrotic syndrome would be at risk for accelerated atherosclerosis, but the data are inconsistent.[176-179] Part of the problem may be the frequent presence of other risk factors for coronary disease such as hypertension, corticosteroid therapy, and chronic renal failure itself. Nevertheless, recent studies in patients with hypercholesterolemia have demonstrated that lowering the plasma cholesterol level has a beneficial effect on the morbidity and mortality from coronary disease.[180,181] Thus, the institution of a low saturated fat diet seems prudent in nephrotic patients in whom the glomerular disease cannot be corrected. The possible role of medications (such as cholestyramine or nicotinic acid) in this setting remains to be determined.

HYPERCOAGULABLE STATE

An increased frequency of arterial and venous thrombosis, particularly deep vein and renal vein thrombosis (RVT), has been described in the nephrotic syndrome.[182-187] An average of 20 to 40 percent of patients may be affected, although it is uncertain how this hypercoagulable state occurs.[183] Perhaps of greatest importance is a low plasma concentration (less than 70 percent of normal) of antithrombin III, an enzyme which antagonizes the action of thrombin as well as activated factors IX, X, and XI.[185,188] The decreased availability of antithrombin III (molecular weight about 65,000) appears to result from increased filtration across the more permeable glomerular capillary wall. Levels low enough to promote spontaneous clotting are found primarily in patients excreting more than 10 g of protein per day with a plasma albumin concentration under 2 g/dL.[185] The renal loss of antithrombin III would also explain the propensity to RVT since the renal venous blood would be the most hypercoagulable.

Other factors also may contribute to the thrombotic tendency in the nephrotic syndrome. These include an elevated plasma fibrinogen level, which could enhance red cell aggregation, and increased activation of platelets.[183,189–191] The mechanism by which these changes might occur is not known.[183]

RVT may be unilateral or bilateral and may extend into the inferior vena cava. It has been described in all forms of the nephrotic syndrome, but most commonly in patients with membranous nephropathy and membranoproliferative glomerulonephritis.[182–186] In some prospective studies, the incidence of RVT has reached 25 to 50 percent in membranous nephropathy,[182,187] but a lower incidence has been found elsewhere.[192] The reasons for the apparent propensity of membranous nephropathy to induce RVT are unclear.

RVT may develop concurrent with the nephrotic syndrome or later in the course of the disease. The presenting symptoms are variable.[182] Flank pain, hematuria (which may be macroscopic), decreased urine output, renal insufficiency (due in part to areas of infarction), and an increase in renal size on radiographic study all may result from acute RVT.

However, the development of RVT is more often insidious with *no symptoms referable to the kidney*.[182,186,187,193] In this setting, the GFR is usually unaffected and renal size is normal because of the formation of collateral vessels. As a result, the only clue pointing toward the presence of RVT may be a pulmonary embolus or, if the inferior vena cava is also involved, edema out of proportion to the degree of hypoalbuminemia or renal failure. RVT should also be suspected if, on renal biopsy, the glomeruli show congestion with red cells and margination of leukocytes, both of which are due to vascular stasis.[184,192]

When suspected clinically because of flank pain, acute renal failure, or pulmonary embolism, the diagnosis of RVT can be confirmed by an inferior vena cavagram and selective renal venogram. It has also been suggested that this study be part of the routine evaluation of all patients with membranous nephropathy since asymptomatic cases of RVT may be discovered.[182,187] In two prospective studies in which routine renal venography was performed in nephrotic patients, eight of 42 patients with RVT had had clinically apparent pulmonary emboli and three had had other thromboembolic events.[182,187] When ventilation-perfusion lung scans were performed in asymptomatic patients, four of 20 were compatible with pulmonary emboli.[182] In comparison, the incidence of pulmonary emboli was much lower (6 percent) in patients without RVT. Anticoagulation completely prevented new thromboembolic episodes.

Despite this data, no study has compared the risk of untreated asymptomatic RVT to the risk of long-term anticoagulation. This issue is further complicated by the observation that patients with an initially negative renal venogram may develop RVT at some later time.[182] As a result, a definitive recommendation cannot now be made. However, it may be justified to perform a renal venogram in patients with membranous nephropathy and proteinuria exceeding 10 g/day, since this does appear to represent a group at relatively high risk for thromboembolic disease.[185]

If given, anticoagulation generally consists of heparin and then warfarin. This therapy should minimize both the frequency of pulmonary emboli and the formation of new thrombi.[182,187,194] It may also promote recanalization of the preexisting thrombus, occasionally leading to improved renal function.[195] Warfarin should probably be continued as long as the patient remains nephrotic to prevent recurrent thromboembolic disease. Patients with *acute* RVT and acute renal failure may benefit from early fibrinolytic therapy to dissolve the clot, followed by conventional anticoagulation.[196,197]

Surgical thrombectomy has also been associated with some improvement in renal function,[198] but there is no evidence that this procedure is more effective than chronic anticoagulation. However, surgery may be considered in the rare patient who develops advanced renal failure that does not respond to anticoagulation.

MISCELLANEOUS

In addition to albumin and antithrombin III, other proteins may be lost in the urine in the nephrotic syndrome including 25-hydroxycholecalciferol (primarily bound to a circulating globulin which is normally not filtered), thyroxine (bound to both thyroxine-binding prealbumin and globulin), IgG, factors B and D of the alternate complement pathway and transferrin-bound iron.[199-206,]* Although the loss of thyroxine does not appear to alter thyroid function,[201] the other changes may be important. Signs of vitamin D deficiency, such as decreased intestinal calcium absorption, a fall in the plasma concentration of ionized calcium, osteomalacia, and secondary hyperparathyroidism, may all be present.[199,208,209] These changes are reversed with remission of the nephrotic syndrome as abnormal urinary protein loss ceases.

The low circulating levels of IgG and factors B (which plays an important role in opsonization) and D could be responsible for the increased incidence of infection, particularly pneumococcal pneumonia or peritonitis.[203,204,210] For example, the mortality rate from infection in children with the nephrotic syndrome was approximately 20 percent before the availability of antimicrobials and corticosteroids (the latter to treat the glomerular disease).[210] Pneumococcal vaccine offers partial but not complete protection against this complication.[211]

The loss of transferrin-bound iron is rarely of clinical importance. However, hypochromic

*Increased filtration of these compounds may not always be reflected by enhanced urinary losses. Factor D, for example, is filtered and then largely taken up by and metabolized in the proximal tubular cells. As a result, the plasma level may fall but factor D may not be demonstrable in the urine.[204,207]

anemia with low plasma iron and transferrin levels (but greater than 90 percent saturation) can occur.[205,206] Iron supplementation is without effect in this setting because of the hypotransferrinemia.

DIFFERENTIAL DIAGNOSIS AND CLASSIFICATION

The diagnosis of most glomerular diseases can be made only by renal biopsy unless the patient has an underlying systemic disease such as diabetes mellitus. However, findings on history, physical examination, and laboratory data frequently provide clues to the correct diagnosis.

HISTORY AND PHYSICAL EXAMINATION

The following information should be obtained from the history and physical examination:

1. Are there signs of a systemic disease associated with a glomerulopathy such as diabetes mellitus, SLE, amyloidosis, bacterial endocarditis, Goodpasture's syndrome, or malignancy (the last disorder may be associated with the nephrotic syndrome, due primarily to membranous nephropathy or minimal change disease)?
2. Is there a history of a recent upper respiratory infection? The latent period between the infection and the onset of glomerular disease (which may be characterized by gross hematuria) is usually 7 to 21 days in poststreptococcal glomerulonephritis but only 1 to 3 days with viral infections as in IgA nephropathy or benign hematuria. The last two disorders may also be associated with recurrent episodes of postinfectious hematuria.
3. Is the patient taking a drug that has been associated with glomerular disease, such as the nephrotic syndrome due to penicillamine or gold?

4. Is the patient pregnant? Proteinuria beginning in the third trimester is suggestive of preeclampsia. In addition, pregnancy can lead to the exacerbation of other renal diseases, particularly SLE.
5. Is the patient edematous or hypertensive, and how long have these findings been present?
6. Has the patient had a previous urinalysis or measurement of the BUN and P_{cr}? If available, this information may help in determining the duration of the disease.

LABORATORY DATA AND CLASSIFICATION

The routine laboratory evaluation of a glomerulopathy is depicted in Table 5–4. Of particular importance are the urinalysis, 24-h urinary protein excretion, and P_{cr}, which allow the different glomerular diseases to be subgrouped into separate categories on clinical grounds.

URINARY CHANGES

As described above, the urinary findings are variable in glomerular disease. In general, three different patterns may be seen, each typically associated with different disorders (Table 5–5).

Nephrotic Sediment. A *nephrotic* sediment is characterized primarily by heavy proteinuria (usually more than 2.5 g/day) and lipiduria.

TABLE 5–4. Laboratory Evaluation of Glomerular Disease

Routine	Optional
Urinalysis	Plasma
24-h urine for protein, creatinine	Albumin
	Glucose
	Complement
	Cholesterol
Hematocrit	Antinuclear antibody titer
BUN	Anti-DNAase B titer (and throat culture)
Plasma creatinine	
	Immunoelectrophoresis of the serum and urine

Although mild microscopic hematuria may also be present, marked hematuria and cellular casts are not typically seen. The reason for the relatively benign sediment is that the diseases associated with these findings (Table 5–6) have increased glomerular permeability but minimal cell proliferation, leukocyte infiltration, or necrosis. Notice that none of these disorders is called glomerulonephr*itis*, a reflection of the general lack of inflammatory change in the glomeruli. For the same reason, acute renal failure is unusual in this setting in the absence of some superimposed problem such as diuretic-induced hypovolemia, the use of nephrotoxins (such as nonsteroidal antiinflammatory drugs; see p. 82), or rarely RVT.

It is important to note that a nonglomerular disease, such as benign nephrosclerosis, can also lead to nephrotic range protein-

TABLE 5–5. The Urinalysis in Various Types of Glomerular Disease

Nephrotic	Nephritic	Chronic
Heavy proteinuria	Red cells	Less proteinuria and hematuria
Free fat droplets	Red cell casts	Broad, waxy casts
Oval fat bodies	Variable proteinuria	Pigmented granular casts
Fatty casts	Frequent white cell and granular casts	
Variable hematuria		

SOURCE: Adapted from G. E. Schreiner, *Arch. Intern. Med.*, 99:356, 1957. Copyright 1957, American Medical Association.

TABLE 5-6. Classification of Major Glomerular Diseases

Nephritic Sediment	Nephritic Sediment	
	Focal	Diffuse
Membranous nephropathy	Benign hematuria	Hypocomplementemic disorders
Minimal change disease	IgA nephropathy	Postinfectious glomerulonephritis
Focal glomerulosclerosis	SLE (focal and mesangial forms)	SLE (diffuse proliferative form)
Diabetes mellitus	Henoch-Schönlein purpura and	Membranoproliferative glomerulonephritis
Amyloidosis	other vasculitides	Mixed cryoglobulinemia
Preeclampsia	Mild forms of diffuse	Rapidly progressive (crescentic)
Benign nephrosclerosis	glomerulonephritis	glomerulonephritis—including anti-GBM
	Hereditary nephritis	disease
		Vasculitis
		Nonsteroidal anti-inflammatory drugs

uria.[212] This generally occurs in older patients with a long history of hypertension in whom renal insufficiency is already present. These patients, however, do not usually demonstrate the other findings of the nephrotic syndrome such as hypoalbuminemia and edema, probably because the glomerular damage is relatively mild. (Remember that a hypoalbuminemic patient with the same degree of proteinuria has a more severe glomerular leak; see p. 160). Similar findings can also occur with the secondary focal glomerulosclerosis induced by hemodynamically mediated glomerular injury (see Chap. 4).

Nephritic Sediment. In contrast, a *nephritic* sediment may contain hematuria, pyuria, cellular and granular casts, and a variable degree of proteinuria. The nephrotic syndrome may occur, but the active sediment distinguishes these disorders from those with a nephrotic sediment (Table 5-6). These urinary changes usually correlate with more marked abnormalities on renal biopsy: cell proliferation and occasionally leukocyte infiltration, crescent formation, or areas of necrosis.

The nephritic disorders can frequently be subdivided on clinical grounds into conditions characterized by *focal* or *diffuse* glomerular involvement since focal diseases tend to produce less severe abnormalities (Table 5-7). Thus, focal glomerulonephritis is usually associated with a normal or only mildly reduced GFR, nonnephrotic proteinuria, a normal plasma albumin concentration and blood pressure, and no edema.[24,213] Many of these patients present with asymptomatic hematuria and/or proteinuria which therefore must be distinguished from nonglomerular disorders such as polycystic kidney disease, which can cause similar findings. Dysmor-

TABLE 5-7. Clinical Characteristics of Focal and Diffuse Glomerulonephritis

Abnormality	Focal	Diffuse
Decreased GFR	Absent or mild	Usually present; may be severe
Nephrotic syndrome	Unusual	May occur
Hypertension	Unusual	Common
Edema	Unusual	Common

phic red cells or red cell casts point strongly toward glomerular disease in this setting.

Diffuse glomerulonephritis, on the other hand, is typically accompanied by renal insufficiency, hypertension, edema, and in some cases, the nephrotic syndrome.[24] The causes of diffuse glomerulonephritis include rapidly progressive (crescentic) glomerulonephritis, vasculitis, and the only glomerulopathies regularly accompanied by hypocomplementemia: postinfectious glomerulonephritis (including bacterial endocarditis and infected ventriculoatrial shunts), SLE, membranoproliferative glomerulonephritis, and mixed cryoglobulinemia.[214]

Several factors appear to be responsible for the development of hypocomplementemia in these disorders, including deposition in the kidney, decreased synthesis, and direct cleavage of C3 by circulating factors.[27] Since complement is fixed to deposited immune complexes, hypocomplementemia in acute, diffuse glomerulonephritis is in part due to increased utilization. In contrast, the rate of complement breakdown is not sufficient to lower the plasma level when a smaller number of immune complexes is present (as in focal glomerulonephritis) or the rate of complex deposition is relatively slow (as in membranous nephropathy).

Direct cleavage of C3 also may be important, particularly in membranoproliferative glomerulonephritis and poststreptococcal glomerulonephritis. In at least some of these patients, a circulating autoantibody is present, directed against the C3 convertase of either the alternate (C3bBb) or classsic pathway (C$\overline{42}$) (see Fig. 5–9).[215-217] These antibodies bind to the C3 convertase, making it less susceptible to inactivation and allowing continued C3 breakdown. The pathogenetic importance of this abnormality is uncertain since it does not correlate with the activity of the glomerular disease.[218,219]

One disorder that may be confused with diffuse glomerulonephritis is acute, usually drug-induced interstitial nephritis (see Chap. 8). Acute renal failure with hematuria, pyuria, and white cell casts are typical manifestations, but proteinuria and red cell casts are generally absent. An exception is the nephrotoxicity occasionally seen with nonsteroidal anti-inflammatory drugs, particularly fenoprofen.[220-222] In this setting, the nephrotic syndrome due to minimal change disease usually accompanies the interstitial nephritis. The interstitial infiltrate is primarily composed of T cells which may also be responsible for the proteinuria via the release of a lymphokine that could increase glomerular permeability.

The hemolytic-uremic syndrome and thrombotic thrombocytopenic purpura also may have renal manifestations compatible with diffuse glomerulonephritis. However, the concurrent presence of thrombocytopenia and microangiopathic hemolytic anemia point strongly toward one of these disorders (see Chap. 7).

Although this approach of differentiating between nephrotic and nephritic, focal and diffuse glomerular diseases correlates relatively well with the histologic findings, exceptions do occur and, therefore, the clinical impression cannot usually substitute for renal biopsy. As an example, up to 10 percent of children with membranous nephropathy (a nephrotic disorder) present with gross hematuria as well as proteinuria, suggesting a nephritic disorder.[223] In addition, a generally focal disease such as IgA nephropathy can present with a more diffuse picture.[224]

Chronic Sediment. Many glomerular diseases progress to advanced renal failure, which is characterized by scarring of most of the glomeruli. As a result of the decreases in GFR and active inflammation, the urinalysis becomes less abnormal with reduced proteinuria and hematuria and with broad waxy ("renal failure") casts being a prominent finding in the sediment (see p. 27). It may be difficult at this time to be certain that the patient has a primary glomerulopathy unless a past history is available or there are persistent findings characteristic of glomerular disease such as dysmorphic red cells, red cell casts, or heavy proteinuria.

OTHER TESTS

In addition to the urinary findings, appropriate laboratory tests can establish the diagnosis of a systemic disease (Table 5–4). Included in this group are antinuclear antibodies and DNA binding in SLE, plasma glucose concentration in diabetes mellitus, throat culture and anti-DNAase B titer in poststreptococcal glomerulonephritis (the latter is more often positive than the antistreptolysin O titer),[225] blood cultures in bacterial endocarditis, and immunoelectrophoresis of the serum and urine to look for a paraprotein in primary amyloidosis.

AGE

The patient's age also may be helpful diagnostically. Although most of the disorders listed in Table 5–6 can occur at any age, many of them are more prevalent in certain age groups. For example, benign hematuria is primarily a disease of children, SLE of 15 to 40-year-old women, and primary amyloidosis of adults over the age of 40. Thus, the clinical differential diagnosis can frequently be narrowed further when the patient's age is considered along with the findings on the urinalysis and blood tests (Table 5–8).

CLINICAL EXAMPLES

The use of the approach outlined above in the differential diagnosis of glomerular disease can be illustrated by the following examples.

TABLE 5–8. Major Causes of Glomerular Disease According to Age

Urinalysis	Age		
	< 15 Years	15–40 Years	> 40 Years
Nephrotic pattern	Minimal change disease Focal glomerulosclerosis	Focal glomerulosclerosis Minimal change disease Membranous nephropathy (including SLE) Diabetes mellitus Preeclampsia	Membranous nephropathy Diabetes mellitus Primary amyloidosis Minimal change disease Benign nephrosclerosis

Nephritic pattern
  Focal disease
	Benign hematuria
	IgA nephropathy
	Henoch-Schönlein
	  purpura
	Mild postinfectious GN*
	Hereditary nephritis
		IgA nephropathy
		SLE
		Hereditary nephritis
			IgA nephropathy

Diffuse disease	Membranoproliferative GN Postinfectious GN	Membranoproliferative GN SLE Hereditary nephritis	Rapidly progressive GN Vasculitis

*Glomerulonephritis.

Case History 5-1. A 32-year-old man is found to have microscopic hematuria on a routine examination. Lipiduria is also present, but there are no casts and 24-h protein excretion is 620 mg. The P_{cr} is 1.6 mg/dL. Other laboratory data include a normal hematocrit, plasma C3 level, and ANA (antinuclear antibody) and anti-DNAase B titers.

There is no personal or family history of renal disease, prior urinalysis, preceding upper respiratory infection, or symptoms suggestive of a systemic disease. On physical examination, the blood pressure is normal and there is no edema or skin rash.

Comment. Although hematuria and mild proteinuria may be seen with nonglomerular diseases, the presence of lipiduria is diagnostic of a glomerular lesion. The urinary findings are more consistent with a nephritic disorder, and the mild renal insufficiency and absence of edema, hypertension, and heavy proteinuria are suggestive of focal disease (Table 5-7). Lack of a family history, systemic symptoms, or elevated anti-DNAase B or ANA titer tend to exclude hereditary nephritis, the focal form of SLE, Henoch-Schönlein purpura, and mild poststreptococcal glomerulonephritis.

The increase in the P_{cr} and the patient's age are inconsistent with benign hematuria. Thus, the most likely diagnosis is IgA nephropathy. This was confirmed by renal biopsy.

Case History 5-2. A 14-year-old boy presents with pedal and periorbital edema increasing over 1 week. He denies gross hematuria, a recent upper respiratory infection, arthralgias, or skin rash.

The physical examination is normal except for the presence of edema. Laboratory evaluation reveals hypoalbuminemia (plasma albumin concentration 2.4 g/dL) and a normal hematocrit, P_{cr}, complement, and ANA titer. The urinalysis shows 4^+ proteinuria, oval fat bodies, free fat droplets but no casts or hematuria; 24-h urinary protein excretion is 8.4 g.

Comment. This patient has the nephrotic syndrome with a nephrotic sediment. In this age group, the most likely diagnoses are minimal change disease and focal glomerulosclerosis (Table 5-8). The patient failed to respond to an 8-week trial of corticosteroids. A renal biopsy was then performed and revealed focal glomerulosclerosis.

REFERENCES

1. Rose, B. D.: *Clinical Physiology of Acid-Base and Electrolyte Disorders,* 2d ed., McGraw-Hill, New York, 1984, chap. 3.
2. Bohman, S-O., G. Jaremko, A-B. Bohlin, and U. Berg: Foot process fusion and glomerular filtration rate in minimal change nephrotic syndrome, *Kidney Int.,* 25:696, 1984.
3. Venkatachalam, M. A., and H. G. Rennke: The structure and molecular basis of glomerular filtration, *Circ. Res.,* 43:337, 1978.
4. Brenner, B. M., T. H. Hostetter, and H. D. Humes: Molecular basis of proteinuria of glomerular origin, *N. Engl. J. Med.,* 298:826, 1978.
5. Kerjaschki, D., A. T. Vernillo, and M. G. Farquhar: Reduced sialation of podocalyxin—the major sialoprotein of rat kidney glomerulus—in aminonucleoside nephrosis, *Am. J. Pathol.,* 118:343, 1985.
6. Vogt, A., R. Rohrbach, F. Shimizu, H. Takamiya, and S. Batsford: Interaction of cationized antigen with rat glomerular basement membrane: In situ immune complex formation, *Kidney Int.,* 22:27, 1982.
7. Myers, B. D., T. B. Okarma, S. Friedman, C. Bridges, J. Ross, S. Asseff, and W. M. Deen: Mechanisms of proteinuria in human glomerulonephritis, *J. Clin. Invest.,* 70:732, 1982.

8. Robson, A. M., J. Giangiacomo, R. A. Kienstra, S. T. Naqvi, and J. R. Ingelfinger: Normal glomerular permeability and its modification by minimal change nephrotic syndrome, *J. Clin. Invest.,* 54:1190, 1974.

9. Vernier, R. L., D. J. Klein, S. P. Sisson, J. D. Mahan, T. R. Oegema, and D. M. Brown: Heparan sulfate-rich anionic sites in the human glomerular basement membrane. Decreased concentration in congenital nephrotic syndrome, *N. Engl. J. Med.,* 309:1001, 1983.

10. Sharon, Z., M. M. Schwartz, B. U. Pauli, and E. J. Lewis: Kinetics of glomerular visceral epithelial cell phagocytosis, *Kidney Int.,* 14:526, 1978.

11. Kreisberg, J. I., and M. J. Karnovsky: Glomerular cells in culture, *Kidney Int.,* 23:349, 1983.

12. Striker, G. E., M. Mannik, and M. Y. Tung: The role of marrow-derived monocytes and mesangial cells in removal of immune complexes from renal glomeruli, *J. Exp. Med.,* 149:127, 1979.

13. Scharschmidt, L. A., and M. J. Dunn: Prostaglandin synthesis by rat glomerular mesangial cells in culture. Effects of angiotensin II and arginine vasopressin, *J. Clin. Invest.,* 71:1756, 1983.

14. MacCarthy, E. P., A. Hsu, Y. M. Ooi, and B. S. Ooi: Evidence for a mouse mesangial cell-derived factor that stimulates lymphocyte proliferation, *J. Clin. Invest.,* 76:426, 1985.

15. Dworkin, L. D., I. Ichikawa, and B. M. Brenner: Hormonal modulation of glomerular function, *Am. J. Physiol.,* 244:F95, 1983.

16. Wilson, C. B., and F. J. Dixon: Diagnosis of immunopathologic renal disease, *Kidney Int.,* 5:389, 1974.

17. Hyman, L. R., J. P. Wagnild, G. J. Beirne, and P. M. Burkholder: Immunoglobulin A distribution in glomerular disease: Analysis of immunofluorescence localization and pathogenetic significance, *Kidney Int.,* 3:397, 1973.

18. Baart de la Faille-Kuyper, E. H., L. Kater, R. H. Kuijten, C. J. Kooiker, S. S. Wagenaar, S. van der Zouwen, and E. J. Dorhout Mees: Occurrence of vascular IgA deposits in clinically normal skin of patients with renal disease, *Kidney Int.,* 9:424, 1976.

19. Wilson, C. B., and F. J. Dixon: Renal response to immunological injury, in B. M. Brenner and F. C. Rector, Jr (eds.), *The Kidney,* 3d ed., Saunders, Philadelphia, 1986.

20. Cameron, J. S., and W. F. Clark: A role for insoluble antibody-antigen complexes in glomerulonephritis?, *Clin. Nephrol.,* 18:55, 1982.

21. Couser, W. G., and D. J. Salant: In situ immune complex formation and glomerular injury, *Kidney Int.,* 17:1, 1980.

22. Dixon, F. J., J. D. Feldman, and J. J. Vazquer: Experimental glomerulonephritis: The pathogenesis of a laboratory model resembling the spectrum of human glomerulonephritis, *J. Exp. Med.,* 113:899, 1961.

23. Germuth, F. G., Jr., J. J. Taylor, S. Y. Sidiqui, and E. Rodriquez: Immune complex disease, VI: Some determinants of the varieties of glomerular lesions in the chronic bovine serum albumin-rabbit system, *Lab. Invest.,* 37:162, 1977.

24. Baldwin, D. S., M. C. Gluck, J. Lowenstein, and G. R. Gallo: Lupus nephritis: Clinical course as related to morphologic forms and their transitions, *Am. J. Med.,* 62:12, 1977.

25. Couser, W. G.: Mechanisms of glomerular injury in immune-complex disease, *Kidney Int.,* 28:569, 1985.

26. Inman, R. D., and N. K. Day: Immunologic and clinical aspects of immune complex disease, *Am. J. Med.,* 70:1097, 1981.

27. Wilson, C. B., and F. J. Dixon: Immunologic mechanisms in nephritogenesis, *Hosp. Pract.,* 14(4):57, 1979.

28. Wiggins, R. C., and C. G. Cochrane: Immune-complex mediated biologic effects, *N. Engl. J. Med.,* 304:518, 1981.

29. Agodoa, L. Y. C., V. J. Gauthier, and M. Mannik: Precipitating antigen-antibody systems are required for the formation of subepithelial electron-dense immune deposits in rat glomeruli, *J. Exp. Med.,* 158:1259, 1983.

30. Friend, P. S., Y. Kim, A. F. Michael, and J. V. Donadio: Pathogenesis of membranous nephropathy in systemic lupus erythematosus: Possible role of nonprecipitating DNA antibody, *Br. Med. J.,* 1:25, 1977.

31. Neilson, E. G., and B. Zakheim: T cell regulation, anti-idiotypic immunity, and the nephritogenic immune response, *Kidney Int.,* 24:289, 1983.

32. Goldman, M., L. M. Rose, A. Hochmann, and P. H. Lambert: Deposition of idiotype-anti-idiotype immune complexes in renal glomeruli after polyclonal B cell activation, *J. Exp. Med.,* 155:1385, 1982.

33. Zanetti, M., and C. B. Wilson: Participation of auto-anti-idiotypes in immune complex glomerulonephritis in rabbits, *J. Immunol.,* 131:2781, 1983.

34. McIntosh, R. M., R. Garcia, L. Rubio, D. Rabideau, J. E. Allen, R. I. Carr, and B. Rodriguez-Iturbé: Evidence for an autologous immune complex

pathogenic mechanism in acute poststreptococcal glomerulonephritis, *Kidney Int.,* 14:501, 1978.

35. Stobo, J. D.: The influence of immune response genes on the expression of disease, *J. Lab. Clin. Med.,* 100:822, 1982.

36. Steinberg, A. D., E. S. Raveché, C. A. Laskin, H. R. Smith, T. Santoro, M. L. Miller, and P. H. Plotz: Systemic lupus erythematosus: Insights from animal models, *Ann. Intern. Med.,* 100:714, 1984.

37. Schwartz, R. S.: Immunologic and genetic aspects of systemic lupus erythematosus, *Kidney Int.,* 19:474, 1981.

38. Frank, M. M., M. I. Hamburger, T. J. Lawley, R. P. Kimberly, and P. H. Plotz: Defective reticuloendothelial system Fc-receptor function in systemic lupus erythematosus, *N. Engl. J. Med.,* 300:518, 1979.

39. Lockwood, C. M., S. Worlledge, A. Nicholas, C. Cotton, and D. K. Peters: Reversal of impaired splenic function in patients with nephritis or vasculitis (or both) by plasma exchange, *N. Engl. J. Med.,* 300:524, 1979.

40. Nicholls, K., and P. Kincaid-Smith: Defective in vivo Fc- and C3b-receptor function in IgA nephropathy, *Am. J. Kid. Dis.,* 4:128, 1984.

41. Miyazaki, S., K. Kawasaki, E. Yaoita, T. Yamamoto, and I. Kihara: Bovine serum albumin (BSA) nephritis in rats. III. Antigen distribution in various organs, *Clin. Exp. Immunol.,* 59:293, 1985.

42. Lawley, T. J., R. P. Hall, A. S. Fauci, S. I. Katz, M. I. Hamburger, and M. M. Frank: Defective Fc-receptor function associated with the HLA-B8/DRw3 haplotype, *N. Engl. J. Med.,* 304:185, 1981.

43. Wilson, J. G., W. W. Wong, P. H. Schur, and D. T. Fearon: Mode of inheritance of decreased C3b receptors on erythrocytes of patients with systemic lupus erythematosus, *N. Engl. J. Med.,* 307:981, 1982.

44. Schifferli, J. A., Y. C. Ng, and D. K. Peters: The role of complement and its receptors in the elimination of imune complexes, *N. Engl. J. Med.,* 315:488, 1986.

45. Schifferli, J. A., G. Steiger, G. Hauptmann, P. J. Spaeth, and A. G. Sjoholm: Formation of soluble immune complexes in sera of patients with various hypocomplementemic states. Difference between inhibition of immune precipitation and solubilization, *J. Clin. Invest.,* 76:2127, 1985.

46. Agnello, V.: Complement deficiency states, *Medicine,* 57:1, 1978.

47. Barcelli, U., R. Rademacher, Y. M. Ooi, and B. S. Ooi: Modification of glomerular immune complex deposition in mice by activation of the reticuloendothelial system, *J. Clin. Invest.,* 67:20, 1981.

48. Fleuren, G., J. Grond, and P. J. Hoedemaker: In situ formation of subepithelial glomerular immune complexes in passive serum sickness, *Kidney Int.,* 17:631, 1980.

49. Kerjaschki, D., and M. G. Farquhar: Immunocytochemical localization of the Heymann nephritis antigen (GP330) in glomerular epithelial cells of normal Lewis rats, *J. Exp. Med.,* 157:667, 1983.

50. Van Damme, J. C., G. J. Fleuren, W. W. Bakker, R. L. Vernier, and Ph. J. Hoedemaker: Experimental glomerulonephritis in the rabbit induced by antibodies directed against tubular antigens, V: Fixed glomerular antigens in the pathogenesis of heterologous immune complex glomerulonephritis, *Lab. Invest.,* 38:502, 1978.

51. Sharon, Z., M. M. Schwartz, B. U. Pauli, and E. J. Lewis: Impairment of glomerular clearance of macroaggregates in immune complex glomerulonephritis, *Kidney Int.,* 22:8, 1982.

52. Ooi, Y. M., B. S. Ooi, and V. E. Pollak: Relationships of levels of circulating immune complexes to histologic patterns of nephritis: A comparative study of membranous glomerulonephropathy and diffuse proliferative glomerulonephritis, *J. Lab. Clin. Med.,* 90:891, 1977.

53. Abrass, C. K., C. L. Hall, W. A. Border, C. A. Brown, R. J. Glassock, and C. H. Coggins: Circulating immune complexes in adults with idiopathic nephrotic syndrome, *Kidney Int.,* 17:545, 1980.

54. Mauer, S. M., D. E. R. Sutherland, R. J. Howard, A. J. Fish, J. S. Najarian, and A. F. Michael: The glomerular mesangium, III. Acute immune mesangial injury: A new model of glomerulonephritis, *J. Exp. Med.,* 137:553, 1973.

55. Golbus, S. M., and C. B. Wilson: Experimental glomerulonephritis induced by in situ formation of immune complexes in glomerular capillary wall, *Kidney Int.,* 16:148, 1979.

56. Tan, E. M., P. H. Schur, R. I. Carr, and H. G. Kunkel: Deoxyribonucleic acid (DNA) and antibodies to DNA in the serum of patients with systemic lupus erythematosus, *J. Clin. Invest.,* 45:1732, 1966.

57. Izui, S., P.-H. Lambert, and P. A. Miescher: In vitro demonstration of a particular affinity of glomerular basement membrane and collagen for DNA: A possible basis for a local formation of DNA-anti-DNA complexes in systemic lupus erythematosus, *J. Exp. Med.,* 144:428, 1976.

58. Gilliam, J. N., D. E. Cheatum, E. R. Hurd, P. Stastny, and M. Ziff: Immunoglobulin in clinically uninvolved skin in systemic lupus erythematosus: Association with renal disease, *J. Clin. Invest.,* 53:1434, 1974.

59. Brentjens, J. R., M. Sepulveda, T. Baliah, C. Bentzel, B. F. Erlanger, C. Elwood, M. Montes, K. C. Hsu, and G. A. Andres: Interstitial immune complex nephritis in patients with systemic lupus erythematosus, *Kidney Int.,* 7:342, 1975.

60. Mannik, M., L. Y. C. Agodoa, and K. A. David: Rearrangement of immune complexes in glomeruli leads to persistence and development of electron-dense deposits, *J. Exp. Med.,* 157:1516, 1983.

61. Gallo, G. R., T. Caulin-Glaser, and M. E. Lamm: Charge of circulating immune complexes as a factor in glomerular basement membrane localization in mice, *J. Clin. Invest.,* 67:1305, 1981.

62. Border, W. A., H. J. Ward, E. S. Kamil, and A. H. Cohen: Induction of membranous nephropathy in rabbits by administration of an exogenous cationic antigen, *J. Clin. Invest.,* 69:451, 1982.

63. Vogt, A.: New aspects of the pathogenesis of immune complex glomerulonephritis: Formation of subepithelial deposits, *Clin. Nephrol.,* 21:15, 1984.

64. Gauthier, V. J., G. E. Striker, and M. Mannik: Glomerular localization of preformed immune complexes prepared with anionic antibodies or with cationic antigens, *Lab. Invest.,* 50:636, 1984.

65. Caulin-Glaser, T., G. R. Gallo, and M. E. Lamm: Nondissociating cationic immune complexes can deposit in glomerular basement membrane, *J. Exp. Med.,* 158:1561, 1983.

66. Vogt, A., S. Batsford, B. Rodriguez-Iturbé, and R. Garcia: Cationic antigens in poststreptococcal glomerulonephritis, *Clin. Nephrol.,* 20:271, 1983.

67. Raij, L., S. Azar, and W. Keane: Role of hypertension in progressive glomerular immune injury, *Hypertension,* 7:398, 1985.

68. Neugarten, J., H. D. Feiner, R. G. Schacht, G. R. Gallo, and D. S. Baldwin: Aggravation of experimental glomerulonephritis by superimposed clip hypertension, *Kidney Int.,* 22:257, 1982.

69. Palmer, J. M., S. L. Eversole, and T. A. Stanley: Unilateral glomerulonephritis: Virtual absence of nephritis in a kidney with partial occlusion of the main renal artery, *Am. J. Med.,* 40:816, 1966.

70. Neugarten, J., B. Kaminetsky, H. Feiner, R. G. Schacht, D. T. Liu, and D. S. Baldwin: Nephrotoxic serum nephritis with hypertension: Amelioration with antihypertensive therapy, *Kidney Int.,* 28:135, 1985.

71. Sakai, T., F. H. Harris, D. J. Marsh, C. M. Bennett, and R. J. Glassock: Extracellular fluid expansion and autoregulation in nephrotoxic serum nephritis in rats, *Kidney Int.,* 25:619, 1984.

72. Steblay, R. W.: Glomerulonephritis induced in sheep by injections of heterologous glomerular basement membrane and Freund's complete adjuvant, *J. Exp. Med.,* 116:253, 1962.

73. Lerner, R. A., R. J. Glassock, and F. J. Dixon: The role of antiglomerular basement membrane antibody in the pathogenesis of human glomerulonephritis, *J. Exp. Med.,* 126:989, 1967.

74. Westberg, N. G., and A. F. Michael: Immunohistopathology of diabetic glomerulosclerosis, *Diabetes,* 21:163, 1972.

75. Gallo, G. R.: Elution studies in kidneys with linear deposition of immunoglobulin in glomeruli, *Am. J. Pathol.,* 61:337, 1970.

76. Madaio, M. P., D. J. Salant, S. Adler, C. Darby, and W. G. Couser: Effect of antibody charge and concentration on deposition of antibody to glomerular basement membrane, *Kidney Int.,* 26:397, 1984.

77. Bhan, A. K., E. E. Schneeberger, A. B. Collins, and R. T. McCluskey: Evidence for a pathogenic role of a cell-mediated immune mechanism in experimental glomerulonephritis, *J. Exp. Med.,* 148:246, 1978.

78. Bolton, W. K., F. L. Tucker, and B. C. Sturgill: New avian model of experimental glomerulonephritis consistent with mediation by cellular immunity, *J. Clin. Invest.,* 73:1263, 1984.

79. Tipping, P. G., T. J. Neale, and S. R. Holdsworth: T lymphocyte participation in antibody-induced experimental glomerulonephritis, *Kidney Int.,* 27:530, 1985.

80. Neild, G. H., K. Ivory, M. Hiramatsu, and D. G. Williams: Cyclosporin A inhibits acute serum sickness nephritis in rabbits, *Clin. Exp. Immunol.,* 52:586, 1983.

81. Shalhoub, R. J.: Pathogenesis of lipoid nephrosis: A disorder of T-cell function, *Lancet,* 2:556, 1974.

82. Couser, W. G., M. M. Stilmant, and N. B. Jermanovich: Complement-independent nephrotoxic nephritis in the guinea pig, *Kidney Int.,* 11:170, 1977.

83. Salant, D. J., M. P. Madaio, S. Adler, M. M. Stilmant, and W. G. Couser: Altered glomerular permeability induced by F (ab')$_2$ and Fab' antibodies to rat renal tubular epithelial antigen, *Kidney Int.,* 21:36, 1982.

84. Couser, W. G., P. J. Baker, and S. Adler: Comple-

ment and the direct mediation of glomerular injury: A new perspective, *Kidney Int.,* 28:879, 1985.

85. Schreiber, R. D., M. K. Pangburn, P. H. Lesabre, and H. J. Müller-Eberhard: Initiation of the alternate pathway of complement: Recognition of activators by bound C3b and assembly of the entire pathway from six isolated proteins, *Proc. Nat. Acad. Sci. (U.S.A.),* 75:3948, 1978.

86. Fearon, D. T., and K. F. Austen: The alternative pathway of complement—A system for host resistance to microbial infection, *N. Engl. J. Med.,* 303:259, 1980.

87. Adler, S., P. J. Baker, R. J. Johnson, R. F. Occhi, P. Pritzl, and W. G. Couser: Complement membrane attack complex stimulates production of reactive oxygen metabolites by cultured rat mesangial cells, *J. Clin. Invest.,* 77:762, 1986.

88. Biesecker, G., S. Katz, and D. Koffler: Renal localization of the membrane attack complex in systemic lupus erythematosus nephritis, *J. Exp. Med.,* 154:1779, 1981.

89. Adler, S., P. J. Baker, P. Pritzl, and W. G. Couser: Detection of terminal complement components in experimental immune glomerular injury, *Kidney Int.,* 26:830, 1984.

90. Perkinson, D. T., P. J. Baker, W. G. Couser, R. J. Johnson, and S. Adler: Membrane attack complex deposition in experimental glomerular injury, *Am. J. Pathol.,* 120:21, 1985.

91. Salant, D. J., S. Adler, C. Darby, N. J. Capparell, G. C. Groggel, I. D. Feintzeig, H. G. Rennke, and J. E. Dittmer: Influence of antigen distribution on the mediation of immunological glomerular injury, *Kidney Int.,* 27:938, 1985.

92. Yoshizawa, N., G. Treser, I. Sagel, A. Ty, U. Ahmed, and K. Lange: Demonstration of antigenic sites in glomeruli of patients with acute poststreptococcal glomerulonephritis by immunofluorescein and immunoferritin technics, *Am. J. Pathol.,* 70:131, 1973.

93. Fligiel, S. E. G., P. A. Ward, K. J. Johnson, and G. O. Till: Evidence for a role of hydroxyl radical in immune-complex-induced vasculitis, *Am. J. Pathol.,* 115:375, 1984.

94. Cochran, C. G., E. R. Unanue, and F. J. Dixon: A role of polymorphonuclear leukocytes and complement in nephrotoxic nephritis, *J. Exp. Med.,* 122:99, 1965.

95. Tucker, B. J., L. C. Gushwa, C. B. Wilson, and R. C. Blantz: Effect of leukocyte depletion on glomerular dynamics during acute glomerular injury, *Kidney Int.,* 28:28, 1984.

96. Holdsworth, S. R., and R. Bellomo: Differential effects of steroids on leukocyte-mediated glomerulonephritis in the rabbit, *Kidney Int.,* 26:162, 1984.

97. Thomson, N. M., S. R. Holdsworth, E. F. Glasgow, and R. C. Atkins: The macrophage in the development of experimental crescentic glomerulonephritis, *Am. J. Pathol.,* 94:223, 1979.

98. Holdsworth, S. R., T. J. Neale, and C. B. Wilson: Abrogation of macrophage dependent injury in experimental glomerulonephritis in the rabbit. Use of an anti-macrophage serum, *J. Clin. Invest.,* 66:686, 1981.

99. Ferrario, F., A. Castiglione, G. Colasanti, G. B. di Belgioroso, S. Bertoli, and G. D'Amico: The detection of monocytes in human glomerulonephritis, *Kidney Int.,* 28:513, 1985.

100. Hooke, D. H., W. W. Hancock, D. C. Gee, N. Kraft, and R. C. Atkins: Monoclonal antibody analysis of glomerular hypercellularity in human glomerulonephritis, *Clin. Nephrol.,* 22:163, 1984.

101. Atkins, R. C., E. F. Glasgow, S. R. Holdsworth, and F. E. Matthews: The macrophage in human rapidly progressive glomerulonephritis, *Lancet,* 1:830, 1976.

102. Schreiner, G. F., R. S. Cotran, V. Pardo, and E. R. Unanue: A mononuclear cell component in experimental immunological glomerulonephritis, *J. Exp. Med.,* 147:369, 1978.

103. Cole, E. H., J. Schulman, M. Urowitz, E. Keystone, C. Williams, and G. A. Levy: Monocyte procoagulant activity in glomerulonephritis associated with systemic lupus erythematosus, *J. Clin. Invest.,* 75: 861, 1985.

104. Wiggins, R. C., A. Glatfelter, and J. Brukman: Procoagulant activity in glomeruli and urine of rabbits with nephrotoxic nephritis, *Lab. Invest.,* 53:156, 1985.

105. Duffus, P., A. Parbtani, G. Frampton, and J. S. Cameron: Intraglomerular localization of platelet related antigens, platelet factor 4 and β-thromboglobulin in glomerulonephritis, *Clin. Nephrol.,* 17:288, 1982.

106. George, C. R. P., S. J. Slichter, L. J. Quadrucci, G. E. Striker, and L. A. Harker: A kinetic evaluation of hemostasis in renal disease, *N. Engl. J. Med.,* 291:1111, 1974.

107. Donadio, J. V., Jr., C. F. Anderson, J. C. Mitchell, III, K. E. Holley, D. M. Ilstrup, V. Fuster, and J. H. Cheesebro: Membranoproliferative glomerulonephritis. A prospective clinical trial of platelet-inhibitor therapy *N. Engl. J. Med.,* 310:1421, 1984.

108. Cochrane, C. G.: Mechanisms involved in deposi-

tion of immune complexes in tissue, *J. Exp. Med.,* 134(suppl.):75s, 1971.

109. Barnes, J. L., S. P. Levine, and M. A. Venkatachalam: Binding of platelet factor four to glomerular polyanion, *Kidney Int.,* 25:759, 1984.

110. Barnes, J. L., and M. A. Venkatachalam: Enhancement of glomerular immune complex deposition by a circulating polycation, *J. Exp. Med.,* 160:286, 1984.

111. McCluskey, R. T., P. Vassalli, G. Gallo, and D. S. Baldwin: An immunofluorescent study of pathogenic mechanisms in glomerular diseases, *N. Engl. J. Med.,* 274:695, 1966.

112. Kincaid-Smith, P.: Anticoagulants are of value in the treatment of renal disease, *Am. J. Kid. Dis.,* 3:299, 1984.

113. Hoyer, J. R., A. F. Michael, and L. W. Hoyer: Immunofluorescent localization of antihemophilic factor antigen and fibrinogen in human renal disease, *J. Clin. Invest.,* 53:1375, 1974.

114. Kant, K. S., V. E. Pollak, M. A. Weiss, H. I. Glueck, M. A. Miller, and E. V. Hess: Glomerular thrombosis in systemic lupus erythematosus: Prevalence and significance, *Medicine,* 60:71, 1981.

115. Border, W. A., C. B. Wilson, and F. J. Dixon: Failure of heparin to affect two types of experimental glomerulonephritis in rabbits, *Kidney Int.,* 8:140, 1975.

116. Clamon, H. N.: Glucocorticosteroids, I: Anti-inflammatory mechanisms, *Hosp. Pract.,* 18(7):123, 1983.

117. Strom, T. B.: Immunosuppressive agents in renal transplantation, *Kidney Int.,* 26:353, 1984.

118. Gershwin, M. E., E. J. Goetzl, and A. D. Steinberg: Cyclophophamide: Use in practice, *Ann. Intern. Med.,* 80:531, 1974.

119. Feehally, J., T. J. Beattie, P. E. C. Brenchley, B. M. Coupes, I. B. Houston, N. P. Mallick, and R. J. Postlethwaite: Modulation of cellular immune function by cyclophosphamide in children with minimal-change nephropathy, *N. Engl. J. Med.,* 310: 415, 1984.

120. Tipping, P. G., and S. R. Holdsworth: The mechanism of action of corticosteroids on glomerular injury in acute serum sickness in rabbits, *Clin. Exp. Immunol.,* 59:555, 1985.

121. Vassalli, P., and R. T. McCluskey: The pathogenic role of the coagulation process in rabbit Masugi nephritis, Am. J. Pathol., 45:653, 1964.

122. Border, W. A.: Anticoagulants are of little value in the treatment of renal disease, *Am. J. Kid. Dis.,* 3:308, 1984.

123. Cattran, D. C., C. J. Cardella, J. M. Roscoe, R. C.

Charron, P. C. Rance, S. M. Ritchie, and P. N. Corey: Results of a controlled drug trial in membranoproliferative glomerulonephritis, *Kidney Int.,* 27:436, 1985.

124. Frye, K. H., D. Hancock, H. Moutsopoulos, H. D. Humes, and A. I. Arieff: Low-dosage heparin in rapidly progressive glomerulonephritis, *Arch. Intern. Med.,* 136:995, 1976.

125. Thomson, N. M., J. Moran, I. J. Simpson, and D. K. Peters: Defibrination with ancrod in nephrotoxic nephritis in rabbits, *Kidney Int.,* 10:343, 1976.

126. Thomson, N. M., I. J. Simpson, D. J. Evans, and D. K. Peters: Defibrination with ancrod in experimental chronic immune complex nephritis, *Clin. Exp. Immunol.,* 20:527, 1975.

127. Kant, K. S., V. E. Pollak, A. Dosekun, P. Glas-Greenwalt, M. A. Weiss, and H. I. Glueck: Lupus nephritis with thrombosis and abnormal fibrinolysis: Effect of ancrod, *J. Lab. Clin. Med.,* 105:77, 1985.

128. Lee, H. S., S. K. Mujais, B. S. Kasinath, B. H. Spargo, and A. I. Katz: Course of renal pathology in patients with systemic lupus erythematosus, *Am. J. Med.,* 77:612, 1984.

129. Fairley, K. F., and D. F. Birch: Hematuria: A simple method for identifying glomerular bleeding, *Kidney Int.,* 21:105, 1982.

130. Fassett, R. G., B. Horgan, D. Gove, and T. H. Mathew: Scanning electron microscopy of glomerular and nonglomerular red blood cells, *Clin. Nephrol.,* 20:11, 1983.

131. Min, K. W., F. Gyorkey, P. Gyorkey, J. Y. Yium, and G. Eknoyan: The morphogenesis of glomerular crescents in rapidly progressive glomerulonephritis, *Kidney Int.,* 5:47, 1974.

132. Kaysen, G. A., B. D. Myers, W. G. Couser, R. Rabkin, and J. M. Felts: Mechanisms and consequences of proteinuria, *Lab. Invest.,* 54:479, 1986.

133. Martin, R. S., and D. M. Small: Physicochemical characterization of the urinary lipid from humans with nephrotic syndrome, *J. Lab. Clin. Med.,* 103: 798, 1984.

134. Chang, R. L. S., W. M. Deen, C. R. Robertson, C. M. Bennett, R. J. Glassock, and B. M. Brenner: Permselectivity of the glomerular capillary wall: Studies of experimental glomerulonephritis in the rat using neutral dextran, *J. Clin. Invest.,* 57:1272, 1976.

135. Sakai, T., F. H. Harris, D. J. Marsh, C. M. Bennett, and R. J. Glassock: Extracellular fluid expansion and autoregulation in nephrotoxic serum nephritis in rats, *Kidney Int.,* 25:619, 1984.

136. Allison, M. E. M., C. B. Wilson, and C. W. Gott-

schalk: Pathophysiology of experimental glomerulonephritis in rats, *J. Clin. Invest.,* 53:1402, 1974.

137. Bohman, S-O., G. Jaremko, A-B. Bohlin, and U. Berg: Foot process fusion and glomerular filtration rate in minimal change nephrotic syndrome, *Kidney Int.,* 25:696, 1984.

138. Kaizu, K., D. Marsh, R. Zipser, and R. J. Glassock: Role of prostaglandins and angiotensin II in experimental glomerulonephritis, *Kidney Int.,* 28:629, 1985.

139. Meltzer, J. I., H. J. Keim, J. H. Laragh, J. E. Sealey, K-M. Jan, and S. Chien: Nephrotic syndrome: Vasoconstriction and hypervolemic types indicated by renin-sodium profiling, *Ann. Intern. Med.,* 91:688, 1979.

140. Garnet, E. S., and C. E. Webber: Changes in blood volume produced by treatment in the nephrotic syndrome, *Lancet,* 2:798, 1967.

141. Miller, T. R., R. J. Anderson, S. L. Linas, W. L. Henrich, A. S. Berns, P. A. Gabow, and R. W. Schrier: Urinary diagnostic indices in acute renal failure: A prospective study, *Ann. Intern. Med.,* 89:47, 1978.

142. Wagnild, J. P., and F. D. Gutmann: Functional adaptation of nephrons in dogs with acute progressing to chronic experimental glomerulonephritis, *J. Clin. Invest.,* 57:1575, 1976.

143. Ichikawa, I., H. G. Rennke, J. R. Hoyer, K. F. Badr, N. Schor, J. L. Troy, C. P. Lechene, and B. M. Brenner: Role for intrarenal mechanisms in the impaired salt excretion of experimental nephrotic syndrome, *J. Clin. Invest.,* 71:91, 1983.

144. Bourgoignie, J. J., K. H. Hwang, E. Ipakchi, and N. S. Bricker: The presence of a natriuretic factor in urine of patients with chronic uremia: The absence of the factor in nephrotic uremic patients, *J. Clin. Invest.,* 53:1559, 1974.

145. Kaysen, G. A., T. T. Paukert, D. J. Menke, W. G. Couser, and M. H. Humphreys: Plasma volume expansion is necessary for edema formation in the rat with Heymann nephritis, *Am. J. Physiol.,* 248:F247, 1985.

146. Brown, E. A., N. Markandu, G. A. Sagnella, B. E. Jones, and G. A. MacGregor: Sodium retention in nephrotic syndrome is due to an intrarenal defect: Evidence from steroid-induced remission, *Nephron,* 39:290, 1985.

147. Dorhout Mees, E. J., J. C. Roos, P. Boer, O. H. Yoe, and T. A. Simatupang: Observations on edema formation in the nephrotic syndrome in adults with minimal lesions, *Am. J. Med.,* 67:378, 1979.

148. Geers, A. B., H. A. Koomans, J. C. Roos, and E. J. Dorhout Mees: Preservation of blood volume during edema removal in nephritic subjects, *Kidney Int.,* 28:652, 1985.

149. Kumagai, H., K. Onoyama, D. Iseki, and T. Omae: Role of renin angiotensin aldosterone on minimal change nephrotic syndrome, *Clin. Nephrol.,* 23:229, 1985.

150. Yamauchi, H., and J. Hopper: Hypovolemic shock and hypotension as a complication in the nephrotic syndrome. Report of ten cases, *Ann. Intern. Med.,* 60:242, 1964.

151. Zarins, C. K., C. L. Rice, R. M. Peters, and R. W. Virgilio: Lymph and pulmonary response to isobaric reduction in plasma oncotic pressure in baboons, *Circ. Res.,* 43:925, 1978.

152. Taylor, A. E.: Capillary fluid filtration: Starling forces and lymph flow, *Circ. Res.,* 49:557, 1981.

153. Rodriguez-Iturbé, B., B. Baggio, J. Colina-Chourio, S. Favaro, R. García, F. Sussana, L. Castillo, and A. Borsatti: Studies on the renin-aldosterone system in the acute nephritic syndrome, *Kidney Int.,* 19:445, 1981.

154. Powell, H. R., R. Rotenberg, A. L. Williams, and D. A. McCredie: Plasma renin activity in acute poststreptococcal glomerulonephritis and the hemolytic-uraemic syndrome, *Arch. Dis. Child.,* 49:802, 1974.

155. Stockigt, J. R., D. J. Topliss, and M. J. Hewett: High-renin hypertension in necrotizing vasculitis, *N. Engl. J. Med.,* 300:1218, 1979.

156. Acosta, J. H.: Hypertension in chronic renal disease, *Kidney Int.,* 22:702, 1982.

157. Ishii, M., T. Ikeda, M. Takagi, T. Sugimoto, K. Atarashi, T. Igori, Y. Vehara, H. Matsuoka, Y. Hirata, K. Kimura, T. Takeda, and S. Murao: Elevated plasma catecholamines in hypertensives with primary glomerular diseases, *Hypertension,* 5:545, 1983.

158. Ginsberg, J. M., B. S. Chang, R. A. Matarese, and S. Garella: Use of single voided urine samples to estimate quantitative proteinuria, *N. Engl. J. Med.,* 309:1543, 1983.

159. Hardwicke, J., and J. R. Squire: The relationship between plasma albumin concentration and protein excretion in patients with proteinuria, *Clin. Sci.,* 14:509, 1955.

160. Shemesh, O., W. M. Deen, B. M. Brenner, E. McNeely, and B. D. Myers: Effect of colloid volume expansion on glomerular barrier size-selectivity in humans, *Kidney Int.,* 29:916, 1986.

161. Kaysen, G. A., J. Gambertoglio, I. Jimenez, H. Jones, and F. N. Hutchison: Effect of dietary pro-

tein intake on albumin homeostasis in nephrotic patients, *Kidney Int.,* 29:572, 1986.

162. Rothchild, M. A., M. Oratz, and S. S. Schreiber: Albumin synthesis, *N. Engl. J. Med.,* 286:748, 816, 1972.

163. Kaysen, G. A., and P. Y. Schoenfeld: Albumin homeostasis in patients undergoing continuous ambulatory peritoneal dialysis, *Kidney Int.,* 25:107, 1984.

164. Jenson, H., N. Rossing, S. B. Andersen, and J. Jarnum: Albumin metabolism in the nephrotic syndrome in adults, *Clin. Sci.,* 33:445, 1967.

165. Kaysen, G. A., W. G. Kirkpatrick, and W. G. Couser: Albumin homeostasis in the nephrotic rat: Nutritional considerations, *Am. J. Physiol.,* 247:F192, 1984.

166. Newmark, S. R., C. F. Anderson, J. V. Donadio, Jr., and R. D. Ellefson: Lipoprotein profiles in adult nephrotics, *Mayo Clin. Proc.,* 50:359, 1975.

167. Rose, B. D.: *Clinical Physiology of Acid-Base and Electrolyte Disorders,* 2d ed., McGraw-Hill, New York, 1984, pp. 311–315.

168. Barter, J. H.: Hyperlipoproteinemia in nephrosis, *Arch. Intern. Med.,* 109:742, 1962.

169. Goldberg, A. C. K., F. G. Eliaschewitz, and E. C. R. Quintao: Origin of hypercholesterolemia in chronic experimental nephrotic syndrome, *Kidney Int.,* 12:23, 1977.

170. Marsh, J. B., and C. E. Sparks: Hepatic secretion of lipoproteins in the rat and the effect of experimental nephrosis, *J. Clin. Invest.,* 64:1229, 1979.

171. Appel, G. B., C. B. Blum, S. Chien, C. L. Kunis, and A. S. Appel: The hyperlipidemia of the nephrotic syndrome: Relation to plasma albumin concentration, oncotic pressure, and viscosity, *N. Engl. J. Med.,* 312:1544, 1985.

172. Cormode, E. J., D. M. Lyster, and S. Israels: Analbuminemia in a neonate, *J. Pediatr.,* 86:862, 1975.

173. Baxter, J. H., H. C. Goodman, and J. C. Allen: Effects of infusions of serum albumin on serum lipids and lipoproteins in nephrosis, *J. Clin. Invest.,* 40:490, 1961.

174. Allen, J. C., J. H. Baxter, and H. C. Goodman: Effects of dextran, polyvinylpyrrolidone, and gamma globulin on the hyperlipidemia of experimental nephrosis, *J. Clin. Invest.,* 40:499, 1961.

175. Kaysen, G. A., B. D. Myers, W. G. Couser, R. Rabkin, and J. M. Felts: Mechanisms and consequences of proteinuria, *Lab. Invest.,* 54:479, 1986.

176. Mallick, N. P., and C. D. Short: The nephrotic syndrome and ischemic heart disease, *Nephron,* 27:54, 1981.

177. Wass, V., and J. S. Cameron: Cardiovascular dis-

ease and the nephrotic syndrome: The other side of the coin, *Nephron,* 27:58, 1981.

178. Curry, R. C., Jr.: Status of the coronary arteries in the nephrotic syndrome: Analysis of 20 necropsy patients aged 15 to 35 years to determine if coronary atherosclerosis is accelerated, *Am. J. Med.,* 63:183, 1977.

179. Wass, V. J., C. Chilvers, R. J. Jarrett, and J. S. Cameron: Does the nephrotic syndrome increase the risk of cardiovascular disease?, *Lancet,* 2:664, 1979.

180. The Lipid Research Clinics Coronary Primary Prevention Trial Results: II. The relationship of reduction in incidence of coronary heart disease to cholesterol lowering, *J. Am. Med. Assoc.,* 251:365, 1984.

181. Arntzenius, A. C., D. Kromhout, J. D. Barth, J. H. C. Reiber, A. V. G. Bruschke, B. Buis, C. M. van Gent, N. Kempen-Voogd, S. Strikwerda, and E. A. van der Velde: Diet, lipoproteins, and the progression of coronary atherosclerosis. The Leiden Intervention Trial. *N. Engl. J. Med.,* 312:805, 1985.

182. Llach, F., S. Papper, and S. G. Massry: The clinical spectrum of renal vein thrombosis: Acute and chronic, *Am. J. Med.,* 69:819, 1980.

183. Llach, F.: Hypercoagulability, renal vein thrombosis, and other thrombotic complications of nephrotic syndrome, *Kidney Int.,* 28:429, 1985.

184. Rosenmann, E., V. E. Pollak, and C. Pirani: Renal vein thrombosis in the adult: A clinical and pathologic study on renal biopsies, *Medicine,* 47:269, 1968.

185. Kauffmann, R. H., J. J. Veltkamp., N. H. Tilburg, and L. A. van Es: Acquired antithrombin III deficiency and thrombosis in nephrotic syndrome, *Am. J. Med.,* 65:607, 1978.

186. Llach, F., A. Koffler, E. Fink, and S. G. Massry: On the incidence of renal vein thrombosis in the nephrotic syndrome, *Arch. Intern. Med.,* 137:333, 1977.

187. Wagoner, R. D., A. W. Stanton, K. E. Holley, and C. S. Winter: Renal vein thrombosis in idiopathic membranous glomerulopathy and nephrotic syndrome: Incidence and significance, *Kidney Int.,* 23:368, 1983.

188. Vaziri, N. D., P. Paule, J. Toohey, E. Hung, S. Alikhani, R. Darwish, and M. V. Pahl: Acquired deficiency and urinary excretion of antithrombin III in nephrotic syndrome, *Arch. Intern. Med.,* 144:1802, 1984.

189. Ozanne, P., R. B. Francis, and H. J. Meiselman: Red blood cell aggregation in nephrotic syndrome, *Kidney Int.,* 23:519, 1983.

190. Schieppati, A., P. Dodesini, A. Benigni, M. Massazza, G. Mecca, G. Remuzzi, M. Livio, G. deGaetano, and E. C. Rossi: The metabolism of arachidonic acid by platelets in nephrotic syndrome, *Kidney Int.,* 25:671, 1984.

191. Kuhlmann, U., J. Steurer, K. Rhyner, A. von Felten, J. Briner, and W. Siegenthaler: Platelet aggregation and β-thromboglobulin levels in nephrotic patients with and without thrombosis, *Clin. Nephrol.,* 15:229, 1981.

192. Trew, P. A., C. G. Biava, R. P. Jacobs, and J. Hopper, Jr.: Renal vein thrombosis in membranous glomerulonephropathy: Incidence and association, *Medicine,* 57:69, 1978.

193. Kauffman, R. H., J. de Graeff, G. B. de la Riviere, and L. A. van Es: Unilateral renal vein thrombosis and nephrotic syndrome: Report of a case with protein selectivity and antithrombin III clearance studies, *Am. J. Med.,* 60:1048, 1976.

194. Ross, D. L., and H. Lubowitz: Anticoagulation in renal vein thrombosis, *Arch. Intern. Med.,* 138:1349, 1978.

195. Balabanian, M. B., D. E. Schnetzler, and G. E. Kaloyanides: Nephrotic syndrome, renal vein thrombosis and renal failure: Report of case with recovery of renal function, loss of proteinuria and dissolution of thrombus after anticoagulant therapy, *Am. J. Med.* 54:768, 1973.

196. Burrow, C. R., W. G. Walker, W. R. Bell, and O. B. Gatewood: Streptokinase salvage of renal function after renal vein thrombosis, *Ann. Intern. Med.,* 100:237, 1984.

197. Rowe, J. M., R. L. Rasmussen, S. L. Mader, P. L. Dimarco, A. T. K. Cockett, and V. J. Marder: Successful thrombolytic therapy in two patients with renal vein thrombosis, *Am. J. Med.,* 77:1111, 1984.

198. Duffy, J. L., J. Letteri, T. Cinque, P. P. Hsu, L. Molho, and J. Churg: Renal vein thrombosis and the nephrotic syndrome, *Am. J. Med.,* 54:663, 1973.

199. Goldstein, D. A., Y. Oda., K. Kurokawa, and S. G. Massry: Blood levels of 25-hydroxyvitamin D in nephrotic syndrome: Studies in 26 patients, *Ann. Intern. Med.,* 87:664, 1977.

200. Korkor, A., J. Schwartz, M. Bergfeld, S. Teitelbaum, L. Avioli, S. Klahr, and E. Slatopolsky: Absence of metabolic bone disease in adult patients with the nephrotic syndrome and normal renal function, *J. Clin. Endocrinol. Metab.,* 56:496, 1983.

201. Afrasiabi, M. A., N. D. Vaziri, G. Gwinup, D. M. Mays, C. H. Barton, R. L. Ness, and L. J. Valenta: Thyroid function studies in the nephrotic syndrome, *Ann. Intern. Med.,* 90:335, 1979.

202. Giangiacomo, J., T. G. Cleary, B. R. Cole, P. Hoffsten, and A. M. Robson: Serum immunoglobulins in the nephrotic syndrome: A possible cause of minimal-change nephrotic syndrome, *N. Engl. J. Med.,* 293:8, 1975.

203. Speck, W. T., S. S. Dresdale, and R. W. McMillan: Primary peritonitis and the nephrotic syndrome, *Am. J. Surg.,* 127:267, 1974.

204. Ballow, M., T. L. Kennedy, III, K. M. Gaudio, N. J. Siegel, and R. H. McLean: Serum hemolytic factor D values in children with steroid-responsive idiopathic nephrotic syndrome, *J. Pediatr.,* 100:192, 1982.

205. Ellis, D.: Anemia in the course of the nephrotic syndrome secondary to transferrin depletion, *J. Pediatr.,* 90:953, 1977.

206. Hancock, D. E., J. W. Onstad, and P. L. Wolf: Transferrin loss into the urine with hypochromic, microcytic anemia, *Am. J. Clin. Pathol.,* 65:73, 1976.

207. Volanakis, J. E., S. R. Barnum, M. Giddens, and J. H. Galla: Renal filtration and catabolism of complement protein D, *N. Engl. J. Med.,* 312:395, 1985.

208. Maluche, H. H., D. A. Goldstein, and S. G. Massry: Osteomalacia and hyperparathyroid bone disease in patients with nephrotic syndrome, *J. Clin. Invest.,* 63:494, 1979.

209. Goldstein, D. A., B. Haldimann, D. Sherman, A. W. Norman, and S. G. Massry: Vitamin D metabolites and calcium metabolism in patients with nephrotic syndrome and normal renal function, *J. Clin. Endocrinol. Metab.,* 52:116, 1981.

210. Arneil, G. C.: 164 children with nephrosis, *Lancet,* 2:1103, 1961.

211. Wilkes, J. C., J. D. Nelson, H. G. Worthen, M. Morris, and R. J. Hogg: Response to pneumococcal vaccination in children with nephrotic syndrome, *Am. J. Kid. Dis.,* 2:43, 1982.

212. Mujais, S. K., D. S. Emmanouel, B. S. Kasinath, and B. H. Spargo: Marked proteinuria in hypertensive nephrosclerosis, *Am. J. Nephrol.,* 5:190, 1985.

213. Rapoport, A., D. A. Davidson, G. A. Deveber, G. N. Ranking, and C. R. McLean: Idiopathic focal proliferative nephritis associated with persistent hematuria and normal renal function, *Ann. Intern. Med.,* 73:921, 1970.

214. Lewis, E. J., C. B. Carpenter, and P. H. Schur: Serum complement levels in human glomerulonephritis, *Ann. Intern. Med.,* 75:555, 1971.

215. Daha, M. R., K. F. Austen, and D. T. Fearon: Heterogeneity, polypeptide chain composition, and antigenic reactivity of C3 nephritic factor, *J. Immunol.,* 120:1389, 1978.

216. Halbwachs, L., M. Leveille, Ph. Lesavre, S. Wattel, and J. Leibowitch: Nephritic factor of the classical pathway of complement. Immunoglobulin G autoantibody directed against the classical pathway C3 convertase enzyme, *J. Clin. Invest.,* 65:1249, 1980.

217. Meri, S.: Complement activation by circulating serum factors in human glomerulonephritis, *Clin. Exp. Immunol.,* 59:276, 1985.

218. Vallota, E. H., J. Forristal, N. C. Davis, and C. D. West: The C3 nephritic factor and membranoproliferative nephritis: Correlation of serum levels of the nephritic factor with C3 levels, with therapy and with progression of the disease, *J. Pediatr.,* 80:947, 1972.

219. West, C. D., and A. J. McAdams: Serum β_{1C} globulin levels in persistent glomerulonephritis with low serum complement: Variability unrelated to clinical course, *Nephron,* 7:193, 1970.

220. Finkelstein, A., D. S. Fraley, I. Stachura, H. A. Feldman, D. R. Gandy, and E. Bourke: Fenoprofen nephropathy: Lipoid nephrosis and interstitial nephritis. A possible T-lymphocyte disorder, *Am. J. Med.,* 72:81, 1982.

221. Stachura, I., S. Jayakumar, and E. Bourke: T and B lymphocyte subsets in fenoprofen nephropathy, *Am. J. Med.,* 75:9, 1983.

222. Clive, D. M., and J. S. Stoff: Renal syndromes associated with nonsteroidal antiinflammatory drugs, *N. Engl. J. Med.,* 310:563, 1984.

223. Habib, R., C. Kleinknecht, and M.-C. Gubler: Extramembranous glomerulonephritis in children: Report of 50 cases, *J. Pediatr.,* 82:754, 1973.

224. Namato, Y., Y. Asano, K. Dohi, M. Fujioka, H. Iida, Y. Kibe, N. Hattori, and J. Takeuchi: Primary IgA glomerulonephritis: Clinicopathological and immunohistological characteristics, *Q. J. Med.,* 47:495, 1978.

225. Dillon, H. C., and M. S. Avery: Streptococcal immune response in nephritis after skin infection, *Am. J. Med.,* 56:333, 1974.

6

NEPHROTIC SYNDROME AND GLOMERULO-NEPHRITIS

Burton D. Rose
Jerome B. Jacobs

Indications for Renal Biopsy
Disorders Usually Associated with a Nephrotic Sediment
   Membranous Nephropathy
   Minimal Change Disease
   Focal Glomerulosclerosis
   Diabetes Mellitus
   Amyloidosis and Light Chain Deposition Disease
   Other
Disorders Usually Associated with Focal Glomerulonephritis
   IgA Nephropathy
   Benign Hematuria
   Hereditary Nephritis
   Other
Disorders Usually Associated with Diffuse Glomerulonephritis
   Acute Postinfectious Glomerulonephritis
   Bacterial Endocarditis or Infected Ventriculoatrial Shunt
   Membranoproliferative Glomerulonephritis
   Lupus Nephritis
   Rapidly Progressive Glomerulonephritis
Chronic Glomerulonephritis

The pathogenesis, clinical manifestations, and approach to the differential diagnosis of glomerular diseases were discussed in the preceding chapter. This chapter will review the individual disorders, grouping them according to the typical findings on the urinalysis—nephrotic, focal nephritic, and diffuse nephritic (see p. 164) (Table 6–1).

INDICATIONS FOR RENAL BIOPSY

Establishment of the correct diagnosis (usually by renal biopsy) is essential in view of the variable prognoses and responses to treat-

ment. As an example, consider the different therapeutic regimens in the nephrotic syndrome in adults: prednisone with or without chlorambucil in membranous nephropathy, prednisone alone in minimal change disease or focal glomerulosclerosis, and possibly prednisone and melphalan in primary amyloidosis.

Assuming that there are no contraindications to biopsy (such as a bleeding disorder,*

*Advanced acute or chronic renal failure can impair platelet function, leading to a prolonged bleeding time. This can usually be normalized with dialysis, cryoprecipitate, dDAVP (an analog of antidiuretic hormone), blood transfusions, and/or estrogen (see p. 101).

TABLE 6–1. Major Causes of Glomerular Disease

Disorders usually presenting with a nephrotic sediment
    Membranous nephropathy
    Minimal change disease
    Focal glomerulosclerosis
    Diabetes mellitus
    Amyloidosis and light chain deposition disease
    Benign nephrosclerosis (see Chap. 11)
    Other
Disorders usually presenting with focal
        glomerulonephritis
    IgA nephropathy
    Benign hematuria
    Hereditary nephritis
    SLE (mesangial and focal forms)
    Henoch-Schönlein purpura*
    Other
Disorders usually presenting with diffuse
        glomerulonephritis
    Hypocomplementemic disorders
        SLE (diffuse form)
        Postinfectious glomerulonephritis
            Poststreptococcal infection
            Bacterial endocarditis or infected ventriculoatrial
                shunts
        Membranoproliferative glomerulonephritis
        Mixed cryoglobulinemia*
    Rapidly progressive (crescentic) glomerulonephritis
    Vasculitis*
Chronic glomerulonephritis

*The different types of vasculitis are reviewed in the following chapter.

severe hypertension, or a single functioning kidney), there are still several settings in which a renal biopsy is not necessary:

1. The presence of an underlying systemic disorder that allows the diagnosis to be made on clinical grounds or by a less invasive procedure. Examples include poststreptococcal glomerulonephritis, bacterial endocarditis, diabetes mellitus, amyloidosis, and the use of a drug known to cause glomerular damage such as gold or penicillamine. On the other hand, a biopsy is usually performed in SLE since treatment varies with the different forms of lupus nephritis.
2. Children with the nephrotic syndrome and a nephrotic sediment most likely have minimal change disease. In this setting, a biopsy is performed only if there is no response to an 8-week course of corticosteroids.
3. Patients with isolated glomerular hematuria frequently have focal glomerulonephritis and a benign prognosis, particularly if the urinalysis reveals no cellular or granular casts.[1] The modes of presentation in this setting include recurrent episodes of gross hematuria or the incidental discovery of microscopic hematuria on a routine urinalysis. However, potentially progressive disorders such as IgA nephropathy, membranoproliferative glomerulonephritis, and hereditary nephritis can also present in a similar fashion. Therefore, a renal biopsy is indicated when there is evidence suggesting more serious glomerular involvement including an elevated P_{cr},* hypocomplementemia, more than 1 g of proteinuria per day, or the concurrent development of hypertension.
4. Patients under the age of 25 with isolated proteinuria should be evaluated for orthostatic proteinuria, a benign disorder that does not require renal biopsy (see p. 52).
5. Adults with mild isolated proteinuria (1 to 2.5 g/day) may not have glomerular disease. Chronic pyelonephritis, nephrosclerosis, or polycystic kidney disease, for example, can all present with similar findings. As a result, a renal ultrasound should be performed first looking for decreased kidney size, asymmetric scarring, or the presence of cysts.
6. A biopsy is usually not performed in patients with renal insufficiency and small kidneys, since marked scarring is undoubtedly present and there is little hope of finding a reversible disease.

*It is important to remember that a stable P_{cr} in the normal or near normal range does not necessarily imply stable disease since compensatory hyperfiltration in relatively uninvolved nephrons can initially mask continuing glomerular damage (see Chap. 4). In this setting, an increase in proteinuria, in the activity of the urinary sediment, or in blood pressure may be the only sign of progressive disease.

DISORDERS USUALLY ASSOCIATED WITH A NEPHROTIC SEDIMENT

MEMBRANOUS NEPHROPATHY

Membranous nephropathy* (MN) is the most common cause of the idiopathic nephrotic syndrome in adults, accounting for 30 to 50 percent of cases.[2,3] Although it may occur at any age,[4,5] it is responsible for fewer than 2 percent of cases in children because of the prevalence of minimal change disease.[6,7]

PATHOLOGY

Although MN is associated with characteristic changes on light microscopy (LM), electron microscopy (EM), and immunofluorescent microscopy (IF), several stages that are thought to reflect differences in severity and in the evolutionary phase of the disease have been identified (Fig. 6–1).[4,6,8] In stage I, the glomeruli usually appear normal on LM. However, the findings of small, subepithelial (epimembranous) dense deposits on EM (Fig. 6–1a) and diffuse, granular deposition in the capillary loops of IgG, C3, and less frequently IgA and IgM on IF (Fig. 5–6b) are diagnostic of MN.

More commonly, the changes are more severe (stage II). Light microscopy shows a diffuse, uniform thickening of the glomerular basement membrane (GBM) which may be associated with mild, focal mesangial proliferation (Fig. 6–2). More and larger deposits are present, and EM reveals growth of the GBM between and around the deposits, resulting in the characteristic spike-and-dome pattern on silver stain (Figs. 6–1b and 6–1c). Fusion of the epithelial foot processes is often present, particularly over the deposits.

In stage III, which may reflect a later phase of the disease, the GBM is irregularly thickened on LM. Discrete deposits may not be detected on EM since the complexes appear to become incorporated into the GBM, occasionally resulting in the appearance of intramembranous lucent areas (Fig. 6–1d). At this time, IF may be less positive, a finding consistent with the lack of discrete deposits.

Finally, diffuse mesangial sclerosis with obliteration of the capillary lumen occurs in patients who progress to renal failure. However, lesions typical of MN can usually be found in some glomeruli even at this time.

The clinical importance of these stages is uncertain. With the exception of diffuse sclerotic changes, the course of the disease is not closely related to the histologic pattern, although stage I may have a somewhat better prognosis.[4,5] Furthermore, classification into a single stage may be difficult in some patients. For example, normal glomeruli on LM (stage I) may be associated with stage II or III changes on EM.[8] It may be that these patients do not deposit enough complexes to produce detectable thickening of the GBM on LM. Nevertheless, eventual incorporation of the deposits into the GBM does occur.

PATHOGENESIS

As described in the preceding chapter, the subepithelial deposits in MN probably occur via an in situ mechanism with circulating antibody reacting with antigen already present in or deposited in the glomerular capillary wall (see p. 149ff.).[9,10] For example, an antigen, called renal tubular epithelial antigen (RTE), normally is present in the brush border of the proximal tubule and in the cell membrane of the glomerular epithelial cells, as they abut the GBM. In animals, either the passive administration of anti-RTE antibodies or the induction of endogenous antibodies by the injection of RTE in adjuvant can produce a lesion similar to MN.[11,12] The role of RTE in idiopathic human MN is uncertain,

---

*Synonyms include membranous glomerulonephritis or glomerulopathy, epimembranous glomerulonephritis, and extramembranous glomerulonephritis.

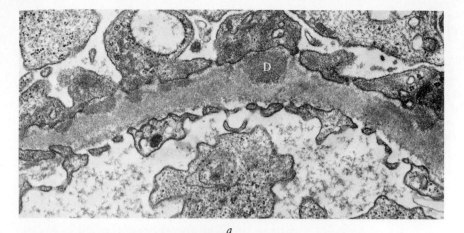

a

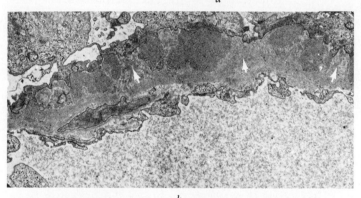

b

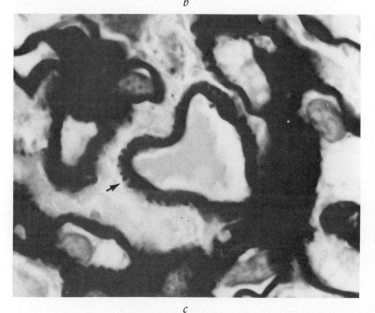

c

FIG. 6-1. Electron microscopy in membranous nephropathy. In each case, as in the other electron micrographs in this chapter, the epithelial cell is on top followed by the GBM, endothelial cell, and capillary space. (*a*) Amorphous, frequently small subepithelial deposits are seen in the early stage (stage I) of the disease. (*b*) In stage II, more and larger deposits are present, and there is growth of the basement membrane between and around the deposits (arrows), resulting in thickening of the capillary wall. Fusion of the foot processes is frequently present, particularly over the deposits. (*c*) This growth of the basement membrane between the deposits results in the characteristic appearance of spikes on silver stain (arrow).

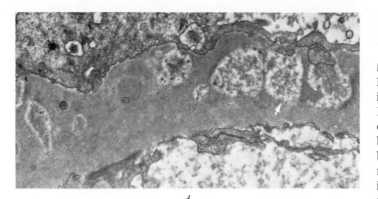

FIG. 6-1 (Continued). (*d*) In stage III, the basement membrane is irregularly and markedly thickened. Discrete deposits may not be detected since they seem to become incorporated into the basement membrane, occasionally resulting in the appearance of intramembranous lucent areas (arrow).

d

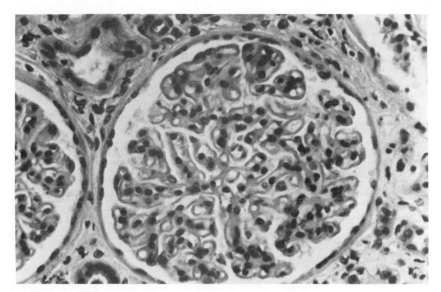

FIG. 6-2. Light microscopy in membranous nephropathy. Prominent thickening of the basement membrane is present in all capillary loops. Glomerular cellularity is relatively normal.

as RTE antigen-antibody complexes cannot be demonstrated in the great majority of patients.[13-16] In some secondary forms of MN (see Table 6-2), however, it is possible that primary damage to the proximal tubule results in the release of RTE into the circulation, leading to antibody production and subsequent complex formation in the glomeruli. This sequence could occur in de novo MN in renal transplants, in sickle cell disease, and following gold therapy for rheumatoid arthritis.[17-21]

When MN is due to extrarenal antigens being deposited in the glomeruli, experimental studies suggest that only cationic antigens (or possibly intact cationic complexes) are able to overcome the charge barrier in the GBM and enter the subepithelial space (see Fig. 5-8).[22-24] Although a variety of endogenous and exogenous antigens can lead

TABLE 6-2. Antigens and Disorders Associated with Membranous Nephropathy (MN)

Endogenous antigens
   DNA (SLE)[*,36]
   Tumor[*,37]
   Thyroglobulin[38]
   ?Renal tubular epithelial
      Idiopathic[15,16]
      Sickle cell disease[19]
      Chronic transplant rejection[17,18,39]
      ?Gold therapy[21]
Exogenous antigens
   Medications
      Gold[*,21,32,40,41]
      Penicillamine[*,41-43]
      Captopril[44,45]
      Mercury[46,47]
      Mercaptopropionylglycine[48]
   Infections
      Hepatitis B virus[*,49-51]
      Syphilis
         Secondary[52,53]
         Congenital[53,54]
      Quartan malaria[55]
      Echinococcal infection[56]
Antigen or inciting agent unidentified
   Most cases of idiopathic MN[*]
   Rheumatoid arthritis[57]
   Superimposition on other glomerulopathy[58,59]
   Weber-Christian disease[60]
   Dermatitis herpetiformis[61]
   Sarcoidosis[62]

[*]Most common causes of MN.

---

to MN, it remains to be proven that they are cationic.

Once subepithelial deposits are formed, damage to the GBM occurs by activation of C3 and then the terminal complement components of the membrane attack complex (see p. 153).[25,26] These changes lead to the creation of larger pores that allow proteinuria to occur.[27] However, C3 deposition is not always demonstrable by IF in humans even though C3d, an inactive fragment can be found.[28] It may be that these patients have relatively quiescent disease.

Genetic factors affecting the immune response appear to affect the susceptibility to MN. White patients with idiopathic or gold-induced MN have a marked increase in the frequency of the HLA-DR3/B8 and DR3/B18 haplotypes.[29-32] HLA-DR3, for example, is frequently associated with decreased removal of circulating complexes by the reticuloendothelial system.[31-33] This abnormality could explain the propensity both to MN and to other autoimmune diseases (including systemic lupus erythematosus and Graves' disease).[34] In comparison, MN in Japanese adults is associated with a different haplotype, HLA-DR2.[30] The mechanism by which this predisposes to MN is not known.

ETIOLOGY AND DIAGNOSIS

Approximately two-thirds of cases of MN are currently idiopathic (and diagnosable only by renal biopsy), with some identifiable cause being present in the remaining one-third (Table 6-2).[4,5,35] Among the more common causes, *malignancies* have been estimated to be responsible for approximately 10 percent of cases of idiopathic nephrotic syndrome in adults.[37] Although a variety of histologic patterns may be found (including amyloidosis), most tumors are associated with MN with the exception of lymphoma, which is usually associated with minimal change disease. The conclusion that a tumor can lead to the nephrotic syndrome is based upon observations such as remission of the nephrotic syndrome following removal of the tumor,[63] the elution of antibodies from the glomerulus that react with the underlying malignancy,[64] and the identification of tumor antigens in the glomerulus.[65,66]

In the majority of patients, the tumor has already been diagnosed or is clinically apparent at the time of onset of the nephrotic syndrome. Only 15 percent of tumor-related MN, or *1.5 percent* of all adults with MN, have an occult malignancy.[37] As a result, an extensive evaluation for an underlying tumor is not indicated in the absence of suggestive signs or symptoms such as unexplained anemia, heme-positive stools, or weight loss.

MN represents 10 to 20 percent of cases of *lupus nephritis* (see "Lupus Nephritis," below). Some patients present with only the nephrotic syndrome, with extrarenal and serologic manifestations not appearing for up to 3 years.[67-69] Nevertheless, there may be electron microscopic findings on the biopsy that are suggestive of underlying SLE.[67,70] These include tubuloreticular structures in the glomerular endothelial cells (see Fig. 6–19) and deposits in the mesangium, subendothelial space, or the tubular basement membranes in addition to those in the subepithelial space. The presence of hypocomplementemia is also suggestive of SLE.[67]

The incidence of MN following *drugs* is variable, averaging 1 to 3 percent with gold,[21,41] probably under 1 percent with captopril,[44,45] and about 7 percent with penicillamine in rheumatoid arthritis[41] but much lower when penacillamine is used in Wilson's disease.[43] The onset of proteinuria in this setting is usually 1 week to 12 months after the drug has been started; discontinuation of the drug usually leads to resolution of the proteinuria within 12 months. Rechallenge may or may not lead to recurrent proteinuria.[21,41]

MN due to hepatitis B virus* occurs primarily in children, many of whom have normal liver function tests and no prior history of hepatitis.[35,50,51,71] The serum is surface-antigen-positive but it appears that it is the *e* antigen that is deposited in the glomeruli.[50] Spontaneous resolution of the proteinuria is common in this setting.[51]

De novo MN may occur in patients with *renal transplants* who had a different primary renal disease.[17,18,39] This complication may be related to chronic transplant rejection in which glomerular or tubular damage leads to the release of native or altered RTE antigens into the circulation, resulting in anti-RTE antibody production, and in situ complex

---

*Hepatitis B virus is also associated with other renal diseases such as membranoproliferative glomerulonephritis, mesangial proliferative glomerulonephritis, and systemic vasculitis.

formation in the glomeruli (see "Pathogenesis," above).

Finally, MN may be superimposed upon *other glomerulopathies,* leading to focal or diffuse subepithelial deposits.[58,59] This is most likely to occur in diabetic nephropathy (a finding confirmed in animals)[72] and may be related to increased glomerular permeability from the primary disease, a change that could promote the formation of subepithelial deposits.

CLINICAL PRESENTATION AND COURSE

The major presenting complaints in MN are edema and proteinuria. Approximately 75 to 85 percent of patients will have the nephrotic syndrome, with the remainder having only nonnephrotic proteinuria.[4,5,34,73,74] Other findings which may be present at the time of diagnosis include hypertension (25 to 40 percent), microscopic (40 to 60 percent) or gross (5 to 10 percent) hematuria, and, in almost all patients, a normal serum complement (except for underlying SLE or hepatitis B infection in which hypocomplementemia may be present),[51] and a normal or only mildly elevated P_{cr}.

The course of MN is variable. Complete recovery within weeks to 1 year is the rule in MN due to drugs or infection when the offending agent is removed. However, mild proteinuria may persist in some patients for more than 2 years.[75] This response to removal of the antigen indicates that persistent disease (as in idiopathic MN) requires the continued formation of antigen-antibody complexes. Clearly, the prognosis is much worse for patients with malignancies, most of whom die from the tumor.

The natural history of the renal disease is frequently not so benign in idiopathic MN. In children, approximately 50 percent have a spontaneous remission which is frequently permanent, 40 percent have persistent proteinuria, and 10 percent progress to end-stage renal failure.[74]

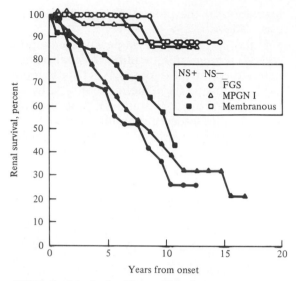

FIG. 6–3. Survival without dialysis or transplantation in patients with membranous nephropathy, focal segmental glomerulosclerosis (FGS), and type I membranoproliferative glomerulonephritis (MPGN I). Life table analysis shows a much better prognosis in those patients without the nephrotic syndrome (NS−). (*From J. S. Cameron, Am. J. Kid. Dis., 1:371, 1982.*)

The prognosis of untreated MN is somewhat worse in adults. At 5- to 10-year follow-up, 20 to 25 percent will have progressed to end-stage renal failure,* 20 to 25 percent will be in remission (some of whom may relapse), and the remainder will have either persistent proteinuria or the nephrotic syndrome.[5,34,73]

It is possible, however, to identify at presentation subgroups with good or bad prognostic findings. Progression to renal failure in 5 to 10 years appears to occur in only about

*Renal failure is generally slowly progressive and associated with increasing glomerular sclerosis. Acute renal failure suggests a superimposed problem such as diuretic-induced hypovolemia, nonsteroidal anti-inflammatory drugs, renal vein thrombosis, or, rarely, a new glomerular lesion such as crescentic glomerulonephritis.[76]

10 percent of women or patients with nonnephrotic proteinuria (less than 2 to 2.5 g/day) (Fig. 6–3).[34,73,77-79] In contrast, there is a high risk of developing renal failure in men with nephrotic range proteinuria (over 50 percent) or patients with an elevated P_{cr} at onset, particularly if over the age of 50.[77,78] In addition, almost all patients who deteriorate will begin to do so within 2 to 3 years. Thus, the maintenance of a normal P_{cr} at 3 years is another indicator of a good prognosis.[73,77] The course of the disease is not as closely related to the findings on renal biopsy (assuming no glomerular sclerosis is present), although remissions are more likely and renal failure less likely in stage I disease (Fig. 6–1a).[5,80]

The course of MN also may be influenced by the presence of renal vein thrombosis, which may occur in up to 25 to 50 percent of cases.[81,82] Renal failure [with acute renal vein thrombosis (RVT)] or pulmonary emboli are the most serious potential complications. The evaluation and treatment of this problem are discussed on p. 161.

TREATMENT

The evaluation of therapy in idiopathic MN is difficult because of relatively frequent spontaneous remissions and the generally slow rate of progression in those who ultimately develop renal failure. Uncontrolled studies have usually suggested a beneficial response to corticosteroids.[80,83-85] This trend has been confirmed in two randomized trials in which prednisone therapy (2 mg/kg up to a maximum of 120 mg every other day for 2 to 3 months or 45 mg/m² daily for 6 months) minimized the deterioration in renal function but did not significantly affect the degree of proteinuria.[86,87] In one study, for example, an increase in the P_{cr} to more than 5 mg/dL (within a mean of 2 years) developed in 10 or 38 controls but only 1 of 34 treated patients.[86]

Even more impressive results have been obtained with an unusual 6-month regimen consisting of corticosteroids (1 g of methylprednisolone intravenously for 3 days, followed by 0.5 mg/kg per day of prednisone in months 1, 3, and 5) and chlorambucil (0.2 mg/kg per day in months 2, 4, and 6).[88,89] At 2 years in the 38 treated patients, 15 were in complete remission (versus only 2 of 35 untreated controls), 11 were in partial remission, and all patients had a stable P_{cr} (versus a 50 percent increase in 10 of 35 controls).[89] Although chlorambucil can be carcinogenic, the total dose with this regimen is well below that generally received by patients described in the literature who subsequently developed a malignancy.[88-91]

Despite these impressive results, the potential toxicity of both prednisone and chlorambucil suggests that immunosuppressive therapy may be initially withheld in those subgroups that are more likely to do well: children, women, and patients excreting less than 2 g of protein per day.[34,73,74,77-79] On the other hand, treatment is probably indicated in men with nephrotic range proteinuria, in patients with a rise in the P_{cr} that appears to be due to the underlying disease, and in markedly nephrotic patients whose edema is difficult to control with diuretics. The relative efficacy of prednisone alone or with chlorambucil is currently unanswered, although the latter seems to be more effective in causing remission of the proteinuria,[86,88] particularly if therapy is begun within 8 months of the onset of disease.[89] Thus, chlorambucil (or cyclophosphamide) should probably be used in markedly nephrotic patients and in those whose P_{cr} begins to rise despite an initial trial of 2 to 3 months of alternate-day prednisone.

Those patients who develop progressive renal insufficiency despite immunosuppressive therapy can be given a trial of antihypertensive agents (particularly using a converting enzyme inhibitor) and possibly dietary protein restriction (the safety of which is uncertain in nephrotic patients; see p. 130) in an attempt to minimize hemodynamically mediated glomerular injury (see Chap. 4). There is one other potential therapy in patients who are markedly symptomatic from nephrotic edema due to severe hypoalbuminemia. Indomethacin and meclofenamate (and probably most other prostaglandin synthesis inhibitors) can substantially reduce the degree of proteinuria and raise the plasma albumin concentration by diminishing both the capillary leak and, in some patients, the GFR.[27,92] The fall in GFR is generally mild and not a contraindication to continued therapy.

Dialysis or renal transplantation can be instituted in those patients who progress to end-stage renal failure. Recurrent MN can develop in the transplant but is typically mild and does not usually lead to loss of the graft.[18,39] (This entity should be distinguished from de novo MN, which is probably a manifestation of chronic rejection in patients who had a different primary renal disease.[17,18,39])

MINIMAL CHANGE DISEASE

Minimal change disease (MCD)* is the major cause of the nephrotic syndrome in children, accounting for 85 to 90 percent of cases under the age of 6 and more than 50 percent in older children.[6,7,93] It is not, however, limited to children as it is responsible for approximately 10 to 20 percent of cases of idiopathic nephrotic syndrome in adults of all ages.[2,94]

PATHOLOGY

The names *minimal change disease* and *nil disease* are derived from the findings on LM,

---

*Minimal change disease has also been called nil disease, lipoid nephrosis, epithelial cell disease, and foot process disease.

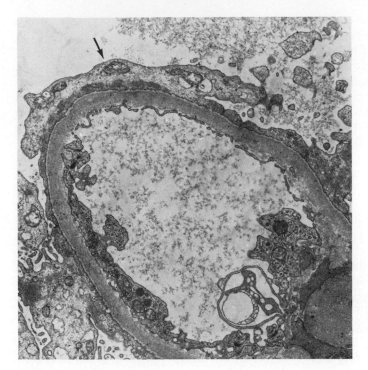

FIG. 6-4. Electron microscopy in minimal change disease revealing only diffuse fusion of foot processes (arrow). The basement membrane is normal, and no deposits are present.

which usually reveals normal glomeruli (see Fig. 5-4), although occasional areas of mild, mesangial hypercellularity may be present.[2,95] IF is usually negative for immunoglobulins and complement but may demonstrate mild, focal deposits of IgM or C3 in the mesangium that probably represent nonspecific trapping.[96] The major histologic change in MCD is fusion of the epithelial cell foot processes on EM (Fig. 6-4). The basement membrane is unaffected and electron-dense deposits are absent. Foot process configuration returns to normal with spontaneous or corticosteroid-induced remission of the disease.

ETIOLOGY

Although MCD is most often idiopathic, a specific cause can sometimes be identified (Table 6-3). *Malignancies* appear to account for approximately 10 percent of cases of idi-

opathic nephrotic syndrome in adults, with solid tumors usually causing membranous nephropathy and lymphomas and leukemias, particularly Hodgkin's disease, typically causing MCD.*[37,97-99] Both the lymphoma and the nephrotic syndrome generally present simultaneously or within a few months of each other. Late development of the nephrotic syndrome (more than 12 months after diagnosis of the lymphoma) is more often due to secondary amyloidosis.[37] The course of the nephrotic syndrome usually parallels that of the lymphoma: effective treatment of the lymphoma (with chemotherapy, surgical excision, or local irradiation) results in remission

---

*This distinction is not absolute since solid tumors can, on occasion, produce MCD, and the hematologic malignancies can produce other lesions such as membranous nephropathy, focal glomerulosclerosis, and a proliferative glomerulonephritis.[99,100]

TABLE 6-3. Etiology of Minimal Change Disease

Idiopathic
Malignancy, particularly Hodgkin's disease
Nonsteroidal anti-inflammatory drugs
IgA nephropathy
Gold
Lithium
Mercaptoproprionylglycine

of the proteinuria; relapse of the lymphoma may then lead to recurrent proteinuria.[37,97,98]

Nonsteroidal anti-inflammatory drugs (NSAID), particularly fenoprofen, may be associated with the unusual combination of acute interstitial nephritis (characterized by hematuria, pyuria, and acute renal failure) and the nephrotic syndrome due to MCD (see p. 391).[101,102] Similar findings have also been reported with ampicillin and recombinant leukocyte interferon in isolated patients.[103,104] The entire picture is not present in all patients, however, as NSAID can produce MCD without interstitial nephritis.[105]

Steroid-responsive nephrotic syndrome with diffuse foot process fusion may occur in association with *IgA nephropathy*.[106-108] In some patients, the MCD (proven by biopsy) preceded the onset of IgA nephropathy, but the reverse sequence may also occur. The factors responsible for this relationship are not known.

Reversible MCD has also been reported with the use of *gold, lithium,* and *mercaptoproprionylglycine* (used primarily in the treatment of cystinuria).[40,48,109,110] Although gold-induced nephrotic syndrome is characteristically due to membranous nephropathy,[21,41] an MCD pattern may occur.[40]

PATHOGENESIS

The pathogenesis of MCD is not well understood. The only experimental model of this disorder involves the administration of the aminonucleoside puromycin,[111] which is spe-cifically toxic to the glomerular epithelial cells.[112] These cells appear to be responsible for the synthesis of the negatively charged sialoproteins and proteoglycans (such as heparan sulfate), which coat the foot processes and are present in the GBM.[113] Thus, epithelial cell injury could lead to reduced production of this glomerular polyanion, an effect which could explain the two characteristic findings of MCD: foot process fusion and proteinuria.

The normal separation of adjacent foot processes appears to be maintained by electrostatic repulsion induced by these anionic charges. The importance of charge has been demonstrated by the following experiment.[114] If the polycation protamine sulfate is infused into the renal artery of a rat, foot process fusion occurs within minutes, presumably owing to neutralization of the glomerular polyanion. This change can be reversed, also within minutes, by counteracting the effect of protamine with supraphysiologic doses of heparin. Thus, foot process fusion in MCD (and other proteinuric states) could be a consequence of the loss of glomerular polyanion induced by epithelial cell damage.

The negative charges in the GBM also appear to contribute to the normally limited filtration of anionic albumin, again acting by electrostatic repulsion (see Fig. 5-3). Thus, decreased glomerular polyanion could lead to increased albumin filtration and subsequent excretion.[115] Studies in humans with MCD are compatible with this hypothesis, indicating that loss of the charge barrier to filtration is responsible for the proteinuria.[116,117]

However, even if epithelial cell damage leading to diminished polyanion production is the primary event, the mechanisms responsible for cell injury are not known. In contrast to the animal model, toxins do not appear to play an important role, at least in idiopathic MCD. The positive response to corticosteroids and cytotoxic drugs in over

90 percent of patients with this disorder suggests that immune mechanisms, either cellular or humoral, may be of primary importance.

It has been postulated that MCD represents a defect in the function of thymus-derived lymphocytes (T cells).[118] A variety of observations are consistent with this hypothesis, including (1) the demonstration of increased lymphocyte reactivity to renal antigens in some patients,[119] (2) the associations of MCD with Hodgkin's disease (in which T-cell function is abnormal) and NSAID-induced interstitial nephritis (in which T cells constitute most of the infiltrating interstitial cells),[97,98,101,120] and (3) the generally excellent response of MCD to cyclophosphamide, a lymphocytotoxin which depletes the number of circulating T cells.[121] If T cells are important, they might act by releasing soluble factors (lymphokines) that damage either the glomerular epithelial cell or the GBM itself.[122] However, nephrotoxic lymphokines have not always been demonstrated in this disorder[123] and, when found, are not specific for MCD.[124] Direct, cell-mediated effects are unlikely since lymphocyte infiltration of the glomerulus does not occur.

As an alternative, MCD could be an immune complex disease. Circulating immune complexes have been found during the active phase but not when the disease is in remission.[125-127] Also supporting the possible role of a humoral mechanism are the associations in some patients of MCD with pollen or milk allergies or elevated plasma IgE levels (although IgE cannot be demonstrated in the kidney).[128-130] Furthermore, the negative histologic findings do not necessarily exclude an antigen-antibody-mediated disorder since small complexes in animals can lead to glomerular disease without demonstrable deposits on IF or EM.[131]

In summary, a large body of indirect evidence supports a possible immunologic abnormality in MCD. Nevertheless, the exact cause of this disorder remains unknown. Whatever the stimulus, genetic factors may also play an important role by determining the susceptibility to MCD. For example, HLA-DQw3 appears to be associated with an elevenfold increase in risk in Japanese adults.[132] How this haplotype might predispose to MCD is not known.

CLINICAL PRESENTATION

Patients with MCD typically present with edema, heavy proteinuria,* and the chemical findings of the nephrotic syndrome.[94,133] The onset of the disease is usually acute and frequently follows a viral upper respiratory infection. The degree of fluid retention is variable, occasionally resulting in ascites as well as pedal and periorbital edema. Hypertension or hematuria occur in only 20 to 30 percent of children[7,133] but are somewhat more prevalent in adults.[94] However, cellular and granular casts typical of a nephritic sediment (see Table 5-5) are absent. The plasma complement levels are normal in virtually all patients.[133]

The GFR is usually normal or mildly reduced.[94,133,134] However, moderate to severe renal failure can occur, particularly in older patients.[94] Three factors can contribute to the fall in GFR: aggressive diuretic therapy[135,136]; severe interstitial edema, leading

---

*The proteinuria in MCD in children is, in general, highly selective.[3,133] Selectivity is measured by comparing the clearance of IgG (MW 170,000) to that of transferrin (MW 88,000). A patient with highly selective proteinuria has a ratio of 0.1 or less, indicating a relatively moderate increase in glomerular permeability with primarily smaller macromolecules (such as transferrin and albumin) being filtered; a value above 0.20 is called nonselective, as more of the larger IgG molecules are filtered. The usefulness of this test, however, is limited. Highly selective proteinuria in a young child is strongly suggestive of MCD, but this makes up 85 to 90 percent of cases to begin with. The selectivity index is much less specific in adults: a value below 0.1 occurring in only 25 percent of patients with MCD,[94] with considerable overlap with other causes of the nephrotic syndrome such as membranous nephropathy or amyloidosis.[3,4]

to tubular collapse[137]; and a decrease in glomerular permeability, resulting from loss of the epithelial cell slit pores (see Fig. 6–4) due to foot process fusion.[134] Each of these forms of renal failure is responsive to therapy: fluids for excessive diuresis, diuretics for interstitial edema, and corticosteroids to restore glomerular function.

DIAGNOSIS

Minimal change disease cannot be definitely differentiated from other causes of the nephrotic syndrome on clinical grounds. Although hypertension, hematuria, and azotemia are more common in other disorders such as membranous nephropathy, focal glomerulosclerosis, and membranoproliferative glomerulonephritis, there is considerable overlap.[133] Thus, renal biopsy is required to make the diagnosis in adults.

The situation is somewhat different in children since MCD is responsible for most cases of the nephrotic syndrome. In this setting, treatment with corticosteroids is usually initiated on empirical grounds and renal biopsy performed only if an 8-week trial is ineffective in inducing a remission. MCD accounts for approximately 50 percent of corticosteroid-resistant cases under the age of 6 but *only about 4 percent* of such cases in older children.[93] The remaining cases have focal glomerulosclerosis, diffuse mesangial proliferation (see p. 195), or membranoproliferative glomerulonephritis.[6,7,93] The last disorder typically presents with a nephritic sediment (containing cellular and granular casts) and is infrequently confused with MCD.[133]

COURSE AND TREATMENT

The availability of antimicrobials and corticosteroids has dramatically altered the course of MCD. Prior to the use of these agents, the 5-year mortality rate in children was as high as 67 percent with the remaining cases undergoing spontaneous remission.[138] The ma-

jor causes of death were infection, particularly peritonitis and pneumonia, and renal failure. Low plasma levels of IgG and factors B and D of the alternate complement pathway may have been responsible for the propensity to infection (see p. 163).

The morbidity from infection was largely ameliorated with the introduction of penicillin and other antimicrobials, and the 5-year mortality rate fell to 35 percent.[138] A further beneficial alteration in the course was achieved with corticosteroids, which induce permanent or transient remissions in most patients. The current long-term mortality rate is probably under 2 percent.[139,140] Infection remains the major (and potentially avoidable) cause, with corticosteroids or other immunosuppressive therapy possibly contributing in some cases.

A standard prednisone regimen in children* consists of 60 mg/m^2 (daily in 3 divided doses) for 4 weeks and then 40 mg/m^2 as a single morning dose on alternate days for 4 more weeks.[141] The effects of prednisone in this setting may be summarized as follows (Fig. 6–5)[93,138,140,142]:

1. Approximately 5 percent will be nonresponders.
2. The remaining 95 percent will undergo complete remission of the proteinuria and edema: 70 percent within 2 weeks, 90 percent by 4 weeks, and 100 percent by 8 weeks.[93]

In those who respond, the remission is permanent in only about 20 percent.[140,142,143] The rest of the patients will have either infrequent or frequent relapses (the latter is defined as two relapses in 6 months or four in 1 year). The initial relapse usually occurs within 2 years, with those destined to be frequent relapsers (about 40 to 50 percent of patients) generally having at least one relapse in the first 6 months.[144] Patients in remission for at least 4 years are typically cured, with

---

*Treatment in adults is somewhat different and is discussed separately below.

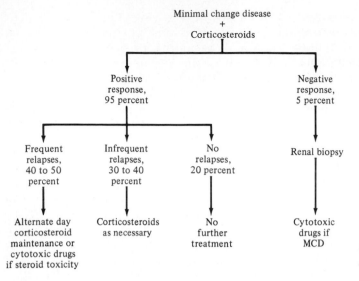

FIG. 6-5. Course and treatment in children with minimal change disease.

relapses being uncommon beyond the age of 20. However, regular relapses can continue into adulthood[145] and rarely can be seen as late as 15 to 25 years after apparently permanent remission.[142,146]

Relapses may occur while the prednisone dose is being lowered or after the drug has been discontinued. In addition to reactivation of the disease, it has been suggested that many relapses, particularly those occurring within 3 to 6 months, are due to posttreatment adrenal insufficiency.[147,148] In this setting, slow tapering of prednisone over 6 to 12 months may reduce the rate of future relapses. Hypoadrenalism with an inadequate stress response also could explain the observation that many relapses appear to follow small stresses such as an upper respiratory infection.[148]

Frequently relapsing MCD is a particular problem in children because chronic or recurrent corticosteroid therapy can lead to a number of serious side effects including infection, osteopenia, decreased growth, hypertension, and cataracts.[148,149] As a result, cytotoxic agents have been evaluated in this disorder. Azathioprine appears to be without

benefit,[150] but cyclophosphamide markedly reduces the frequency of subsequent relapses to approximately 10 percent at 2 years and 50 percent at 7 years (Fig. 6-6).[151-153] Chlorambucil may be even more effective than cyclophosphamide with the relapse rate being as low as 5 percent at 1 year and 20 percent at 4 years.[154,155] These drugs may be more effective in patients who relapse after corticosteroids have been discontinued than in those who are corticosteroid-dependent and relapse while still on prednisone treatment.[155,156]

However, the efficacy of cytotoxic agents must be weighed against their potential toxicity, *particularly in a disease which ultimately remits in almost all patients.*[142,145] Cyclophosphamide can induce hemorrhagic cystitis, and both drugs can cause bone marrow suppression, infection, testicular and less commonly ovarian fibrosis which can lead to sterility, and neoplasia.[90,157-162] However, gonadal fibrosis and neoplasia are highly unlikely if the total dose is less than 300 mg/kg for cyclophosphamide (2 to 2.5 mg/kg for 8 weeks) and less than 8 mg/kg for chlorambucil (0.15 mg/kg for 8 weeks).[90,140,158,159] Furthermore, boys who develop oligospermia may recover relatively normal testicular function over a period of years.[163]

In view of these potential problems, the following recommendations seem prudent in children with MCD. Infrequent relapsers can be treated with short courses of prednisone. More aggressive therapy is indicated only in frequently relapsing disease. Once a remission is induced with prednisone, the patient should be switched to 40 mg/m² given on alternate days (a dose at which normal growth may occur).[149,164] This dose can be reduced at a rate of 5 to 10 mg per month, aiming for a maintenance dose as low as 10 to 15 mg every other day. If the child relapses, daily prednisone should be reinstituted and, after the proteinuria remits, the alternate-day dose then tapered to 5 to 10 mg higher than that at which the relapse occurred. It should be noted that some infection-induced relapses *may remit spontaneously.* Therefore, increased corticosteroid therapy can be delayed for 10 to 14 days, unless the patient is very symptomatic.[140,165]

The use of cytotoxic drugs is indicated *only* in children who demonstrate unacceptable corticosteroid toxicity. Low-dose prednisone is usually continued during the course of cytotoxic therapy to minimize the incidence of leukopenia. In general, treatment should be limited to 8 weeks at the dosage described above to minimize the risk of sterility and neoplasia. Although safer, shorter courses of therapy tend to be less effective.[140,166] One exception to this general rule is patients who relapse while still on prednisone. These corticosteroid-dependent children have a relatively high relapse rate on cytotoxic therapy (22 of 34 in one study) and may benefit from extending the course of cyclophosphamide to 10 to 12 weeks,[140,156] since the total dose will still be below 300 mg/kg.[158] This cannot be done as safely with chlorambucil, since 8 weeks of treatment is already near the relatively safe upper limit (in terms of gonadal toxicity) of 8 mg/kg.[156] For similar reasons, a second course of cytotoxic therapy should probably be avoided if the patient continues to relapse.

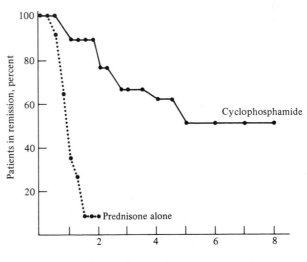

FIG. 6-6. Percentage of children with frequently relapsing minimal change disease remaining in remission after discontinuation of therapy with either prednisone or cyclophosphamide. (*From J. Chiu and K. N. Drummond, J. Pediatr., 84:825, 1974.*)

Corticosteroid Resistance. Two types of corticosteroid resistance occur in MCD. Approximately 5 percent are resistant to the initial course of therapy and should have a renal biopsy to establish the correct diagnosis. About one-half of children up to the age of 6 but very few older children will have MCD in this setting.[93] Those with MCD are at increased risk of ultimately developing focal glomerulosclerosis and renal failure (see below), but some undergo a spontaneous remission.[167] If the nephrotic syndrome persists, cyclophosphamide or chlorambucil can both induce a remission and make the patient corticosteroid-sensitive if a relapse occurs.[152,159,168]

Corticosteroid resistance also may occur as a secondary event in approximately 5 to 15 percent of corticosteroid-responsive frequently relapsing patients.[140,143] Biopsy at this time may show focal glomerulosclerosis.[143,169] Cyclophosphamide or chlorambucil will frequently induce a remission in this setting[169,170] but progression to renal failure may occur.[169-171]

Adults. Prednisone (beginning with 1 mg/kg per day in divided doses) is also effective in inducing a remission in adults.[94,172] The response, however, tends to be slower than in children: 90 to 95 percent of children are in remission by 8 weeks[93] versus only about 60 percent of adults, with some patients not responding until as late as 16 weeks.[94] Both frequent relapses and corticosteroid resistance may occur in adults, settings in which cyclophosphamide and less often azathioprine have been successfully used.[94,173] However, the benefits of such aggressive therapy (amelioration of edema and prevention of nephrotic complications such as thrombotic episodes)[94] must be weighed against the side effects of these medications and the observation that the disease tends to remit *spon-*

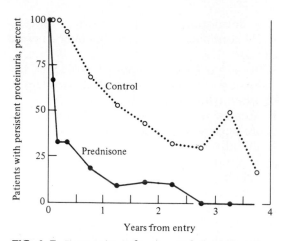

FIG. 6–7. Proportion of untreated control and prednisone-treated adults with minimal change disease having more than 1 g of proteinuria per day. (*From D. A. Black, G. Rose, and D. B. Brewer, Br. Med. J., 3:421, 1970. By permission of the British Medical Journal.*)

taneously within 4 years in most adults* (Fig. 6–7). It is probably reasonable to treat patients who relapse with marked symptoms with a repeat course of prednisone followed, if they are frequent relapsers, by low-dose alternate day maintenance prednisone therapy for about 1 year. A trial of cyclophosphamide should be limited to patients who are corticosteroid-resistant or who develop corticosteroid toxicity.[94]

RELATION TO OTHER DISEASES

Minimal change disease appears to be related in pathogenesis and clinical characteristics to other glomerular disorders, including focal glomerulosclerosis (FGS; see below), diffuse mesangial proliferation (DMP), and IgM nephropathy. As an example, children with cor-

*A short duration of disease is also typical of older children, as most children with a prolonged, frequently relapsing course have their initial episode before the age of 7.[145]

ticosteroid-responsive, frequently relapsing nephrotic syndrome are considered on clinical grounds to have MCD. However, in one series of 38 patients who were biopsied after a mean disease duration of 6 years, only 18 had MCD: the remaining children had FGS or DMP.[174] The clinical importance of these findings is uncertain: in this study, all patients responded to cyclophosphamide and had normal renal function at 11- to 14-year follow-up, although those patients with FGS or DMP were somewhat more likely to have a relapse after cytotoxic therapy. In another series, however, transition to FGS was associated with a relatively high risk of progressive renal insufficiency.[175]

Diffuse Mesangial Proliferation. Approximately 3 to 5 percent of patients with the nephrotic syndrome have mild, diffuse mesangial cell proliferation but no focal sclerosis

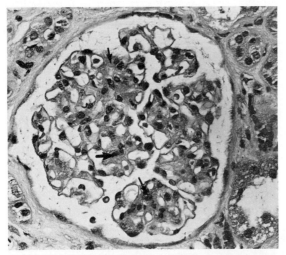

FIG. 6–8. Light microscopy in diffuse mesangial proliferation, demonstrating mesangial hyperplasia, increased mesangial matrix (arrow), but no segmental sclerosis.

on LM (Fig. 6–8).[96,143,176–178] IF may reveal scattered deposition of IgM and C3; EM demonstrates foot process fusion and occasional mesangial deposits. More than one-half of patients appear to respond initially to prednisone in most studies.[96,143,176,177] Even those who are nonresponders at 8 weeks frequently go into remission by 1 year, and most maintain a relatively normal glomerular filtration rate (GFR).[143,177] This had led to the suggestion that DMP may be a more severe form of MCD in which the initial injury was greater, leading to mesangial dysfunction and a slower rate of recovery.[143] The observation that as many as 25 percent of patients with frequently relapsing corticosteroid-responsive nephrotic syndrome show this histologic pattern is consistent with this hypothesis.[175]

The prognosis is not so good in all patients, however. Ten to thirty percent may develop progressive renal insufficiency, and many of those show FGS on repeat renal biopsy.[96,176,178] The response to cyclophosphamide or chlorambucil in this setting is variable,[176,177] but an 8-week trial of these drugs may be reasonable in those patients with persistent nephrotic syndrome who have a rising P_{cr}.

IgM Nephropathy. Some nephrotic patients have diffuse IgM deposition on IF, may have mesangial deposits on EM, and have a variable response to corticosteroids.[179,180] These characteristics led to the suggestion that *IgM nephropathy* might be a disorder that is different from the other causes of the nephrotic syndrome. However, IgM deposition has been found with roughly equal incidence in MCD, FGS, and DMP, with the prognosis correlating with the findings on LM.[96] Thus, it is likely that IgM nephropathy is not a specific entity; the IgM deposition may simply reflect nonspecific adsorption onto an abnormal GBM rather than the local formation of immune complexes.[96,181]

SUMMARY

Minimal change disease is a common cause of the nephrotic syndrome (and a nephrotic sediment) in all age groups, particularly children. The diagnosis is established by biopsy in adults and by inference in children unless prednisone is ineffective. Initial therapy consists of a course of prednisone which induces a remission in about 95 percent of patients. Approximately one-half of responders will have frequent relapses. These patients can frequently be maintained in remission on low-dose, alternate day corticosteroid therapy. In children, a short course of cyclophosphamide or chlorambucil should be used only if corticosteroid resistance or signs of corticosteroid toxicity develop. Because of the high frequency of spontaneous resolution within 4 years in adults (Fig. 6–7), only patients with severe refractory edema should be treated with repeated courses of prednisone or cytotoxic agents.

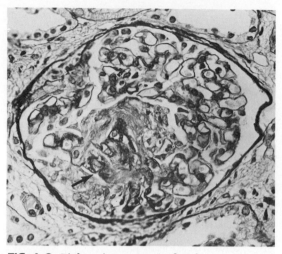

FIG. 6–9. Light microscopy in focal glomerulosclerosis. The characteristic change is segmental mesangial sclerosis with collapse of the capillary loops (arrow). The rest of the glomerulus is normal in this patient, but mild mesangial hyperplasia may occasionally be seen.

FOCAL GLOMERULOSCLEROSIS

Focal glomerulosclerosis (FGS)* is the third most common form of the idiopathic nephrotic syndrome after membranous nephropathy and minimal change disease (MCD), accounting for approximately 10 to 15 percent of cases in both children and adults.[2,6,7] Although most cases of this disorder occur before the age of 50, FGS has been described occasionally in patients over 70 years old.[182]

PATHOLOGY

The characteristic histologic change in FGS is the presence in some but not all glomeruli (hence the term *focal*) of areas of mesangial sclerosis with collapse of the capillary loops (Fig. 6–9). The sclerotic lesions usually spread

*Synonyms for focal glomerulosclerosis include focal segmental sclerosis with hyalinosis and focal sclerosing glomerulonephritis.

out from the central region of the tuft and may be associated with adhesions to Bowman's capsule.[183,184] Other changes which may be present include mild, mesangial hypercellularity and occlusion of the capillary lumina in these areas by eosinophilic, hyaline deposits. These deposits are thought to represent the insudation of plasma proteins into the abnormally permeable glomerular wall.

The degree of change in involved glomeruli is variable, as either segmental (affecting only part of the tuft) or global (affecting the entire glomerulus) lesions may be found. As described below, focal global sclerosis tends to have a more favorable prognosis.

Immunofluorescent microscopy may reveal IgM and C3, mostly within the sclerotic areas. The primary changes on EM are mesangial sclerosis in affected glomeruli and foot process fusion in all glomeruli. The latter finding, which is similar to that in MCD, indicates that

FGS is actually a diffuse disease even though only a small number of glomeruli may be abnormal on light microscopy.

In the early stages of the disease, only a few glomeruli may show segmental sclerosis, primarily in the juxtamedullary rather than the outer cortical glomeruli. Thus, differentiation from MCD may not be possible on histologic grounds if the biopsy does not contain affected glomeruli. One clue may be the presence of areas of tubulointerstitial damage (tubular atrophy, interstitial infiltrate, and edema), which is presumably secondary to glomerular injury and suggests FGS rather than MCD.[183] It is easier to make the diagnosis with more advanced disease, since greater than 50 to 70 percent of the glomeruli may be abnormal on light microscopy.

It should be emphasized that the finding of focal segmental sclerosis on LM is not specific for idiopathic FGS. Similar changes may be seen with nephrosclerosis, the healing phase of disorders such as poststreptococcal or focal glomerulonephritis, and hemodynamically mediated injury as occurs in chronic pyelonephritis or sickle cell disease (see Chap. 4).[185-187] The differentiation between these disorders and idiopathic FGS can usually be made on clinical and histologic grounds. Although distinguishing between FGS and healing glomerulonephritis may be difficult on LM alone, the latter disorder is usually associated with mesangial or loop immune complex deposition that can be detected by IF and EM.[185] The glomerular damage in nephrosclerosis is thought to result from chronic glomerular ischemia and, in contrast to idiopathic FGS, primarily involves the outer cortical glomeruli, usually affects patients older than 50 with a prior history of hypertension, and does not result in the nephrotic syndrome. Chronic pyelonephritis is associated with marked renal scarring and blunting of the calyces that can be detected on an intravenous pyelogram or renal ultrasound.

ETIOLOGY

Although most cases of FGS are idiopathic, an identifiable cause is occasionally present (Table 6-4). Chronic intravenous *heroin* use can lead to the nephrotic syndrome and FGS.[188-190] The mechanism by which this occurs is not known, but a toxic contaminant in the diluent may be involved.[188,189] A genetic predisposition may also play a role since this disorder occurs almost exclusively in black patients.[188,189] It should be noted that other glomerular lesions can also be seen in this setting, particularly secondary amyloidosis in patients with chronic, suppurative subcutaneous infections.[190]

The nephrotic syndrome can develop in 10 percent or more of patients with the *acquired immune deficiency syndrome*.[191-193] Renal biopsy generally reveals FGS and/or mesangial proliferation (which may be a precursor of FGS).[192] Since T-cell function is markedly abnormal in this disorder, release of a toxic lymphokine could be responsible for the glomerular injury (see "Pathogenesis," below).

Malignancy in adults accounts for approximately 10 percent of cases of the idiopathic nephrotic syndrome.[37,99] Membranous nephropathy is most often found with solid tumors and MCD with hematologic malignancies, particularly Hodgkin's disease. However, FGS may also occur with lymphomas, with the course of the glomerular disease paralleling that of the malignancy.[194]

FGS may also be associated with *chronic transplant rejection*.[195-197] Vascular damage lead-

TABLE 6-4. Etiology of Focal Glomerulosclerosis

Idiopathic
  Including progression from minimal change disease
Heroin
Acquired immune deficiency syndrome
Malignancy
Chronic transplant rejection
Massive obesity

ing to glomerular ischemia is probably responsible for the glomerulosclerosis in this setting. This disorder is different from FGS in the transplant that is due to recurrence of the primary disease (see "Course and Treatment," below).

Nephrotic syndrome is an uncommon complication of *massive obesity* and is most often due to FGS or diabetes mellitus.[198] Obesity is often associated with an elevation in GFR, suggesting that hemodynamically mediated injury (similar to that seen in many forms of progressive renal disease; see Chap. 4) may be playing an important role.

PATHOGENESIS

The pathogenesis of idiopathic FGS is incompletely understood. The observation that this disorder may recur within hours to weeks after renal transplantation[18,199,200] suggests that FGS is a systemic disease with circulating factors capable of damaging the kidney.[201]

Experimental models of FGS,[202,203] as well as studies in humans,[204] suggest that the initial site of damage may be the *glomerular epithelial cell.* Since the epithelial cells are responsible for the synthesis of the anionic sialoproteins and proteoglycans in the glomerular capillary wall,[112] injury to these cells could decrease the net anionic charge, producing both proteinuria (due to loss of the charge barrier to filtration) and foot process fusion (see "Minimal Change Disease: Pathogenesis" above).[113,205] The sclerotic lesions could eventually result from healing of the initial damage or overloading of the mesangium with macromolecules (due to the enhanced glomerular permeability).[203]

An understanding of FGS requires an appreciation of the experimental and clinical similarities between FGS and MCD:

1. The administration of the aminonucleoside puromycin, an epithelial cell toxin,[112] to experimental animals can result in either MCD (low-dose)[111] or FGS.[202,203]

2. Both disorders are characterized by diffuse foot process fusion and proteinuria that is due to loss of the anionic charge barrier rather than increased pore size.[116,205]

3. Some patients with initial, biopsy-proven MCD progress to FGS.[142,169,171,206] Other patients with a steroid-responsive, frequently relapsing course typical of MCD have FGS when finally biopsied.[174] It is possible that an earlier biopsy would have shown MCD, but FGS could have been present from the beginning.

In summary, at least some cases of FGS appear to represent either a more severe stage of MCD (as with puromycin) or a consequence of recurrent proteinuria in MCD (perhaps due to mesangial overloading).[203] It is also likely that, as nephrons become damaged, hyperfiltration injury contributes to the glomerular sclerosis. As described above in the section on MCD, the release of a lymphokine from activated T cells or small immune complexes could be responsible for initiating the glomerular damage in these disorders.

This hypothesis may not apply to all patients, however. Many patients, particularly adults, are corticosteroid-resistant from the onset, progress to renal failure relatively quickly, and may have early, recurrent proteinuria in the transplant without a prior stage of MCD. It is possible that this represents a different entity from MCD-related FGS, but a similar, more severe initial insult can also explain these findings.[206]

CLINICAL PRESENTATION

Most patients with idiopathic FGS present with the clinical and chemical findings of the nephrotic syndrome, although some patients have only nonnephrotic proteinuria.[170,207,208] Hypertension, hematuria (which is occasionally macroscopic), and mild azotemia are present in approximately one-half of children and a somewhat higher proportion of adults.[7,133,208] In those patients with prior

MCD, the late onset of corticosteroid resistance is the primary clue suggesting the development of FGS.[169,171,206]

In some patients, a precipitating factor such as an upper respiratory infection precedes the onset of disease, although it is not clear if or how this induces glomerular damage. In addition, FGS may first become clinically apparent during or be exacerbated by pregnancy, suggesting that pregnancy might have a deleterious effect on the course of the disease.[209,210] This is in contrast to most other glomerular disorders (excluding SLE), which are usually not adversely affected by pregnancy in the absence of renal insufficiency or severe hypertension (see p. 348).

DIAGNOSIS

The diagnosis of idiopathic FGS is made by renal biopsy. In children, this procedure is performed only after there has been no response to 8 weeks of prednisone therapy, thereby tending to exclude MCD, which is more common. Although this protocol will not diagnose those cases of FGS that are corticosteroid-responsive, establishing the correct diagnosis is not important as long as patients behave as if they have MCD.[174]

COURSE AND TREATMENT

Focal glomerulosclerosis appears to progress to end-stage renal failure in most patients.[207,208,211,212] The time required for this to occur is variable, ranging from 1 to more than 20 years. The course tends to be more indolent in patients with nonnephrotic proteinuria (see Fig. 6–3),[213] previous corticosteroid-responsive MCD,[174,175,206] and focal *global* sclerosis which tends to behave more like MCD.[96,214,215]

The response to treatment is variable in children. Some children respond to corticosteroids, although the biopsy diagnosis of FGS will usually not be made at this time because it will be assumed that MCD is present.[142,174,206,215] The presence of FGS (or progression of MCD to FGS) will be confirmed only when a biopsy is performed because of the development of late corticosteroid resistance. These initially responsive patients frequently have a complete or partial remission of proteinuria after cyclophosphamide (2 to 2.5 mg/kg per day for 8 weeks),[170,174,206,215] although ultimate progression to renal failure may still occur.[175,206] (Chlorambucil has been less extensively evaluated in FGS than in MCD). Repeated or prolonged courses of cyclophosphamide should be avoided because of the risks of gonadal fibrosis and neoplasia (see p. 192).

The proper therapeutic regimen is less clear in children who are initially resistant to corticosteroids. Most studies have shown a low response to cyclophosphamide in this setting.[170,206,215] However, one recent report described a complete or partial remission in 12 of 20 nephrotic children: only 1 of these 12 progressed to end-stage renal failure versus 7 of 8 who had no response.[216] Those children with FGS and *nonnephrotic* proteinuria had a lesser response to cyclophosphamide but generally ran a more benign course (see Fig. 6–3).[216] Considering the typically grim prognosis of this disease if untreated, a trial of cyclophosphamide is probably reasonable.

Adults have been considered to be unresponsive to both prednisone and cyclophosphamide,[170,208,217] and many physicians have chosen not to try these drugs, considering their potential toxicity. As in children, however, recent uncontrolled studies suggest that up to 40 percent of adults may undergo a complete or partial remission of proteinuria following a standard course of prednisone.[218,219] Furthermore, responders appear to have a much better long-term prognosis with less progression to renal failure.[218] Thus, it seems reasonable to try prednisone and, if necessary, cyclophosphamide in this usually progressive disorder. Prolonged therapy, however, is not warranted.

Another potential therapy consists of the use of meclofenamate (and probably other prostaglandin synthesis inhibitors except sulindac; see pp. 82–83). Some patients with FGS will respond with a marked reduction in proteinuria, a rise in the plasma albumin concentration, and a mild reduction in GFR which tends to be self-limited and stable.[92] Similar changes have been demonstrated in patients with membranous nephropathy, in whom a decrease in both the glomerular leak and the GFR appears to be responsible for the antiproteinuric effect.[27] Discontinuing therapy leads to rapid recurrence of the proteinuria. Although the use of meclofenamate may aid in the control of severe hypoalbuminemic edema, it is not yet known if this agent alters the usually progressive course of the disease.

In those patients who show evidence of progressive disease, an effort should be made to minimize hemodynamic injury in relatively undamaged nephrons. This can be attempted by rigorous control of the blood pressure and institution of a low-protein diet (see Chap. 4). It is not yet proven, however, that this regimen will preserve renal function in FGS.

Those patients who progress to end-stage renal failure are generally young and good candidates for renal transplantation. FGS presents some relatively unique problems in this setting, however, because approximately 20 to 30 percent will develop recurrent disease in the transplant, with proteinuria usually reappearing within 1 month.[197,199,200] This will ultimately lead to loss of transplant function in one-third to one-half of these patients. One group appears to be at greatest risk of recurrent FGS: those whose initial disease progressed to renal failure within 3 years.[197,199] The incidence of recurrent disease is about 50 percent in these patients versus 10 to 20 percent in those with more indolent primary disease.

These data should not discourage an attempt at transplantation since one-half of

high-risk patients will not develop recurrent disease. However, patients who do lose their first transplant to recurrent FGS probably should be treated with chronic dialysis because the incidence of recurrent disease in the second transplant approaches 80 percent.[199]

DIABETES MELLITUS

Glomerular disease due to diabetes mellitus, particularly type 1, is one of the more common causes of the nephrotic syndrome in adults. It is also a major cause of morbidity and mortality, as approximately 40 to 50 percent of type 1 (insulin-dependent) and 6 percent of type 2 (non-insulin-dependent) diabetics develop renal failure.[220] The reason for this difference in severity between the two types of diabetes is discussed below.

In addition to the glomerular changes, a variety of other renal lesions also may occur in diabetes, including nephrosclerosis due to accelerated arterial and arteriolar sclerosis, pyelonephritis (perhaps due in part to decreased bladder tone, which enhances the susceptibility to infection), papillary necrosis due both to infection and reduced blood flow (see Chap. 8), and acute renal failure following the injection of radiocontrast media (see Chap. 3).

PATHOLOGY

The primary glomerular changes of diabetes mellitus are diffuse and nodular glomerulosclerosis (Fig. 6–10).[221,222] The diffuse lesion, which may occur with or without the nodular change, is characterized on LM and EM by a uniform increase in the mesangial matrix (which represents basement membrane-like material) (Fig. 6–10). The basement membrane is also eventually affected, as it may be thickened to 5 or 10 times its normal width. These changes on LM are not specific and may also be seen with arteriolar nephrosclerosis or membranous nephropathy.

Nodular glomerulosclerosis (the Kimmel-stiel-Wilson lesion) tends to occur at a later stage of the disease and is always accompanied by the diffuse changes. It is considered to be virtually pathognomic of diabetic glomerulopathy, although similar lesions on LM can be seen with light chain deposition disease (see "Amyloidosis and Light Chain Deposition Disease," below). The nodules are acellular, hyaline masses of varying size, which appear to represent an extension of the diffuse process from the mesangium into the capillary loops (Fig. 6–10). As the diffuse and nodular lesions progress, there is compression and narrowing of the capillary loops, eventually resulting in obliteration of the capillaries and destruction of the glomerulus.[223]

Hyaline, acellular deposits are also frequently found in the afferent and particularly the efferent glomerular arterioles. The latter change is relatively specific for diabetes and may be one of the earliest signs of recurrent disease in the transplant.[224] These lesions are thought to represent plasma proteins trapped in the abnormally permeable vascular wall. If they are severe, glomerular ischemia can ensue, potentially contributing to the glomerular damage. Similar hyaline masses may also be found along the periphery of the capillary loops (as a crescent-shaped fibrin cap) and just inside Bowman's space (as a capsular drop).[183]

Other findings that are commonly present are narrowing of the small arteries by diffuse, subintimal thickening (arteriosclerosis) and tubulointerstitial changes (tubular atrophy, interstitial fibrosis, and focal mononuclear cell infiltrate), which are in part secondary to the glomerular and vascular disease.

Immunofluorescent microscopy in diabetic glomerulosclerosis frequently demonstrates linear deposition of immunoglobulins similar to that seen in anti-GBM antibody disease (see Fig. 5–6a).[225] However, circulating anti-GBM antibodies are not present, and the immunoglobulin deposition probably represents nonspecific protein adsorption onto the abnormal GBM.[226] The observation of concurrent linear deposition of albumin is consistent with this hypothesis.[225] Similar protein deposition can be demonstrated in the dermal capillaries,[227] indicating a more generalized capillary abnormality that may be due to glycosylation of capillary basement membrane proteins.[226] Leaky capillaries also explain the greater predisposition of diabetic patients to develop edema.[228]

PATHOGENESIS

An increasing body of evidence supports a primary role for hyperglycemia (or insulin deficiency), as opposed to a separate underlying vascular abnormality, in the genesis of diabetic nephropathy (and other microvascular complications). This includes the following observations:

1. Thickening of the GBM and proteinuria can be demonstrated in both experimental animals with chemical-induced diabetes and humans with secondary diabetes due to pancreatic disease or toxic exposure.[229-231] Furthermore, retinopathy and widening of the muscle capillary basement membranes can also be seen in secondary diabetes.[231]

2. These changes can be reversed in animals by maintaining normoglycemia with insulin.[229]

3. Transplantation of kidneys with mild diabetic glomerulosclerosis into a nondiabetic recipient results in almost complete resolution of the sclerotic changes.[232]

4. Transplantation of a kidney from a nondiabetic donor into a diabetic recipient can result in recurrent diabetic nephropathy,[224,233] a change that may be preventable with maintenance of normoglycemia.[234]

In the past, a major argument in favor of a separate vascular abnormality was the occasional demonstration of classic nodular glo-

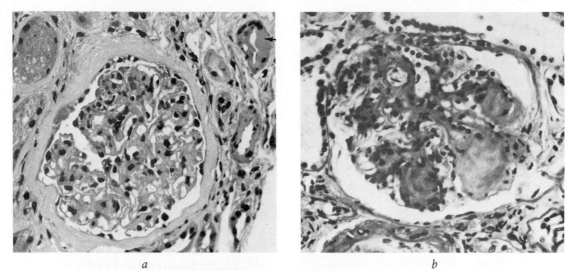

a

b

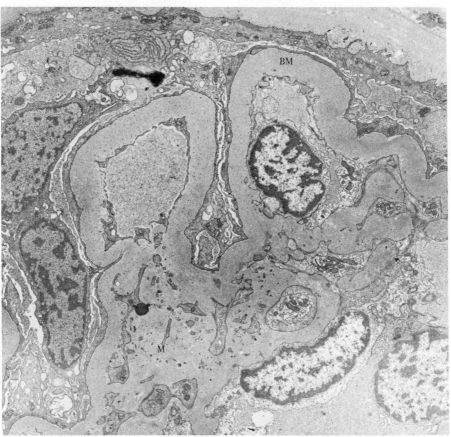

c

merulosclerosis in patients with normal glucose tolerance.[235] It is probable, however, that at least some of these patients had light chain deposition disease, not minimal diabetes mellitus.[236]

The primary role of hyperglycemia is also supported by the observation that the incidence of diabetic nephropathy is related to the degree of diabetic control.[237] Nevertheless, other factors also must be important, since only 35 to 50 percent of type 1 diabetics develop clinical glomerular disease.[220,237] Genetic susceptibility,[238] dietary protein intake, and the level of the systemic blood pressure all may contribute to this process (see "Treatment," below).

Sequential renal biopsies in patients with type 1 diabetes have revealed a normal GBM and mesangium at the time of diagnosis. Within 1 to 2 years, however, the initial increment in GBM thickness is evident, well before the onset of clinically detectable proteinuria.[239] Increases in RNA production and in the activity of enzymes regulating basement membrane synthesis can be demonstrated relatively early in the course of the disease.[240,241]

Several, not mutually exclusive theories have been proposed to explain how hyperglycemia produces these changes. According to one theory, glycosylation of mesangial and GBM proteins (similar to that which occurs with hemoglobin) promotes trapping of circulating macromolecules in the glomerular capillary wall, which then causes mesangial hyperplasia and increased production of GBM-like material.[226] The same net effect could also result from glycosylation of circulating plasma proteins, which could preferentially accumulate in the mesangium.[242]

Another major theory proposes an essential role for a *hyperglycemia-induced alteration in renal hemodynamics.*[243,244] Early in the course of type 1 diabetes and persisting for 5 to 10 years, many patients have a 25 to 50 percent increase in GFR[222,245-248] that appears to result from renal vasodilation and a subsequent rise in intraglomerular pressure.[243] According to the hemodynamic theory, the glomeruli are unable to tolerate these high pressures in the long-term, leading to progressive glomerulosclerosis and a reduction in GFR.[243] Many observations are consistent with this hypothesis. In diabetic animals, for example, correcting the intraglomerular hypertension by restricting dietary protein intake or by lowering the systemic blood pressure with a converting enzyme inhibitor (see Chap. 4) can prevent the glomerulosclerosis even though hyperglycemia persists.[249,250] Similar results have been obtained in preliminary studies in humans as control of the systemic blood pressure appears to slow the progression of established diabetic nephropathy.[251-253] Furthermore, those patients who hyperfilter early in the course of their disease (and presumably have intraglomerular hypertension) seem to be at much greater risk of developing progressive renal disease than those patients whose GFR remains within the normal range.[254]

The factors responsible for the glomerular

FIG. 6-10. Histologic changes in diabetic nephropathy. (*a*) Diffuse glomerulosclerosis occurs first and is characterized by a uniform increase in mesangial matrix (or basement membrane-like material), thickening of the basement membrane, but no increase in cellularity. Subintimal hyaline thickening of the arterioles also may be seen (arrow). (*b*) Nodular lesions may occur at a later stage and consist of hyaline, acellular masses extending out from the mesangium into the capillary loops. A rim of compressed glomerular cells can be seen around the nodules. (*c*) Electron microscopy reveals marked, uniform thickening of the basement membrane (BM) (approximately 5 to 10 times normal) and increased mesangial matrix (M).

hyperfiltration are incompletely understood. One important factor may be increased production of basement membrane-like material, thereby enhancing the surface area available for filtration.[246,255] However, restoration of normoglycemia in early diabetes lowers the GFR toward normal before changing glomerular or kidney size,[246,255] indicating that increased surface area may be necessary but is not sufficient for hyperfiltration to occur.[243]

It is likely that arteriolar dilation, leading to enhanced glomerular pressure and flow, also plays an important role.*,[243,256] However, the mechanisms by which this occurs are not known. The following neurohumoral changes all have been described in diabetes, each of which could contribute to renal vasodilation.[244]

1. Decreased plasma renin activity and presumably plasma angiotensin II levels, effects which could be due to diabetic autonomic neuropathy or reduced conversion of inactive into active renin.[262]
2. Diminished response to angiotensin II due to a decrease in hormone receptor density.[263]
3. Diminished response to norepinephrine, also due to a reduction in receptor density, an abnormality that is reversed by insulin.[264,265]
4. Extracellular volume expansion, as hyperglycemia-induced hyperosmolality causes fluid movement from the cells into the extracellular space.[256,266] However, raising the extracellular osmolality and volume

with hypertonic mannitol does not lead to a similar increase in GFR.[267]
5. Increased renal production of vasodilator prostaglandins[268] since inhibiting prostaglandin synthesis minimizes the vasodilation and hyperfiltration.[267]
6. Enhanced secretion of glucagon,[269] which also can promote renal vasodilation.[270]

It is also possible that moderate hyperglycemia itself increases renal perfusion and the GFR.[271,272] One mechanism by which this might occur is related to the increased filtered load and proximal tubular reabsorption of glucose, effects that are independent of the availability of insulin. The associated increase in oxygen consumption could then promote renal vasodilation in an attempt to enhance oxygen delivery.[273]

CLINICAL PRESENTATION AND COURSE

The various stages in the course of the nephropathy in type 1 diabetes are depicted in Table 6–5.[248,274] The initial stage consists of an increase in GFR as described above. Some increase in albumin excretion is demonstrable at this time and may be due to the high GFR or to enhanced filtration of glycosylated (as opposed to native) albumin.[274,275] Nevertheless, total protein excretion and the urinalysis remain normal.

Stage II is characterized by progressive mesangial expansion and thickening of the GBM but still no clinical evidence of disease. Albumin excretion is relatively normal at rest but may show an increase with exercise.[276] The hemodynamic stress associated with exercise probably unmasks the occult changes in the GBM.

The third stage, clinically incipient disease, begins after 10 or more years. This stage is associated with progressive glomerulosclerosis and a gradual reduction in GFR from the initially high level down toward normal. Thus, marked histologic changes are present

---

*This microvascular dilation is not limited to the kidney, as similar changes occur in the retina and skeletal muscle.[244,257,258] Thus, diabetic retinopathy, like the nephropathy, could be explained in part by local vasodilation, leading sequentially to increased capillary hydrostatic pressure, capillary damage as evidenced by enhanced permeability,[259] marked thickening of the capillary basement membrane, and eventual vascular occlusion and microaneurysm formation. The observation that hypertension exacerbates the retinopathy also is compatible with the importance of local hemodynamics.[260,261]

TABLE 6-5. Stage of Nephropathy in Type 1 Diabetes Mellitus*

Stage	Characteristic	Time after Onset	GFR	Albumin Excretion	Blood Pressure	Reversibility with Insulin
I	Renal enlargement and hyperfiltration	Days to weeks	Markedly increased	Slightly increased owing to elevation in GFR; total protein excretion remains normal	Normal	Yes with strict control
II	Glomerular lesions without clinical signs of disease	2 years and progressively thereafter	Markedly increased	Normal if good control but may increase with exercise	Normal	Initially reversible with strict control
III	Clinically incipient disease	10 to 15 years with great variation	Normal to increased	Progressive microalbuminuria, increases with exercise	Normal to increased	Strict control can reduce microalbuminuria and may minimize further reduction in GFR
IV	Clinical disease	5 to 10 years after stage III with variation	Normal to progressive decrease	Clinically evident: total protein excretion initially exceeds 500 mg/day	Increased	Not reversible with insulin; strict control of hypertension can minimize further deterioration

*Adapted from C. E. Mogensen, *Kidney Int.*, 21:673, 1982. Reprinted by permission from *Kidney International.*

at a time when the GFR is still in the normal range.

The development of *microalbuminuria* also occurs at this time. This is defined as the excretion of albumin in excess of 15 μg/min on a resting sample or 30 μg/min on an overnight collection (normal less than 5 μg/min, which is equivalent to 7 mg/day).[277,278] Total protein excretion, however, remains normal (less than 150 mg/day). Microalbuminuria can be detected only by special assay, since the dipstick is not generally positive until total protein excretion reaches 400 to 500 mg/day.[274]

Microalbuminuria is both indicative of glomerular damage and highly predictive of subsequent clinical nephropathy. In two studies in which patients with type 1 diabetes were followed for 7 to 14 years, clinically evident proteinuria developed in 19 of 22 (86 percent) with initial microalbuminuria but in only 2 of 84 (2.5 percent) without this abnormality.[277,278] The patients with microalbuminuria, who also developed more severe retinopathy, began with a higher GFR and systemic blood pressure, findings which are compatible with the deleterious effects of intraglomerular hypertension.[278]

Clinically detectable proteinuria (stage IV) usually occurs within 15 to 25 years of the onset of diabetes and is typically followed by increasing proteinuria and hypertension as well as progressive renal failure.[237,248,274] Nephrotic range proteinuria ultimately develops in up to 40 percent of patients.[279] The proteinuria at this time is primarily due to the presence of large pores in the GBM, with some contribution from loss of the anionic charge barrier.[274,280] In general, the GFR falls at a rate of 10 to 15 mL/min per year,[252,253] usually leading to end-stage renal failure within 3 to 10 years after the onset of detectable proteinuria.[237,281]

Type 2 Diabetes. The course of the nephropathy in type 2 diabetics appears to be more indolent.[279] Although proteinuria occurs in more than one-third (and is usually preceded by microalbuminuria),[282] it is typically mild and the GFR may remain stable for many years. Thus, only 4 percent of patients develop the nephrotic syndrome[279] and 6 percent progress to end-stage renal failure.[220]

The relatively benign course of the nephropathy in type 2 diabetes may be related to the older age of the patients. If all diabetics are considered, the incidence of renal failure is dependent upon the age of onset of the diabetes: approximately 40 percent if below 20, 9 percent between 20 and 40, and less than 3 percent over the age of 40.[279] It may be that increasing age limits the hyperfiltration response that ultimately damages the glomeruli, since the rise in GFR that typically occurs in type 1 diabetes cannot usually be demonstrated in type 2.[248]

DIAGNOSIS

Although the diagnosis of diabetic glomerulosclerosis can be made definitively only by renal biopsy, this procedure is usually unnecessary because the combination of longstanding diabetes mellitus, proteinuria with a benign sediment, and renal insufficiency is so characteristic of this disorder. Most patients also have evidence of retinopathy, since this complication generally occurs earlier and is more common that the renal disease.[283] Nevertheless, diabetic nephropathy can occur in the absence of clinically evident retinal disease.[284]

However, there are several potential diagnostic problems. First, diabetics may develop some other form of glomerular disease that may be treatable. For example, membranous nephropathy, minimal change disease, and proliferative glomerulonephritis all have been found in diabetic patients.[285-287] Clues suggesting the possible presence of some non-diabetes-related disorder are known duration of diabetes of less than 10 years, per-

sistent microscopic hematuria (particularly if accompanied by red cell casts), the development of acute renal failure, and in type 1 diabetes, the nephrotic syndrome with a persistently normal GFR since renal insufficiency is almost always present in diabetic nephropathy in this setting.[286,288]

Second, reversible causes for a deterioration in renal function should always be excluded rather than assuming irreversible progression of diabetic glomerulosclerosis. Possible causes include prerenal disease due to heart failure or the use of diuretics, postrenal disease due to papillary necrosis, or a reaction to radiocontrast media.[289]

Third, nephrosclerosis due to atherosclerotic vascular disease is a common cause of renal insufficiency in older patients with diabetes. This disorder is differentiated clinically from diabetic nephropathy by the degree of proteinuria, which is usually under 1.5 g/day in nephrosclerosis. This distinction is largely academic, however, since the basic therapy is the same: control of the blood pressure and the plasma glucose concentration.

TREATMENT

The optimal treatment of type 1 diabetic nephropathy varies with the stage of the disease. Early in the course, the restoration of normoglycemia with intensive insulin therapy can lower the GFR toward normal[246,255] and reverse exercise-induced albuminuria.[290] Later on, in stage III disease, insulin can reduce the degree of microalbuminuria[291] and prevent or minimize the progressive decline in GFR.[292] Mild to moderate glomerulosclerosis also may be reversed, as evidenced by the use of these kidneys for renal transplantation.[232]

However, strict control of the plasma glucose concentration is usually ineffective in maintaining the GFR once there is intermittent or persistent clinically detectable proteinuria (by dipstick).[293-295] At this time, daily protein excretion usually exceeds 400 to 500 mg/day (the threshold level that can be detected by the dipstick), and advanced glomerulosclerosis is already present.* Hemodynamic factors now appear to be of primary importance due to several factors including the initial hyperfiltration, superimposed systemic hypertension, and the compensatory response in relatively unaffected glomeruli. As a result, correction of systemic hypertension (which will also reduce the intraglomerular pressure) is the only therapeutic modality that has been shown to preserve renal function in this setting.[251-253] The aim should be to reduce the diastolic pressure to 80 mmHg, if possible, preferentially using a converting enzyme inhibitor which directly lowers the intraglomerular pressure (see p. 123). In some patients with advanced disease, for example, captopril can reduce proteinuria by about 50 percent.[297] This effect presumably reflects a change in intrarenal hemodynamics since it can occur with little change in the systemic blood pressure.

Lowering the systemic blood pressure, even if initially normal, also may prove to be beneficial earlier in the course of the disease, e.g., when microalbuminuria is discovered, since this appears to be a marker for progressive disease.[277,278] Minimizing the intraglomerular hypertension at this time may prevent or delay the development of glomerulosclerosis.[249]

Dietary protein restriction also may reduce the glomerular hyperperfusion and delay the progression to renal failure (see Chap. 4).[250] This regimen is somewhat less desirable than antihypertensive therapy, however, since diabetics already limit carbohydrate and fat intake, and the safety of protein restriction in proteinuric patients has not been definitely established.[298]

*Relative maintenance of normoglycemia is also ineffective in reversing already established diabetic retinopathy.[291,296]

In addition to the use of converting enzyme inhibitors, antihypertensive therapy in established diabetic nephropathy also may require weight reduction (if the patient is obese), a diuretic, and dietary sodium restriction.[266] The efficacy of this regimen reflects the importance of volume expansion in this setting, due both to renal insufficiency and to hyperglycemia-induced movement of water from the cells into the extracellular fluid. In refractory cases, an attempt should be made to achieve "dry weight," which is defined as that weight at which the blood pressure is normalized or signs of hypovolemia appear (such as cramps, weakness, or increasing azotemia).[288] If necessary, a calcium channel blocker or a direct vasodilator can then be added. However, sympathetic blockers such as methyldopa or clonidine should generally be avoided because underlying diabetic neuropathy can increase the incidence of sexual dysfunction and postural hypotension.[266] Beta-adrenergic blockers also have potential disadvantages in that they can exacerbate peripheral vascular disease and, in patients who become hypoglycemic, mask the early symptoms, delay recovery, and cause a marked increase in blood pressure (as epinephrine-induced α-receptor-mediated vasoconstriction is now unopposed by β-receptor-mediated vasodilation).[299-302]

It is likely that the same therapeutic principles apply to the nephropathy in type 2 diabetes. However, confirmatory evidence is lacking, in part because of the much lower rate of progression to renal insufficiency.

END-STAGE RENAL FAILURE

Those patients who progress to end-stage renal failure can be treated with dialysis or transplantation.[281] Regardless of which modality is ultimately chosen, dialysis is frequently begun relatively early, before the onset of uremic symptoms, e.g., when the P_{cr} exceeds 7 to 8 mg/dL.[281,303] The rationale for this approach is that waiting for uremia to develop can exacerbate the retinopathy (due to hypertension and decreased platelet function), the neuropathy (due to uremic neuropathy), and the vascular disease (due to metastatic calcification).

The optimal treatment of end-stage diabetic nephropathy is uncertain. Although early studies showed very poor survival on hemodialysis (as low as 25 percent at 3 years), this has improved to about 50 percent at 3 years, still 20 to 30 percent below that in nondiabetics.[281,304] The major causes of death are atherosclerotic complications such as a myocardial infarction. Even those who survive do not do very well, however, since progressive retinopathy, neuropathy, and vascular disease is common and return to work is infrequent.[305]

It has been suggested that diabetic patients may do subjectively better on continuous ambulatory peritoneal dialysis, with insulin added to the dialysate to control the plasma glucose concentration.[306,307] This modality has the advantages of no heparin (which could exacerbate the retinopathy), easier control of fluid balance and hypertension, and more efficient removal of middle molecules which may play a role in uremic neuropathy.[308] However, improved survival as compared to hemodialysis has not yet been demonstrated.[305]

The best results appear to be attained with renal transplantation.[281,304,305,309] In addition to the improved lifestyle with a successful transplant, patient survival is higher, approaching 85 percent at 2 to 3 years with a living related donor and somewhat lower with a cadaver donor. Although these findings may in part reflect the selection of healthier patients, patients with a functioning transplant appear to not be better than those on dialysis since the neuropathy tends to improve and the retinopathy to remain stable.[281,305] However, the morbidity rate from vascular disease remains high, as 15 to 20 percent of

patients require amputation of one or more extremities.[309]

In general, transplantation is the treatment of choice in patients under the age of 45 to 50 without advanced vascular disease, particularly if a living related donor is available.[281] Diabetic glomerulosclerosis may recur in the transplant, but progression to renal failure is rare.[224,233] Combined renal and segmental pancreatic transplantation has been tried with varying success in an attempt to normalize glucose balance; this remains at present an experimental procedure.[234,310,311]

AMYLOIDOSIS AND LIGHT CHAIN DEPOSITION DISEASE

Renal involvement occurs in over 90 percent of patients with either primary or secondary amyloidosis.[312-314] The primary form, which now accounts for more than 90 percent of cases, is a plasma cell dyscrasia and may be associated with multiple myeloma. It is a disease of adults, almost always occurring in patients over the age of 40.[313] Light chain deposition disease (LCDD) is a disorder of similar pathogenesis except that the abnormal proteins do not form the β-pleated amyloid fibrils.[236]

In comparison, secondary amyloidosis is a consequence of chronic inflammatory diseases such as rheumatoid arthritis, some neoplasias (particularly renal cell carcinoma and Hodgkin's disease), Crohn's disease, chronic skin or decubitus ulcer infections in intravenous drug abusers or paraplegics, osteomyelitis, bronchiectasis, and familial Mediterranean fever.[37,190,312,315-320] Secondary amyloidosis is not age-related since the duration and activity of the underlying disease are the main determinants of amyloid formation.

PATHOLOGY

The primary change on LM in amyloidosis is the diffuse deposition of amorphous hyaline material first in the mesangium and then in the capillary loops (Fig. 6–11a). These deposits may also be seen in the arterioles, small arteries, and tubular basement membranes.[314,321] Progressive deposition leading to narrowing of the arteriolar and capillary lumens is primarily responsible for the common development of renal failure.

Amyloid deposition in the glomeruli can result in the formation of nodules that, on LM, resemble those in diabetic nephropathy (see Fig. 6-10b).[321] As a result, special stains and

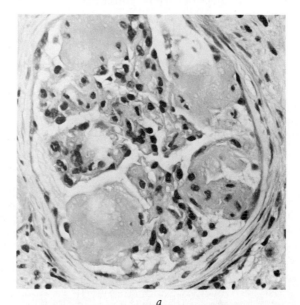

a

FIG. 6–11. Pathologic findings in renal amyloidosis. (*a*) Light microscopy demonstrates diffuse deposition of the hyaline material in the mesangium and capillary loops. These changes may resemble those in diabetic glomerulosclerosis (see Fig. 6–10). (*b*) Definitive confirmation of the diagnosis is made by electron microscopy, which shows widening of the mesangium (M) and then the subendothelial space by characteristic amyloid fibrils (inset).

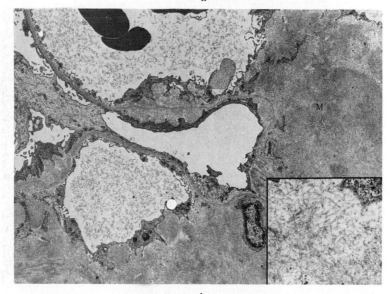

b

EM are required to establish the diagnosis of amyloidosis. For example, thioflavine-T produces an intense yellow-green fluorescence, whereas Congo red induces green birefringence when viewed under polarized light.[312,314] However, misleading results can be obtained with these tests, and the only diagnostic finding is the demonstration of characteristic amyloid fibrils in the glomeruli on EM (Fig. 6-11b).

Immunofluorescent microscopy for immunoglobulins and complement is generally negative or minimally positive (due to non-specific uptake of circulating macromolecules by the abnormal glomerular capillary wall). IF may be weakly positive for monoclonal λ or κ light chains, but the results are less prominent than in LCDD.[322]

Light Chain Deposition Disease. The histologic changes on LM in LCDD resemble those in amyloidosis except for the more frequent prominence of glomerular nodules and bright, refractile ribbonlike thickening of the *tubular* basement membranes (TBM).[236,322,323] The diagnosis, however, is established by IF and EM. IF is strongly positive for a monoclonal light chain (κ much more often than λ) in the TBM and usually in the glomeruli. EM reveals finely granular material (not fibrillar as in amyloidosis) along the basement membranes.[236,323] This material may be dense enough to suggest membranoproliferative glomerulonephritis, type 2 (dense deposit disease; see Fig. 6-18), but the positive IF for light chains establishes the correct diagnosis.[324,325]

PATHOGENESIS

Immunochemical studies have revealed that the composition of the amyloid deposits differs in the various forms of the disease: fragments of monoclonal light chains in primary amyloidosis and LCDD; amyloid A protein in secondary amyloidosis; prealbumin in several disorders that do not affect the kidney, such as familial polyneuropathy; and an unidentified protein in a rare familial disorder that does involve the kidney.[326,327] Each of these proteins has the ability to form the β-pleated fibrils that are characteristic of amyloid deposits.[326]

Primary Amyloidosis. The fibrils in primary amyloidosis consist of segments of the variable portions of monoclonal light chains* (molecular weight between 5000 and 18,000).[326] Thus, primary amyloidosis (also called AL amyloidosis) is a plasma cell dyscrasia in which the malignant characteristics of multiple myeloma are usually absent. Circulating light chains are frequently demonstrable and have a composition that is identical with the amyloid deposits.[326]

However, only a minority of patients who produce an excessive amount of light chains (such as those with multiple myeloma) develop amyloidosis,[328] indicating that additional factors must be important. The excess light chains must be able to be taken up and degraded by circulating macrophages, which then secrete the preamyloid fragments (Fig. 6-12).[329] The light chains must also have the appropriate chemical properties since in vitro incubation with proteolytic enzymes reveals that only some light chains are able to form amyloid fibrils.[330] For example, λ light chains, particularly those containing the λ_{VI} variable region, are much more likely to produce amyloidosis than κ light chains.[326,331]

Similar principles apply to LCDD, except that κ light chains are more often involved and the fragments contain the constant region.[236,322] In addition, the light chains may be abnormal, being secreted by the plasma cells as polymers or in a glycosated form.[236]

It is also important to note that patients

---

*The presence of the *variable* portion of light chains probably explains why immunofluorescent microscopy with anti-light chain antisera is usually only weakly positive.[322] In comparison, IF is markedly positive in LCDD in which the deposited light chain fragments contain at least part of the *constant* region.[236,322]

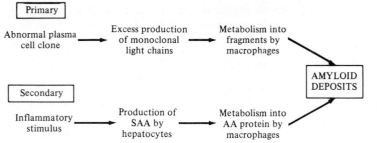

FIG. 6-12. Pathogenesis of the primary and secondary forms of amyloidosis.

with primary amyloidosis and LCDD generally excrete a relatively small amount of light chains in the urine and rarely develop myeloma kidney with intratubular cast formation (see Chap. 8).[236,326,332] Conversely, patients with myeloma kidney do not typically have amyloid deposits.[332] The reason for these differences may once again relate to the chemical properties of the light chains that are produced, particularly the isoelectric point (pI).[332] Light chains with a low pI are highly anionic and less able to be filtered across the anionic charge barrier in the GBM (see Fig. 5–3), particularly if their molecular size is increased by polymerization. As a result, the nonexcreted light chains accumulate in the plasma, thereby promoting tissue deposition. On the other hand, monomeric light chains with a relatively high pI are less anionic or even cationic. Thus, they are more easily filtered, potentially leading to myeloma kidney but not amyloidosis or LCDD since plasma accumulation does not occur.

Another possible contributing factor is the ability of the light chains to be taken up by and metabolized in macrophages. The deposits in primary amyloidosis and LCDD are fragments of light chains, which even if filtered, may be less likely to promote intratubular obstruction than the intact light chains seen in myeloma kidney.[326]

Secondary Amyloidosis. As described above, secondary amyloidosis is associated with a variety of chronic inflammatory disorders. In this setting, activated macrophages release a soluble factor that stimulates the production of serum amyloid A protein (SAA) by hepatocytes.*,[333] SAA is an acute phase reactant, similar to C-reactive protein,[335] and its plasma levels are markedly elevated in inflammatory states.[315,336,337] It is taken up by circulating monocytes/macrophages, where it may then be cleaved to a smaller fragment called AA protein (MW 5000 to 8000), which is the major component of the deposited amyloid fibrils (Fig. 6–12).[326,338]

The mechanism responsible for the formation of AA protein and its subsequent tissue deposition are incompletely understood. Factors other than increased SAA production must also be important since only some patients with chronic inflammatory diseases develop amyloidosis. For example, SAA levels in rheumatoid arthritis patients without amyloidosis are elevated to the same degree as in those who have the disease.†,[339] Genetic differences either in AA degradation (within monocytes or in the circulation) or in the amyloidogenic potential of this protein have been proposed to explain these findings.[316,338–340]

---

*SAA also may be produced by neutrophils.[334] The mechanism by which this is regulated and its clinical relevance are not known since hepatic production is thought to be of primary importance.

†It is of interest that SAA levels are only mildly elevated in SLE, a disorder in which secondary amyloidosis is rare.[315,326]

CLINICAL PRESENTATION

Patients with amyloidosis most often present with either nonspecific symptoms such as fatigue and weight loss or signs of renal disease such as proteinuria or edema.[312-314] In addition, the history and physical examination may reveal evidence of multisystem involvement including congestive heart failure, the carpal tunnel syndrome, peripheral neuropathy, hepatomegaly, splenomegaly, or macroglossia. These findings can occur with either the primary or secondary forms of the disease. Extrarenal involvement also can occur in LCDD, with hepatic and cardiac abnormalities being most common.[236] However, lack of *clinically apparent* extrarenal involvement is frequent and therefore does not exclude the diagnosis of these disorders.[236,314] Signs of an underlying inflammatory disease should be present in patients with secondary amyloidosis.

Renal insufficiency, as evidenced by an elevated P_{cr}, is present at the time of diagnosis in up to one-half of patients with amyloidosis and even more commonly in LCDD.[236,313,314] The urine sediment typically reveals few cells or casts. Proteinuria occurs in almost all patients and is frequently in the nephrotic range. However, minimal proteinuria may be present when the deposits are primarily in the blood vessels[341] or tubules,[236] not in the glomeruli. Prominent tubular deposits also can lead to a variety of tubular abnormalities such as renal tubular acidosis, nephrogenic diabetes insipidus, and hyperkalemia due to diminished distal potassium secretion.[342,343]

Another common abnormality in primary amyloidosis and LCDD is the finding of a paraprotein in the serum (as an M spike on protein electrophoresis) or urine (as monoclonal light chains) in over 85 percent of patients with these disorders.[236,313] Malignant transformation of the plasma cell clone into multiple myeloma occurs in about 20 percent of patients with primary amyloidosis[313] and more than 50 percent of those with LCDD who may also have lymphoma or Waldenström's macroglobulinemia.[236]

DIAGNOSIS

The diagnosis of amyloidosis can be made only by the demonstration of tissue deposition of amyloid fibrils. Although kidney or liver biopsy may be positive in over 90 percent of patients, similar results may be obtained with less invasive procedures such as biopsy of the abdominal fat pad (80 to 90 percent), rectum (50 to 80 percent), gingiva (60 percent), or skin (50 percent).[313,344] LCDD is diagnosed primarily by renal biopsy.[236]

Since amyloidosis is an infrequent cause of the nephrotic syndrome, only those patients in whom there is some suspicion of this disorder should undergo fat pad or rectal biopsy prior to renal biopsy. Clues suggesting amyloidosis include the presence of a chronic inflammatory disease or characteristic multisystem abnormalities. In addition, all nephrotic patients over the age of 50 (up to 20 percent of whom may have amyloidosis)[345] should have plasma and urine immunoelectrophoresis in view of the high incidence of paraprotein production in primary amyloidosis.

Once the diagnosis of primary amyloidosis or LCDD is made, the patient should be evaluated for multiple myeloma. Findings suggestive of myeloma include hypercalcemia, anemia out of proportion to the degree of renal failure, back pain, and lytic bone lesions on x-ray. The diagnosis can be confirmed by bone marrow examination. On the other hand, the findings of albuminuria and hypoalbuminemia in a patient with multiple myeloma suggests the concurrent presence of amyloidosis or LCDD.[328]

COURSE AND TREATMENT

Prognosis and therapy are dependent upon the type of amyloidosis that is present. Patients with multiple myeloma do very poorly, having a mean survival rate of as low as 4 months.[312] Comparable figures for primary amyloidosis without myeloma are only slightly better with a mean survival of 12 to 15 months.[312,313] The major causes of death are cardiac or renal failure, infection, and progression of the myeloma. However, occasional long-term survival may occur.[314]

The nephropathy in primary amyloidosis and LCDD usually progresses slowly to renal failure if the patient survives long enough.[236,313,345] Although transient remissions in proteinuria may occur, this does not seem to be associated with either regression of amyloid deposits or prevention of progression to renal insufficiency.[346,347] More commonly, heavy proteinuria persists even with advanced renal failure.[314] This is in contrast to most other nephrotic states in which a very low GFR is typically associated with reductions in albumin filtration and excretion.

The combination of melphalan and prednisone (as used in multiple myeloma) is the major mode of therapy that has been tried in primary amyloidosis. A stable or increased creatinine clearance and a reduction in proteinuria have been described in some patients treated with these drugs,[347-350] although this is probably not accompanied by a reduction in renal amyloid deposition.[347] In the only controlled study, a decrease in proteinuria was noted in almost 40 percent of treated patients, although there was no increase in survival rate as compared with the control group.[350] In addition, melphalan has been associated with the development of acute leukemia.[351] Thus, the decision to institute a trial of melphalan, the effectiveness of which remains unproven, should be undertaken only with the patient's complete understanding of the potential toxicity of this drug. Uncontrolled observations suggest that melphalan and prednisone may be more beneficial in LCDD.[236]

Other therapeutic modalities that have been tried in primary amyloidosis include colchicine (because of its effect in some forms of secondary amyloidosis) and dimethylsulfoxide (DMSO), which may cause dissociation of the amyloid fibrils. However, the efficacy of these drugs remains unproven in this setting.[352-354]

The prognosis in secondary amyloidosis is dependent upon the ability to control the underlying inflammatory disease since plasma SAA levels correlate both with disease activity[315] and roughly with the severity of renal involvement.[355] Although measurement of circulating SAA levels is not widely available, there is a reasonably close correlation between this parameter and C-reactive protein, the other major acute phase reactant. Thus, monitoring C-reactive protein levels allows assessment of the degree of inflammation.[355] When the inflammation can be reduced, the renal disease stabilizes or improves and the amyloid deposits may or may not resolve over several years.[356-358]

Colchicine (in a dose of 1 to 2 mg/day) and DMSO also have been used in some patients with secondary amyloidosis. The rationale for the use of colchicine is based upon the *experimental* observations that it blocks SAA release from hepatocytes and neutrophils[333,334] and that it prevents casein-induced secondary amyloidosis.[359] In familial Mediterranean fever, colchicine markedly reduces the frequency of attacks (in which abdominal pain and neutrophilic accumulation in the peritoneum are prominent), substantially diminishes the incidence of renal disease, and can stabilize the GFR in patients who have moderate (nonnephrotic proteinuria) but not advanced renal involvement.[320,356] Colchicine also can prevent or delay recurrent amyloidosis in the renal transplant.[360]

The possible role of colchicine in other forms of secondary amyloidosis has not been proven. It is difficult to extrapolate from the results with familial Mediterranean fever since the beneficial effect of the drug in this disorder may be related to decreased neutrophilic chemotaxis or phagocytosis, thereby decreasing the inflammatory process, not a direct reduction in SAA release.[361]

Uncontrolled studies in a small number of patients suggest that DMSO may be effective in secondary amyloidosis if given before the onset of severe renal failure.[353,354] However, these results are preliminary, and use of this drug may be limited by the associated offensive breath odor.

Both dialysis and transplantation have been used in patients with amyloidosis or LCDD who progress to end-stage renal failure. Patient survival is well below that of other causes of renal failure, due primarily to complications arising from cardiac involvement or underlying multiple myeloma.[313,362,363] Recurrent amyloid or light chain deposition is relatively common in the transplant[364,365] with the possible exception of colchicine therapy in familial Mediterranean fever.[360]. Although these deposits can lead to the nephrotic syndrome, the GFR is reasonably well maintained in most patients.

IMMUNOTACTOID GLOMERULOPATHY

Another disorder that can simulate amyloidosis histologically has recently been described: immunotactoid glomerulopathy.[366,367] This condition is characterized by mesangial expansion and fibrillar deposits on electron microscopy. In contrast to amyloidosis, the fibrils in immunotactoid glomerulopathy are larger and do not stain with Congo red or thioflavine-T. The origin of these deposits is uncertain; immunofluorescent microscopy is generally positive for IgG, suggesting that immunoglobulins are involved. There is, however, usually no evidence of a circulating or urinary paraprotein, and long-term follow-up has not revealed an association with multiple myeloma or any other malignancy.

Patients with this disorder typically present with proteinuria which is usually in the nephrotic range, microscopic hematuria, renal insufficiency which may be acutely progressive, and hypertension. Progression to end-stage renal failure has occurred in over 50 percent of patients. There is no known therapy in this disorder.

OTHER

A variety of disorders with histologic patterns somewhat different from the diseases described above are uncommon causes of the nephrotic syndrome with a nephrotic sediment.[368] Included in this group are preeclampsia (see Chap. 7), massive obesity in which an elevation in GFR may be the major abnormality and can lead to focal glomerulosclerosis similar to that seen in other hyperfiltration states (see Chap. 4),[369,370] rare patients with renal artery stenosis in whom angiotensin II-mediated hemodynamic changes appear to be of primary importance,[371,372] chronic hypertensive nephrosclerosis,[373] congenital and hereditary diseases (congenital nephrotic syndrome, nail-patella syndrome),[374-376] infections (quartan malaria, schistosomiasis),[377,378] dermatitis herpetiformis,[379] drugs (probenecid, nifedipine),[380,381] allergens (bee sting, snake bite, poison oak),[368] and renal transplantation.[382] In addition, those disorders usually associated with a nephritic sediment (such as membranoproliferative glomerulonephritis and IgA nephropathy) may occasionally present only with the nephrotic syndrome (see individual disorders, below).

DISORDERS USUALLY ASSOCIATED WITH FOCAL GLOMERULONEPHRITIS

Focal glomerulonephritis is typically manifested by hematuria, which may be macroscopic. Proteinuria also may be present but is generally mild. Findings characteristic of either the nephrotic states (heavy proteinuria and edema) or diffuse glomerulonephritis (hypertension, edema, and renal insufficiency) are usually absent in focal disease.[383,384] The term *focal* in this discussion is primarily based upon the relatively mild clinical and light microscopic abnormalities since IF and EM frequently reveal diffuse involvement.

Although a variety of disorders can cause focal glomerulonephritis (see Table 6-1), only IgA nephropathy, benign hematuria, and hereditary nephritis are discussed in detail in this section. Other causes of focal disease such as SLE, poststreptococcal glomerulonephritis (both of which are frequently associated with diffuse involvement), and Henoch-Schönlein purpura will be discussed below and in Chap. 7.

Presentation with hematuria is not limited to glomerulonephritis, as a variety of extraglomerular disorders (such as stones, tumors, and prostatic disease) can lead to urinary bleeding. Clues suggesting the presence of glomerular disease include brown urine, dysmorphic red cells, red cell casts, and protein excretion exceeding 500 mg/day (see p. 44). The degree of bleeding is not of diagnostic value since microscopic or macroscopic hematuria can occur with lesions anywhere in the urinary tract.

IgA NEPHROPATHY

IgA nephropathy (Berger's disease) is one of the most common causes of primary glomerular disease.[385-388] It can occur at any age, but most patients present between the ages of 10 and 50.

PATHOLOGY

The pathologic changes in IgA nephropathy are primarily located in the mesangium.[386-388] Light microscopy usually reveals mild to moderate mesangial hypercellularity and increased mesangial matrix, occurring in seg-

ments of some or all glomeruli, i.e., either focal or diffuse disease may be present (Fig. 6-13a). Crescent formation and areas of fibrinoid necrosis also may occur but are uncommon. In the later stages of the disease, healing can lead to glomerular sclerosis.

Electron microscopy characteristically demonstrates globular deposits in the mesangium (see Fig. 5-5c) and much less often in the subendothelial or subepithelial space. However, both the LM and EM findings are nonspecific and can be found in many causes of focal glomeruloncphritis.

The *diagnosis of IgA nephropathy is made by IF* which shows mesangial deposition of IgA and C3 (Fig. 6-13b). IgG or IgM also may be found but are less prominent. In contrast to the frequently focal abnormalities on LM, IF typically reveals diffuse involvement.

Although some IgA can be found in a variety of glomerular diseases,[389] prominent mesangial IgA deposits occur in only two other disorders: Henoch-Schönlein purpura, which is histologically indistinguishable from IgA nephropathy[386]; and SLE, in which IgG deposition is typically more pronounced.

PATHOGENESIS

The IF and EM findings indicate that IgA nephropathy is an immune complex disease, with deposition probably occurring by an in situ mechanism (see p. 149). A variety of observations suggest a relatively specific abnormality in IgA-mediated events. These include an elevated plasma IgA level in up to 50 percent of patients,[387] concurrent IgA deposition in the dermal capillaries of normal skin,[390] circulating immune complexes containing IgA that roughly parallel the activity of the renal disease,[391,392] and increased in vitro production of IgA (but not IgG or IgM) by the patient's lymphocytes.[393]

The origin of this IgA, however, is uncertain. The elevated IgA levels in the plasma[394,395] and the IgA that is deposited in the glomeruli are polymeric (subclass A_1),[395,396]

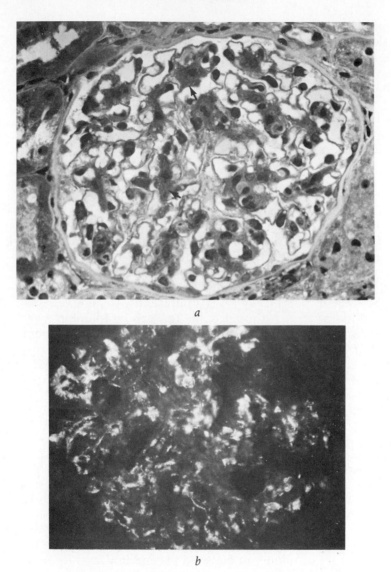

a

b

FIG. 6–13. Histologic changes in IgA nephropathy. (*a*) Light microscopy shows prominence of the mesangial areas with increased cellularity and matrix (arrows). The capillary loops and basement membrane are typically normal. (*b*) Immuno-fluorescent microscopy is diagnostic, revealing prominent IgA deposits that are usually limited to the mesangial areas.

which could be derived from either circulating B cells or mucosal secretory sites. The presence of polymeric IgA is essential since the monomer is unable to form the large antigen-antibody lattices that are required for the development of renal disease (see p. 148).[397]

The association of viral infections with recurrent episodes of gross hematuria has led to the hypothesis that the primary event is mucosal immunization (in the respiratory or intestinal tract), leading to an exaggerated local IgA response.[387] The observation that tonsillar lymphocytes from patients with IgA nephropathy have a higher than normal percentage of cells producing polymeric IgA is consistent with this hypothesis.[398] The rapid recurrence of hematuria within 1 to 3 days of the infection raises the possibility that viral antigens may be chronically sequestered in the mesangium, where they can combine by an in situ mechanism with IgA antiviral antibodies formed during the acute infection.

Intestinal IgA production may also be important in certain cases since gross hematuria can follow an episode of gastroenteritis.[388] There is also experimental support for this possibility. Chronic oral feeding of a foreign protein antigen in adjuvant to animals can induce mucosal IgA synthesis and the subsequent deposition of antigen and IgA in the glomerular mesangium.[399]

Mechanisms other than primary overproduction of mucosal IgA also may be important, particularly in patients with associated underlying diseases. For example, a defect in the mucosal barrier could lead to enhanced antigen exposure to the local IgA-producing cells. This could explain the occasional association of IgA nephropathy with dermatitis herpetiformis or gluten enteropathy (celiac disease).[400]

Another possibility is decreased clearance of IgA-containing immune complexes, a process that normally occurs primarily in the Kupffer cells in the liver.[401] Thus, liver disease could predispose to IgA nephropathy by delaying the clearance of IgA complexes from the circulation. This hypothesis is probably true in at least some cases, since IgA nephropathy, which may be clinically silent, occurs with increased frequency in animals or humans with hepatic cirrhosis.[402-404] IgA deposition also may be present in the hepatic sinusoids and dermal capillaries in this setting.[405]

Another mechanism by which the clearance of IgA complexes might be impaired involves complement. Most antigen-antibody complexes bind C1, leading to the formation of C3b (see Fig. 5–9). C3b then plays an important role in *preventing immune complex disease*, both by limiting growth of the antigen-antibody lattice (thereby minimizing the formation of large precipitating complexes that are more likely to produce tissue damage) and by facilitating delivery of immune complexes (in part via attachment to C3b receptors on erythrocytes) to their site of elimination in the reticuloendothelial system.[405a] In comparison to most subclasses of IgG, IgA is unable to bind C1. This effect could diminish complex elimination, thereby promoting the deposition of IgA-containing complexes in the glomerular mesangium.[405a]

ETIOLOGY

Although IgA nephropathy is most often idiopathic, it can occasionally be found with other disorders (Table 6–6). The mechanism of these associations is not always readily apparent, although possible mucosal abnormalities (dermatitis herpetiformis, gluten enteropathy, tuberculosis, pulmonary diseases) or hepatic disease may be present. In addition, genetic factors, which could influence any of the pathogenetic mechanisms described above, probably affect the susceptibility to developing IgA nephropathy. Famil-

TABLE 6-6. Causes of IgA Nephropathy

Idiopathic
   May be familial[406]
Hepatic cirrhosis[403,404]
Dermatitis herpetiformis and gluten enteropathy[407,408]
Seronegative arthritis, particularly ankylosing
   spondylitis[409,410]
Mycosis fungoides[411]
Disseminated tuberculosis[412]
Pulmonary diseases[413]
Oat cell carcinoma[414]

ial cases may occur[406] and an increased frequency of HLA-DR4 has been described in patients with this disorder.[415,416]

CLINICAL PRESENTATION AND COURSE

The major modes of presentation of IgA nephropathy are macroscopic hematuria or the incidental finding of hematuria and proteinuria (usually less than 1 g/day) on a routine urinalysis.[386-388] Although the P_{cr}, blood pressure, and complement levels are typically normal, some patients with gross hematuria develop transient acute renal failure (without hypertension or edema) that may be due primarily to red cell obstruction of the tubules.[417]

The episodes of macroscopic hematuria may be recurrent, occurring 1 to 3 days after an upper respiratory infection (or, less commonly, gastroenteritis). This is in contrast to poststreptococcal glomerulonephritis which most often has a latent period exceeding 7 days. The gross bleeding in IgA nephropathy lasts only a few days, although microscopic hematuria generally persists.

Less frequently, IgA nephropathy presents with the nephrotic syndrome or a picture similar to acute, diffuse glomerulonephritis, with hypertension and renal insufficiency accompanying the urinary abnormalities and diffuse glomerular involvement, often with crescents, found on renal biopsy.[386-388,418,419] Early nephrotic syndrome occurs in 5 to 10 percent of patients.[388,420] This is generally a bad prognostic sign with a high risk of eventual progression to renal failure.[388,420] However, there appears to be a subgroup of patients who present with the acute nephrotic syndrome and *no hematuria*. These patients may behave as if they have minimal change disease with a corticosteroid-responsive, frequently relapsing course and a potentially persistent remission of the proteinuria after a course of cyclophosphamide.[420,421]

The prognosis in IgA nephropathy is frequently good, although the microscopic hematuria or episodes of gross hematuria may persist for many years. However, this disorder is not always benign, since end-stage renal disease occurs in about 10 percent of patients at 10 years and 20 percent at 20 years.[387,388] In addition, another 20 to 30 percent may have some decline in renal function by 20 years.[387] Thus, slowly progressive disease may ultimately develop in up to one-half of patients.

As with other glomerulopathies, relatively bad prognostic signs include proteinuria exceeding 1 g/day, hypertension, an elevated P_{cr}, and, on biopsy, glomerulosclerosis, tubulointerstitial disease, or diffuse proliferation with prominent crescent formation.[388,418,422-424] Some patients with crescents may have an acutely progressive course, similar to that with other forms of rapidly progressive glomerulonephritis.[419]

DIAGNOSIS

IgA nephropathy should be suspected in patients presenting with either macroscopic or microscopic hematuria and proteinuria. The absence of hypocomplementemia, the lack of evidence of an antecedent streptococcal infection, and a negative family history of renal disease tend to exclude other disorders that may present in a similar fashion, such as membranoproliferative or poststreptococcal glomerulonephritis or hereditary nephritis. Similarly, the absence of purpura and abdominal or joint pain tends to exclude Henoch-Schönlein purpura, a multisystem disorder associated with the same renal findings as IgA nephropathy.[386]

However, IgA nephropathy cannot usually be differentiated on clinical grounds from benign hematuria when the presenting problem is glomerular hematuria with no or only mild (less than 1 g/day) proteinuria. In this setting, approximately 20 to 40 percent of patients will have IgA nephropathy with the remainder showing other, usually nonspecific pathologic findings (see "Benign Hematuria," below).[425-428]

Since the prognosis of IgA nephropathy and benign hematuria is generally benign, renal biopsy to confirm the diagnosis should be performed only when there is some suggestion that a progressive disease may be present. Thus, indications for biopsy in a patient presenting with hematuria of glomerular origin include hypocomplementemia (if there is no antecedent streptococcal infection), protein excretion persistently greater than 1 g/day, persistent hypertension (assuming the onset of hypertension was coincident with the renal disease), and renal insufficiency.

TREATMENT

There is no therapy that has been shown to alter the course of IgA nephropathy.[387,388] Prednisone and cytotoxic agents are generally ineffective both in the primary disease and in the renal transplant where the rate of recurrent IgA nephropathy may be as high as 50 percent despite the use of prednisone and azathioprine.[18,429] However, the latter finding should not preclude renal transplantation since recurrent disease does not usually lead to a progressive impairment in renal function.[18]

One apparent exception to the ineffectiveness of immunosuppressive therapy occurs in patients who present with the nephrotic syndrome and no hematuria. In this setting, prednisone (and cyclophosphamide if there are frequent relapses) can induce a remission similar to that seen in minimal change disease.[420,421]

A more specific form of therapy that has been tried is the administration of phenytoin, which has been shown to lower the plasma IgA concentration. When given to patients with IgA nephropathy, phenytoin reduces the circulating level of IgA and IgA-containing immune complexes but does not appear to alter the course of the renal disease.[430,431] These findings raise the possibility that nonimmunologic factors (such as hyperfiltration and systemic hypertension) may play an important role in progressive disease. Thus, strict control of the blood pressure and dietary protein restriction should be instituted in patients with deteriorating renal function (see Chap. 4).

BENIGN HEMATURIA

Benign hematuria refers to a variety of disorders that have similar clinical manifestations to IgA nephropathy: recurrent episodes of gross hematuria shortly after a viral upper respiratory infection or occasionally after severe exercise; or asymptomatic microscopic hematuria.[425-428,432-437] The blood pressure, P_{cr}, and plasma complement levels typically remain within normal limits, and protein excretion is usually less than 1 g/day.

Benign hematuria is a common cause of hematuria in children, but it may also be seen in adults. Most cases are sporadic, but familial cases may occur.[432,438,439] Although a viral infection frequently precedes the episodes of hematuria, it is not known why affected patients are prone to developing hematuria in this setting.

Renal biopsy reveals a variety of histologic changes, a finding which is consistent with the heterogeneous nature of this disorder. Light microscopy usually shows minimal to moderate mesangial cell proliferation with increased mesangial matrix, a pattern similar to that in IgA nephropathy (see Fig. 6-13).[433-435] However, several different abnormalities have been described on IF and EM: scattered, IgG or IgM with mesangial deposits,[425,426,437] thinning of the GBM ("thin membrane disease"), a disorder that is usually familial[428,438,439]; and focal deposits of C3 in the glomeruli or blood vessels.[428,440] In addition, some biopsies will be normal, indicating either nonglomerular bleeding or minimal, nondetectable glomerular disease.[428,441]

Regardless of the histology, no therapy is indicated since the long-term prognosis is excellent with only rare, probably hemodynamically mediated progression to renal failure (see Chap. 4).[442] The differential diagnosis and indications for renal biopsy are the same as in IgA nephropathy.

HEREDITARY NEPHRITIS

A variety of rare heredofamilial disorders can cause glomerular disease, including the congenital nephrotic syndrome,[374,375] the nail-patella syndrome,[376] Fabry's disease,[443] and amyloidosis due to familial Mediterranean fever.[320] More common than these disorders is hereditary nephritis (Alport's syndrome), which is frequently accompanied by hearing loss and anterior lenticonus.[444-446] These abnormalities appear to result from the production of abnormal basement membranes.

PATHOLOGY

The pathologic changes in hereditary nephritis increase in severity with age, with the diagnostic findings being present only on EM.[445-447] Light microscopy initially reveals only focal increases in mesangial cellularity and matrix.[448] With time, these lesions progress to glomerular sclerosis (infrequently seen before the age of 10) with associated tubular atrophy and interstitial fibrosis. An interstitial infiltrate which includes foam cells (large cells of uncertain origin with foamy, lipid-containing cytoplasm) is characteristic of but not specific for this disorder. Immunofluorescent microscopy is usually negative, although nonspecific trapping of C3 and IgM may be seen.

The diagnostic histologic change in hereditary nephritis is found on EM, which shows longitudinal splitting of the glomerular and occasionally the tubular basement membranes with clear areas in between, resulting in a laminated appearance (Fig. 6–14).[447,449] There may also be some thinning of the GBM[447,450] similar to that seen in some cases of benign hematuria in which laminations and progressive renal failure do not occur.[438,439]

The number of glomeruli showing splitting of the GBM is age- and sex-dependent. In males, this change can usually be demonstrated in about 30 percent of the glomeruli by age 10, 70 percent by age 20, and more than 90 percent by age 30.[450] Thus, early renal biopsy in a young boy could, by sampling error, be nondiagnostic. In comparison, less than 30 percent of the glomeruli are usually affected in females, and there is

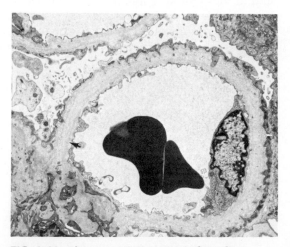

FIG. 6–14. Electron microscopy in hereditary nephritis reveals the characteristic split or laminated appearance of the glomerular basement membrane (arrow).

typically no or only slow progression with age. This finding is consistent with the generally benign course in females.

Rarely, patients with progressive renal disease will have a normal GBM on EM.[446] In this setting, the diagnosis cannot be definitively made by renal biopsy. However, the lack of immunologic activity on IF and EM, a positive family history of renal failure, and concurrent hearing loss usually allow a presumptive diagnosis of hereditary nephritis to be made.

INHERITANCE

Three modes of inheritance have been described in different kindreds: X-linked dominant; autosomal dominant, which may preferentially segregate with the X chromosome; and, less commonly, autosomal recessive.[451] In most families, the disease is not transmitted from affected fathers to their sons.[451] This finding could be explained by either of the first two mechanisms since the father would be passing on only the unaffected Y chromosome. X-linked inheritance could also account for the more benign course in females by the Lyon hypothesis.[444] Since only one of the two X chromosomes is active per cell, roughly half the cells would be normal in females (who have one normal and one abnormal X chromosome), thereby minimizing the renal and extrarenal manifestations of the disease.

PATHOGENESIS

It is presumed that hereditary nephritis represents a disorder of basement membrane synthesis in the kidney, inner ear, and eye.[444,445] Analysis of the GBM reveals several abnormalities including decreased content of hydroxyproline (a component of the collagenous part of the GBM)[452] and lack of normal GBM antigen(s). In some, but not all, families, the GBM does not bind anti-GBM antibodies from patients with Goodpasture's syndrome (see "Rapidly Progressive Glomerulonephritis," below).[453-457] The GBM does, however, bind antibodies derived from rabbits who are immunized with human GBM.[454] This finding suggests that some patients with hereditary nephritis lack the specific nephritogenic antigen, possibly in the noncollagenous domain of type IV collagen,[457] against which antibodies are directed in Goodpasture's syndrome. This antigen is also normally present in the membranes of the lens, eye, and organ or Corti in the ear, suggesting that its absence could also explain the extrarenal manifestations of the disease.[456]

The absence of normal GBM antigen(s) may be clinically important in patients who undergo renal transplantation. In this setting, anti-GBM disease can occur in the transplant, presumably because the normal antigen is recognized as foreign.[454,457] Fortunately, this complication, which can lead to loss of the graft, is uncommon.

Another question that arises is, Why should a basement membrane abnormality lead to glomerular sclerosis and renal failure? One likely possibility is that hereditary nephritis represents a form of hemodynamic injury (see Chap. 4). Although the glomerular pressure and flow are initially "normal," they may be too high for the weakened basement membrane in this disorder. This can lead to cycles of damage and then repair which are manifested by the laminations in the GBM. As some glomeruli become sclerotic, the adaptive hyperfiltration in the less affected glomeruli will accelerate the hemodynamic injury.

CLINICAL PRESENTATION AND COURSE

The most common abnormalities in hereditary nephritis are renal disease (which may occasionally occur alone), sensorineural hearing loss (primarily high-tone), and eye changes such as anterior lenticonus, cataracts, and whitish perimacular lesions in the retina.[444-446,458] Other less common disturbances which are present in some kindreds include peripheral neuropathy, retinitis pigmentosa, and platelet dysfunction.

The initial renal manifestations are similar to other focal nephritides: recurrent episodes of gross hematuria or microscopic hematuria with mild proteinuria. The blood pressure, P_{cr}, and serum complement are usually normal at the time of presentation. Although hematuria begins early in boys (being detectable in almost one-half before the age of 5),[445] it may not be discovered until early adulthood unless the patient is routinely examined because of the positive family history. Similarly, hearing loss, can be detected by audiometry in children but may not become clinically important for many years. There is no necessary relationship between the degrees of renal disease and hearing loss.

Characteristically, males are affected more frequently, more severely, and earlier than females.[444-446] Renal disease in males is usually progressive with the nephrotic syndrome and hypertension ultimately developing in many patients. End-stage renal failure typically occurs between the ages of 16 and 35, but occasionally is delayed until the patient is 45 or older.[445,451] Despite this interfamilial variability, the age at which renal failure is seen is relatively constant within a given kindred. Hearing loss is also typically progressive, frequently leading to deafness. The presence of whitish, perimacular lesions appears to be a bad prognostic sign, being associated with an increased incidence of early renal failure and hearing loss.[458]

On the other hand, uremia is rare in females and does not usually develop until the patient is more than 45 years old.[445,459] However, exceptions do occur in some families as renal failure can be seen below the age of 25.[459] Hearing impairment is also typically less common and less severe in females.[445]

DIAGNOSIS AND TREATMENT

The diagnosis of hereditary nephritis can be made from the family history, presence of extrarenal manifestations, and renal biopsy. Hereditary nephritis can usually be easily differentiated from the benign form of familial hematuria in which there is only thinning of the GBM and no family history of renal failure.[438,439]

There is no proven therapy that will alter the course of the disease. However, lowering the intraglomerular pressure may be beneficial by minimizing hemodynamic damage to the GBM. This can be achieved by restricting dietary protein intake and by reducing the systemic blood pressure (even if initially normal) with a converting enzyme inhibitor (see p. 123). Since the efficacy of this regimen is at present unproven, it should be reserved for patients at high risk, e.g., males with an already elevated P_{cr} or a family history of the early development of renal failure.

Dialysis or transplantation can be used when end-stage renal failure occurs. Although recurrent disease does not develop in the transplant (since the donor GBM is normal),[460] some patients are at risk of developing anti-GBM antibody disease due to exposure to previously unseen GBM antigen(s).[454,457]

OTHER

Occasional patients develop focal glomerulonephritis that does not fit into any of the specific disease states described above. In many cases, an infectious process initiates the disease, which is typically short-lived and characterized by microscopic hematuria and mild proteinuria.[461] Among the infectious agents that may be involved are bacteria (streptococci, pneumococci, salmonella),[462-464] viruses (Epstein-Barr virus, influenza, measles, hepatitis B virus),[465-468] mycoplasma,[469] and parasites (trichinosis).[470]

Occult postinfectious focal glomerulonephritis is more common than is generally appreciated. In one prospective study of 240 patients with a nonstreptococcal upper respiratory infection and no urinary symptoms, nine (3.8 percent) had microscopic hematuria and red blood cell casts which cleared in 2 to 7 months.[466] Similar findings have been reported after group A beta-hemolytic streptococcal infection as 20 of 248 patients (8 percent) developed both asymptomatic urinary abnormalities and hypocomplementemia.[462]

Not all cases of focal glomerulonephritis are postinfectious. As an example, a patient with Graves' disease developed microscopic hematuria and mild proteinuria due to apparent deposition of thyroglobulin and antithyroglobulin antibodies in the glomeruli.[471]

DISORDERS USUALLY ASSOCIATED WITH DIFFUSE GLOMERULONEPHRITIS

Diffuse forms of glomerulonephritis are commonly associated with edema, hypertension, a nephritic urinary sediment, cell proliferation in all glomeruli on renal biopsy, and, with the exception of rapidly progressive glomerulonephritis, hypocomplementemia. Other than the glomerular diseases listed in Table 6-1 and systemic vasculitis, the major disorder that may present with similar clinical findings is acute interstitial nephritis, e.g., due to methicillin (see Chap. 8). The history of drug administration, the usual absence of red cell casts and heavy proteinuria, and the common findings of fever, eosinophilia, and eosinophiluria usually suggest the presence of interstitial nephritis.[472] One exception may occur with the interstitial nephritis associated with nonsteroidal anti-inflammatory drugs (or rarely other drugs) in which the nephrotic syndrome due to minimal change disease may also be present.[102] This diagnosis is suggested by the history of drug use and, if necessary, can be confirmed by renal biopsy.

ACUTE POSTINFECTIOUS GLOMERULONEPHRITIS

A variety of infections can lead to a diffuse proliferative glomerulonephritis. Streptococcal pharyngitis or pyoderma is the most common and will be discussed in detail in this section. Other infections that can on occasion lead to a similar picture include bacterial endocarditis or an infected ventriculoatrial shunt, visceral abscesses,[473] *Streptococcus pneumoniae*,[474] and rarely other bacterial infections (salmonella, corynebacteria) or viral diseases such as varicella or the Guillain-Barré syndrome.[475-478] Each of these infections, including that with group A streptococci, can also produce milder, focal glomerular lesions (see "Focal Glomerulonephritis: Other," above).

PATHOLOGY

The pathologic changes in poststreptococcal glomerulonephritis (PSGN) vary with the severity of the disease. In patients with mild, frequently subclinical disease, LM reveals only minimal to moderate mesangial cell proliferation and increased mesangial matrix.[462] With more severe disease, diffuse endothelial cell and mesangial proliferation plus infiltration of circulating macrophages result in narrowing or closure of the capillary lumens (Fig. 6-15a).[183,479,480] Neutrophilic infiltration in the glomeruli and interstitial edema are also frequently prominent. Other less common changes which may be found include crescent formation and focal areas of necrosis. Basement membrane thickening, however, is usually absent. If present, glomerular sclerosis, tubular atrophy, and interstitial fibrosis suggest that the patient has an acute exacerbation of chronic glomerulonephritis.[481]

Electron microscopy typically reveals mesangial deposits and characteristic subepithelial "humps" (Fig. 6-15b) in the peripheral capillary loops. Immunofluorescent micros-

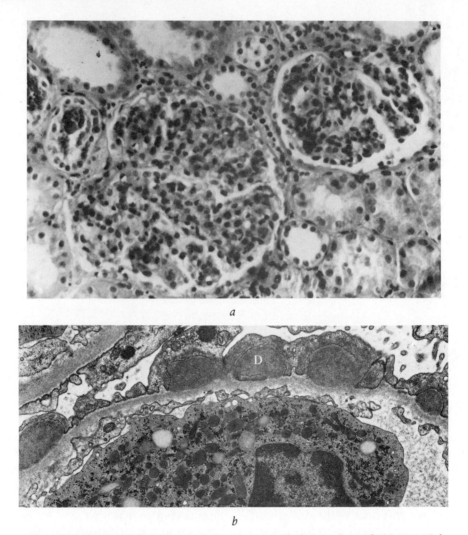

FIG. 6-15. Histologic findings in poststreptococcal glomerulonephritis. (*a*) Light microscopy demonstrates diffuse endothelial and mesangial cell proliferation with neutrophilic infiltration. The result is narrowing or closure of capillary lumens and enlargement of the capillary tuft so that Bowman's space is almost obliterated. (*b*) Electron microscopy shows the hump-shaped subepithelial deposits (D) that are characteristic of this disease. A neutrophil is present in the capillary lumen.

copy usually demonstrates irregular, granular deposits containing IgG, C3, and frequently fibrin in the glomerular capillary wall and mesangium. Streptococcal antigens also may be found in the glomerulus early in the course of the disease.[482]

These histologic changes tend to resolve in almost all patients. The deposits on EM and IF begin to decrease in number within 1 to 2 months and disappear by 9 to 12 months.[483,484] The light microscopic changes regress more slowly. Although the neutrophilic infiltration and most of the cell proliferation begin to improve within 6 weeks, mild mesangial cell proliferation and increased mesangial matrix persist in some patients for more than 4 years.[479,485,486] Segmental areas of glomerular sclerosis may be seen and may represent either healing of damage that occurred during the acute episode[479] or progressive glomerular injury due to hemodynamic factors (see "Course and Prognosis," below).[487]

PATHOGENESIS

With some rare exceptions,[488] PSGN follows infection only with group A beta-hemolytic streptococci. There must be some specific property of the bacterium involved since only certain strains produce glomerular disease, particularly type 12 with pharyngitis and type 49 with pyoderma.[489-492] This is in contrast to acute rheumatic fever which can be induced by almost any group A beta-hemolytic streptococcus.[493] These two post-streptococcal diseases only rarely occur together.[494,495]

The IF and EM findings indicate that immune mechanisms are responsible for the glomerular disease. It is not clear, however, what the offending antigen is. In some patients with PSGN, a unique streptococcal antigen has been identified in the glomeruli early in the course of the disease,[482] and probably in circulating immune complexes.[496] On the other hand, glomeruli and streptococci from patients without PSGN do not appear to have this antigen.*

How such an antigen would predispose to the development of glomerular disease is uncertain. One possible explanation is antigenic charge since cationic antigens have been eluted from the glomeruli of patients with PSGN.[498] This would promote both antigen binding to the negative charges in the GBM (where complexes can initially form in the sub*endo*thelial space)[499] and subsequent antigen movement across the GBM. In experimental animals, only cationic antigens are able to form subepithelial deposits as occur in PSGN (see p. 150).

Mechanisms other than the direct renal deposition of streptococcal antigens also may play a role in this disorder. Circulating antibodies against proteoglycans in the GBM (such as heparan sulfate) have been demonstrated which cross react with streptococcal hyaluronidase.[500] These antibodies could contribute either to the primary disease or to persistent injury after the streptococcal antigens have been removed. It is also possible, however, that they are merely a secondary phenomenon, as the initial inflammatory damage leads to exposure of GBM antigens to the systemic circulation.

Another hypothesis proposes that nephritogenic streptococci produce an enzyme, neuraminidase, which alters endogenous IgG, making it immunogenic. As a result, anti-IgG antibodies would be formed and IgG-anti-IgG complexes deposited in the kidney producing a proliferative glomerulonephritis.[501,502] In support of this theory, antibodies to IgG have been found in the circulation and glomeruli of patients with PSGN. These autoantibodies (which result in elevated rheumatoid factor titers) first appear 10 or more days after the streptococcal infection, the same time as the onset of the glomerular disease.[501] There is also confirmatory experimental evidence since injection of neuraminidase-altered, autologous IgG in rabbits can lead to anti-IgG antibody formation and an immune complex glomerulonephritis.[503]

Abnormalities in cellular immunity are also present as lymphocytes from patients with PSGN show increased reactivity to antigens from both streptococcal and damaged glomerular basement membranes.[504,505] The pathogenetic significance of these findings is uncertain since lymphocytes cannot be dem-

---

*Other investigators have claimed to identify a different nephritogenic antigen,[497] but its pathogenetic importance is uncertain.[496]

onstrated in the glomeruli.[480] It is possible, however, that activated T cells against glomerular bound antigen are present very early in the disease, a time at which renal biopsy is not performed.[506] These T cells could release lymphokines that promote the accumulation of macrophages, which then produce the glomerular damage (see p. 155).[506,507]

CLINICAL PRESENTATION

PSGN may follow an episode of either pharyngitis or pyoderma (impetigo) in children or, less commonly, in adults.[479,481,489,491,508–510] This may occur either with epidemics or in sporadic cases. Epidemic PSGN may occur with pharyngitis[489] but is most often associated with skin infection, particularly with type 49, group A streptococci.[491,508,509]

Even within epidemics, only a minority of infected patients develop glomerular disease, the attack rates being about 25 percent with pyoderma and 5 to 10 percent following throat infections.[489,491] These findings suggest that host factors (such as the nature and intensity of the immune response) play a role in the susceptibility to PSGN.[511]

The latent period between the onset of infection and evidence of renal disease is dependent upon the site of infection, with a mean of 10 days with pharyngitis and 21 days with pyoderma.[510] A latent period of less than 5 days suggests that the patient either has a virus-activated disease such as IgA nephropathy or benign hematuria (see "IgA Nephropathy," above), or an exacerbation of underlying chronic glomerulonephritis due to streptococcal or nonstreptococcal infection.

The typical presenting symptoms of classic PSGN include the acute onset of macroscopic hematuria ("Coca Cola-colored" urine), oliguria, pedal and periorbital edema, and flank pain due to stretching of the renal capsule.[485,489,510] In addition to peripheral edema, the physical examination may reveal

hypertension and congestive heart failure, both due primarily to sodium and water retention resulting from the low GFR.[512,513] Signs of encephalopathy (lethargy, confusion) may be present in patients with advanced renal failure or severe hypertension. It should be noted that the normal diastolic pressure in children is usually less than 70 mmHg. Thus, a diastolic pressure exceeding 100 mmHg, which represents only mild hypertension in adults, can cause hypertensive encephalopathy in children.

The laboratory data at the time of presentation most often reveal elevations in the blood urea nitrogen (BUN) and P_{cr}. The degree of renal insufficiency is relatively mild in most patients, with the P_{cr} usually being under 3 mg/dL. However, more severe disease which may require dialysis also may occur.[481,485,514] The plasma C3 level is reduced in the first week in over 90 percent of patients.[515,516] This may reflect activation by both alternate and classic pathways. In addition to deposition in the glomeruli, direct cleavage of C3 may occur in the systemic circulation.[517–519] This appears to be mediated in at least some cases by an autoantibody directed against the C3 convertase of the classic pathway (C$\overline{42}$) (see Fig. 5–9).[518] This antibody binds to the C3 convertase, making it less susceptible to inactivation and allowing continued C3 breakdown. Elevated rheumatoid factor titers (representing antibody to IgG) and circulating cryoglobulins are also found in most patients.[501,520] The mechanisms responsible for the production of these autoantibodies are incompletely understood.

The urinalysis in PSGN is characterized by a high specific gravity, a nephritic sediment, and proteinuria. There is frequently marked pyuria, a probable reflection of neutrophilic infiltration in the glomeruli. Although the nephrotic syndrome may occur, protein excretion is usually less than 2 g/day.[485]

In addition to this classic presentation, prospective studies of patients with group A beta-hemolytic streptococcal infections have revealed that subclinical disease characterized by microscopic hematuria, mild proteinuria, or hypocomplementemia may occur in as many as 20 percent of patients.[462,490] Renal biopsy in these patients demonstrates mild mesangial changes rather than a diffuse proliferative glomerulonephritis. Subclinical disease may also occur in family members of affected patients[521] and during epidemics.[491]

DIAGNOSIS

The diagnosis of PSGN may be suspected from the history, urinary findings, and presence of hypocomplementemia. Evidence of a recent streptococcal infection is best obtained by serologic tests since culture of the throat or skin may be negative, especially if antimicrobials have already been administered. Approximately 75 to 80 percent of patients with pharyngitis have an elevated plasma antistreptolysin O (ASO) titer.[511] The frequency of positive tests can be increased to 90 percent or more if antihyaluronidase and anti-DNAase B titers are also measured. In contrast, the ASO titer is elevated in only 50 percent of patients with pyoderma and glomerulonephritis,[511] perhaps due to inactivation of this antigen by skin lipids.[522] In this setting, evidence of a recent streptococcal infection can be better demonstrated by measuring the anti-DNAase B titers, which are elevated in more than 90 percent of patients.[492,511] Screening with the streptozyme test is useful because it includes antibodies to multiple streptococcal antigens.[492]

Although these serologic tests may be of diagnostic importance, there is no correlation between the severity of the renal disease and the level of circulating antistreptococcal antibodies. In addition, antibody titers can be reduced with early antibiotic therapy without affecting the course of the glomerulonephritis.[490,523]

The differential diagnosis in the patient with hypocomplementemia includes the other hypocomplementemic glomerulopathies, particularly membranoproliferative glomerulonephritis (MPGN). Clues suggesting the diagnosis of PSGN rather than MPGN are improvement in renal function usually beginning within 1 to 2 weeks[485] and return of the complement level to normal within 6 weeks.[515] On the other hand, the persistence of renal insufficiency, hypocomplementemia, or the nephrotic syndrome are unusual in PSGN and suggest the possible presence of MPGN. In this setting, a renal biopsy (which is not necessary in classic PSGN) should be performed to ascertain the correct diagnosis. Other hypocomplementemic disorders such as systemic lupus erythematosus, bacterial endocarditis, and mixed cryoglobulinemia can usually be excluded by appropriate laboratory tests and the lack of evidence of multisystem disease.

In those patients with normal complement levels, other diseases which should be considered are IgA nephropathy, rapidly progressive glomerulonephritis, and vasculitis. Renal biopsy is indicated if there is no evidence of an antecedent streptococcal infection or if there is persistent renal insufficiency.

TREATMENT

The treatment of PSGN is essentially supportive. Since volume overload is largely responsible for the development of edema and hypertension, these problems should be treated with loop diuretics to remove the excess fluid.[510,512] Dialysis is indicated in those patients who have fluid overload that is refractory to diuretics or who become clinically uremic.

Appropriate antimicrobials (penicillin in nonallergic patients) should be administered to control the local symptoms and to prevent spread of a potentially nephritogenic infection to close contacts. In contrast to its effectiveness in rheumatic fever, penicillin does not appear to prevent the development of glomerulonephritis,[490,523] with the possible exception of extremely early administration (within 36 h of the onset of infection).[489] This suggests that the pathogenetic events of PSGN are initiated very early in the course of the disease, even though clinical abnormalities do not usually occur for 7 to 21 days.

Bed rest is necessary only if symptoms are severe. Full ambulation can be started without deleterious effects once improvement begins.[524]

Specific measures directed against the renal disease are not effective. Corticosteroids, immunosuppressive agents, and anticoagulants have not been shown to be beneficial and are not necessary since almost all patients recover spontaneously, including those with severe renal failure.[514,525,526]

COURSE AND PROGNOSIS

The ultimate prognosis of PSGN is controversial and appears to be somewhat different in children and adults. Almost all children recover from the acute episode. In general, a diuresis begins within 1 week, and the P_{cr} returns to normal by 3 to 4 weeks.[485,527] The urinary changes tend to resolve more slowly. Microscopic hematuria usually disappears within 6 months, but proteinuria is still present in 15 percent of patients at 3 years, 5 percent at 5 years, and 2 percent at 7 to 10 years.[481,527,528] Persistent proteinuria is typically associated with mesangial hypercellularity and increased mesangial matrix, findings which have been referred to as *latent glomerulonephritis*. However, rather than representing continued disease activity, latent glomerulonephritis may reflect slow healing since the incidence of proteinuria falls with each succeeding year of observation during the first 7 to 10 years.

The results are not quite so good with longer follow-up. At 11 to 17 years in children who recovered from the initial episode

of PSGN (either epidemic or endemic), proteinuria is present in 4 to 11 percent and a new decline in renal function in up to 5 percent.[528,529] These changes may reflect hemodynamically mediated injury.[487]

Severe renal failure, frequently associated with crescents or a membranoproliferative pattern on biopsy, develops in the acute stage in less than 5 percent of children.[481,485,525] However, spontaneous recovery is commonly seen even in this group.[525,526] With current methods of therapy, death during the acute episode or irreversible renal failure probably occurs in less than 1 percent of children (excluding those with exacerbations of underlying chronic glomerulonephritis).[510]

In contrast, the prognosis appears to be less benign in adults. This may be due in part to a higher frequency of severe acute disease characterized by renal insufficiency or the nephrotic syndrome.[479,530] Even patients who partially or completely recover from the acute episode may subsequently develop proteinuria, hypertension, or renal insufficiency as long as 40 years after the acute episode.[487,530,531] This progression is associated with glomerular and vascular sclerosis on renal biopsy and is thought to reflect damage induced by intraglomerular hypertension (see Chap. 4).[487] According to this theory, some glomeruli are irreversibly injured during the acute illness, but the GFR initially remains in the normal range because of hyperfiltration in the less affected glomeruli. This adaptive response is ultimately maladaptive since the high intraglomerular pressure damages the glomerular capillary wall.

It has been suggested that evidence of irreversible disease may occur in more than one-half of adults with PSGN.[530] However, this conclusion has been challenged on several grounds.[532,533] Most importantly, these studies were performed only on hospitalized patients who had relatively severe acute disease. Consequently, adults with milder disease may have a better prognosis.

Nevertheless, it seems prudent to consider

PSGN a potentially progressive disease in adults, even though the frequency with which this occurs is probably well under 50 percent.[529,534] As a result, these patients should be followed at regular intervals after the acute episode, looking for the late development of hypertension, proteinuria, or renal insufficiency. If these complications occur, restricting dietary protein intake and lowering the blood pressure (even if still normal) with a converting enzyme inhibitor may help preserve renal function by minimizing hemodynamic injury (see Chap. 4).

BACTERIAL ENDOCARDITIS OR INFECTED VENTRICULOATRIAL SHUNT

A postinfectious glomerulonephritis also may occur with bacterial endocarditis[535-537] or an infected ventriculoatrial shunt.[538] Although a variety of organisms may be involved, the most common are *Staphylococcus aureus* and *Streptococcus viridans* in acute and subacute endocarditis, respectively, and *Staphylococcus epidermidis* with an infected shunt.

PATHOLOGY

The major pathologic change on LM in these disorders is mesangial and endothelial cell proliferation which, depending upon the severity of the disease, can be either focal or diffuse (similar to Figs. 6-13 and 6-15).[535-539] Basement membrane thickening also may be present in shunt nephritis, producing a histologic picture similar to membranoproliferative glomerulonephritis (see "Membranoproliferative Glomerulonephritis," below).[538] Focal areas of necrosis or crescent formation can be seen in some patients as well as glomerular sclerosis in prolonged, untreated disease.

Immunofluorescent microscopy usually reveals granular deposition of IgG and C3 in the mesangium and capillary loops. Mesangial and subendothelial deposits or subepithelial humps may be seen on EM.[535-539] These pathologic findings are not specific and resemble those found in PSGN or SLE.

PATHOGENESIS

The renal lesion in endocarditis was at one time attributed to focal emboli from vegetations on the diseased valve. Although emboli can occur,[536] the development of glomerular disease in patients with right-sided endocarditis (which should be associated with pulmonary not systemic emboli) and in patients with no demonstrable emboli on examination of the kidney indicates that other factors are of primary importance. The findings on IF and EM plus the demonstration of circulating immune complexes[540] suggest that immune complex deposition is the primary event in both endocarditis and shunt nephritis. These complexes appear to represent bacterial antigen and antibacterial antibodies in at least some patients.[541-544]

CLINICAL PRESENTATION

Most patients present with symptoms and physical findings due to the endocarditis or infected shunt including fever, weakness, heart murmur, and hepatosplenomegaly. The manifestations of the renal disease are variable.[535-538] In some patients, microscopic hematuria and mild proteinuria are incidentally discovered on a routine urinalysis. In this setting, the P_{cr} is usually normal and only focal changes are seen on renal biopsy.

On the other hand, a picture similar to diffuse PSGN also may be seen as a nephritic urinary sediment is accompanied by renal insufficiency. For reasons that are unclear, edema and hypertension appear to be less common than in PSGN.[537] The nephrotic syndrome is unusual in endocarditis but is present in about 30 percent of patients with shunt nephritis.[538] The C3, C4, and C2 levels are reduced in both disorders, suggesting that activation of complement has occurred by the classic pathway.[535,538,545] Rheumatoid factor is often present (being proportional to the duration of the disease), and circulating cryoglobulins may be found.[535,536,544]

The severity of the renal disease is primarily related to the duration of infection prior to the institution of antibiotic therapy.[535,537] Thus, glomerular disease is most likely to occur in patients who do not seek medical attention early in the course of the disease or in whom the diagnosis is delayed, e.g., due to culture-negative or right-sided endocarditis. Patients who do not have evidence of renal disease at the time of diagnosis are not likely to subsequently develop glomerulonephritis because of the ability of antimicrobials to markedly reduce the incidence of glomerular involvement.[546]

DIAGNOSIS

The history (including the presence of a ventriculoatrial shunt), physical examination, and positive blood cultures usually allow the diagnosis of bacterial endocarditis or an infected shunt to be made. However, glomerulonephritis must be differentiated from acute interstitial nephritis resulting from a reaction to antimicrobial therapy (see Chap. 8) and, in endocarditis, from infected or sterile emboli. The glomerulonephritis is typically present at or near the peak of severity before antimicrobials are begun. In contrast, acute interstitial nephritis usually does not become apparent until more than 10 days after the onset of treatment.[547] Eosinophilia, eosinophiluria, and recurrence of fever are also suggestive of this disorder.[472]

Renal emboli may occur at any time, even months after bacteriologic cure had been effected. As with the glomerular disease, hematuria, mild proteinuria, and, with bilateral involvement, renal insufficiency may be present. Clues favoring the diagnosis of renal emboli are unilateral flank pain, evidence of other systemic emboli, e.g., to the brain, and an elevated lactate dehydrogenase with normal or only mildly elevated transaminases (see Chap. 7). In patients with large or multiple emboli, a radioisotope renogram usually demonstrates localized defects in renal perfusion.

TREATMENT AND COURSE

The mainstays of therapy are appropriate antimicrobials and removal of the infected shunt. This should lead to recovery of renal function, even in most patients with advanced renal failure.[535-538] However, persistent hypertension, proteinuria, or rarely irreversible renal failure (associated with glomerular sclerosis on biopsy) may occur in patients with severe acute disease (initial P_{cr} greater than 4 mg/dL), particularly if there has been a long delay between the onset of infection and antimicrobial therapy.[537,548,549]

MEMBRANOPROLIFERATIVE GLOMERULONEPHRITIS

Membranoproliferative glomerulonephritis* (MPGN) is an infrequent cause of glomerular disease in both children and adults.[550-555] This disorder primarily occurs between the ages of 8 and 30 but it can affect patients of any age. Although no apparent cause can be identified in the majority of cases, a variety of underlying diseases have on occasion been associated with MPGN (Table 6–7).

PATHOLOGY

Three major forms of MPGN have been identified with different histologic findings, particularly on EM and IF (Table 6–8).[551,554,568]

*This disorder has also been called mesangiocapillary, lobular, and chronic hypocomplementemic glomerulonephritis.

Light microscopy is similar in each type, typically showing diffuse (or less commonly focal)[569,570] mesangial hypercellularity and increased mesangial matrix. The net result is a lobular appearance of the glomerular tufts and compression of the capillary lumens (Fig. 6–16a).

An additional characteristic of MPGN is extension of the mesangial cell cytoplasm between the basement membrane and the endothelial cell (mesangial interposition) with subsequent deposition of new basement membrane-like material. The result is a double-contour ("tram-track") appearance of the capillary wall, which can be seen on LM,

particularly with periodic acid Schiff (PAS) or silver stain (Fig. 6–16b). This change plus immune complex deposition results in thickening of the basement membrane which can be appreciated on LM or EM (Fig. 6–16c). Neutrophilic infiltration or focal crescent formation may also be seen.

In type 1 MPGN, IF is positive for C3, IgG, and occasionally IgM or IgA, usually in a lobular or fringe pattern (Fig. 6–17). In addition to mesangial interposition, EM reveals mesangial and subendothelial deposits.

In comparison, the characteristic change in type 2 MPGN (also called dense deposit disease) is found on EM, which demonstrates continuous dense deposits in the basement membranes of the glomerulus, tubules, and Bowman's capsule (Fig. 6–18).[551,571] Mesangial deposits also may be present. Immunofluorescent microscopy is positive for C3 but usually negative or only mildly positive for immunoglobulins.

Type 3 MPGN is characterized by mesangial and contiguous subendothelial and subepithelial deposits.[551,568] Immunofluorescent microscopy again shows C3 but no or minimal deposition of immunoglobulins.

Despite their histologic differences on EM and IF, these disorders are all considered variants of MPGN because of similar findings on LM, a typical, slowly progressive clinical course, and usually persistent hypocomplementemia.

TABLE 6–7. Causes of Membranoproliferative Glomerulonephritis

Idiopathic
Partial lipodystrophy (only with type 2)[556]
Complement deficient states[557,558]
Hepatitis B virus[468,559]
Visceral abscesses[473]
Chronic lymphocytic leukemia[99]
Heroin or pentazocine abuse[560,561]
Infected ventriculoatrial shunt[538]
Mixed cryoglobulinemia[562]
Chronic transplant rejection[563]
Malignant melanoma[564]
α_1-Antitrypsin deficiency[565]
Chlorpropamide[566]
Schistosomiasis[567]

TABLE 6–8. Different Histologic Characteristics of Major Types of MPGN

Type	Location of Deposits on EM	IF	Primary Complement Pathway Activated
1	Mesangial and subendothelial	IgG and C3 in fringe pattern	Classic
2	Mesangial and dense intra-membranous deposits	C3 and negative or mildly positive for IgG	Alternate
3	Mesangial, subepithelial, and subendothelial	C3 and negative or mildly positive for IgG	Alternate

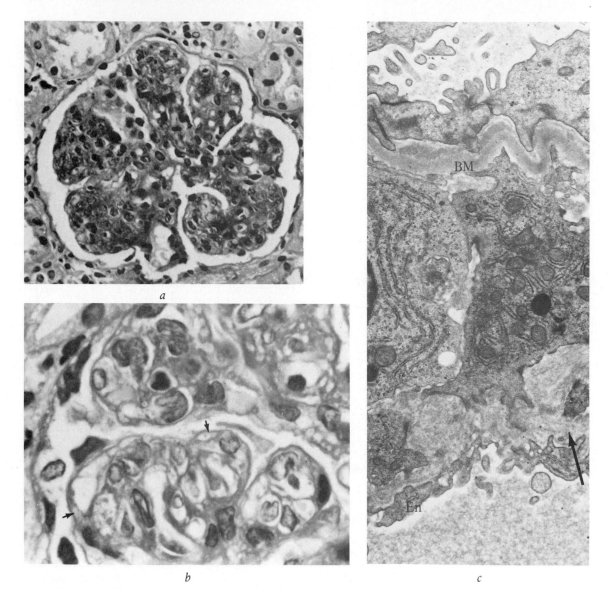

FIG. 6–16. Histologic findings in membranoproliferative glomerulonephritis. (*a*) Light microscopy reveals cellular proliferation, basement membrane thickening, and frequently a lobular appearance of the glomerular tuft. (*b*) Higher power demonstrates splitting of the basement membrane due to interposition of mesangial cytoplasm, resulting in double-contour appearance of the capillary wall (arrows). (*c*) Electron microscopy shows that widening of the basement membrane is primarily due to growth of the mesangial cytoplasm between the basement membrane (BM) and fenestrated endothelium (En). New basement membrane-like material, which is responsible for the double-contour appearance of the capillary wall on light microscopy, can be seen just above the endothelium (arrow).

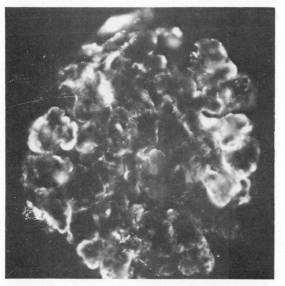

FIG. 6–17. Lobular or fringe pattern of immuno-fluorescence for C3 in membranoproliferative glomerulonephritis.

PATHOGENESIS

The pathogenesis of MPGN is poorly understood. In type 1, which is the most common, the findings of IF and EM are compatible with the glomerular deposition of immune complexes. The demonstration of circulating complexes which appear to correlate roughly with the severity of the glomerular disease is also consistent with this hypothesis.[572,573] However, the identity of the antigen is not known. It is of interest that patients with this disorder have elevated circulating levels of IgG3 (a subclass of IgG)[574] and, in the few patients studied, seven of seven have had IgG3 as the predominant or only IgG deposited in the glomeruli.[575,576] Since IgG3 is the primary antiviral IgG,[577] these findings suggest a viral etiology may be involved. The identification of hepatitis B virus in a few patients with this disorder is consistent with this hypothesis.[468,559]

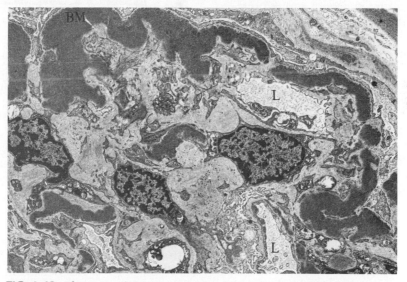

FIG. 6–18. Electron microscopy in type 2 membranoproliferative glomerulonephritis (or dense-deposit disease) reveals dense, continuous ribbonlike deposits in the basement membrane (BM). Mesangial proliferation and increased mesangial matrix are also present, resulting in marked narrowing of the capillary lumen (L). (*Courtesy of Dr. Robert Colvin.*)

In contrast, immune complexes may not be important in type 2 MPGN, since immunoglobulins are frequently absent on IF and the dense deposits on EM do not have the appearance of the discrete deposits usually seen with immune complex-mediated diseases (see Fig. 5–5). A primary abnormality in the basement membrane also does not appear to play a role since recurrent dense deposits are found in almost all patients who receive a transplant.[18,571] As a result of these findings, it has been suggested that type 2 MPGN is a systemic disorder, which in an unknown manner damages the renal basement membranes, and that the dense deposits represent aggregation of basement membrane-like material.[571] The complement deposition that is demonstrable on IF may simply reflect binding to the abnormal GBM.[578] However, immune mechanisms may contribute in some patients as evidenced by the elution from the glomeruli of melanoma antigen and antimelanoma antibody in a patient with type 2 MPGN and malignant melanoma.[564]

Little is known about the pathogenesis of type III MPGN. The presence of discrete deposits on EM suggests an immune complex mechanism, although there is no or only minimal IgG deposited by IF.[568]

Platelets, perhaps activated by the initial tissue damage, may be an important secondary mediator of glomerular injury in MPGN. This possibility is supported by the findings of increased platelet consumption[579] and an apparently positive response to therapy with antiplatelet agents.[580,581] How platelets might act in this setting is reviewed on p. 155.

CLINICAL PRESENTATION

Patients with MPGN usually present in one of four ways, with (1) the insidious onset of edema due to the nephrotic syndrome; (2) recurrent episodes of gross hematuria, frequently associated with an antecedent upper respiratory infection (similar to IgA nephropathy or benign hematuria); (3) an acute nephritic syndrome as seen with poststreptococcal glomerulonephritis—macroscopic or microscopic hematuria, edema, and hypertension preceded by symptoms of pharyngitis; or (4) the incidental discovery of hematuria and proteinuria on a routine urinalysis.[552-555]

At the time of presentation, the BUN and P_{cr} are usually normal or only mildly elevated. However, advanced renal failure may occur in patients presenting with an acute nephritic syndrome. The urinalysis in MPGN reveals hematuria, cellular and granular casts, and proteinuria that is in the nephrotic range in over one-half of patients.[552-554]

Hypocomplementemia is present initially in approximately 70 percent and at some time in the course of the disease in 85 percent of patients, particularly those with type 2 MPGN.[553,554] The mechanism by which this occurs is complex. In type 1, complement activation occurs primarily by the classic pathway (see Fig. 5–9) in a reaction presumably initiated by antigen-antibody complexes.[582] In this setting, there is usually only a moderate reduction in the plasma C3 level, which may be normal on some measurements.[554]

In contrast, the alternate pathway is involved in type 2 MPGN and persistent and frequently marked hypocomplementemia is typically found.[554,582] This appears to be due in part to a circulating IgG, called *C3 nephritic factor* (C3NeF), which induces the cleavage of C3. This factor, which is of extrarenal origin, can be demonstrated in the plasma of most patients with type 2 and some patients with type 1 and is apparently absent in type 3 MPGN.[551,554,568] The occasional persistence of both C3NeF and hypocomplementemia after nephrectomy suggests that peripheral catabolism and perhaps reduced synthesis might be more important than renal deposition in the production of low C3 levels in this disorder.[583]

C3NeF is a conformational autoantibody that is directed against and binds to C3bBb, the C3 convertase of the alternate pathway (see Fig. 5–9).[584,585] The C3bBb in this complex is protected against inactivation, thereby allowing continued C3 breakdown. Both the source of this antibody and its pathogenetic importance are unknown. Disease activity does not correlate with either C3NeF or C3 levels,[586] as progressive renal failure can occur even in patients who remain normocomplementemic.[587]

DIAGNOSIS

Because of its differing modes of presentation, MPGN may simulate either focal (recurrent hematuria) or diffuse (acute nephritic syndrome) glomerulopathies. The major clinical clue suggesting idiopathic MPGN in an adolescent or young adult is the presence of hypocomplementemia. In this setting, MPGN must be differentiated from PSGN and lupus nephritis. (Bacterial endocarditis and mixed cryoglobulinemia are much less common and are associated with characteristic physical and laboratory findings.)

In addition to renal biopsy, there are certain clinical clues that may be of help in suggesting the correct diagnosis. SLE, which may histologically be similar to type 1 MPGN, can usually be diagnosed by the concurrent clinical and serologic abnormalities (see "Lupus Nephritis," below). The distinction of MPGN from PSGN may be more difficult since both disorders can be initiated by an upper respiratory infection. With PSGN, however, the nephrotic syndrome is less common, renal insufficiency is usually transient, beginning to improve within 1 to 2 weeks, and complement levels return to normal within 6 to 8 weeks (see "Poststreptococcal Glomerulonephritis," above). Thus, persistence of these abnormalities favors the diagnosis of MPGN.

COURSE

Most patients with MPGN have progressive disease. The course is usually slow with the total GFR being relatively well maintained in many patients for 3 or more years. By 10 years, however, approximately one-half have reached end-stage renal failure.[552,554,555] In general, the disease is more severe in adults (particularly men) who tend to present with more marked renal dysfunction.[588] Other signs that suggest an increased likelihood of early progression include renal insufficiency (especially if associated with crescent formation), hypertension, the nephrotic syndrome, and type 2 disease.[554,555]

On the other hand, the prognosis is not always grim, as some patients follow an indolent course. This is most likely to occur in patients with a normal P_{cr}, no hypertension, nonnephrotic proteinuria (see Fig. 6–3), and a biopsy showing focal rather than diffuse disease.[589–591]

TREATMENT

A variety of different therapeutic regimens have been tried in MPGN with conflicting results. This is not particularly surprising in view of the chronic nature of the disease and the long period in which renal function may remain stable.

Uncontrolled studies using corticosteroids have given conflicting results.[553,592–594] In one long-term study, for example, prednisone was given in a dose of 2 mg/kg to a maximum of 80 mg every other day for 1 year, followed by slow tapering to a maintenance dose of 20 mg every other day which was continued for 3 to 10 years.[553,594] This appeared to result in stabilization of renal function and decreased cellular proliferation but some glomerular sclerosis on repeat biopsy. At 15 years, only 10 percent had progressed to end-stage renal failure versus 50 percent or more from historic controls. Type 1 seemed to show the best response.[553]

The efficacy of this regimen has been best evaluated by a controlled trial performed by the International Study of Kidney Disease in Children.[595] In type 1 MPGN, the prednisone-treated group (2 mg/kg to a maximum of 40 to 60 mg every other day) had a substantially lower incidence of a decline in GFR (5 versus 43 percent). This benefit, however, was offset by corticosteroid toxicity, particularly marked exacerbation of hypertension with its attendant complications such as seizures. A similar study has not been performed in adults.

Controlled trials also suggest that antiplatelet agents may be beneficial in MPGN. In one, aspirin (975 mg/day) and dipyridamole (225 mg/day) were administered *for 1 year.*[580] This regimen usually reversed the increase in platelet consumption that was present in many patients. It also significantly slowed the rate of fall in GFR (1.3 versus 19.6 mL/min per 1.73 m^2 per year in the control group) and decreased the incidence of progression to renal failure (14 versus 47 percent at 3 to 5 years). Another study utilizing dipyridamole and warfarin also reported positive results, but almost 40 percent of patients had some bleeding complication.[581]

These positive results must be weighed against a third controlled study in which a regimen of cyclophosphamide, warfarin, and dypyridamole had no benefit after 2 years of treatment.[596] There was also a substantial incidence of side effects requiring discontinuation of therapy. It is difficult to reconcile this trial with the positive findings described above. One possibility is that the period of follow-up was too short, although this remains unproven.

Cytotoxic agents, particularly cyclophosphamide, have also been tried in MPGN. Although they seem to be without benefit in most patients,[596] anecdotal reports suggest some improvement (when given with prednisone, warfarin, and dipyridamole) in patients with acutely progressive renal insufficiency.[597,598] However, the potential toxicity remains high, and only a minority of these patients maintained renal function in the long term.[554,598]

In summary, the optimal treatment of MPGN is uncertain. Therapy can probably be withheld in patients who appear to be at low risk of progressive disease, i.e., those with a normal P_{cr}, normal blood pressure, nonnephrotic proteinuria, and frequently focal changes on renal biopsy.[554,589,591]

Treatment is probably indicated in other patients since the likelihood of developing renal failure is so high. Children, particularly with type 1 disease, can be tried on the alternate day prednisone regimen.[553,595] The blood pressure must be carefully monitored since marked hypertension can be induced in this setting. Children who fail on prednisone and adults can be treated with aspirin and dipyridamole.[580] Warfarin seems to add little other than an increased risk of bleeding.[581,596]

The treatment of rapidly progressive disease, usually with crescent formation on biopsy, is unclear. Adding cyclophosphamide to prednisone and dipyridamole may be of benefit in some patients.[554,598] Considering the risks of the prolonged administration of cyclophosphamide (see p. 192), it may be safer to switch to azathioprine at 3 months if the patient has had a positive response.

Dialysis or transplantation can be used in those patients who progress to end-stage renal failure. The incidence of recurrent disease in the transplant is quite high, averaging 30 percent in type 1 and almost 90 percent in type 2 MPGN.[18,571,599] This does not preclude transplantation however, since most cases are asymptomatic and loss of transplant function due to recurrent disease is uncommon, occurring in only about 10 percent of all transplanted patients.[18] Those patients whose initial disease rapidly progressed to renal failure appear to be more likely to develop severe recurrence in the transplant.[600] In this setting, it may be desirable to delay transplantation for about 1 year to possibly allow the activity of the underlying disease to diminish.

LUPUS NEPHRITIS

Renal disease is extremely common in patients with SLE. The frequency with which it can be demonstrated depends upon how completely the patient is evaluated. Clinical evidence of renal involvement (abnormal urinalysis, elevated P_{cr}) is present at onset in approximately 50 percent and eventually develops in 70 to 75 percent of patients.[601] If, however, renal biopsy is performed even in the absence of urinary abnormalities, typical changes of lupus nephritis will be found in over 95 percent of patients.[602-604]

Both glomerular and tubular involvement may occur in SLE. Tubulointerstitial disease (perhaps due to immune complex deposition in the tubular basement membranes) is less common and is almost always seen in patients who also have glomerular disease.[605] Rarely, tubulointerstitial damage may be the only manifestation of lupus nephritis.[606,607] This entity is suggested by the finding of renal insufficiency in a patient with SLE and a relatively normal urinalysis.

Four distinct types of glomerular disease have been identified in SLE: mesangial, focal proliferative, diffuse proliferative, and membranous.[36,608,609] Although these disorders have different histologic changes, clinical characteristics, responses to therapy, and prognoses (Table 6-9), they are not strictly separate since 15 to 40 percent of patients evolve from one form to another.[36,608-610] Thus, a patient with the usually benign mesangial form still requires careful follow-up because of the not infrequent transition to diffuse proliferative lupus nephritis. On the other hand, therapy can convert the diffuse

nephritis into the less severe mesangial or membranous forms.[609,610]

PATHOLOGY

The histologic changes in the different forms of SLE resemble those found in other glomerular diseases.[36,608,609] Although there are no findings which are diagnostic of SLE, the presence of hematoxylin bodies are very suggestive of this disorder.[609] Hematoxylin bodies, which are found in only some patients, are basophilic, amorphous masses located in peripheral portions of the capillary loops. They are thought to represent the staining of nuclear components from damaged cells, perhaps as an in vivo manifestation of the LE cell phenomenon.

A second change which is found on EM in virtually all patients with lupus nephritis but may also occasionally be seen in other connective tissue diseases is intraendothelial, tubuloreticular structures (Fig. 6-19).[67,611] Although these particles have the appearance of viral inclusions, they appear to be induced by interferon and may represent interferon aggregates.[612] Another distinctive change in lupus is a "fingerprint" pattern seen in the electron-dense deposits.[609] This finding, however, may reflect the deposition of cryoglobulins[613] and is probably not specific for lupus.

The *mesangial* form is the mildest and probably earliest type of lupus nephritis.[36,608,609] Light microscopy may be normal or show mild, mesangial cell proliferation and increased mesangial matrix. Even when LM is normal, IF reveals granular deposits confined to the mesangium, containing primarily IgG and C3. Electron microscopy shows an expanded mesangium with increased cellularity and matrix and mesangial deposits.

Light microscopy in *focal proliferative* lupus nephritis reveals mesangial *and* endothelial proliferation in a focal, segmental distribution, i.e., involving portions of less than

TABLE 6-9. Characteristics of Different Types of Lupus Glomerular Disease

	Mesangial	Focal Proliferative	Diffuse Proliferative	Membranous
Approximate incidence, percent of patients	10–20	10–20	40–60	10–20
LM	Normal, or mild, mesangial proliferation	Focal segmental mesangial and endothelial proliferation. Areas of necrosis may also be seen.	Diffuse proliferative and necrotizing lesions. "Wire-loop" changes and crescents may be found	Diffuse basement membrane thickening as in other forms of membranous nephropathy
IF	IgG, C3, and sometimes IgA, IgM in granular pattern in mesangial areas even if LM is normal	Diffuse mesangial and occasionally capillary wall granular deposition of IgG, C3, C4, and less commonly IgM, IgA	Diffuse granular staining throughout glomeruli for IgG, C3, C4, IgM, and occasionally IgA	Diffuse granular deposition in capillary walls of IgG, C3, and less commonly IgA
EM (Intraendothelial viruslike particles may be seen in all forms)	Deposits only in mesangium	Deposits in mesangium and in subendothelial and subepithelial areas	Deposits in all sites, larger and more numerous than focal form, especially mesangial and subendothelial	Subepithelial and occasionally mesangial deposits
Clinical presentation	No clinical abnormalities in some. Others have mild proteinuria and/or hematuria. Nephrotic syndrome, hypertension, and renal insufficiency absent	Proteinuria and hematuria in almost all. Nephrotic syndrome, mild renal insufficiency, hypertension uncommon but may occur	Proteinuria, hematuria in all. Nephrotic syndrome, hypertension, renal insufficiency common and may be severe	Proteinuria in all. Nephrotic syndrome initially in 50 percent, eventually in 90 percent. Microscopic hematuria and hypertension may occur. Mild renal insufficiency may be present at onset
Renal prognosis	Excellent unless patient develops diffuse proliferative or membranous forms	Renal insufficiency does not develop unless there is transition to diffuse proliferative glomerulonephritis	If untreated, common progression to end-stage renal failure in 2 to 4 years. Commonly associated with severe extrarenal lupus. With remission, may develop mesangial or membranous forms	May see slow progression to renal failure in patients with persistent nephrotic syndrome. Remission in one-third. May rarely develop diffuse proliferative form
Treatment for renal disease	None required	None required unless chronic changes or transition to diffuse proliferative form	Prednisone and add cyclophosphamide or azathioprine if chronic changes or progressive increase in P_{cr}. Pulse methylprednisolone for severe acute disease	Probably none if normal renal function. Prednisone with cytotoxic agents if progressive disease or severe nephrosis

50 percent of the glomeruli (Fig. 6–20). Neutrophilic infiltration, fibrinoid necrosis, and focal thickening of the basement membrane may be found in the affected areas, changes clearly more severe than those in mesangial lupus. Healing of these lesions can lead to segmental areas of glomerular sclerosis.[614]

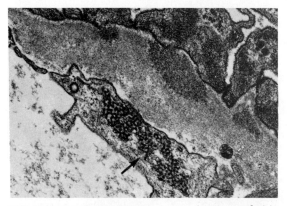

FIG. 6–19. Electron microscopy in lupus nephritis shows intraendothelial, tubuloreticular particles (arrow). Occasional subepithelial deposits can also be seen in the basement membrane.

Immunofluorescent microscopy shows granular deposits of IgG, C3, C4, and less often IgM and IgA in the mesangium and occasionally in the capillary loops. Electron microscopy demonstrates deposits in the mesangium and in the subendothelial and subepithelial areas.

The histologic changes in the *diffuse proliferative* form are similar to but more severe than those in focal proliferative lupus nephritis. Mesangial and endothelial cell proliferation is generalized but may vary in intensity among glomeruli (Fig. 6–21*a*). Crescent formation also may occur, a finding usually associated with severe renal disease. Basement membrane thickening is common, due primarily to deposition of immune complexes in the capillary wall. Characteristic eosinophilic "wire loop" lesions may be seen when the basement membrane is markedly thickened by extensive subendothelial deposits (Fig. 6–21*b*). Areas of intense neutrophilic infiltration and fibrinoid necrosis also may be found, occasionally resulting in the appearance of hematoxylin bodies.

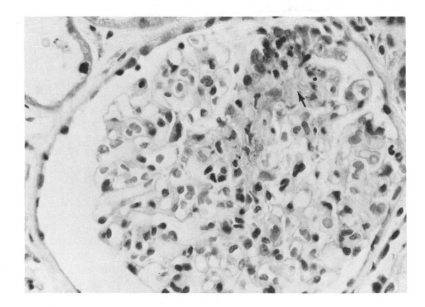

FIG. 6–20. Light microscopy in focal proliferative lupus nephritis reveals segmental cellular proliferation and a small area of fibrinoid necrosis (arrow) with the remainder of the glomerulus appearing to be normal.

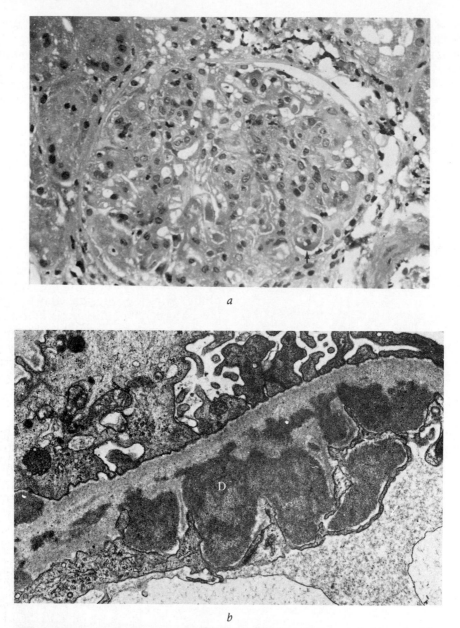

FIG. 6-21. Histologic changes in diffuse proliferative lupus nephritis. (*a*) Light microscopy shows hypercellularity, increased mesangial matrix, basement membrane thickening with wire-loop formation (arrow), and enlargement of the tuft, filling Bowman's space. (*b*) Electron microscopy demonstrates prominent subendothelial and, on the left side of the diagram, subepithelial deposits.

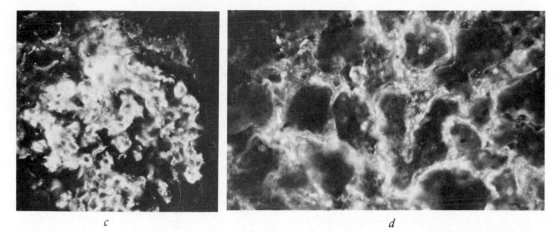

c   *d*

FIG. 6-21 (Continued).   (*c*) and (*d*) Immunofluorescent microscopy reveals intense granular deposition of IgG in the glomerular and occasionally along the tubular basement membranes, respectively.

In some patients, lobular accentuation of the glomerular capillaries can lead to an appearance similar to that of membranoproliferative glomerulonephritis (see Fig. 6–16*a*). Other changes that may be found include an arteritis affecting the afferent arterioles and interlobular arteries, and hyaline thrombi in the capillary loops. Both of these abnormalities are associated with a relatively poor long-term prognosis.[615,616]

Immunofluorescent microscopy shows diffuse granular staining for IgG, IgM, C3, C4, and infrequently IgA in the glomeruli and occasionally along the tubular basement membranes (Fig. 6–21*c* and *d*).[605] Fibrin may also be found, particularly in areas of crescent formation. Electron microscopy reveals mesangial, subendothelial, and less often, subepithelial deposits (Fig. 6–21*b*), which are larger and more numerous than in the focal form. These EM changes are required to make the diagnosis of diffuse proliferative disease. If the deposits are limited to the mesangium, the patient is considered to have mesangial lupus even if there are diffuse changes on LM.

The pathologic changes in the *membranous* form of lupus are similar to those produced by other causes of membranous nephropathy: diffuse, uniform basement membrane thickening without much hypercellularity on LM; granular deposits of primarily IgG and C3 in the capillary loops in IF; and subepithelial deposits on EM (Figs. 6–1 and 6–2).[67-69] Histologic findings which suggest SLE in this setting include intraendothelial tubuloreticular structures, marked mesangial or subendothelial deposits, and, on IF, immunoglobulin and complement deposition on the tubular basement membranes.[67,70]

Chronic Changes. The histologic findings described above review the acute changes seen with the different forms of lupus nephritis. In addition, signs of "chronic" disease such as glomerular sclerosis, tubular atrophy, and interstitial fibrosis also may be present. These changes, which occur most often in the diffuse proliferative form, are very important prognostically since they appear to best identify those patients who are likely to have progressive disease and who may be most likely to benefit from the use of cytotoxic drugs such as cyclophosphamide or azathioprine (see "Treatment," below).[617,618]

PATHOGENESIS OF SLE

Many of the clinical changes in SLE are due to the production of autoantibodies against a variety of constituents of the cells and cell membranes including double-stranded (native) and single-stranded DNA (dsDNA and ssDNA), RNA, histones, Sm antigen (a small ribonucleoprotein particle), and cardiolipin.[619-621] The deposition of DNA-anti-DNA complexes in the glomeruli with subsequent activation of the complement pathway appears to be of primary importance in the development of glomerular disease.[622-625]

A complete review of the pathogenesis of SLE is beyond the scope of this discussion. Nevertheless, a brief review of some pertinent aspects may be helpful.

Autoantibodies. Although the autoantibodies in SLE react against native antigens, this does not necessarily mean that a large number of different antibodies is being produced. Studies with experimental and human hybridomas* have shown that a single autoantibody is usually *polyspecific*, reacting with multiple antigens such as dsDNA, ssDNA, RNA, and cardiolipin.[627-629] Thus the antibodies appear to be directed against an antigen (perhaps part of the sugar-phosphate backbone of DNA and RNA) that is present in a variety of cellular constituents.[629,630]

These observations do not explain why autoantibodies are formed in SLE. However, autoantibody formation itself may not be an abnormal event. Studies with normal tonsil-

---

*A hybridoma refers to the fusion of a single antibody-producing cell with a tumor cell. The hybridoma has the properties of both parent cells: it produces a single antibody, and it can replicate continuously in vitro so that large amounts of antibody can be harvested.[626]

lar lymphocytes indicate that autoantibody production is relatively common, with up to 12 percent of cells producing anti-DNA antibodies.[629] Furthermore, analysis of anti-DNA antibodies in SLE frequently demonstrates areas of homology with antibodies directed against common bacterial antigens.[630,631] These findings suggest that autoantibodies are encoded in the gene pool[630,631a] and that it is the regulation of their synthesis that is abnormal in SLE.

Autoantibody Production. The overproduction of antibodies in SLE reflects B-cell activation, a change that could represent an abnormality in either the B cell itself or in its regulation by T cells. Studies in humans and animals indicate that *SLE is a heterogeneous disease in which different abnormalities may be of primary importance in different individuals*.[632,633] For example, suppressor T cells (T_s) are a subset of thymus-derived lymphocytes that suppress immune responsiveness. In many patients with active SLE, T_s activity is reduced.[634-636] The potential importance of this finding is suggested by the observation that the in vitro production of anti-dsDNA antibodies by B cells from patients with active SLE can be diminished by the addition of T cells from normal subjects.[635]

If decreased T_s activity is important, it is not clear if this represents a primary or secondary event. Autoantibodies directed against T_s are frequently present, a finding which could cause a secondary decrease in circulating T_s.[637,638] Furthermore, T_s number returns to normal in many patients with inactive SLE.[634] However, abnormal T_s function may be a primary event in some cases. For example, asymptomatic first-degree relatives of SLE patients may have a reduced number of circulating T_s, suggesting an inherited defect.[636] It may be that a viral infection (or some other insult) is required to initiate autoantibody production in such a genetically susceptible host.

In other patients, primary B-cell activation or a defect in anti-idiotypic antibody formation may be present. The latter is a second major pathway that suppresses the immune response. Antibodies contain unique determinants within the antigen-binding region that are called *idiotypes.* As these antibodies are produced, the idiotype itself is perceived as a new antigen, since it has not previously been seen by the immune system. This leads to the formation of anti-idiotypic antibodies that usually serve to suppress further antibody production.[639] Some patients with active SLE do not appear to make anti-idiotypic antibodies directed against the anti-dsDNA antibody, an abnormality that could contribute to the continued autoantibody production.[640]

In addition to enhanced antibody production, acquired and inherited defects in immune complex removal can also contribute to the development of SLE. Complex elimination is normally mediated by C3b and Fc receptors on macrophages in the liver and spleen. Decreased complex clearance has been described in patients with SLE,[641] an effect which is probably due in part to saturation of the receptors by the high level of circulating complexes.[642] However, an inherited defect also may play a role. Some patients, for example, have decreased C3b receptors on their erythrocytes;[643] these receptors normally transport antigen-antibody-complement complexes to their site of elimination in the liver and spleen.[405a]

Reduced complex elimination also may explain the markedly increased incidence of SLE in patients with inherited complement deficiences (up to 50 percent in some disorders).[405a,644–646] Complement normally plays an important role in limiting growth of the antigen-antibody lattice and in clearing immune complexes, thereby preventing the formation of insoluble immune precipitates that are responsible for glomerular disease (see page 149).[647,648] A possible alternative expla-nation for the association with SLE is that complement deficiency is simply a marker for abnormal immune responsiveness, since the genes governing the immune response on the short arm of the sixth chromosome are located near those responsible for the synthesis of several complement components (C2, C4, C6, and factor B of the alternate pathway).[649] However, the development of SLE in patients with deficiencies of C1 or C3 makes this "marker" hypothesis less likely,[647] since the genes for these proteins are not on the sixth chromosome.

Genetic Factors. The importance of genetic factors can be illustrated by the concordance for SLE in approximately two-thirds of monozygotic twins,[650] the increased incidence of SLE in patients with the HLA-DR3 and -DR2 genotypes,[646,651] and the enhanced incidence of other autoimmune diseases in close relatives of patients with SLE.[652]

There is, however, a difference between susceptibility to autoantibody production and the development of SLE. In one study of first-degree relatives of lupus patients, 16 percent had an elevated ANA (antinuclear antibody) titer but only 2 percent had SLE.[650] Similar results have been obtained in murine lupus. The NZB mouse has only a positive ANA and a hemolytic anemia, the NZW mouse is clinically normal, but the NZB/W female offspring develop severe lupus with marked glomerulonephritis.[650] These findings indicate that multiple genetic abnormalities underlie the susceptibility to SLE.[632,650] It may be, for example, that the NZW mouse has a defect in complex removal but has no disease since it does not form an excessive amount of immune complexes. However, severe lupus ensues when it is mated with the auto-antibody-producing (but normal complex-removing) NZB mouse.

Other Factors. In addition to genetic regulation of antibody formation (including the amount, avidity, and type of antibody produced) and of complex removal, other factors are also important in the development of SLE. In both humans and the NZB/W mouse, SLE occurs more commonly in females, an effect that appears to be mediated by estrogens, plus the absence of a possible protective effect of androgens.[653,654] As illustrated in Fig. 6–22, the administration of androgen to a prepubertally castrated NZB/W female results in a dramatic increase in survival, which is associated with a decline in circulating anti-DNA antibody levels. On the other hand, castrated males given estrogens show poor survival, approximating that in intact females.

Findings compatible with these results have been obtained in some humans, as affected males frequently have abnormal estrogen metabolism.[655-657] It is not clear, however, how these hormones act to affect the susceptibility to SLE.

Sex hormones cannot be implicated in all forms of SLE. In another mouse model, the B X SB, males are more severely affected. This tendency appears to be related to some factor on the Y chromosome but is not hormonally mediated.[632,658] A possible human counterpart has been described in families with predominant male involvement and father-to-son transmission.[659]

Summary. Animal and human studies have shown that SLE is a heterogeneous disorder characterized by a variety of different genetic and acquired abnormalities. The inherited component involves the susceptibility to produce an excessive amount of autoantibodies and then deposit immune complexes in the tissues. Multiple genes affecting immune responsiveness, T_s function and number, complement production, complex removal, and hormone production all appear to be involved. In addition, an acquired inciting factor such as a viral or bacterial infection or drug or chemical exposure is probably also important since not all susceptible subjects develop the disease.

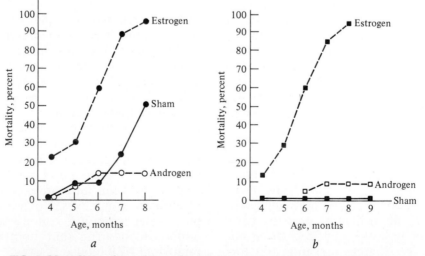

FIG. 6–22. Effect of prepubertal castration and sex hormone treatment on cumulative mortality rates of female (*a*) and male (*b*) NZB/W mice. (*From J. R. Roubinian, N. Talal, J. S. Greenspan, J. R. Goodman, and P. K. Sitteri, J. Exp. Med., 147:1568, 1978.*)

PATHOGENESIS OF LUPUS NEPHRITIS

The mechanisms involved in immune-mediated glomerular damage are discussed in detail in Chap. 5. Nevertheless, it is instructive to review how these principles apply to the patient with SLE. The primary antigens deposited in the kidney are dsDNA or ssDNA.[622-624] It is unclear if it is the intact DNA molecule or a smaller circulating fragment that is actually involved.[660] In contrast, patients who produce only antibodies to RNA have a low incidence of clinically important renal disease.[661] One possible reason for this difference in susceptibility is that free DNA has a high affinity for binding to basement membranes, thereby promoting its trapping in the glomeruli.[662]

In many animal models, marked glomerular disease is produced more easily by in situ complex formation (the separate deposition of free antigen and then free antibody) than by deposition of the intact complex (see p. 149). The demonstration of free DNA and anti-DNA antibody in the circulation[663,664] and the affinity of DNA for basement membranes are consistent with this hypothesis. Further indirect supporting evidence has come from the observation that free IgG anti-dsDNA antibody can be demonstrated in the serum but not in the urine, despite a generalized increase in IgG excretion because of the glomerular leak.[625] This finding suggests that the anti-dsDNA antibody is being trapped in the kidney, presumably by bound antigen.

Once complex formation and growth of the lattice occur, the complement system becomes activated and is presumably responsible for at least part of the ensuing glomerular damage. In both the kidney and skin, the deposition of the membrane attack complex (C5b-C9) is closely correlated with tissue injury.[665,666] Plasma C5b-C9 levels also parallel the activity of the disease.[667]

If we again extrapolate from animal models, the type of lupus nephritis that occurs is dependent upon the characteristics and quantity of the antigens and antibodies that are involved (see p. 146). The immune complexes initially form in the mesangium, producing disease that is limited to that area. If, however, a large amount of complexes is formed, the capacity of the mesangium is overwhelmed, leading to accumulation in the subendothelial space and focal or diffuse proliferative glomerulonephritis.

Membranous lupus appears to have a somewhat different pathogenesis. Experimental studies indicate that only cationic antigens or cationic intact complexes are able to cross the negatively charged GBM and form subepithelial deposits (see p. 150). Such cationic antigens have yet to be isolated in SLE, and an alternative possibility may exist. Patients with membranous lupus form fewer autoantibodies (the ANA titer may initially be negative in 20 to 50 percent of patients),[608,668] and the antibodies that are produced tend to be of low affinity.[669,670] These findings may reflect genetic differences in the intensity of the immune response. Regardless of the mechanism, the net effect may be the production of relatively small complexes that can traverse the GBM.

Thrombus Formation. In addition to immune complex deposition and complement activation, thrombus formation may contribute to glomerular injury.[616] The mechanism by which this occurs is uncertain since fibrin but not factor VIII deposition may be present, suggesting that fibrin formation may occur independent of the clotting cascade.[671] This could be mediated by circulating monocytes which have been shown to possess prothrombinase activity in patients with active SLE.[672]

PATHOGENESIS OF DRUG-INDUCED LUPUS

A variety of drugs can induce a lupuslike syndrome. This is most likely to occur with drugs that are metabolized by hepatic acetylation such as hydralazine, procainamide, and less often isoniazid.[673-676] It may also be seen, however, with other agents including quinidine, penicillamine, beta-adrenergic blockers, and methyldopa.[677-681]

The pathogenesis of drug-induced lupus has been best studied with hydralazine and procainamide. Immunologic studies with these agents reveal that the autoantibodies are predominantly directed against nuclear histones (or a drug-histone complex) rather than against DNA, as in idiopathic lupus.[682-684] These findings suggest that the drug may combine with histones, resulting in the generation of an immunogenic complex.

Total drug exposure is also important, as the incidence of lupus is increased in patients taking higher doses and occurs more often, earlier, and at lower doses in slow acetylators who metabolize the drug more slowly.[673,685-687] Women and patients with the HLA-DR4 genotype are also at increased risk.[688,689] With hydralazine, for example, it was initially thought that only patients taking high doses (300 mg per day or more) were likely to develop the disease. However, even patients taking lower doses are at risk with the incidence of disease in slow acetylators being as high as 5 percent at 100 mg/day, 10 percent at 200 mg/day, 19 percent in *women* taking 200 mg/day[688] and, in one small study, in 13 of 13 women taking 200 mg/day with the HLA-DR4 genotype.*[689] Similarly, up to 30 percent of patients taking procainamide may become symptomatic.[676] The incidence of an elevated ANA titer is substantially higher than that of symptomatic disease, reaching in slow acetylators 50 to 80 percent with procainamide and 50 percent with hydralazine.[676,687]

---

*The genetic susceptibility to drug-induced disease is different from that to idiopathic lupus in which the HLA-DR3 and -DR2 genotypes are more prevalent.[646,651]

CLINICAL PRESENTATION

Lupus primarily affects females (9:1 female/male ratio), with the onset of the disease most often occurring between the ages of 15 and 40. Patients may present with a variety of symptoms and signs including arthralgias, arthritis, fever, malaise, malar rash, pleuritis, or pericarditis. Renal involvement is most often evident within the first year, although it may be delayed for 3 or more years in some patients.[36]

The manifestations of lupus nephritis are dependent upon the type of disease that is present since the severity of the urinary and renal functional changes is often proportional to the severity of the histologic changes (see Table 6–9).[36,690] Thus, mild proteinuria and/or microscopic hematuria and red cell casts are typically the only abnormalities in mesangial lupus. Similar urinary findings are frequently present in the focal proliferative form, although one-fourth to one-third of patients also have the nephrotic syndrome, hypertension, or mild renal insufficiency. As with other causes of membranous nephropathy, patients with lupus have either asymptomatic proteinuria or more commonly the nephrotic syndrome and edema. Mild microscopic hematuria may be present, but the P_{cr} is initially normal or only slightly increased.

The changes in diffuse proliferative lupus are variable, ranging at the time of presentation from findings similar to the focal proliferative form to acute renal failure with a nephritic sediment, nephrotic range proteinuria, edema, and hypertension.[36,608,690] However, diffuse (or focal) proliferative glomerulonephritis with mesangial and subendothelial deposits are also found in some lupus patients who present with no evidence of renal disease (normal urinalysis and GFR).[602-604] Although it is unclear why this occurs, the long-term prognosis is better than in those patients with clinically evident disease. Furthermore, urinary abnormalities ultimately develop before any substantial decline in GFR.[603,604]

Hyperkalemia out of proportion to the degree of renal insufficiency also may occur in lupus nephritis. This is presumably due to a selective defect in distal potassium secretion (induced by tubular damage) since both aldosterone secretion and the sodium reabsorptive response to aldosterone are normal (the latter excludes simple aldosterone resistance).[691]

DIAGNOSIS

Patients with lupus nephritis generally have clinically apparent extrarenal involvement and one or more of the characteristic serologic manifestations of this disorder: an elevated ANA titer, circulating antibodies to DNA, and hypocomplementemia.[608,692] When hypocomplementemia is present, both C3 and C4 levels are usually reduced, suggesting activation of the classic pathway.[692] Measurement of the individual complement components should also be obtained in patients with a family history of SLE or other connective tissue disease in an attempt to detect an underlying complement deficiency state. C2 deficiency is the most common,[647] and low C3 levels in this setting must be due to activation of the alternate pathway since C2 is an essential component of the classic pathway (see Fig. 5–9).[644,647]

Another test that may be helpful in questionable cases is a biopsy of normal skin. Immunofluorescent studies frequently show immunoglobulin and C3 deposition along the dermal-epidermal junction, usually of the same class as deposited in the glomeruli (Fig. 6–23).[693-695] This "lupus band" is most likely to be present in patients who are hypocomplementemic.[693]

Some patients, however, present with renal disease but initially no serologic or extrarenal evidence of SLE. This almost always occurs with membranous lupus,[67-69] a setting in which 20 to 50 percent of patients have a negative ANA titer and normal plasma complement level.[608,668] The histologic findings which suggest underlying SLE rather than idiopathic membranous nephropathy are described above.[67,70]

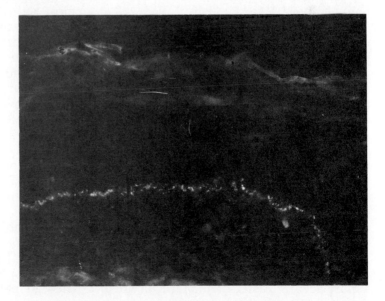

FIG. 6–23. Immunofluorescent microscopy of a biopsy specimen of clinically uninvolved skin from a patient with lupus. A band of IgG deposition is seen along the basement membrane at the dermal-epidermal junction.

Idiopathic SLE must also be differentiated from drug-induced disease in patients taking the appropriate drugs. Most patients with drug-induced lupus do not have hypocomplementemia, anti-DNA antibodies, or clinically important renal disease. However, exceptions do occur[679,683,696-700] and, therefore, the presence or absence of these findings is of limited diagnostic importance. The demonstration that the antinuclear antibodies are predominantly directed against histones is strong evidence in favor of drug-induced disease,[682-684] but this test is not widely available. Thus, the major way to diagnosis drug-related lupus is to demonstrate resolution of the disease within 1 to 7 months after the drug has been discontinued.

An uncommon disorder that may simulate SLE is mixed connective tissue disease, which is associated with clinical findings suggestive of scleroderma and polymyositis as well as lupus, elevated ANA titers (with a speckled pattern), and occasionally renal involvement.[701,702] However, hypocomplementemia is unusual, and the antinuclear antibodies in this disorder are against extractable nuclear antigen (containing both RNA and Sm protein) and not DNA.

Once the presence of idiopathic SLE is established, a renal biopsy should be performed in patients with evidence of kidney disease. The type of lupus nephritis cannot always be predicted from the laboratory findings (see Table 6–9),[703] and documenting the correct diagnosis is required for the development of an appropriate therapeutic regimen.

One possible exception to early biopsy is the patient who presents with only mild proteinuria or a few red or white cells in the urine. Biopsy at this time will most likely show mesangial lupus which, in some patients, is just the earliest stage of some more significant lesion. Delaying the renal biopsy for several months or until the urinary changes become more prominent will allow a more accurate assessment of the nature of the glomerular disease.

COURSE AND THERAPY

Recent advances in therapy (antimicrobials, dialysis, immunosuppressives) and earlier diagnosis of milder cases have improved the 5-year survival rate for all patients with SLE from approximately 70 percent (before 1968) to over 90 percent.[650,704,705] The major causes of death in the first few years are infection (perhaps due in part to the use of prednisone and other immunosuppressive agents) and renal failure, whereas late mortality is primarily due to atherosclerotic heart disease.[706] Hypertension, renal insufficiency, and prolonged corticosteroid therapy all may contribute to the increase in atherogenesis.

The patient's prognosis and the necessity for therapy in SLE are determined by both the extrarenal and renal manifestations of the disease. In terms of the renal changes, the prognosis for preservation of renal function and the kind of therapy that may be needed vary with the type of disease that is present.

DIFFUSE PROLIFERATIVE NEPHRITIS

Diffuse proliferative glomerulonephritis is the most serious form of renal disease in SLE. Studies performed before 1970 revealed that 50 percent of patients developed renal failure within 2 years and that only 25 percent survived for 5 years because severe extrarenal changes were also frequently present.[707] However, more recent studies of patients treated with prednisone and frequently cytotoxic agents have found the incidence of progressive renal disease to be much lower and the patient survival rate to be 65 to 80 percent at 5 years.[608,704,708,709]

The optimal treatment of diffuse proliferative lupus nephritis is uncertain. High-dose prednisone (1 mg/kg per day) appears to stabilize or improve renal function in many patients.[36,710] Cytotoxic agents, particularly cyclophosphamide or azathioprine, have been tried in patients with corticosteroid resistance or toxicity. However, the use of these drugs has produced both positive[617,618,711-713] and negative results.[710,714-716]

One possible reason for this conflicting data is the lack of identification of specific subgroups that would benefit from cytotoxic therapy. Such a group could be hidden by the inclusion of patients with a benign prognosis who will do well with prednisone alone and those with a poor prognosis who will not respond to any conventional therapy.[717] In this setting, the number of patients required to demonstrate a positive effect of therapy is larger than the studies denoted above. When these studies are combined to markedly increase the size of the patient population, it appears that the addition of cyclophosphamide or azathioprine to pred-

nisone decreases the incidence of progressive renal disease by about 40 percent.[718] However, it may take 5 years or more before the benefit of adding a cytotoxic agent becomes evident (Fig. 6–24a)[617]

An example of this problem of subgroup identification is illustrated in Fig. 6–24b. In the past, the renal prognosis was thought to correlate with the activity of the disease as manifested in part by the presence of crescents, fibrinoid necrosis, and subendothelial deposits.[711,719] Although these findings are important, recent studies suggest that the best long-term prognostic indicator is the presence or absence of irreversible "chronic" changes such as glomerular sclerosis, fibrous crescents, tubular atrophy, and interstitial

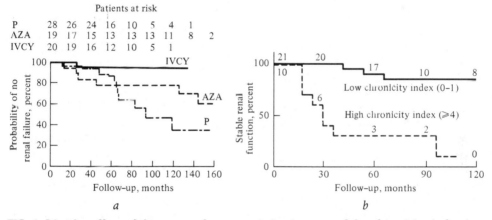

FIG. 6-24. The effect of therapy and prognostic importance of the chronicity index in patients with diffuse proliferative lupus nephritis. (*a*) The probability of not progressing to end-stage renal failure versus time in patients treated with intravenous pulses of cyclophosphamide (IVCY), oral azathioprine (AZA), or oral prednisone (P). Despite the apparent trends, the relatively small number of patients meant that a statistically significant improvement over prednisone alone was seen only with IVCY at 120 months. Oral cyclophosphamide (not shown here) appeared to be as effective as oral azathioprine. (*b*) The likelihood of having stable renal function (defined as less than a twofold elevation in the plasma creatinine concentration) versus time according to the degree of chronic changes. Those patients with a high chronicity index had a much worse prognosis, regardless of therapy. (*Adapted from H. A. Austin, III, J. H. Klippel, J. E. Balow, N. G. H. leRiche, A. D. Steinberg, P. H. Plotz, and J. L. Decker, N. Engl. J. Med., 314:614, 1986, reprinted by permission from the New England Journal of Medicine; and S. Carette, J. H. Klippel, J. L. Decker, H. A. Austin, P. H. Plotz, A. D. Steinberg, and J. E. Balow, Ann. Intern. Med., 99:1, 1983.*)

fibrosis (Fig. 6–24b).[617,618,719] Patients with none or few of these changes fall into a low-risk group that responds well to prednisone alone. In contrast, patients with prominent glomerular sclerosis and tubulointerstitial damage have advanced disease that does not appear to respond to any form of anti-inflammatory or immunosuppressive therapy.[617] Only those patients with intermediate chronicity (some but not marked sclerotic changes) are likely to benefit from the addition of cyclophosphamide or azathioprine.[617]

Another confounding factor that could have hidden or minimized the beneficial effect of cytotoxic agents is using the GFR or P_{cr} as the measure of therapeutic effect. Maintenance of the GFR does not necessarily mean stable disease because compensatory hyperfiltration can initially mask nephron loss (see p. 9). When repeat renal biopsy is used to assess therapeutic efficacy, progressive glomerular and tubulointerstitial scarring are much more common in those patients treated only with prednisone.[618]

The mechanism by which cytotoxic therapy might be more beneficial than prednisone alone is not well understood. It has been assumed that cyclophosphamide acts by producing more potent immunosuppression. An alternative explanation, however, is that prednisone has a deleterious hemodynamic effect. High doses of corticosteroids lead to renal vasodilatation and an elevation in the glomerular capillary pressure. This intraglomerular hypertension has been shown to exacerbate experimental renal disease[720] and could limit the effectiveness of prednisone in lupus nephritis.

However, the positive effects of cyclophosphamide, and to a lesser degree azathioprine,[617] must be weighed against their potential side effects. This is particularly true of cyclophosphamide which can induce bone marrow suppression, infection (both of which can also occur with azathioprine), alopecia, gonadal fibrosis, hemorrhagic cystitis, and neoplasia (particularly cancer of the bladder).[157–163,721–723]

In an attempt to minimize the incidence of these complications, it has been suggested that cyclophosphamide be administered intravenously in 5 to 7 monthly boluses (0.75 to 1.0 g per square meter of body surface area) rather than daily in a dose of 2.5 mg/kg per day (Fig. 6–24a).[617,724] This regimen results in less total drug exposure in terms of both time and quantity. Although the incidence of hemorrhagic cystitis is markedly reduced, it is not known if similar protection is afforded against malignancy.[617] In any case, the risk is probably relatively small. Extrarenal mortality does not seem to be significantly increased,[709,718] perhaps because cytotoxic agents allow lower doses of prednisone to be used, thereby minimizing the more severe forms of chronic steroid toxicity, such as ischemic necrosis of bone.[725]

To summarize, the treatment of diffuse proliferative lupus nephritis is dependent upon the histologic and clinical findings (Table 6–10). Patients with few or no chronic changes should be started on prednisone (1 mg/kg per day) in divided doses. Patients who respond show stable or improved renal function and a less active urine sediment (fewer casts and cells). At this point, prednisone can be slowly tapered to the minimal effective dose. Alternate-day prednisone may be able to sustain a

TABLE 6-10. Treatment of Diffuse Proliferative Lupus Nephritis

Histologic and Clinical Findings	Treatment
Chronic changes	
Few or none	Prednisone
Moderate	Cyclophosphamide (or azathioprine) plus prednisone
Advanced	Control of systemic blood pressure and dietary protein restriction
Acute renal failure	Pulse methylprednisolone ? Plasmapheresis

remission with a lesser incidence of toxicity, although many patients require a small dose (2.5 to 7.5 mg) on the alternate day for control of arthralgias.

Cyclophosphamide should probably be administered to patients with moderate chronic changes on biopsy but only after all the potential side effects have been carefully explained. Low-dose prednisone (0.5 mg/kg per day) should also be given and then tapered to an alternate-day dose. To minimize the long-term risk, it may be safer to administer oral cyclophosphamide for only 3 to 4 months and then switch to azathioprine (2 mg/kg per day). (This regimen has been successfully used in Wegener's granulomatosis).[726] Azathioprine can also be given to patients who refuse or cannot tolerate cyclophosphamide. The role of intravenous pulses of cyclophosphamide remains to be defined, although the initial results are encouraging, in terms of both efficacy and safety.[617]

Patients with advanced glomerular sclerosis generally do poorly (Fig. 6–24b), and aggressive therapy with prednisone or cytotoxic agents is likely to do more harm than good. In this setting, control of the compensatory hemodynamic changes that can exacerbate the glomerular damage is probably of primary importance. This can be achieved by lowering the systemic blood pressure (preferably with a converting enzyme inhibitor) and restricting dietary protein intake (see Chap. 4). Prevention of hypertension should also be an *essential component of therapy* in all forms of lupus nephritis since the associated elevation in intraglomerular pressure can exacerbate the immunologically mediated glomerular injury.[727,728]

More aggressive initial therapy may be required in patients who develop acute renal failure. This is frequently associated with high levels of circulating immune complexes,[729,730] and an arteritis may be found on renal biopsy. These patients may not respond to conventional doses of prednisone,

and it takes 1 to 2 weeks before an effect is seen with cytotoxic agents. In this setting, pulse methylprednisolone therapy has been effective in improving the renal and extrarenal manifestations of the disease.[729-732] This response can then be maintained with conventional doses of prednisone and a cytotoxic drug.

The mechanisms responsible for the enhanced effectiveness of pulse therapy are incompletely understood. The excess steroid, which is derived from cholesterol, may intercalate into the lipid bilayer of target cell membranes.[733] The ensuing decrease in membrane fluidity (a change not seen with conventional corticosteroid doses) may then cause a marked reduction in inflammatory cell function. The plasma levels achieved with pulse therapy also can inhibit complement activation,[734] another effect that could decrease disease activity.

The optimal dose of methylprednisolone is also uncertain. The standard regimen, which was initially used to treat acute transplant rejection, consists of 1 g given intravenously over 30 min on three successive days. However, this regimen has, on occasion, been associated with sudden cardiac arrest or a marked elevation in blood pressure.[735-737] Since a "minipulse" of 250 mg appears to be just as effective in reversing transplant rejection,[738,739] it may be advisable initially to try this lower dose in SLE. Prolonged or multiple courses of pulse therapy should be avoided because of an increased incidence of infection.[740]

Plasmapheresis has also been used in patients with severe lupus nephritis.[729,741,742] Although it may be effective (in part by removing the circulating immune reactants), plasmapheresis is more difficult to perform than minipulse therapy and is associated with a variety of potential side effects.[743] Thus, the role of this modality in the treatment of lupus nephritis is at present uncertain; its use should currently be limited to patients with acute disease that is refractory to other forms of treatment.*

Regardless of which therapy is used, a positive therapeutic response is typically characterized by stabilization or improvement in the P_{cr}, a decreased number of cells and casts in the urine sediment, and, on renal biopsy, decreased activity of the disease with occasional conversion to a more benign histologic pattern.[609,610] This is usually accompanied by the return of plasma C3 levels and DNA binding titers toward the normal range. Patients with persistent hypocomplementemia are at increased risk of progressive renal insufficiency.[746]

Once improvement has occurred, the patient should be followed carefully both for side effects resulting from the medications (particularly leukopenia and infection) and for evidence of reactivation of the disease. Serial measurement of the plasma C3 level and/or DNA binding titer may be particularly helpful since the development of hypocomplementemia or increased DNA binding may precede clinical evidence of disease activity by 1 to 3 months.[747,748] However, this is not an absolute rule since hypocomplementemia may be found only with extrarenal disease[749] and some patients may have persistent abnormalities in complement and DNA binding for as long as 4 or more years without any clinical disturbances.[750] For these reasons, the efficacy of increasing the dose of prednisone for an asymptomatic fall in the plasma C3 level has not been proven. Nevertheless, patients with this finding should be followed carefully and treatment instituted if signs or symptoms of active disease ensue.

The optimal duration of therapy is not known. Patients are generally maintained on low-dose alternate-day prednisone and, if

indicated, a cytotoxic agent. Although cyclophosphamide is preferable initially, long-term maintenance may be safer with azathioprine. Consideration can be given to stopping therapy in patients who have been in clinical and serologic remission for 2 years, particularly if repeat renal biopsy shows resolution of active immunologic disease.[711] Although a high incidence of reactivation has been reported to follow cessation of azathioprine,[751] this was probably due to premature discontinuation.[711]

Despite the above therapies, up to 20 to 35 percent of patients will still develop progressive renal insufficiency. In addition to those patients with chronic changes on renal biopsy, the risk of renal failure appears to be increased in children, males, blacks, and hispanics.[752-754] On the other hand, patients over the age of 50 generally have more indolent disease.[753,755]

An interesting finding in those patients who progress to renal failure is the common (but not universal) disappearance of the extrarenal and serologic manifestations of the disease.[756,757] The lupus usually remains inactive with the institution of dialysis or transplantation,[758,759] and recurrent nephritis in the transplant is rare.[18,756,759,760] The factors responsible for this change are incompletely understood. It may reflect the reduction in immune responsiveness that is induced by end-stage renal failure.[761] If so, this effect must be long-lasting since reversal of the azotemia by spontaneous recovery of renal function or by transplantation does not usually reactivate the disease.[756,761] However, recurrent symptoms may occur, in some cases after a remission of more than 12 months.[760]

Between 10 and 40 percent of patients who require dialysis recover enough renal function to allow dialysis to be discontinued.[758,759,762] This is most likely to occur in patients with acute renal failure who may respond to immunosuppressive therapy or plasmapheresis. In this setting, therefore,

---

*Other experimental regimens that are currently being evaluated include the administration of eicosapentaenoic acid and defibrination (to prevent fibrin deposition) with pit-viper venom.[744,745]

renal transplantation should be delayed for 1 year to see if renal function will improve.

FOCAL PROLIFERATIVE AND MESANGIAL NEPHRITIS

The focal proliferative form of lupus nephritis has generally been considered to have a benign prognosis and not to require specific therapy.[36] However, 20 to 30 percent of patients develop progressive disease.[690,708] This should not be surprising since the distinction between the focal and diffuse forms is somewhat arbitrary (less than or more than 50 percent of glomeruli involved). Furthermore, transformation to diffuse proliferative disease occurs in 15 to 20 percent of cases.[36,609,610,763] This change can be diagnosed only by repeat renal biopsy, a procedure that should be considered when focal lupus nephritis shows clinical evidence of increasingly severe disease.

It is likely that patients with focal disease who have the chronic changes described above are at higher risk of developing renal failure and probably should be treated with prednisone and a cytotoxic agent.[617,618] It has also been suggested that the presence of subendothelial deposits is another bad prognostic finding.[711] However, this association is uncertain since many such patients follow a relatively benign course.[690,763]

Mesangial lupus, which typically has mild histologic and clinical findings, usually follows a benign course and requires no therapy. However, it is probable that most forms of lupus nephritis begin with mesangial changes, and transformation to diffuse proliferative disease with more prominent clinical abnormalities may occur.[609,610]

MEMBRANOUS NEPHROPATHY

The renal prognosis in the membranous form of lupus is relatively good.[36,668] Most patients have the nephrotic syndrome at some point, but partial or complete remissions in proteinuria are common. The majority of patients maintain a relatively normal GFR for 5 or more years, particularly those with nonnephrotic proteinuria. However, progression to renal failure may occur, particularly in patients with chronic sclerotic changes or those who transform to diffuse proliferative disease.[36,609,668] In either of these settings, therapy with a cytotoxic agent and prednisone (as described above) may be beneficial.[617,618]

OTHER FACTORS

In addition to the type of renal disease, other factors may affect renal function in SLE. A modest reversible reduction in GFR of about 15 percent may be induced by the use of aspirin (or other nonsteroidal anti-inflammatory drug).[764,765] This effect appears to be mediated by a reduction in the renal synthesis of vasodilator prostaglandins, which may be mildly increased in SLE. Although the GFR is decreased in this setting, it should not be assumed that this change is necessarily deleterious in the long term. The associated reductions in glomerular plasma flow and hydrostatic pressure could actually be beneficial by diminishing the severity both of immune-mediated damage and of hemodynamic injury (see Chap. 4).[727,728]

Another potential problem in women with lupus nephritis is pregnancy. This is associated with an increased incidence of fetal loss and exacerbation of both the renal and extrarenal abnormalities in 25 to 45 percent of patients.[766-769] Worsening of the lupus usually occurs in the first 8 weeks postpartum but may also be seen during the pregnancy. Because of these problems, women should be encouraged to delay pregnancy until the disease can be rendered inactive (if possible) for at least 6 months, a setting in which the risk of complications is reduced.[766,769] It has also been suggested that the frequency of postpartum flares can be diminished by increasing the corticosteroid dose for 4 to 5 days after delivery.[767-769]

RAPIDLY PROGRESSIVE GLOMERULONEPHRITIS

Rapidly progressive (or crescentic) glomerulonephritis (RPGN) is characterized morphologically by extensive crescent formation in the glomeruli and clinically by progression to end-stage renal failure in most untreated patients within weeks to months. Crescent formation may occur in virtually any form of proliferative glomerulonephritis or vasculitis.[770] Less commonly, RPGN is not associated with any identifiable underlying disease or is accompanied by pulmonary hemorrhage and anti-GBM antibodies (Goodpasture's syndrome). These latter disorders will be discussed in this section.

PATHOLOGY

Idiopathic RPGN may be associated with the deposition of antigen-antibody complexes, anti-GBM antibodies, or with no apparent antibody involvement.[771-774] Regardless of the underlying mechanism, LM reveals similar findings.[770,775] Crescents that fill and obliterate Bowman's space are the hallmark of the disease. They may partially or totally encircle the glomerular tuft and are present in more than 50 to 60 percent of the glomeruli (Fig. 6-25). (A smaller number of crescents may be seen in many diseases which generally lack the progressive course of RPGN.)

Mesangial or endothelial cell proliferation is typically minimal or absent, although hypercellularity may appear to be present because of compression of the tuft by the crescent. The compressed capillary lumens are usually closed and bloodless, changes which undoubtedly contribute to the development of renal insufficiency. Other findings which may be seen are areas of necrosis in the glomeruli and tubulointerstitial changes such as edema, mononuclear cell infiltration, and tubular dilatation. If the course of the disease is not altered by therapy, there is rapid

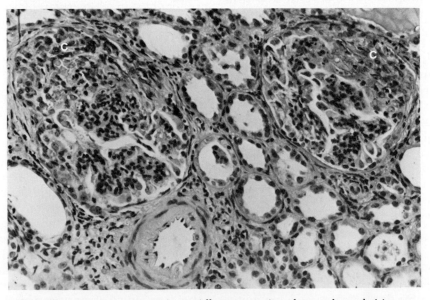

FIG. 6-25. Light microscopy in rapidly progressive glomerulonephritis demonstrates cellular crescents (C) filling Bowman's space and encircling and compressing the glomerular tufts.

progression of these lesions, characterized by fibrosis of the crescents, eventual hyalinization of the entire glomerular tuft, interstitial fibrosis, and marked tubular atrophy.

Crescents appear to consist of both proliferating epithelial cells (lining the glomerulus and Bowman's capsule)[775,776] and infiltrating macrophages.[777-779] Multiple factors may be responsible for the influx of macrophages including complement-mediated chemotaxis or attraction by thrombin or tissue breakdown products. In experimental anti-GBM disease, for example, neutrophils are responsible for the initial glomerular damage, followed by the entry of macrophages at a time when neutrophils can no longer be found.[780]

The pathologic differentiation between the different types of idiopathic RPGN is made by IF and EM.[771-774] Anti-GBM antibody disease is characterized on IF by diffuse linear deposition of IgG and less often C3 along the GBM (Fig. 6–26) and on EM by a nonspecific increase in granularity of the GBM without evident deposits. Linear IgG deposition may also be found along the basement membranes of the tubules[781] and, in Goodpasture's syndrome, along the alveolar capillaries.[782] These antibodies may contribute to the development of tubulointerstitial disease and pulmonary hemorrhage, respectively.

In contrast, RPGN due to immune complexes is characterized by granular deposition of IgG, IgM, and C3 on IF, and mesangial, subendothelial or subepithelial deposits on EM.[770,771] In the third type of RPGN, there is no evidence of immune deposits on either IF or EM.[773]

In addition to these specific changes, fibrin can be demonstrated within the crescents on IF and EM (Fig. 6–27) in all patients with RPGN.[783,784] Disruptions in the GBM are essential for this to occur by allowing fi-

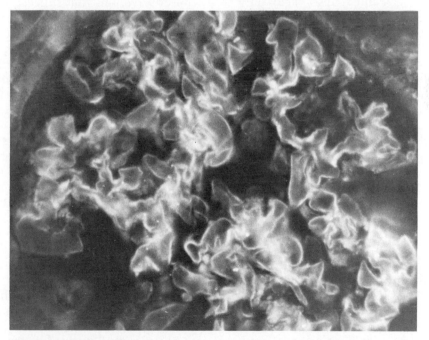

FIG. 6–26. Immunofluorescent microscopy demonstrating linear deposition of IgG in anti-GBM disease.

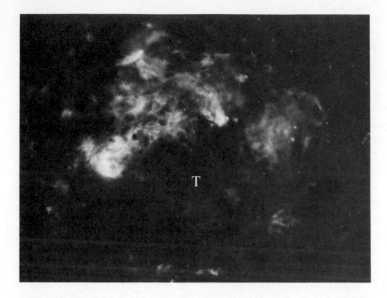

FIG. 6–27. Immunofluorescence in rapidly progressive glomerulonephritis shows the deposition of fibrin within the crescent but not the glomerular tuft (T).

brinogen or fibrin (molecular weight about 400,000) to pass through the GBM into Bowman's space (see "Pathogenesis," below).[785,786]

Pathologic changes also may be present, which suggest that the patient has an underlying glomerular or vascular disease rather than idiopathic RPGN.[770] Mesangial hypercellularity is suggestive of secondary RPGN and may be accompanied by subepithelial humps on EM in poststreptococcal glomerulonephritis, mesangial interposition or dense deposits on EM in membranoproliferative glomerulonephritis, prominent IgA deposition on IF in Henoch-Schönlein purpura or IgA nephropathy, or subendothelial deposits and intraendothelial tubuloreticular structures in SLE (see individual diseases above). Finally, the combination of focal areas of glomerular necrosis on LM with no deposits on EM or IF is suggestive of some form of vasculitis, even if vascular involvement cannot be demonstrated on LM.[787]

PATHOGENESIS

Since RPGN may be seen with virtually any form of glomerulonephritis, it is likely that crescents represent a nonspecific response to severe glomerular injury. There are several observations that suggest that the entry of fibrinogen or fibrin into Bowman's space, presumably through disruptions in the GBM, is the initiating event in crescent formation. These include the uniform finding of fibrin in the crescents,[783,784] the prevention of experimental RPGN by the prior or concurrent administration of anticoagulants,[788] and the reversal of experimental RPGN with defibrination.[789,790] However, the mechanism by which fibrin is formed is unclear. The observation that the deposition of fibrin is not accompanied by that of factor VIII suggests that the intrinsic clotting pathway is not involved.[784] Other possibilities include activation of the extrinsic clotting pathway or of prothrombin directly by the release of procoagulant material from activated macrophages.[791,792]

The mechanism by which fibrin in Bowman's space stimulates crescent formation is also not known. It may be that phagocytosis of fibrin by infiltrating macrophages is of primary importance.[777-779] The macrophages may both comprise part of the crescent and release factors which promote epithelial cell proliferation and therefore enlargement of the crescent.

ANTI-GBM ANTIBODY DISEASE

Experimental models have demonstrated that anti-GBM antibodies can lead to glomerulonephritis.[793,794] That this also occurs in humans is suggested by the linear IgG deposition on IF and the observation that glomerulonephritis can be induced in animals by the administration of anti-GBM antibodies obtained from the plasma or eluted from the glomeruli of patients with Goodpasture's syndrome.[772,795]

However, the mechanisms responsible for anti-GBM antibody formation are uncertain. In patients with Goodpasture's syndrome who also have antibodies against lung capillaries, immunoglobulins eluted from the lung or kidney bind to both lung and kidney but not to other tissues.[796,797] This suggests the presence of cross-reacting antigens limited to these organs.

Several theories have been proposed to explain the initial event in anti-GBM antibody formation.[798] These include viral or bacterial antigens cross-reacting with lung and kidney (for which there is little evidence) and primary damage to the lung or kidney, leading to basement membrane antigens being exposed to the circulation or made immunogenic. In addition, genetic factors (particularly the presence of HLA-DR2) may be important in predisposing to the development of anti-GBM antibodies after a given stimulus.[799,800]

It is likely that pulmonary damage is the inciting event in at least some cases of anti-GBM antibody disease. In experimental animals, for example, the administration or induction of antilung antibodies can induce both pulmonary and glomerular disease.[801,802] These findings may apply to humans since Goodpasture's syndrome is occasionally preceded by primary pulmonary disorders such as influenza or smoke inhalation.[803,804] In

these settings, the lung disease occurs before and tends to be more severe than the renal changes. The possible association of Goodpasture's syndrome with hydrocarbon exposure[771,805] could also be due to lung damage induced by vapor inhalation.

On the other hand, antibodies directed against renal basement membrane antigens also may initiate the disease. As an example, some patients with hereditary nephritis have an abnormal GBM that lacks one or more normal antigens.[454] Renal transplantation supplies these antigens which may be recognized as foreign, occasionally resulting in the development of anti-GBM antibody disease.[454,457]

Studies in hereditary nephritis have also shed some light on the antigen(s) against which anti-GBM antibodies are directed. The glomeruli from some patients with this disorder will not bind anti-GBM antibodies from humans with Goodpasture's syndrome but will bind antibodies derived from rabbits immunized with normal human GBM.[454] These results suggest that the antibodies in Goodpasture's syndrome are directed against a specific antigen[456,806] that may be missing in hereditary nephritis.

Approximately 60 to 80 percent of patients with anti-GBM antibody disease have pulmonary hemorrhage.[772,774] However, the relationship between Goodpasture's syndrome and anti-GBM antibody disease without lung involvement is unclear.[771,807] The observations that patients with isolated anti-GBM disease tend to be older (mean age 50 versus 33 years) and do not show the marked male predominance seen with Goodpasture's syndrome[771] are compatible with the hypothesis that these may be different disorders (such as primary pulmonary damage in Goodpasture's syndrome and primary renal damage in isolated anti-GBM antibody disease).

However, the presence or absence of pulmonary disease could also be due to changes in lung permeability that affect the access of circulating antibodies to the alveolar basement membrane. A history of cigarette smoking may be particularly important in this regard. In one study, 37 of 39 patients with pulmonary hemorrhage smoked as compared to no smokers in eight patients with isolated anti-GBM antibody disease.[808]

IMMUNE COMPLEX DEPOSITION

Rapidly progressive glomerulonephritis with discrete immune deposits on IF and EM is typically associated with immune complexes in the circulation.[809] Although the inciting antigen is usually unknown, penicillamine, syphilis, and possibly malignancies have been implicated in isolated cases.[99,324,810,811]

NONANTIBODY RPGN

Immunofluorescent and electron microscopy do not reveal immune deposits in 15 to 40 percent of patients with idiopathic RPGN.[771,773,774] Two hypotheses have been proposed to account for these findings. First, the patient may have an underlying vasculitis.[787] Glomerular IF is usually negative in vasculitis,[770] and there may initially be no clinical evidence of extrarenal involvement.

Second, the glomerular damage may be due to cell-mediated immunity.[774] An experimental model of this mechanism has been described.[812] Chickens were bursectomized (to remove humoral immunity) and then immunized with bovine GBM. A severe crescentic glomerulonephritis ensued that was presumably mediated by cellular mechanisms since no glomerular antibody deposition could be demonstrated. Although glomerular lymphocytic infiltration is not present in human RPGN, it is possible that activated T cells against glomerular bound antigen are present early in the disease, a time at which renal biopsy is not performed.[813] These T cells could release lymphokines that promote the accumulation of macrophages, which then produce further glomerular damage.[813]

CLINICAL PRESENTATION

Idiopathic RPGN primarily affects adults (mean age about 50 years) with a slight male predominance.[771,773] An exception occurs in Goodpasture's syndrome in which 75 to 85 percent of patients are men with an average age of 20 to 30 years.[771,772] Although RPGN can occur in children, there is usually an identifiable cause such as an antecedent streptococcal infection, Henoch-Schönlein purpura, or membranoproliferative glomerulonephritis.[814]

The onset of symptoms related to the renal disease may be abrupt and similar to that in poststreptococcal glomerulonephritis with the patient presenting with macroscopic hematuria, decreased urine output, and edema. More commonly, the onset is insidious and the presenting symptoms are due to uremia or fluid retention.[771-774] A preceding upper respiratory or viral infection is present in many patients. This is followed over a period of weeks to months by malaise, weakness, edema, and eventually oliguria or anuria.

Hemoptysis and dyspnea are characteristic of Goodpasture's syndrome but may also be seen with other forms of RPGN, although the mechanism is frequently not apparent in these disorders.[773,774,815] The pulmonary symptoms in Goodpasture's syndrome usually precede or occur together with the renal disease. However, hemoptysis may follow the clinical onset of renal disease by 1 to 12 months in as many as one-fourth of patients.[772] In other patients, the pulmonary abnormalities may predominate with no or only minimal clinical evidence of kidney disease.[803,804]

The physical examination may reveal pallor, peripheral edema, or rales which may be due either to fluid overload or pulmonary hemorrhage. Hypertension is primarily induced by volume expansion and occurs more often in patients with advanced disease.[774,814]

Renal insufficiency is present at the time of diagnosis in virtually all patients with RPGN and is frequently severe with the P_{cr} exceeding 5 mg/dL.[771-774] The urinalysis reveals proteinuria which is usually not in the nephrotic range (probably due to the marked fall in GFR), hematuria, and red cell and other casts. Anemia is common and may be out of proportion to the degree of renal failure even in patients without hemoptysis. This may be accompanied by low plasma iron levels in Goodpasture's syndrome, due in part to iron sequestration in the lungs. The plasma C3 level is normal in idiopathic RPGN. The chest x-ray may reveal congestive heart failure or bilateral pulmonary infiltrates due to hemorrhage.

DIAGNOSIS

Acute oliguric or anuric renal failure with a nephritic sediment may be seen with the other diffuse glomerulonephritides, vasculitis, or allergic interstitial nephritis as well as RPGN. Thus, signs or symptoms of a systemic disease (arthralgias, rash, pharyngitis, heart murmur, hepatosplenomegaly) should be looked for in the history and physical examination. If indicated, appropriate laboratory tests should also be performed, including ANA (antinuclear antibody) or ASO titers, plasma C3 level, blood cultures, or testing the serum for cryoglobulins.

If RPGN is considered likely on clinical grounds, it may be helpful to check for circulating anti-GBM antibodies to allow a rapid diagnosis to be made. This can be done most quickly by indirect immunofluorescence in which the patient's serum is incubated with normal renal tissue; fluorescein-tagged anti-human IgG antibodies are then added to see if IgG deposition has occurred. A positive test is diagnostic of anti-GBM antibody disease, but up to 40 percent of patients have a false-negative result.[774] Radioimmunoassay is much more sensitive and is the preferred test for sequential monitoring of anti-GBM antibody titers.

In general, the diagnosis of RPGN is made by renal biopsy. This should be performed as early as possible to allow therapy to be begun before irreversible renal failure has occurred. Pulmonary hemorrhage does not obviate the need for renal biopsy since this finding is not specific for Goodpasture's syndrome.[773,774,815] It should also be noted that linear deposition of IgG on IF is not diagnostic of anti-GBM antibody disease. A similar finding may occasionally be found in other glomerular disorders, particularly diabetic nephropathy.[225] In these settings, crescents are not seen and the IgG deposition is thought to represent nonspecific absorption onto an abnormal GBM since albumin may also be deposited in a linear pattern and circulating anti-GBM antibodies are not present.[225]

COURSE AND PROGNOSIS

The renal prognosis of untreated RPGN is poor. It has been estimated that 70 to 80 percent of all patients with this disorder and over 90 percent of those who are oliguric or anuric die or require dialysis within weeks to months.[771,772,816] The prognosis and likelihood of a positive response to therapy is primarily related to the severity of the disease at the time treatment is initiated. Bad prognostic signs include anuria, a P_{cr} greater than 6 to 8 mg/dL, crescents involving more than 80 percent of the glomeruli, fibrous crescents, and the presence of anti-GBM antibody disease.[774,816-819]

The prognosis for recovery of renal function is somewhat better in those forms of secondary RPGN for which effective therapy is available such as vasculitis and SLE.[816,818] Even those patients with severe acute renal failure who require dialysis may, in this setting, recover enough function to allow dialysis to be discontinued.[818]

The major disorder in which the prognosis of oliguric RPGN is relatively good is poststreptococcal glomerulonephritis.[525,526,814] Survival without dialysis occurs in most of these patients, many of whom spontaneously regain relatively normal renal function. Thus, it is extremely important to establish the correct diagnosis before unnecessary[525] and potentially dangerous immunosuppressive therapy is begun. An elevated ASO or anti-DNAase B titer, hypocomplementemia, and subepithelial humps (see Fig. 6–15b) are all indicative of underlying PSGN.

TREATMENT

The generally poor prognosis of idiopathic RPGN has led to the use of a variety of therapeutic regimens in an effort to preserve renal function. In general, prednisone alone or in combination with cyclophosphamide or azathioprine has had little effect on the course of the renal disease,[774,820,821] although prednisone may control the pulmonary hemorrhage in Goodpasture's syndrome.[771] In view of the role of fibrin in crescent formation, heparin, warfarin, or a combination of prednisone, cyclophosphamide, warfarin, and dipyridamole have been used with some apparent success, particularly in nonoliguric patients with a GFR exceeding 10 mL/min.[819,822-824] However, the use of these regimens has been limited by their toxicity, the prohibition against administering anticoagulants to patients with pulmonary hemorrhage, their inconsistent benefit, and the greater effectiveness of other modes of therapy.[825] Defibrination with pit-viper venom, which is extremely effective in animals[789,790] has not yet been evaluated in humans with RPGN.

There are, however, two therapeutic modalities that may lead to a dramatic improvement in renal function and regression of many of the histologic changes: pulse methylprednisolone given as an intravenous bolus and plasmapheresis. Methylprednisolone (see p. 251 for a discussion of dosage and possible complications) followed by conventional prednisone therapy (1 mg/kg per day) may be effective even in patients with advanced renal failure.[817,826-828] More than one-half of patients have responded to this regimen with, in some studies, a stable reduction in the P_{cr} from a mean of 10.6 to 2.2 mg/dL.[817,826] Nonresponders are more likely to have irreversible changes such as fibrosis of the crescents and glomerular tufts[826] or anti-GBM antibody disease (see below).[817] The mechanism by which such high doses of corticosteroids act is uncertain (see p. 251).[829]

Plasmapheresis has also been shown to be effective in RPGN, including anti-GBM antibody disease.[774,809,816,830,831] In those patients who respond, renal function begins to improve within 10 days.

Plasmapheresis presumably works by removing circulating free antibody or intact complexes and perhaps by removing mediators of inflammation such as fibrinogen and complement.[830,831] The fall in circulating immune complexes may also have an important secondary effect: previously saturated Fc receptors in the reticuloendothelial system become unblocked, allowing removal of newly formed complexes.[832]

The lowering of plasma antibody levels with plasmapheresis is followed by a rebound increase due both to stimulation of new antibody production[833,834] and to equilibration with the extravascular pool.[830] As a result, prednisone and cyclophosphamide must also be given to minimize the increment in antibody formation.

The optimal frequency and duration of plasma exchange therapy is uncertain. A reasonable regimen is to perform daily 3- to 4-L exchanges for 4 to 6 days and then assess the clinical and laboratory response.

In general, albumin-containing electrolyte solutions are administered to replace the removed plasma. However, the loss of fibrinogen, platelets, and other clotting factors can aggravate the bleeding in patients with pulmonary hemorrhage. Thus, fresh frozen plasma should also be used in this setting.[831]

Plasmapheresis can lead to a variety of complications that are usually reversible.[743] These include bleeding, volume depletion or overload if fluid replacement is inaccurate, citrate toxicity from the replacement fluid, and problems related to vascular access.

The relative efficacy of pulse therapy and plasmapheresis in RPGN is uncertain. With the exception of anti-GBM antibody disease (see below), the data suggest that these two modalities probably produce comparable results. It seems reasonable to initially try high doses of corticosteroids since this regimen is less toxic (cyclophosphamide is not required), simpler to use (vascular access and plasma exchange are not needed), and less expensive.[829] Plasmapheresis can then be added if no improvement is seen within 2 weeks or if progression of the renal failure continues after 1 week. The likelihood of a positive response is increased if treatment is begun as quickly as possible. However, recovery of some renal function can occur (at least in non-anti-GBM antibody disease), even in patients with severe acute renal failure who require early dialysis.[818]

Those patients who respond should, once they are stable, be slowly tapered to a maintenance dose of prednisone (15 to 20 mg every other day) that should be continued for 6 to 9 months. Stable renal function may persist for many years in this group although drug-responsive relapses may occur as late as 2 to 4 years after remission has been induced.[835]

Anti-GBM Antibody Disease. Early treatment is essential in anti-GBM disease since *recovery or preservation of renal function is rare if the P_{cr} exceeds 6 to 8 mg/dL prior to the onset of therapy.*[818,830,836,837] In contrast, survival without dialysis may occur in over 80 percent of patients with less severe disease.[830,836] The early preservation of renal function is particularly important because this disorder tends to be self-limited; anti-GBM antibodies usually disappear spontaneously after 6 to 12 months[772,837] or after as few as 8 weeks with combined plasmapheresis and immunosuppressive therapy.[836]

Thus, the treatment of choice in progressive anti-GBM antibody disease is plasmapheresis;[830,831,833,836] in comparison, pulse methylprednisolone has little effect on the glomerular disease,[817] although it can control the pulmonary hemorrhage.[838] However, it is probably advisable to *withhold therapy* for the renal disease if the P_{cr} is above 6 to 8 mg/dL since the risks outweigh the small likelihood of benefit.[818,836,837]

The optimal duration of therapy is uncertain. In general, the patient should be reevaluated clinically and serologically after the first 4- to 6-day course of plasmapheresis. If the pulmonary and renal manifestations have improved and the plasma anti-GBM antibody titers (as assessed by radioimmunoassay) are markedly reduced, further plasmapheresis may be unnecessary and the patient can be maintained on prednisone and cyclophosphamide. During the maintenance phase, serial anti-GBM antibody titers should be obtained to ascertain that the disease is remaining quiescent. Infections should be treated as early as possible since they can lead to exacerbation of the pulmonary and renal manifestations, usually *without* any elevation in anti-GBM antibody levels.[839] How infection intensifies the damage produced by a constant level of antibody is unknown.

Immunosuppressive therapy is typically continued for a total of 9 to 12 months, a time at which anti-GBM antibody production usually remits.[772,837,840] In patients who are doing well, it may be possible to switch from cyclophosphamide to the less toxic azathioprine at 3 to 4 months.[836] Cyclophosphamide can then be reinstituted if recurrent disease occurs. This regimen has been used successfully in patients with Wegener's granulomatosis.[726]

The proper therapy is less clear in patients with milder, noncrescentic glomerular lesions who may have minimal urinary findings and normal renal function. In this setting, remissions of the renal disease can occur spontaneously or with only oral corticosteroids.[803,804,841] However, some patients can subsequently progress to crescent formation and renal failure.[842] Thus, these patients should be followed carefully (with monitoring of the P_{cr}, urinalysis, and anti-GBM antibody titers) if it is initially decided to withhold plasmapheresis because the disease appears to be following a benign course.

The efficacy of plasmapheresis and corticosteroids in controlling the pulmonary disease has made it unnecessary to consider bilateral nephrectomy for severe uncontrollable pulmonary hemorrhage. In some patients, this procedure has resulted in a dramatic improvement in the pulmonary abnormalities within 24 to 48 h.[843,844] The mechanism by which this occurs is not known, although it has been suggested that the kidneys might release some factor (such as bradykinin) which increases vascular permeability, thereby facilitating antibody deposition in the lungs. However, nephrectomy is frequently ineffective,[772,845] and some patients have had recurrent pulmonary hemorrhage in the late postoperative period.[846]

All patients with anti-GBM antibody disease require long-term follow-up even after the clinical and serologic abnormalities have abated. Although permanent remission usually occurs after 12 months,[772,837] late relapses may rarely be seen as late as 5 years after apparent resolution of the disease.[847]

END-STAGE RENAL DISEASE

Despite the above therapeutic modalities, 40 to 60 percent of patients with idiopathic RPGN will still require dialysis or transplantation for end-stage renal failure.[816,819] This is most likely to occur in oliguric or anuric patients who present with a P_{cr} exceeding 6 to 8 mg/dL.[816,818,819,836]

Anti-GBM antibody disease presents a special problem since early transplantation can lead to recurrence in the graft in 55 to 70 percent of patients.[772] This can be almost entirely prevented if transplantation is deferred (and the patient maintained on dialysis) for 9 to 12 months, a time at which anti-GBM antibody production should cease as evidenced by no demonstrable circulating antibody.[772]

CHRONIC GLOMERULONEPHRITIS

The term chronic glomerulonephritis is nonspecific and refers to a glomerular disease that is characterized by a protracted course, eventually resulting in progressive renal insufficiency. At the time of diagnosis, there may be no prior history of renal disease.

PATHOLOGY

The major pathologic findings in chronic glomerulonephritis are on LM. These include focal or diffuse mesangial cell proliferation, increased mesangial matrix, and segmental or global glomerular scarring (Fig. 6–28).[2,848] The prominence of these changes has led to the term chronic *sclerosing* glomerulonephritis. Secondary tubulointerstitial changes such as tubular dilatation and atrophy and interstitial fibrosis are also present.

Immunofluorescent microscopy frequently shows focal granular deposition of IgM and C3, primarily in areas of glomerular sclerosis.[849] These changes are probably due to

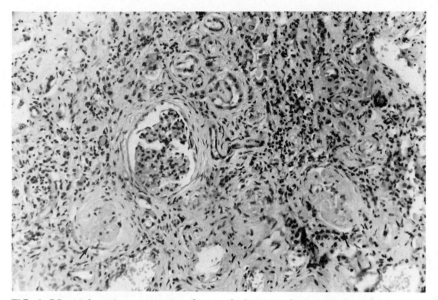

FIG. 6–28. Light microscopy in advanced chronic glomerulonephritis reveals marked tubulointerstitial changes, two hyalinized glomeruli (arrows), and one moderately abnormal but still intact glomerulus. Although these findings are not diagnostic, immunofluorescent or electron microscopy of the intact glomerulus may show changes characteristic of the underlying disease such as IgA nephropathy or type II membranoproliferative glomerulonephritis (dense-deposit disease).

nonspecific absorption onto the damaged GBM since deposits cannot usually be seen on EM. However, complement could contribute to the glomerular injury since damaged renal cells can directly activate the complement pathway.[850]

PATHOGENESIS

It is likely that many of these patients had some identifiable disorder, such as IgA nephropathy, membranoproliferative glomerulonephritis, or membranous nephropathy, which progressed to renal insufficiency after years of asymptomatic hematuria or proteinuria. It may be possible in some patients to establish the underlying diagnosis on renal biopsy by examination of the less severely

damaged glomeruli which may show characteristic changes such as mesangial IgA deposits in IgA nephropathy.

In addition to progressive immunologic injury, hemodynamically mediated damage can also contribute to the glomerular sclerosis (see Chap. 4). Some patients with poststreptococcal glomerulonephritis, for example, completely recover from the acute illness only to develop proteinuria, hypertension, glomerular sclerosis, and renal failure many years later.[487,530,531] It is likely that some nephrons were irreversibly damaged during the initial episode, leading to a compensatory rise in GFR in the relatively normal glomeruli. Although initially adaptive, this hyperfiltration ultimately damages the glomeruli which are not able to handle the associated increase in intraglomerular hydrostatic pressure.

CLINICAL PRESENTATION AND COURSE

Since many patients do not have an episode of symptomatic acute glomerulonephritis, the presence of renal disease is most often discovered incidentally. The findings at the time of diagnosis vary with the severity of the disease.[851] In the early stages, microscopic hematuria or mild proteinuria may be found on a routine urinalysis. The P_{cr} and blood pressure are usually normal at this time. Over the next few years, hypertension and increasing proteinuria may occur, although the P_{cr} tends to remain in or near the normal range. Renal insufficiency, which may not begin for 10 to 20 years, is frequently followed by relatively rapid progression to end-stage renal failure within 1 to 2 years.[851] The urinary changes at this time tend to be less prominent than during the early stages and consist of mild proteinuria, broad, waxy casts, and usually microscopic hematuria.

DIAGNOSIS

The diagnosis of chronic glomerulonephritis can be established only by renal biopsy since vascular or tubulointerstitial disorders such as nephrosclerosis or chronic pyelonephritis can also present with renal insufficiency, hypertension, and nonspecific urinary abnormalities. However, in patients with advanced renal failure and small, scarred kidneys, biopsy is not likely to be helpful regardless of the underlying disease. At this stage, a reversible process is probably not present, and the histologic changes are frequently too severe to allow a specific diagnosis to be made.

TREATMENT

Controlled studies have revealed that prednisone alone or in combination with azathioprine or cyclophosphamide has no effect on the course of chronic glomerulonephritis.[820,821] Thus, there seems to be little justification for the use of these agents in this disorder, particularly when one considers their toxicity, the increased incidence of exacerbation of the disease when cytotoxic agents are discontinued,[852] and the prolonged latent period during which renal function remains relatively normal. The major therapeutic goal in patients with a rising P_{cr} is to minimize hemodynamically mediated injury by the use of a low protein diet and lowering the systemic blood pressure, preferentially with a converting enzyme inhibitor (see Chap. 4).

REFERENCES

1. Györy, A. Z., C. Hadfield, and C. S. Lauer: Value of urine microscopy in predicting histological changes in the kidney: Double blind comparison, *Br. Med. J.,* 288:819, 1984.
2. Glassock, R. J., A. H. Cohen, S. G. Adler and H. J. Ward: Primary glomerular diseases, in B. M. Brenner and F. C. Rector, Jr. (eds.), *The Kidney,* 3d ed., Saunders, Philadelphia, 1986, chap. 22.
3. Cameron, J. S.: Histology, protein clearances and responses to treatment in the nephrotic syndrome, *Br. Med. J.,* 4:352, 1968.
4. Row, P. G., J. S. Cameron, D. R. Turner, D. J. Evans, R. H. R. White, C. S. Ogg, C. Chantler, and C. B. Brown: Membranous nephropathy: Long-term follow-up and association with neoplasia, *Q. J. Med.,* 44:207, 1975.
5. Noel, L. H., M. Zanetti, D. Droz, and C. Barbanel: Long-term prognosis of idiopathic membranous glomerulonephritis: Study of 116 untreated patients, *Am. J. Med.,* 66:82, 1979.
6. Churg, J., R. Habib, and R. H. R. White: Pathology of the nephrotic syndrome in children: A report

from the international study of kidney diseases in children, *Lancet,* 1:1299, 1970.

7. White, R. H. R., E. F. Glasgow, and R. J. Mills: Clinicopathological study of nephrotic syndrome in childhood, *Lancet,* 1:353, 1970.

8. Tornroth, T., G. Talqvist, A. Pasternack, and E. Linder: Nonprogressive histologically mild membranous glomerulonephritis appearing in all evolutionary phases as histologically "early" membranous glomerulonephritis, *Kidney Int.,* 14:511, 1978.

9. Couser, W. G., and D. J. Salant: In situ immune complex formation and glomerular injury, *Kidney Int.,* 17:1, 1980.

10. Vogt, A.: New aspects of the pathogenesis of immune complex glomerulonephritis: Formation of subepithelial deposits, *Clin. Nephrol.,* 21:15, 1984.

11. Van Damme, J. C., G. J. Fleuren, W. W. Bakker, R. L. Vernier, and Ph. J. Hoedemaeker: Experimental glomerulonephritis in the rabbit induced by antibodies directed against tubular antigens, V: Fixed glomerular antigens in the pathogenesis of heterologous immune complex glomerulonephritis, *Lab. Invest.,* 38:502, 1978.

12. Glassock, R. J., T. S. Edgington, J. E. Watson, and F. J. Dixon: Autologous immune complex nephritis induced with renal tubular antigen, II: Pathogenetic mechanism, *J. Exp. Med,* 127:573, 1968.

13. Zager, R. A., W. G. Couser, B. S. Andrews, W. K. Bolton, and M. A. Pohl: Membranous nephropathy: A radioimmunologic search for anti-renal tubular epithelial antibodies and circulating immune complexes, *Nephron* 24:10, 1979.

14. Collins, A. B., G. A. Andres, and R. T. McCluskey: Lack of evidence for a role of renal tubular antigen in human membranous glomerulonephritis, *Nephron,* 27:297, 1981.

15. Naruse, T., K. Kitamura, Y. Miyakawa, and S. Shibata: Deposition of renal tubular epithelial antigen along the glomerular capillary walls of patients with membranous glomerulonephritis, *J. Immunol.,* 110:1163, 1973.

16. Douglas, M. F. S., D. P. Rabideau, M. M. Schwartz, and E. J. Lewis: Evidence of autologous immune-complex nephritis, *N. Engl. J. Med.,* 305:1326, 1981.

17. Cosyns, J-P., Y. Pirson, J-P, Squifflet, G. P. J. Alexandre, C. van Ypersele de Strihou, V. W. Pinn, S. J. Sweet, K. S. Shapiro, S. Cho, and J. T. Harrington: De novo membranous nephropathy in human renal allografts: Report of nine patients, *Kidney Int.,* 22:177, 1982.

18. Cameron, J. S.: Glomerulonephritis in renal transplants, *Transplantation,* 34:237, 1982.

19. Ozawa, T., M. F. Mass, S. Guggenheim, J. Strauss, and R. M. McIntosh: Autologous immune complex nephritis associated with sickle cell trait: Diagnosis of the hemoglobinopathy after renal structural and immunological studies, *Br. Med. J.,* 1:369, 1976.

20. Ueda, S., M. Wakashin, Y. Wakashin, H. Yoshida, K. Iesato, T. Mori, B. Akikusa, and K. Okuda: Experimental gold nephropathy in guinea pigs: Detection of autoantibodies to renal tubular antigens, *Kidney Int.,* 29:539, 1986.

21. Katz, W. A., R. C. Blodgett, and R. G. Pietrusko: Proteinuria in gold-treated rheumatoid arthritis, *Ann. Intern. Med.,* 101:176, 1984.

22. Gallo, G. R., T. Caulin-Glaser, and M. E. Lamm: Charge of circulating immune complexes as a factor in glomerular basement membrane localization in mice, *J. Clin. Invest.,* 67:1305, 1981.

23. Border, W. A., H. J. Ward, E. S. Kamil, and A. H. Cohen: Induction of membranous nephropathy in rabbits by administration of an exogenous cationic antigen, *J. Clin. Invest.,* 69:451, 1982.

24. Gauthier, V. J., M. Mannik, and G. E. Striker: Effect of cationized antibodies in preformed immune complexes on deposition and persistence in renal glomeruli, *J. Exp. Med.,* 156:766, 1982.

25. Couser, W. G., P. J. Baker, and S. Adler: Complement and the direct mediation of glomerular injury: A new perspective, *Kidney Int.,* 28:879, 1985.

26. De Heer, E., M. R. Daha, S. Byakdi, H. Bazin, and L. A. van Es: Possible involvement of terminal complement complex in active Heymann nephritis, *Kidney Int.,* 27:388, 1985.

27. Shemesh, O., J. C. Ross, W. M. Deen, G. W. Grant, and B. D. Myers: Nature of the glomerular capillary injury in human membranous glomerulopathy, *J. Clin. Invest.,* 77:868, 1986.

28. Doi, T., K. Kanatsu, H. Nagai, F. Suehiro, T. Kuwahara, and Y. Hamashima: Demonstration of C3d deposits in membranous nephropathy, *Nephron,* 37:232, 1984.

29. Klouda, P. T., E. J. Acheson, F. S. Goldby, W. Lawler, J. Munos, P. A. Dyer, R. Harris, N. P. Mallick, and G. Williams: Strong association between idiopathic membranous nephropathy and HLA-DRW3, *Lancet* 2:770, 1979.

30. Hiki, Y., Y. Kobayashi, I. Itoh, and N. Kashiwagi: Strong association of HLA-DR2 and MT1 with idiopathic membranous nephropathy in Japan, *Kidney Int.,* 25:953, 1984.

31. Berthoux, F. C., B. Laurent, J.-C. Le Petit, C. Genin, F. Broutin, F. Touraine, A. A. Hassan, and A. Champailler: Immunogenetics and immunopathology of human primary membranous glomerulonephritis: HLA-A, B, DR antigens; functional activity of splenic macrophage Fc-receptors and peripheral blood T-lymphocyte subpopulations, *Clin. Nephrol.,* 22:15, 1984.

32. Wooley, P. H., J. Griffin, G. S. Panayi, J. R. Batchelor, K. I. Welsh, and T. J. Gibson: HLA-DR antigens and toxic reactions to sodium aurothiomalate and D-penicillamine in patients with rheumatoid arthritis, *N. Engl. J. Med.,* 303:300, 1980.

33. Lawley, T. J., R. P. Hall, A. S. Fauci, S. I. Katz, M. I. Hamburger, and M. M. Frank: Defective Fc-receptor function associated with the HLA-B8/DRw3 haplotype, *N. Engl. J. Med.,* 304:185, 1981.

34. Mallick, N. P., C. D. Short, and J. Manos: Clinical membranous nephropathy, *Nephron,* 34:209, 1983.

35. Kleinknecht, C. M., M. Levy, M.-F. Gagnadoux, and R. Habib: Membranous glomerulonephritis with extra-renal disorders in children, *Medicine,* 58:219, 1979.

36. Baldwin, D. S., M. C. Gluck, J. Lowenstein, and G. R. Gallo: Lupus nephritis: Clinical course as related to morphologic forms and their transitions, *Am. J. Med.,* 62:12,1977.

37. Eagen, J. W., and E. J. Lewis: Glomerulopathies of neoplasia, *Kidney Int.,* 11:297, 1977.

38. Horvath, F., Jr., P. Teague, E. F. Gaffney, D. R. Mars, and T. J. Fuller: Thyroid antigen associated immune complex glomerulonephritis in Graves' disease, *Am. J. Med.,* 67:901, 1979.

39. Berger, B. E., F. Vincenti, C. Biava, W. J. Amend, Jr., N. Feduska, and O. Salvatierra, Jr.: De novo and recurrent membranous glomerulopathy following kidney transplantation, *Transplantation,* 35:315, 1983.

40. Tornroth, T., and B. Skrifvars: Gold nephropathy: Prototype of membranous glomerulonephritis, *Am. J. Pathol.,* 75:573, 1974.

41. Adler, S. G., A. H. Cohen, and W. A. Border: Hypersensitivity phenomena and the kidney: Role of drugs and environmental agents, *Am. J. Kid. Dis.,* 5:75, 1985.

42. Bacon, P. A., C. R. Tribe, J. C. Mackenzie, J. Jones, R. H. Cumming, and B. Amer: Penicillamine nephropathy in rheumatoid arthritis: A clinical, pathological and immunological study, *Q. J. Med.,* 45:661, 1976.

43. Editorial: Penicillamine nephropathy, *Br. Med. J.,* 1:761, 1981.

44. Textor, S. C., G. N. Gephardt, E. L. Bravo, R. C. Tarazi, F. M. Fouad, R. Tubbs, and J. T. McMahon: Membranous glomerulopathy associated with captopril therapy, *Am. J. Med.,* 74:705, 1983.

45. Case, D. B., S. A. Atlas, J. A. Mouradian, R. A. Fishman, R. L. Sherman, and J. H. Laragh: Proteinuria during long-term captopril therapy, *J. Am. Med. Assoc.,* 244:346, 1980.

46. Becker, C. G., E. L. Becker, J. F. Maher, and G. E. Schreiner: Nephrotic syndrome after contact with mercury, *Arch. Intern. Med.,* 110:178, 1962.

47. Tubbs, R. R., G. N. Gephardt, J. T. McMahon, M. C. Pohl, D. G. Vidt, S. A. Barenberg, and R. Valenzuela: Membranous glomerulonephritis associated with industrial mercury exposure. Study of pathogenetic mechanisms, *Am. J. Clin. Pathol.,* 77:409, 1982.

48. Lupo, A., T. Faraggiana, C. Loschiavo, C. Parolini, and G. Maschio: Nephrotic syndrome during 2-mercapto-propionyl-glycine (Thiola) therapy, *Nephron,* 28:96, 1981.

49. Kohler, P. F., R. E. Cronin, W. S. Hammond, D. Olin, and R. I. Carr: Chronic membranous glomerulonephritis caused by hepatitis B antigen-antibody immune complexes, *Ann. Intern. Med.,* 81:448, 1974.

50. Hirose, H., K. Udo, M. Kojima, Y. Takahashi, Y. Miyakawa, K. Miyamto, H. Yoshizawa, and M. Mayumi: Deposition of hepatitis B e antigen in membranous glomerulonephritis: Identification by F (ab')$_2$ fragments of monoclonal antibody, *Kidney Int.,* 26:338, 1984.

51. Yoshikawa, N., H. Ito, Y. Yamada, H. Hashimoto, Y. Katayama, S. Matsuyama, O. Hasegawa, S. Okada, H. Hajikano, H. Yoshizawa, M. Mayumi, and T. Matsuo: Membranous glomerulonephritis associated with hepatitis B antigen in children: A comparison with idiopathic membranous glomerulonephritis, *Clin. Nephrol.,* 23:28, 1985

52. Gamble, C. N., and J. B. Reardan: Immunopathogenesis of syphilitic glomerulonephritis: Elution of antitreponemal antibody from glomerular complex deposits, *N. Engl. J. Med.,* 292:449, 1975.

53. O'Regan, S., J. S. C. Fong, J-P. de Chadarévian, J. R. Rishikof, and K. N. Drummond, Treponemal antigens in congenital and acquired syphilitic nephritis. Demonstration by immunofluorescence studies, *Ann. Intern. Med.,* 85:325, 1976.

54. Sanchez-Bayle, M., J. L. Ecija, R. Estepa, M. J. Cambronero, and M. A. Martinez: Incidence of

glomerulonephritis in congenital syphilis, *Clin. Nephrol.,* 20:27, 1983.

55. Hendrickse, R. G., E. F. Glasgow, A. Adeniyi, R. H. R. White, G. M. Edington, and V. Houba: Quartan malarial nephrotic syndrome: Collaborative clinicopathological study in Nigerian children, *Lancet,* 1:1143, 1972.

56. Sánchez Ibarrola, A., B. Sobrini, J. Guisantes, J. Pardo, J. Diez, J. M. Monfá, and A. Purroy: Membranous glomerulonephritis secondary to hydatid disease, *Am. J. Med.,* 70:311, 1981.

57. Samuels, B., J. C. Lee, E. P. Engelman, and J. Hopper, Jr.: Membranous nephropathy in patients with rheumatoid arthritis: Relationship to gold therapy, *Medicine,* 57:319, 1978.

58. Rao, K. V., and J. T. Crosson: Idiopathic membranous glomerulonephritis in diabetic patients. Report of three cases and review of the literature, *Arch. Intern. Med.,* 140:624, 1980.

59. Bertani, T., G. B. Appel, V. D'Agati, M. A. Nash, and C. L. Pirani: Focal segmental membranous glomerulonephropathy associated with other glomerular diseases, *Am. J. Kid. Dis.,* 2:439, 1983.

60. Dupont, A. G., D. L. Verbeelen, and R. O. Six: Weber-Christian panniculitis with membranous glomerulonephritis, *Am. J. Med.,* 75:527, 1983.

61. Editorial: Dermatitis herpetiformis, glomerulonephritis, and HLA-DRw3, *Lancet,* 2:911, 1979.

62. Taylor, R. G., C. Fisher, and B. I. Hoffbrand: Sarcoidosis and membranous glomerulonephritis: A significant association, *Br. Med. J.,* 284:1297, 1982.

63. Cantrell, E. G.: Nephrotic syndrome cured by removal of gastric carcinoma, *Br. Med. J.,* 2:739, 1969.

64. Lewis, M. G., L. W. Loughridge, and T. M. Phillips: Immunologic studies in nephrotic syndrome associated with extrarenal malignant disease, *Lancet,* 2:134, 1971.

65. Costanza, M. E., V. Pinn, R. S. Schwartz, and L. Nathanson: Carcinoembryonic antigen-antibody complexes in a patient with colonic carcinoma and nephrotic syndrome, *N. Engl. J. Med.,* 298:520, 1973.

66. Couser, W. G., J. B. Wagonfeld, B. H. Spargo, and E. J. Lewis: Glomerular deposition of tumor antigen in membranous nephropathy associated with colonic carcinoma, *Am. J. Med.,* 57:962, 1974.

67. Jennette, J. C., S. S. Iskandar, and F. G. Dalldorf: Pathologic differentiation between lupus and nonlupus membranous glomerulonephropathy, *Kidney Int.,* 24:377, 1983.

68. Lebit, S. A., B. Burke, A. F. Michael, and R. L.

Vernier: Extramembranous glomerulonephritis in childhood: Relationship to systemic lupus erythematosus, *J. Pediatr.,* 88:394, 1976.

69. Adu, D., D. G. Williams, D. Taube, A. R. Vilches, D. R. Turner, J. S. Cameron, and C. S. Ogg: Late onset systemic lupus erythematosus and lupus-like disease in patients with apparent idiopathic glomerulonephritis, *Q. J. Med.,* 52:471, 1983.

70. Shearn, M. A., C. Biava, and J. Hopper, Jr.: Mesangial deposits (by electron microscopy) in idiopathic membranous glomerulonephritis, *N. Engl. J. Med.,* 301:212, 1979.

71. Ślusarczyk, J., T. Michalak, T. Nazarewicz-de Mezer, K. Krawczyński, and A. Nowolslawski: Membranous glomerulopathy associated with hepatitis B core antigen immune complexes in children, *Am. J. Pathol.,* 98:29, 1980.

72. Okuda, S., Y. Oh, K. Onoyama, S. Fujumi, and T. Omae: Autologous immune complex nephritis in streptozotocin-induced diabetic rats, *Nephron,* 37:166, 1984.

73. Davison, A. M., J. S. Cameron, D. N. S. Kerr, C. S. Ogg, and R. W. Wilkinson: The natural history of renal function in untreated idiopathic membranous glomerulonephritis in adults, *Clin. Nephrol.,* 22:61, 1984.

74. Habib, R., C. Kleinknecht, and M.-C. Gubler: Extramembranous glomerulonephritis in children: Report of 50 cases, *J. Pediatr.,* 82:754, 1973.

75. Neild, G. H., H.-V. Garter, and A. Bohle: D-penicillamine-induced membranous glomerulonephritis, *Lancet,* 1:1201, 1975.

76. Klassen, J., C. Elwood, A. L. Grossberg, F. Milgrom, M. Montes, M. Sepulveda, and G. A. Andres: Evolution of membranous nephropathy into anti-glomerular-basement-membrane glomerulonephritis, *N. Engl. J. Med.,* 290:1340, 1974.

77. Cameron, J. S.: Membranous nephropathy: The treatment dilemma, *Am. J. Kid. Dis.,* 1:371, 1982.

78. Hopper, J., P. A. Trew, and C. G. Biava: Membranous nephropathy: The relative benignity in women, *Nephron,* 29:18, 1981.

79. Idelson, B. A., N. Smithline, G. W. Smith, and J. T. Harrington: Prognosis in steroid-treated nephrotic syndrome in adults: Analysis of major predictive factors after ten-year follow-up, *Arch. Intern. Med.,* 137:891, 1977.

80. Glassock, R. J.: Corticosteroid therapy is beneficial in adults with idiopathic membranous glomerulopathy, *Am. J. Kid. Dis.,* 1:376, 1982.

81. Llach, F.: Hypercoagulability, renal vein throm-

bosis, and other thrombotic complications of nephrotic syndrome, *Kidney Int.,* 28:429, 1985.

82. Wagoner, R. D., A. W. Stanton, K. E. Holley, and C. S. Winter: Renal vein thrombosis in idiopathic membranous glomerulopathy and nephrotic syndrome: Incidence and significance, *Kidney Int.,* 23:368, 1983.

83. Ehrenreich, T., J. G. Porush, J. Churg, L. Garfinkel, S. Glabman, M. H. Goldstein, E. Grishman, and S. L. Yunis: Treatment of idiopathic membranous nephropathy, *N. Engl. J. Med.,* 295:741, 1976.

84. Bolton, W. K., N. O. Atuk, B. C. Sturgill, and F. B. Westervelt, Jr.: Therapy of the idiopathic nephrotic syndrome with alternate day steroids, *Am. J. Med.,* 62:60, 1977.

85. Hopper, J., Jr., C. G. Biava, and W-H. Tu: Membranous nephropathy: High-dose alternate-day therapy with prednisone, *West. J. Med.,* 135:1, 1981.

86. Collaborative Study of the Adult Idiopathic Nephrotic Syndrome: A controlled study of short-term prednisone treatment in adults with membranous nephropathy, *N. Engl. J. Med.,* 301:1301, 1979.

87. Cattran, D., C. Cardella, R. Charron, J. Roscoe, P. Rance, M. Cusimana, R. Bear, M. Johnson, and P. Corey: Preliminary results of controlled trial of alternate-day prednisone in idiopathic membranous glomerulonephritis (abstract), *Kidney Int.,* 19:388, 1981.

88. Ponticelli, C., P. Zucchelli, E. Imbasciati, L. Cagnoli, C. Pozzi, P. Passerini, C. Grassi, D. Limido, S. Pasquali, T. Volpini, M. Sosdelli, and F. Locatelli: Controlled trial of methyl prednisolone and chlorambucil in idiopathic membranous nephropathy, *N. Engl. J. Med.,* 310:946, 1984.

89. Ponticelli, C.: Prognosis and treatment of membranous nephropathy, *Kidney Int.,* 29:927, 1986.

90. Cameron, J. S.: Chlorambucil and leukemia, *N. Engl. J. Med.,* 296:1065, 1977.

91. Smith, A. G., A. G. Prentice, N. P. Lucie, J. D. Browning, J. H. Dagg, and M. Rowan: Acute myelogenous leukaemia following cytotoxic therapy: Five cases and a review, *Q. J. Med.,* 51:227, 1982.

92. Velosa, J. A., V. E. Torres, J. V. Donadio, Jr., R. D. Wagoner, K. E. Holley, and K. P. Offord: Treatment of severe nephrotic syndrome with meclofenamate: An uncontrolled pilot study, *Mayo Clin. Proc.,* 60:586, 1985.

93. A Report of the International Study of Kidney Disease in Children: The primary nephrotic syndrome in children. Identification of patients with

94. Nolasco, F., J. S. Cameron, E. F. Heywood, J. Hicks, C. Ogg, and D. G. Williams: Adult-onset minimal change nephrotic syndrome: A long-term follow-up, *Kidney Int.,* 29:1215, 1986.

95. Drummond, K. N., A. F. Michael, R. A. Good, and R. L. Vernier: The nephrotic syndrome of childhood: Immunologic, clinical and pathologic correlations, *J. Clin. Invest.,* 45:620, 1966.

96. Ji-Yun, Y., T. Melvin, R. Sibley, and A. F. Michael: No evidence for a specific role of IgM in mesangial proliferation of idiopathic nephrotic syndrome, *Kidney Int.,* 25:100, 1984.

97. Moorthy, A. V., S. W. Zimmerman, and P. M. Burkholder: Nephrotic syndrome in Hodgkin's disease: Evidence for pathogenesis alternative to immune complex deposition, *Am. J. Med.,* 61:471, 1976.

98. Plager, J., and L. Stutzman: Acute nephrotic syndrome as a manifestation of active Hodgkin's disease. Report of four cases and review of the literature, *Am. J. Med.,* 50:56, 1971.

99. Alpers, C. E., and R. S. Cotran: Neoplasia and glomerular injury, *Kidney Int.,* 30:465, 1986.

100. Moorthy, A. V.: Minimal change glomerular disease: A paraneoplastic syndrome in two patients with bronchogenic carcinoma, *Am. J. Kid. Dis.,* 3:58, 1983.

101. Finkelstein, A., D. S. Fraley, I. Stachura, H. A. Feldman, D. R. Gandy, and E. Bourke: Fenoprofen nephropathy: Lipoid nephrosis and interstitial nephritis. A possible T-lymphocyte disorder, *Am. J. Med.,* 72:81, 1982.

102. Clive, D. M., and J. S. Stoff: Renal syndromes associated with nonsteroidal antiinflammatory drugs, *N. Engl. J. Med.,* 310:563, 1984.

103. Rennke, H. G., P. C. Roos, and S. G. Wall: Drug-induced interstitial nephritis with heavy glomerular proteinuria (letter), *N. Engl. J. Med.,* 302:691, 1980.

104. Averbuch, S. D., H. A. Austin, III, S. A. Sherwin, T. Antonovych, P. A. Bunn, Jr., and D. L. Longo: Acute interstitial nephritis with the nephrotic syndrome following recombinant leukocyte A interferon therapy for mycosis fungoides, *N. Engl. J. Med.,* 310:32, 1984.

105. Lomvardias, S., V. W. Pinn, M. L. Wadhwa, K. M. Koshy, and M. Heller: Nephrotic syndrome associated with sulindac (letter), *N. Engl. J. Med.,* 304:424, 1981.

106. Mustonen, J. A., A. Pasternack, and I. Rantala: The nephrotic syndrome in IgA glomerulonephri-

tis: Response to corticosteroid therapy, *Clin. Nephrol.,* 20:172, 1983.

107. Abreo, K., and S-F. Wen: A case of IgA nephropathy with an unusual response to corticosteroid and immunosuppressive therapy, *Am. J. Kid. Dis.,* 3:54, 1983.

108. A Report of the Southwest Pediatric Nephrology Study Group: Association of IgA nephropathy with steroid-responsive nephrotic syndrome, *Am. J. Kid. Dis.,* 5:157, 1985.

109. Richman, A. V., H. L. Masco, S. I. Rifkin, and M. K. Acharya: Minimal-change disease and the nephrotic syndrome associated with lithium therapy, *Ann. Intern. Med.,* 92:70, 1980.

110. Alexander, F., and J. Martin: Nephrotic syndrome associated with lithium therapy, *Clin. Nephrol.,* 15:267, 1981.

111. Michael, A. F., E. Blau, and R. L. Vernier: Glomerular polyanion: Alteration in aminonucleoside nephrosis, *Lab. Invest.,* 23:649, 1970.

112. Kreisberg, J. I., R. L. Hoover, and M. J. Karnovsky: Isolation and characterization of rat glomerular epithelial cells in vitro, *Kidney Int.,* 14:21, 1978.

113. Kerjaschki, D., A. T. Vernillo, and M. G. Farquhar: Reduced sialation of podocalyxin—the major sialoprotein of rat kidney glomerulus—in aminonucleoside nephrosis, *Am. J. Pathol.,* 118:343, 1985.

114. Seiler, M. W., H. G. Rennke, M. A. Venkatachalam, and R. S. Cotran: Pathogenesis of polycation-induced alterations ("fusion") of glomerular epithelium, *Lab. Invest.,* 36:48, 1977.

115. Brenner, B. M., T. H. Hostetter, and H. D. Humes: Molecular basis of proteinuria of glomerular origin, *N. Engl. J. Med.,* 298:826, 1978.

116. Meyers, B. D., T. B. Okarma, S. Friedman, C. Bridges, J. Ross, S. Asseff, and W. M. Deen: Mechanisms of proteinuria in human glomerulonephritis, *J. Clin. Invest.,* 70:732, 1982.

117. Carrie, B. J., W. R. Salyer, and B. D. Myers: Minimal change nephropathy: An electrochemical disorder of the glomerular membrane, *Am. J. Med.,* 70:262, 1981.

118. Shalhoub, R. J.: Pathogenesis of lipoid nephrosis: A disorder of T-cell function, *Lancet,* 2:556, 1974.

119. Moorthy, A. V., S. W. Zimmerman, and P. M. Burkholder: Inhibition of lymphocyte blastogenesis by plasma of patients with minimal-change nephrotic syndrome, *Lancet,* 1:1160, 1976.

120. Stachura, I., S. Jayakumar, and E. Bourke: T and B lymphocyte subsets in fenoprofen nephropathy, *Am. J. Med.,* 75:9, 1983.

121. Feehally, J., T. J. Beattie, P. E. C. Brenchley, B. M. Coupes, I. B. Houston, N. P. Mallick, and R. J. Postlethwaite: Modulation of cellular immune function by cyclophosphamide in children with minimal-change nephropathy, *N. Engl. J. Med.,* 310:415, 1984.

122. Sobel, A., J-M. Heslan, A. Branellec, and G. Lagrue: Vascular permeability factor produced by lymphocytes of patients with nephrotic syndrome, *Adv. Nephrol.,* 100:315, 1981.

123. Couser, W., A. Badger, S. Cooperhead, S. Stilman, J. Jermanovich, S. Aurora, D. Doner, and G. Schmitt: Hodgkin's disease and lipoid nephrosis, *Lancet,* 1:912, 1977.

124. Boulton Jones, J. M., I. Tulloch, B. Dore, and A. McLay: Changes in the glomerular capillary wall induced by lymphocyte products and serum of nephrotic patients, *Clin. Nephrol.,* 20:72, 1983.

125. Levinsky, R. J., P. N. Malleson, T. M. Barrett, and J. F. Soothill: Circulating immune complexes in steroid responsive nephrotic syndrome, *N. Engl. J. Med.,* 298:126, 1978.

126. Poston, R. N., R. Cerio, and J. S. Cameron: Circulating immune complexes in minimal change nephritis, *N. Engl. J. Med.,* 298:1089, 1978.

127. Abrass, C. K., C. L. Hall, W. A. Border, C. A. Brown, R. J. Glassock, and C. H. Coggins: Circulating immune complexes in adults with idiopathic nephrotic syndrome, *Kidney Int.,* 17:545, 1980.

128. Meadow, S. R., and J. K. Sarsfield: Steroid-responsive nephrotic syndrome and allergy: Clinical studies, *Arch. Dis. Child.,* 56:509, 1981.

129. Meadow, S. R., J. K. Sarsfield, D. G. Scott, and S. M. Rajah: Steroid-responsive nephrotic syndrome and allergy: Immunological studies, *Arch. Dis. Child.,* 56:517, 1981.

130. Editorial: Atopy and steroid-responsive childhood nephrotic syndrome, *Lancet,* 2:964, 1981.

131. Germuth, F. G., Jr., A. J. Valdes, J. J. Taylor, O'L. Wise, and E. Rodriguez: Fatal immune complex glomerulonephritis without deposits, *Johns Hopkins Med. J.,* 136:189, 1975.

132. Kobayashi, Y., X-M. Chen, Y. Hiki, K. Fujii, and N. Kashiwagi: Association of HLA-DRw8 and DQw3 with minimal change nephrotic syndrome in Japanese adults, *Kidney Int.,* 28:193, 1985.

133. A Report of the International Study of Kidney Disease in Children: Nephrotic syndrome in children: Prediction of histopathology from clinical and laboratory characteristics at time of diagnosis, *Kidney Int.,* 13:159, 1978.

134. Bohman, S-O., G. Jaremko, A-B. Bohlin, and U. Berg: Foot process fusion and glomerular filtration rate in minimal change nephrotic syndrome, *Kidney Int.,* 25:696, 1984.

135. Connolly, M. E., O. M. Wrong, and N. F. Jones: Reversible renal failure in idiopathic nephrotic syndrome with minimal glomerular changes, *Lancet,* 1:665, 1968.

136. Meltzer, J. I., H. J. Keim, J. H. Laragh, J. E. Sealey, K-M. Jan, and S. Chien: Nephrotic syndrome: Vasoconstriction and hypervolemic types indicated by renin-sodium profiling, *Ann. Intern. Med.,* 91:688, 1979.

137. Lowenstein, J., R. G. Schacht, and D. S. Baldwin: Renal failure in minimal change nephrotic syndrome, *Am. J. Med.,* 70:227, 1981.

138. Arneil, G. C., and C. N. Lam: Long-term assessment of steroid therapy in childhood nephrosis, *Lancet,* 2:819, 1966.

139. A Report of the International Study of Kidney Disease in Children: Minimal change nephrotic syndrome in children: Deaths during the first 5 to 15 years' observation, *Pediatrics,* 73:497, 1984.

140. Grupe, W. E.: Relapsing nephrotic syndrome in childhood, *Kidney Int.,* 16:75, 1979.

141. A Report of "Arbeitgemeinschaft für Pädiatrische Nephrologie": Alternate-day versus intermittent prednisone in frequently relapsing nephrotic syndrome, *Lancet,* 1:401, 1979.

142. Siegel, N. J., B. Goldberg, L. S. Krassner, and J. P. Hayslett: Long-term follow-up of children with steroid responsive nephrotic syndrome, *J. Pediatr.,* 81:251, 1972.

143. A Report of the International Study of Kidney Disease in Children: Primary nephrotic syndrome in children: Clinical significance of histopathologic variants of minimal change and of diffuse mesangial hypercellularity, *Kidney Int.,* 20:765, 1981.

144. A Report of the International Study of Kidney Disease in Children: Early identification of frequent relapsers among children with minimal change nephrotic syndrome, *J. Pediatr.,* 101:514, 1982.

145. Trompeter, R. S., W. B. Lloyd, J. Hicks, R. H. R. White, and J. S. Cameron: Long-term outcome for children with minimal-change nephrotic syndrome, *Lancet,* 1:368, 1985.

146. Pru, C., C. M. Kjellstrand, R. A. Cohn, and R. L. Vernier: Late recurrence of minimal lesion nephrotic syndrome, *Ann. Intern. Med.,* 100:69, 1984.

147. Leisti, S., and O. Koskimies: Risk of relapse in steroid-sensitive nephrotic syndrome: Effect of stage of post-prednisone adrenocortical suppression, *J. Pediatr.,* 103:553, 1983.

148. Arant, B. S., Jr., S. A. Singer, and J. Bernstein: Steroid-dependent nephrotic syndrome, *J. Pediatr.,* 100:328, 1982.

149. Travis, L. B., R. Chesney, P. McEnery, D. Moel, A. Pennisi, D. Potter, Y. B. Talwalkar, and E. Wolff: Growth and glucocorticoids in children with kidney disease, *Kidney Int.,* 14:365, 1978.

150. Abramowicz, M., H. L. Barnett, C. M. Edelmann, Jr., and I. Greifer: Controlled trial of azathioprine in children with nephrotic syndrome, *Lancet* 1:959, 1970.

151. Cameron J. S., C. Chantler, C. S. Ogg, and R. H. R. White: Long-term stability of remission in nephrotic syndrome after treatment with cyclophosphamide, *Br. Med. J.,* 4:7, 1974.

152. Spitzer, A., G. Gordiollo-P., I. B. Houston, and L. B. Travis: Prospective, controlled trial of cyclophosphamide therapy in children with nephrotic syndrome, *Lancet,* 2:423, 1974.

153. McDonald, J., A. V. Murphy, and G. C. Arneil: Long-term assessment of cyclophosphamide therapy for nephrosis in children, *Lancet,* 2:980, 1974.

154. Williams, S. A., S. P. Makker, J. R. Inglefinger, and W. E. Grupe: Long-term evaluation of chlorambucil plus prednisone in the idiopathic nephrotic syndrome of childhood, *N. Engl. J. Med.,* 302:929, 1980.

155. Grupe, W. E.: Cytotoxic drugs for nephrotic syndrome (letter), *N. Engl. J. Med.,* 307:313, 1982.

156. Arbeitgemeinschaft für Pädiatrische Nephrologie: Effect of cytotoxic drugs in frequently relapsing nephrotic syndrome with and without steroid dependence, *N. Engl. J. Med.,* 306:451, 1982.

157. Schein, P. S., and S. H. Winokur: Immunosuppressive and cytotoxic chemotherapy: Long-term complications, *Ann. Intern. Med.,* 82:84, 1975.

158. Etteldorf, J. N., C. D. West, J. A. Pitcock, and D. L. Williams: Gonadal function, testicular histology, and meiosis following cyclophosphamide therapy in patients with nephrotic syndrome, *J. Pediatr.,* 88:206, 1976.

159. Callis, L., J. Nieto, A. Vila, and J. Rende: Chlorambucil treatment in minimal lesion nephrotic syndrome: A reappraisal of its gonadal toxicity, *J. Pediatr.,* 97:653, 1980.

160. Puri, H. C., and R. A. Campbell: Cyclophosphamide and malignancy, *Lancet,* 1:1306, 1977.

161. Decker, J. L.: Azathioprine and cyclophosphamide as slow-acting drugs for rheumatoid arthritis, *Am. J. Med.,* 75(6A):74, 1983.

162. Kleinknecht, C., P. Guesry, G. Lenoir, and M. Broyer: High cost-benefit of chlorambucil in frequently relapsing nephrosis, *N. Engl. J. Med.,* 296:48, 1977.

163. Watson, A. R., C. P. Rance, and J. Bain: Long-term effects of cyclophosphamide on testicular function, *Br. Med. J.,* 291:1457, 1985.

164. McEnery, P. T., L. L. Gonzalez, L. W. Martin, and C. D. West: Growth and development of children with renal transplants. Use of alternate-day steroid therapy, *J. Pediatr.*, 83:806, 1973.

165. Wingen, A. M., D. E. Müller-Wiefel, and K. Schärer: Spontaneous remissions in frequently relapsing and steroid dependent idiopathic nephrotic syndrome, *Clin. Nephrol.*, 23:35, 1985.

166. Barratt, T. M., J. S. Cameron, C. Chantler, C. S. Ogg, and J. F. Soothill: Comparative trial of 2 weeks and 8 weeks cyclophosphamide in steroid-sensitive relapsing nephrotic syndrome of childhood, *Arch. Dis. Child.*, 48:286, 1973.

167. Koskimies, O., J. Vilska, J. Rapola, and N. Hallman: Long-term outcome of primary nephrotic syndrome, *Arch. Dis. Child.*, 57:544, 1982.

168. Siegel, N. J., A. Gur, L. S. Krassner, and M. Kashgarian: Minimal-lesion nephrotic syndrome with early resistance to steroid therapy, *J. Pediatr.*, 87:377, 1975.

169. Hayslett, J. P., L. S. Krassner, K. G. Bensch, M. Kashgarian, and F. H. Epstein: Progression of "lipoid nephrosis" to renal insufficiency, *N. Engl. J. Med.*, 281:181, 1969.

170. Habib, R., and M.-C. Gubler: Focal sclerosing glomerulonephritis, in P. Kincaid-Smith, T. Mathew, and E. L. Becker (eds.), *Glomerulonephritis: Morphology, Natural History and Treatment*, Wiley, New York, 1973.

171. A Report of the Southwest Pediatric Nephrology Study Group: Focal segmental glomerulosclerosis in children with idiopathic nephrotic syndrome, *Kidney Int.*, 27:442, 1985.

172. Black, D. A. K., G. Rose, and D. B. Brewer: Controlled trial of prednisone in adult patients with the nephrotic syndrome, *Br. Med. J.*, 3:421, 1970.

173. Cade, R., D. Mars, M. Privette, R. Thompson, B. Croker, J. Peterson, and K. Campbell: Effect of long-term azathioprine administration in adults with minimal change glomerulonephritis and nephrotic syndrome resistant to corticosteroids, *Arch. Intern. Med.*, 146:737, 1986.

174. Siegel, N. J., K. M. Gaudio, L. S. Krassner, B. M. McDonald, F. P. Anderson, and M. Kashgarian: Steroid-dependent nephrotic syndrome in children: Histopathology and relapses after cyclophosphamide treatment, *Kidney Int.*, 19:454, 1981.

175. Tejani, A.: Morphological transition in minimal change nephrotic syndrome, *Nephron*, 39:157, 1985.

176. A Report of the Southwest Pediatric Nephrology Study Group: Childhood nephrotic syndrome associated with diffuse mesangial hypercellularity, *Kidney Int.*, 24:87, 1983.

177. Brown, E. A., K. Upadhyaya, J. P. Hayslett, M. Kashgarian, and N. J. Siegel: The clinical course of mesangial proliferative glomerulonephritis, *Medicine*, 58:295, 1979.

178. Waldherr, R., M.-C. Gubler, M. Levy, M. Broyer, and R. Habib: The significance of pure diffuse mesangial proliferation in idiopathic nephrotic syndrome, *Clin. Nephrol.*, 10:171, 1978.

179. Cohen, A. H., W. A. Border, and R. J. Glassock: Nephrotic syndrome with glomerular mesangial IgM deposits, *Lab. Invest.*, 38:610, 1978.

180. Bhasin, H. K., J. G. Abuelo, R. Nayak, and A. R. Esparza: Mesangial proliferative glomerulonephritis, *Lab. Invest.*, 39:21, 1978.

181. Pardo, V., I. Riesgo, G. Zillervelo, and J. Strauss: The clinical significance of mesangial IgM deposits and mesangial hypercellularity in minimal change nephrotic syndrome, *Am. J. Kid. Dis.*, 3:264, 1984.

182. Bolton, W. K., F. B. Westervelt, Jr., and B. C. Sturgill: Nephrotic syndrome and focal glomerular sclerosis in aging man, *Nephron*, 20:307, 1978.

183. Kashgarian, M., J. P. Hayslett, and B. H. Spargo: Renal disease, *Am. J. Pathol.*, 89:187, 1977.

184. Hyman, L. R., and P. M. Burkholder: Focal sclerosing glomerulonephropathy with segmental hyalinosis: A clinicopathologic analysis, *Lab. Invest.*, 28:533, 1973.

185. Kincaid-Smith, P.: *The Kidney: A Clinicopathological Study*, Lippincott, Philadelphia, 1975, sec. 6.

186. Bhathena, D. B., J. H. Weiss, N. H. Holland, R. G. McMorrow, J. J. Curtis, B. A. Lucas, and R. G. Luke: Focal and segmental glomerular sclerosis in reflux nephropathy, *Am. J. Med.*, 68:886, 1980.

187. Tejani, A., K. Phadke, O. Adamson, A. Nicastri, C. K. Chen, and D. Sen: Renal lesions in sickle cell nephropathy in children, *Nephron*, 39:352, 1985.

188. Cunningham, E. E., J. R. Brentjens, M. A. Zielezny, G. A. Andres, and R. C. Venuto: Heroin nephropathy. A clinicopathologic and epidemiologic study, *Am. J. Med.*, 68:47, 1980.

189. Cunningham, E. E., M. A. Zielezny, and R. C. Venuto: Heroin-associated nephropathy. A nationwide problem, *J. Am. Med. Assoc.*, 250:2935, 1983.

190. Dubrow, A., N. Mittman, V. Ghali, and W. Flamenbaum: The changing spectrum of heroin-associated nephropathy, *Am. J. Kid. Dis.*, 5:36, 1985.

191. Rao, T. K. S., E. J. Filippone, A. D. Nicastri, S. H. Landesman, E. Frank, C. K. Chen, and E. A. Friedman: Associated focal and segmental glomerulo-

sclerosis in the acquired immunodeficiency syndrome, *N. Engl. J. Med.,* 310:669, 1984.

192. Pardo, V., M. Aldana, R. M. Colton, M. A. Fischl, D. Jaffee, L. Moskowitz, G. T. Hensley, and J. J. Bourgoignie: Glomerular lesions in the acquired immunodeficiency syndrome, *Ann. Intern. Med.,* 101:429, 1984.

193. Gardenswartz, M. H., C. W. Lerner, G. R. Seligson, P. M. Zabetakis, H. Rotterdam, M. L. Tapper, M. F. Michelis, and M. S. Bruno: Renal disease in patients with AIDS: A clinico-pathologic study, *Clin. Nephrol.,* 21:197, 1984.

194. Case Records of the Massachusetts General Hospital (Case 15-1983), *N. Engl. J. Med.,* 308:888, 1983.

195. Cheigh, J. S., J. Mouradian, M. Soliman, L. Tapia, R. R. Riggio, K. H. Stenzel, and A. L. Rubin: Focal segmental glomerulosclerosis in renal transplants, *Am. J. Kid. Dis.,* 2:449, 1983.

196. Ettenger, R. B., E. T. Heuser, M. H. Malekzadeh, A. J. Pennisi, C. H. Uittenbogaart, and R. N. Fine: Focal glomerulosclerosis in renal allografts: Association with the nephrotic syndrome and chronic rejection, *Am. J. Dis. Child.,* 131:1347, 1977.

197. Lewis, E. J.: Recurrent focal sclerosis after renal transplantation, *Kidney Int.,* 22:315, 1982.

198. Kasiske, B. L., and J. T. Crosson: Renal disease in patients with massive obesity, *Arch. Intern. Med.,* 146:1105, 1986.

199. Pinto, J., G. Lacerda, J. S. Cameron, D. R. Turner, M. Bewick, and C. S. Ogg, and the Physicians, Pediatricians, and Pathologists of the Southeast Thames Renal Units: Recurrence of focal segmental glomerulosclerosis in renal allografts, *Transplantation,* 32:83, 1981.

200. Maizel, S. E., R. K. Sibley, J. P. Horstman, C. M. Kjellstrand, and R. L. Simmons: Incidence and significance of recurrent focal segmental glomerulosclerosis in renal allograft recipients, *Transplantation,* 32:512, 1981.

201. Zimmerman, S. W.: Increased urinary protein excretion in the rat produced by serum from a patient with recurrent focal glomerular sclerosis after renal transplantation, *Clin. Nephrol.,* 22:32, 1984.

202. Diamond, J. R., and M. J. Karnovsky: Focal and segmental glomerulosclerosis following a single intravenous dose of puromycin aminonucleoside. *Am. J. Pathol.,* 122:481, 1986.

203. Grond, J., J. Koudstaal, and J. D. Elema: Mesangial function and glomerular sclerosis in rats with aminonucleoside nephrosis, *Kidney Int.,* 27:405, 1985.

204. Schwartz, M. M., and E. J. Lewis: Focal glomerulosclerosis: The cellular lesion, *Kidney Int.,* 28:968, 1985.

205. Winetz, J. A., C. R. Robertson, H. V. Golbetz, B. J. Carrie, W. R. Salyer, and B. D. Myers: The nature of the glomerular injury in minimal change and focal sclerosing glomerulopathies, *Am. J. Kid. Dis.,* 1:91, 1981.

206. Tejani, A., A. D. Nicastri, D. Sen, C. K. Chen, K. Phadke, O. Adamson, and K. M. H. Butt: Long-term evaluation of children with nephrotic syndrome and focal segmental glomerular sclerosis, *Nephron,* 35:225, 1983.

207. Beaufils, H., J. C. Alphonse, J. Guedon, and M. Legrain: Focal glomerulosclerosis: Natural history and treatment: A report of 70 cases, *Nephron,* 21:75, 1978.

208. Jenis, E. H., S. Teichman, W. A. Briggs, P. Sandler, C. E. Hollerman, P. L. Calcagno, M. R. Kneiser, G. E. Jensen, and J. E. Valeski: Focal segmental glomerulosclerosis, *Am. J. Med.,* 57:695, 1974.

209. Taylor, J., R. Novak, R. Christiansen, and E. T. Sorensen: Focal sclerosing glomerulopathy with adverse effects during pregnancy, *Arch. Intern. Med.,* 138:1695, 1978.

210. Sutton, J. M., J. Hopper, Jr., and C. G. Biava: Focal glomerular sclerosis and pregnancy, abstract, *Kidney Int.,* 14:664, 1978.

211. Habib, R.: Focal glomerular sclerosis, *Kidney Int.,* 4:355, 1973.

212. Brown, C. B., J. S. Cameron, D. R. Turner, C. Chantler, C. S. Ogg, D. G. Williams, and M. Bewick: Focal segmental glomerulosclerosis with rapid decline in renal function, *Clin. Nephrol.,* 10: 51, 1978.

213. Velosa, J. A., K. E. Holley, V. E. Torres, and K. P. Offord: Significance of proteinuria on the outcome of renal function in patients with focal segmental glomerulosclerosis, *Mayo Clin. Proc.,* 58: 568, 1983.

214. Nash, M. A., I. Greifer, H. Olbing, J. Bernstein, B. Bennett, and A. Spitzer: The significance of focal sclerotic lesions of glomeruli in children, *J. Pediatr.,* 88:806, 1976.

215. Mongeau, J.-G., L. Corneille, P. Robitaille, S. O'Regan, and M. Pelletier: Primary nephrosclerosis in childhood associated with focal glomerular sclerosis: Is long-term prognosis that severe?, *Kidney Int.,* 20:743, 1981.

216. Geary, D. F., M. Farine, P. Thorner, and R. Baumal: Response to cyclophosphamide in steroid-resistant focal segmental glomerulosclerosis: A reappraisal, *Clin. Nephrol.,* 22:109, 1984.

217. Cameron, J. S., D. R. Turner, and R. O. Weller: Focal glomerulosclerosis, in P. Kincaid-Smith, T. Mathew, and E. L. Becker (eds.), *Glomerulonephritis: Morphology, Natural History and Treatment,* Wiley, New York, 1973.

218. Korbet, S. M., M. M., Schwartz, and E. J. Lewis: The prognosis of focal segmental glomerular sclerosis of adulthood, *Medicine,* 65:304, 1986.

219. Pei, Y., T. Delmore, A. Katz, A. Lange, C. Rance, and D. Cattran: Focal glomerulosclerosis—A comparison between adults and children (abstract), *Kidney Int.,* 29:200, 1986.

220. Knowles, H. C., Jr.: Magnitude of the renal failure problem in diabetic patients, *Kidney Int.,* 6(suppl):2, 1974.

221. Gellman, D. D., C. L. Pirani, J. F. Soothill, R. C. Muehrcke, and R. M. Kark: Diabetic nephropathy: A clinical and pathologic study based on renal biopsies, *Medicine,* 38:321, 1959.

222. Brown, D. M., G. A. Andres, T. H. Hostetter, S. M. Mauer, R. Price, and M. A. Venkatachalam: Kidney complications, *Diabetes,* 31(suppl 1):71, 1982.

223. Mauer, S. M., M. W. Steffes, E. N. Ellis, D. E. R. Sutherland, D. M. Brown, and F. C. Goetz: Structural-functional relationships in diabetic nephropathy, *J. Clin. Invest.,* 74:1143, 1984.

224. Mauer, S. M., J. Barbosa, R. L. Vernier, C. M. Kjellstrand, T. J. Buselmeier, R. L. Simmons, J. S. Najarian, and F. C. Goetz: Development of diabetic vascular lesions in normal kidney transplanted into patients with diabetes mellitus, *N. Engl. J. Med.,* 295:916, 1976.

225. Westberg, N. G., and A. F. Michael: Immunohistopathology of diabetic glomerulosclerosis, *Diabetes,* 21:163, 1972.

226. Brownlee, M., H. Vlassara, and A. Cerami: Nonenzymatic glycosylation and the pathogenesis of diabetic complications, *Ann. Intern. Med.,* 101:527, 1984.

227. Chavers, B., D. Etzwiler, and A. F. Michael: Albumin deposition in dermal capillary basement membrane in insulin-dependent diabetes mellitus. A preliminary report, *Diabetes,* 30:275, 1981.

228. Bollinger, A., J. Frey, K. Jäger, J. Furrer, J. Seglias, and W. Siegenthaler: Patterns of diffusion through skin capillaries in patients with long-term diabetes, *N. Engl. J. Med.,* 307:1305, 1982.

229. Mauer, S. M., M. W. Steffes, A. F. Michael, and D. M. Brown: Studies of diabetic nephropathy in animals and man, *Diabetes,* 25:850, 1976.

230. Ireland, J. T., B. K. Patnark, and L. J. Duncan: Glomerular ultrastructure in secondary diabetes and normal subjects, *Diabetes,* 16:628, 1967.

231. Feingold, K. R., T. H. Lee, M. Y. Chung, and M. D. Siperstein: Muscle capillary basement membrane width in patients with vacor-induced diabetes mellitus, *J. Clin. Invest.,* 78:102, 1986.

232. Abouna, G. M., G. D. Kremer, S. K. Daddah, M. S. Al-Adnani, S. A. Kumar, and G. Kusma: Reversal of diabetic nephropathy in human cadaveric kidneys after transplantation into non-diabetic recipients, *Lancet,* 2:1274, 1983.

233. Mauer, S. M., M. W. Steffes, J. Connett, J. S. Najarian, D. E. R. Sutherland, and J. Barbosa: The development of lesions in the glomerular basement membrane and mesangium after transplantation of normal kidneys to diabetic patients, *Diabetes,* 32:948, 1983.

234. Bohman, S-O., G. Tyden, H. Wilczek, G. Lundgren, G. Jaremko, R. Gunnarsson, J. Östman, and C. G. Groth: Prevention of kidney graft diabetic nephropathy by pancreatic transplantation in man, *Diabetes,* 34:306, 1985.

235. Harrington, A. R., H. G. Hare, W. N. Chambers, and H. Valtin: Nodular glomerulosclerosis suspected during life in a patient without demonstrable diabetes mellitus, *N. Engl. J. Med.,* 275:206, 1966.

236. Ganeval, D., L-H. Noël, J-L. Preud'Homme, D. Droz, and J-P. Grünfeld: Light-chain deposition disease: Its relation with AL-type amyloidosis, *Kidney Int.,* 26:1, 1984.

237. Krolewski, A. S., J. H. Warram, A. Christlieb, E. J. Busick, and C. R. Kahn: The changing natural history of nephropathy in type 1 diabetes, *Am. J. Med.,* 78:785, 1985.

238. Marks, J. F., P. Raskin, and P. Stastny: Increase in capillary basement width in parents of children with type 1 diabetes mellitus. Association with HLA-DR4, *Diabetes,* 30:475, 1981.

239. Osterby, R.: Early phases of the development of diabetic glomerulopathy, *Acta Med. Scand., Suppl.* 574:1, 1975.

240. Cortes, P., F. Dumler, K. K. Venkatachalam, J. Goldman, K. S. S. Sastry, H. Venkatachalam, J. Bernstein, and N. W. Levin: Alterations in glomerular RNA in diabetic rats: Roles of glucagon and insulin, *Kidney Int.,* 20:491, 1981.

241. Spiro, R. G.: Biochemistry of the renal glomerular basement membrane and its alterations in diabetes mellitus, *N. Engl. J. Med.,* 288:1337, 1973.

242. McVerry, B. A., A. Hopp, C. Fisher, and E. R. Huehns: Production of pseudodiabetic renal glo-

merular changes in mice after repeated injections of glucosylated proteins, *Lancet,* 1:738, 1980.

243. Hostetter, T. H., H. G. Rennke, and B. M. Brenner: The case for intrarenal hypertension in the initiation and progression of diabetic and other glomerulopathies, *Am. J. Med.,* 72:375, 1982.

244. Zatz, R., and B. M. Brenner: Pathogenesis of diabetic microangiopathy. The hemodynamic view, *Am. J. Med.,* 80:443, 1986.

245. Mogensen, C. E.: Glomerular filtration rate and renal plasma flow in short-term and long-term juvenile diabetes mellitus, *Scand. J. Clin. Lab. Invest.,* 28:91, 1971.

246. Christiansen, J. S., J. Gammelgaard, B. Tronier, P. A. Svendsen, and H-H. Parving: Kidney function and size in diabetics before and during initial insulin treatment. *Kidney Int.,* 21:683, 1982.

247. Mogensen, C. E., and C. K. Christiansen: Predicting diabetic nephropathy in insulin-dependent patients, *N. Engl. J. Med.,* 311:89, 1984.

248. Mogensen, C. E.: Diabetes mellitus and the kidney, *Kidney Int.,* 21:673, 1982.

249. Zatz, R., B. R. Dunn, S. Anderson, H. G. Rennke, and B. M. Brenner: Prevention of diabetic glomerulopathy by pharmacological amelioration of glomerular capillary hypertension, *J. Clin. Invest.,* 77:1925, 1986.

250. Zatz, R., T. W. Meyer, H. G. Rennke, and B. M. Brenner: Predominance of hemodynamic rather than metabolic factors in the pathogenesis of diabetic nephropathy, *Proc. Natl. Acad. Sci. U.S.A.,* 82:5963, 1985.

251. Mogensen, C. E.: Long-term antihypertensive treatment inhibiting progression of diabetic nephropathy, *Br. Med. J.,* 285:685, 1982.

252. Parving, H-H., U. M. Smidt, A. R. Andersen, and P. A. Svendsen: Early aggressive antihypertensive treatment reduces rate of decline in kidney function in diabetic nephropathy, *Lancet,* 1:1175, 1983.

253. Parving, H-H., A. R. Andersen, E. Hommel, and U. Smidt: Effects of long-term antihypertensive treatment on kidney function in diabetic nephropathy, *Hypertension,* 7(suppl. II):II-114, 1985.

254. Mogensen, C. E.: Early glomerular hyperfiltration in insulin-dependent diabetics and late nephropathy, *Scand. J. Clin. Lab. Invest.,* 46:201, 1986.

255. Wiseman, M. J., A. J. Saunders, H. Keen, and G-C. Viberti: Effect of blood glucose control on increased glomerular filtration rate and kidney size in insulin-dependent diabetes, *N. Engl. J. Med.,* 312:617, 1985.

256. Hostetter, T. H., J. L. Troy, and B. M. Brenner: Glomerular hemodynamics in experimental diabetes mellitus, *Kidney Int.,* 19:410, 1981.

257. Skouborg, F., A. V. Nielsen, E. Lauritzen, and O. Hartkopp: Diameters of the retinal vessels in diabetic and normal subjects, *Diabetes,* 18:292, 1969.

258. Gundersen, H. J. G.: Peripheral blood flow and metabolic control in juvenile diabetes, *Diabetologia,* 10:225, 1974.

259. White, N. H., S. R. Waltman, T. Krupin, and J. V. Santiago: Reversal of abnormalities in ocular fluorophotometry in insulin-dependent diabetes after five to nine months of improved metabolic control, *Diabetes,* 31:80, 1982.

260. Knowler, W. C., P. H. Bennett, and E. J. Ballantine: Increased incidence of retinopathy in diabetes with elevated blood pressure. A six-year follow-up study in Pima Indians, *N. Engl. J. Med.,* 302:645, 1980.

261. Gay, A. J., and A. J. Rosenbaum: Retinal artery pressure in asymmetric diabetic retinopathy, *Arch. Ophthalmol.,* 75:758, 1977.

262. Beretta-Piccoli, C., P. Weidmann, and G. Keusch: Responsiveness of plasma renin and aldosterone in diabetes mellitus, *Kidney Int.,* 20:259, 1981.

263. Ballerman, B. J., K. L. Skorecki, and B. M. Brenner: Reduced glomerular angiotensin II receptor density in early untreated diabetes mellitus in the rat, *Am. J. Physiol.,* 247:F110, 1984.

264. Pfaffman, M. A., C. R. Ball, A. Darby, and R. Hilman: Insulin reversal of diabetes-induced inhibition of vascular contractility in the rat, *Am. J. Physiol.,* 242:H490, 1982.

265. Dighe, R. R., F. J. Rojas, L. Birnbaumer, and A. J. Garber: Glucagon-stimulatable adenyl cylcase in rat liver. The impact of streptozotocin-induced diabetes mellitus, *J. Clin. Invest.,* 73:1013, 1984.

266. Lipson, L. G.: Special problems in treatment of hypertension in the patient with diabetes mellitus, *Arch. Intern. Med.,* 144:1829, 1984.

267. Kasiske, B. L., M. P. O'Donnell, and W. F. Keane: Glucose-induced increases in renal hemodynamic function. Possible modulation by renal prostaglandins, *Diabetes,* 34:360, 1985.

268. Schambelan, M., S. Blake, J. Sraer, M. Bens, M-P. Nivez, and F. Wahbe: Increased prostaglandin production by glomeruli isolated from rats with streptozotocin-induced diabetes mellitus, *J. Clin. Invest.,* 75:404, 1985.

269. Unger, R. H., and L. Orci: Glucagon and the A cell. Physiology and pathophysiology, *N. Engl. J. Med.,* 304:1518, 1575, 1981.

270. Parving, H-H., J. S. Christiansen, I. Noer, B. Tronier, and C. E. Mogensen: The effect of glucagon

infusion on kidney function in short-term insulin-dependent juvenile diabetics, *Diabetologia,* 19:350, 1980.

271. Brøchner-Mortensen, J.: The glomerular filtration rate during moderate hyperglycemia in normal man, *Acta Med. Scand.,* 194:31, 1973.

272. Wiseman, M. J., G-C. Viberti, and H. Keen: Threshold effect of plasma glucose in the glomerular hyperfiltration of diabetes, *Nephron,* 38:257, 1984.

273. Brezis, M., P. Silva, and F. H. Epstein: Amino acids induce renal vasodilation in isolated perfused kidney: Coupling to oxidative metabolism, *Am. J. Physiol.,* 247:H999, 1984.

274. Viberti, G-C., and H. Keen: The patterns of proteinuria in diabetes mellitus. Relevance to pathogenesis and prevention of diabetic nephropathy, *Diabetes,* 33:686, 1984.

275. Ghiggeri, G. M., G. Candiano, G. Delfino, and C. Queirolo: Electrical charge of serum and urinary albumin in normal and diabetic humans, *Kidney Int.,* 28:168, 1985.

276. Mogensen, C. E., E. Vittinghus, and K. Sølling: Abnormal albumin excretion after two provocative renal tests in diabetes: Physical exercise and lysine injection, *Kidney Int.,* 16:385, 1979.

277. Viberti, G-C., R. J. Jarrett, U. Mahmud, R. D. Hill, A. Argyropoulos, and H. Keen: Microalbuminuria as a predictor of clinical nephropathy in insulin-dependent diabetes mellitus, *Lancet,* 1:1430, 1982.

278. Mogensen, C. E., and C. K. Christensen: Predicting diabetic nephropathy in insulin-dependent patients, *N. Engl. J. Med.,* 311:89, 1984.

279. Fabre, J., L. P. Balant, P. G. Dayer, H. M. Fox, and A. T. Vernet: The kidney in maturity onset diabetes mellitus: A clinical study of 510 patients, *Kidney Int.,* 21:730, 1982.

280. Myers, B. D., J. A. Winetz, F. Chui, and A. S. Michaels: Mechanisms of proteinuria in diabetic nephropathy: A study of glomerular barrier function, *Kidney Int.,* 21:633, 1982.

281. Friedman, E. A.: Diabetic nephropathy: Strategies in prevention and management, *Kidney Int.,* 21:780, 1982.

282. Mogensen, C. E.: Microalbuminuria predicts clinical proteinuria and early mortality in maturity-onset diabetes, *N. Engl. J. Med.,* 310:356, 1984.

283. Lestradet, H., L. Papoz, Cl. H. De Menibus, F. Levavasseur, J. Besse, L. Billaud, F. Battistelli, Ph. Tric, and F. Lestradet: Long-term study of mortality and vascular complications in juvenile-onset (type 1) diabetes, *Diabetes,* 30:175, 1981.

284. Heptinstall, R. H.: *Pathology of the Kidney,* 3d ed., Little, Brown, Boston, 1983, chap. 26.

285. Urizar, R. E., A. Schwartz, F. Top, Jr., and R. L. Vernier: The nephrotic syndrome in children with diabetes mellitus of recent onset: Report of five cases, *N. Engl. J. Med.,* 281:173, 1969.

286. Kasinath, B. S., S. K. Mujais, B. H. Spargo, and A. I. Katz: Nondiabetic renal disease in patients with diabetes mellitus, *Am. J. Med.,* 75:613, 1983.

287. Rao, K. V., and J. T. Crosson: Idiopathic membranous glomerulonephritis in diabetic patients. Report of three cases and review of the literature, *Arch. Intern. Med.,* 140:624, 1980.

288. Goldstein, D. A., and S. G. Massry: Diabetic nephropathy: Clinical course and effect of hemodialysis, *Nephron,* 20:286, 1978.

289. Fang, L. S-T.: Contrast medium-induced acute renal failure, *Medical Gr. Rounds,* 2:263, 1983.

290. Vittinghus, E., and C. E. Mogensen: Graded exercise and protein excretion in diabetic man and the effect of insulin treatment, *Kidney Int.,* 21:725, 1982.

291. The Kroc Collaborative Study Group: Blood glucose control and the evolution of diabetic retinopathy and albuminuria. A preliminary multicenter trial, *N. Engl. J. Med.,* 311:365, 1984.

292. Holman, R. R., V. Mayon-White, C. Orde-Peckar, J. Steemson, B. Smith, K. McPherson, C. Rizza, A. H. Knight, T. L. Dornan, J. Howard-Williams, L. Jenkins, R. Rolfe, D. Barbour, P. Y. W. Poon, J. I. Mann, A. J. Bron, and R. C. Turner: Prevention of deterioration of renal and sensory-nerve function by more intensive management of insulin-dependent diabetic patients. A two-year randomised prospective study, *Lancet,* 1:204, 1983.

293. Bending, J. J., G-C. Viberti, P. J. Watkins, and H. Keen: Intermittent clinical proteinuria and renal function in diabetes: Evolution and the effect of glycemic control, *Br. Med. J.,* 292:83, 1986.

294. Steno Study Group: Effect of 6 months of strict metabolic control on eye and kidney function in insulin-dependent diabetics with background retinopathy, *Lancet,* 1:121, 1982.

295. Viberti, G-C., R. W. Bilous, D. Mackintosh, J. J. Bending, and H. Keen: Long term correction of hyperglycaemia and progression of renal failure in insulin dependent diabetes, *Br. Med. J.,* 286:598, 1983.

296. Lauritzen, T., H-W. Larsen, K. Frost-Larsen, T. Deckert, and the Steno Study Group: Effect of 1 year of near-normal blood glucose levels on retinopathy in insulin-dependent diabetics, *Lancet,* 1:200, 1983.

297. Taguma, Y., Y. Kitamoto, G. Futaki, H. Ueda, H. Monma, M. Ishizaki, H. Takahashi, H. Sekino, and Y. Sasaki: Effect of captopril on heavy proteinuria in azotemic diabetics, *N. Engl. J. Med.,* 313:1617, 1985.

298. Kaysen, G. A., J. Gambertoglio, I. Jimenez, H. Jones, and F. N. Hutchison: Effect of dietary protein intake on albumin homeostasis in nephrotic patients, *Kidney Int.,* 29:572, 1986.

299. Vale, J. A., S. J. Van de Pette, and T. M. L. Price: Peripheral gangrene complicating beta-blockade, *Lancet,* 2:412, 1977.

300. Skinner, D. J., and R. I. Misbin: Uses of propranolol, *N. Engl. J. Med.,* 293:1205, 1975.

301. Shepherd, A. M. M., M-S. Lin, and T. K. Keeton: Hypoglycemia-induced hypertension in a diabetic patient on metoprolol, *Ann. Intern. Med.,* 94:357, 1981.

302. Lager, I., G. Blohmé, and U. Smith: Effect of cardioselective and nonselective β-blockade on the hypoglycaemic response in insulin-dependent diabetics, *Lancet,* 1:458, 1979.

303. Massry, S. G., E. I. Feinstein, and D. A. Goldstein: Early dialysis in diabetic patients with chronic renal failure, *Nephron,* 23:2, 1979.

304. Najarian, J. S., D. E. R. Sutherland, R. L. Simmons, R. J. Howard, C. M. Kjellstrand, S. M. Mauer, W. Kennedy, R. Ramsey, J. Barbosa, and F. C. Goetz: Kidney transplantation for the uremic diabetic patient, *Surg. Gynecol. Obstet.,* 144:682, 1977.

305. Shyh, T. P., M. M. Beyer, and E. A. Friedman: Treatment of the uremic diabetic, *Nephron,* 40:129, 1985.

306. Mitchell, J. C., P. P. Frohnert, S. B. Kurtz, and C. F. Anderson: Chronic peritoneal dialysis in juvenile-onset diabetes mellitus: A comparison with hemodialysis, *Mayo Clin. Proc.,* 53:775, 1978.

307. Amair, P., R. Khanna, B. Leibel, A. Pierratos, S. Vas, E. Meema, G. Blair, L. Chisolm, M. Vas, W. Zingg, G. Digenis, and D. Oreopoulos: Continuous ambulatory peritoneal dialysis in diabetics with end-stage renal disease, *N. Engl. J. Med.,* 306:625, 1982.

308. Popovich, R. P., J. W. Moncrief, K. D. Nolph, A. J. Ghods, Z. J. Twardowski, and W. K. Pyle: Continuous ambulatory peritoneal dialysis, *Ann. Intern. Med.,* 88:449, 1978.

309. Peters, C., D. E. R. Sutherland, R. L. Simmons, D. S. Fryd, and J. S. Najarian: Patient and graft survival in amputated versus nonamputated diabetic primary renal allograft recipients, *Transplantation,* 32:498, 1981.

310. Editorial: Transplantation of pancreas with kidney, *Lancet,* 1:720, 1982.

311. Sutherland, D. E. R., F. C. Goetz, B. A. Elick, and J. S. Najarian: Experience with 49 segmental pancreas transplants in 45 diabetic patients, *Transplantation,* 34:330, 1982.

312. Kyle, R. A., and E. D. Bayrd: Amyloidosis: Review of 236 cases, *Medicine,* 54:271, 1975.

313. Kyle, R. A., and P. R. Greipp: Amyloidosis (AL). Clinical and laboratory features in 229 cases, *Mayo Clin. Proc.* 58:665, 1983.

314. Triger, D. R., and A. M. Joekes: Renal amyloidosis—A fourteen-year follow-up, *Q. J. Med.,* 42:15, 1972.

315. de Beer, F. C., R. K. Mallya, E. A. Fagan, J. G. Lanham, G. R. V. Hughes, and M. B. Pepys: Serum amyloid A protein concentration in inflammatory diseases and its relationship to the incidence of reactive systemic amyloidosis, *Lancet,* 2:231, 1982.

316. Pras, M., E. C. Franklin, S. Shibolet, and B. Frangione: Amyloidosis associated with renal cell carcinoma of the AA type, *Am. J. Med.,* 73:426, 1982.

317. Rashid, H., D. Blake, R. Gokal, D. Gooptu, and D. N. S. Kerr: The association of renal amyloidosis with regional enteritis (Crohn's disease)—report of two cases and review of the literature, *Clin. Nephrol.,* 14:154, 1980.

318. Dietrick, R. B., and S. Russi: Tabulation and review of autopsy findings in fifty-five paraplegics, *J. Am. Med. Assoc.,* 166:41, 1958.

319. Meyerhoff, J.: Familial Mediterranean fever: Report of a large family, review of the literature, and discussion of the frequency of amyloidosis, *Medicine,* 59:66, 1980.

320. Petaxas, P.: Familial Mediterranean fever and amyloidosis, *Kidney Int.,* 20:676, 1981.

321. Nakamoto, Y., S. Hamanaka, T. Akihama, A. B. Miura, and Y. Uesaka: Renal involvement patterns of amyloid nephropathy: A comparison with diabetic nephropathy, *Clin. Nephrol.,* 22:188, 1984.

322. Noel, L. H., D. Droz, D. Ganeval, and J. P. Grunfeld: Renal granular monoclonal light chain deposits: Morphological aspects in 11 cases, *Clin. Nephrol.,* 21:263, 1984.

323. Tubbs, R. R., G. N. Gephardt, J. T. McMahon, P. M. Hall, R. Valenzuela, and D. G. Vidt: Light chain nephropathy, *Am. J. Med.,* 71:263, 1981.

324. Lapenas, D. J., S. J. Drewry, R. L. Luke, and D. A. Leeber: Crescentic light-chain glomerulopathy. Report of a case. *Arch. Pathol. Lab. Med.,* 107:319, 1983.

325. Knobler, H., J. Kopolovic, Y. Kleinman, D. Rubinger, J. Silver, M. M. Friedlander, and M. M.

Popovtzer: Multiple myeloma presenting as dense deposit disease. Light chain nephropathy, *Nephron,* 34:58, 1983.

326. Glenner, G. G.: Amyloid deposits and amyloidosis. The β-fibrilloses, *N. Engl. J. Med.,* 302:1283, 1333, 1980.

327. Lanham, J. G., M. L. Meltzer, F. C. de Beer, G. R. V. Hughes, and M. B. Pepys: Familial amyloidosis of Ostertag, *Q. J. Med.,* 51:25, 1982.

328. Stone, M. J., and E. P. Frenkel: The clinical spectrum of light chain myeloma: A study of 35 patients with special reference to the occurrence of amyloidosis, *Am. J. Med.,* 58:601, 1975.

329. Durie, B. G. M., B. Persky, B. J. Soehnlen, T. M. Grogan, and S. E. Salmon: Amyloid production in human myeloma stem-cell culture, with morphologic evidence of amyloid secretion by associated macrophages, *N. Engl. J. Med.,* 307:1689, 1982.

330. Shirahama, T., M. D. Benson, A. S. Cohen, and A. Tanaka: Fibrillar assemblage of variable segments of immunoglobulin light chains: An electron microscopic study, *J. Immunol.,* 110:21, 1973.

331. Solomon, A., B. Frangione, and E. C. Franklin: Bence Jones proteins and light chains of immunoglobulins. Preferential association of the $V_{\lambda VI}$ subgroup of human light chains with amyloidosis AL (λ), *J. Clin. Invest.,* 70:453, 1982.

332. Hill, G. S., L. Morel-Maroger, J-P. Méry, J. C. Brouet, and F. Mignon: Renal lesions in multiple myeloma: Their relationship to associated protein abnormalities, *Am. J. Kid. Dis.,* 2:423, 1983.

333. Sclinger, M. J., K. P. W. J. McAdam, M. M. Kaplan, J. D. Sipe, S. N. Vogel, and D. L. Rosenstreich: Monokine-induced synthesis of serum amyloid A protein by hepatocytes, *Nature,* 285:498, 1980.

334. Rosenthal, C. J., and L. Sullivan: Serum amyloid A: Evidence for its origin in polymorphonuclear leukocytes, *J. Clin. Invest.,* 62:1181, 1978.

335. Kushner, I., H. Gewurz, and M. D. Benson: C-reactive protein and the acute-phase response, *J. Lab. Clin. Med.,* 97:739, 1981.

336. Rosenthal, C. J., and E. C. Franklin: Variation with age and disease of an amyloid A protein-related serum component, *J. Clin. Invest.,* 55:746, 1975.

337. Knecht, A., F. C. de Beer, and M. Pras: Serum amyloid A protein in familial Mediterranean fever, *Ann. Intern. Med.,* 102:71, 1985.

338. Lavie, G., D. Zucker-Franklin, and E. C. Franklin: Degradation of serum amyloid A protein by surface-associated enzymes of human blood monocytes, *J. Exp. Med.,* 148:1020, 1978.

339. Wegelius, O., A-M. Teppo, and C. P. J. Maury: Reduced amyloid degrading activity in serum in amyloidosis associated with rheumatoid arthritis, *Br. Med. J.,* 284:617, 1982.

340. Maury, C. P. J., and A-M. Teppo: Mechanism of reduced amyloid-A-degrading activity in serum of patients with secondary amyloidosis, *Lancet,* 2:234, 1982.

341. Falck, H. M., T. Tornroth, and O. Wegelius: Predominantly vascular amyloid deposition in the kidney in patients with minimal or no proteinuria, *Clin. Nephrol.,* 19:137, 1983.

342. Luke, R. G., M. E. Allison, J. F. Davidson, and W. P. Duguid: Hyperkalemia and renal tubular acidosis due to renal amyloidosis, *Ann. Intern. Med.,* 70:1211, 1969.

343. Carone, F. A., and F. H. Epstein: Nephrogenic diabetes insipidus caused by amyloid disease: Evidence in man of the role of collecting ducts in concentrating urine, *Am. J. Med.,* 29:539, 1960.

344. Westermark, P., and B. Stenkvist: A new method for the diagnosis of systemic amyloidosis, *Arch. Intern. Med.,* 132:522, 1973.

345. Ogg, C. S., J. S. Cameron, D. G. Williams, and D. R. Turner: Presentation and course of primary amyloidosis of the kidney, *Clin. Nephrol.,* 15:9, 1981.

346. Michael, J., and N. F. Jones: Spontaneous remissions of nephrotic syndrome in renal amyloidosis, *Br. Med. J.,* 1:1592, 1978.

347. Kyle, R. A., R. D. Wagoner, and K. E. Holley: Primary systemic amyloidosis. Resolution of the nephrotic syndrome with melphalan and prednisone, *Arch. Intern. Med.,* 142:1445, 1982.

348. Cohen, H. J.: Combination chemotherapy for primary amyloidosis reconsidered, *Ann. Intern. Med.,* 89:572, 1978.

349. Horne, M. K.: Improvement in amyloidosis, *Ann. Intern. Med.,* 83:281, 1975.

350. Kyle, R. A., and P. R. Greipp: Primary systemic amyloidosis: Comparison of melphalan and prednisone versus placebo, *Blood,* 52:818, 1978.

351. Kyle, R. A., R. V. Pierre, and E. D. Bayrd: Primary amyloidosis and acute leukemia associated with melphalan therapy, *Blood,* 44:333, 1974.

352. Ravid, M., M. Robson, and I. Kedar (Keizman): Prolonged colchicine treatment in four patients with amyloidosis, *Ann. Intern. Med.,* 87:568, 1977.

353. Scheinberg, M. A., J. C. Pernambuco, and M. D. Benson: DMSO and colchicine therapy in amyloid disease, *Ann. Rheum. Dis.,* 43:421, 1984.

354. Ravid, M., J. Shapira, R. Lang, and I. Kedar: Prolonged dimethylsulphoxide treatment in 13 pa-

tients with systemic amyloidosis, *Ann. Rheum. Dis.,* 41:587, 1982.

355. Falck, H. M., C. P. J. Maury, A-M. Teppo, and O. Wegelius: Persistently high serum amyloid A protein and C-reactive protein levels correlate with rapid progression of secondary amyloidosis, *Br. Med. J.,* 286:1391, 1983.

356. Zemer, D., M. Pras, E. Sohar, M. Modan, S. Cabili, and J. Gafni: Colchicine in the prevention and treatment of the amyloidosis of familial Mediterranean fever, *N. Engl. J. Med.,* 314:1001, 1986.

357. Dirkman, S. H., T. Kahn, D. Gribetz, and J. Churg: Resolution of renal amyloidosis, *Am. J. Med.,* 63: 430, 1977.

358. Lowenstein, J., and G. Gallo: Remission of the nephrotic syndrome in renal amyloidosis, *N. Engl. J. Med.,* 282:128, 1970.

359. Shirahama, T., and A. S. Cohen: Blockage of amyloid induction by colchicine in an animal model, *J. Exp. Med.,* 140:1102, 1974.

360. Jacob, E. T., N. Bar-Nathan, Z. Shapira, and J. Gafni: Renal transplantation in the amyloidosis of familial Mediterranean fever: Experience in ten cases, *Arch. Intern. Med.,* 139:1135, 1979.

361. Matzner, Y., and A. Brzezinski: C5a-inhibitor deficiency in peritoneal fluids from patients with familial Mediterranean fever, *N. Engl. J. Med.,* 311: 287, 1984.

362. Jones, N. F.: Renal amyloidosis: Pathogenesis and therapy, *Clin. Nephrol.,* 6:459, 1976.

363. Editorial: Treatment of renal amyloidosis, *Lancet,* 1:1062, 1980.

364. Helin, H., A. Pasternack, H. Falck, and B. Kuhlback: Recurrence of renal amyloid and de novo membranous glomerulonephritis after transplantation, *Transplantation,* 32:6, 1981.

365. Case Records of the Massachusetts General Hospital (Case 1-1981), *N. Engl. J. Med.,* 304:33, 1981.

366. Korbet, S. M., M. M. Schwartz, B. F. Rosenberg, R. K. Sibley, and E. J. Lewis: Immunotactoid glomerulopathy, *Medicine,* 64:228, 1985.

367. Alpers, C. E., H. G. Rennke, J. Hopper, Jr., and C. G. Biava: Fibrillary glomerulonephritis: A morphological entity with unusual immunofluorescence features, *Kidney Int.* (in press), 1987.

368. Earley, L. E., and M. Forland: Nephrotic syndrome, in L. E. Earley and C. W. Gottschalk (eds.), *Strauss and Welt's Diseases of the Kidney,* 3d ed., Little, Brown, Boston, 1979.

369. Kasiske, B. L., and J. T. Crosson: Renal disease in patients with massive obesity, *Arch. Intern. Med.,* 146:1105, 1986.

370. Wesson, D. E., N. A. Kurtzman, and J. P. From-

mer: Massive obesity and nephrotic proteinuria with a normal renal biopsy, *Nephron,* 40:235, 1985.

371. Kumar, A., and A. P. Shapiro: Proteinuria and nephrotic syndrome induced by renin in patients with renal artery stenosis, *Arch. Intern. Med.,* 140: 1631, 1980.

372. Takeda, R., S. Morimoto, K. Uchida, T. Kigoshi, T. Sumitami, and F. Matsubara: Effect of captopril on both hypertension and proteinuria: Report of a case of renovascular hypertension associated with nephrotic syndrome, *Arch. Intern. Med.,* 140: 1531, 1980.

373. Mujais, S. K., D. S. Emmanouel, B. S. Kasinath, and B. H. Spargo: Marked proteinuria in hypertensive nephrosclerosis, *Am. J. Nephrol.,* 5:190, 1985.

374. Schneller, M., S. E. Braga, H. Moser, A. Zimmermann, and O. Oetliker: Congenital nephrotic syndrome: Clinicopathological heterogeneity and prenatal diagnosis, *Clin. Nephrol.,* 19:243, 1983.

375. Sibley, R. K., J. Mahan, S. M. Mauer, and R. L. Vernier: A clinicopathologic study of forty-eight infants with nephrotic syndrome, *Kidney Int.,* 27: 544, 1985.

376. Bennett, W. M., J. E. Musgrove, R. A. Campbell, D. Elliot, R. Cox, R. E. Brooks, E. W. Lovrien, R. K. Beals, and G. A. Porter: The nephropathy of the nail-patella syndrome. Clinicopathologic analysis of 11 kindreds, *Am. J. Med.,* 54:304, 1973.

377. Hendrickse, R. G., and A. Adeniyi: Quartan malarial nephrotic syndrome in children, *Kidney Int.,* 16:64, 1979.

378. Andrade, Z. A., and H. Rocha: Schistosomal glomerulopathy, *Kidney Int.,* 16:23, 1979.

379. Gaboardi, F., L. Perletti, M. Cambie, and M. J. Mihatsch: Dermatitis herpetiformis and nephrotic syndrome, *Clin. Nephrol.,* 20:49, 1983.

380. Hertz, P., H. Yager, and J. A. Richardson: Probenecid-induced nephrotic syndrome, *Arch. Pathol.,* 94:241, 1972.

381. Scoble, J. E., J. S. Uff, and J. B. Eastwood: Nifedipine nephritis (letter), *Clin. Nephrol.,* 21:302, 1984.

382. Maryniak, R. K., M. R. First, and M. A. Weiss: Transplant glomerulopathy: Evolution of morphologically distinct changes, *Kidney Int.,* 27:799, 1985.

383. Rapoport, A., D. A. Davidson, G. A. Deveber, G. N. Ranking, and C. R. McLean: Idiopathic focal proliferative nephritis associated with persistent hematuria and normal renal function, *Ann. Intern. Med.,* 73:921, 1970.

384. Baldwin, D. S., M. C. Gluck, J. Lowenstein, and

G. R. Gallo: Lupus nephritis: Clinical course as related to morphologic forms and their transitions, *Am. J. Med.,* 62:12, 1977.

385. Berger, J.: IgA glomerular deposits in renal disease, *Transplant Proc.,* 1:939, 1969.

386. Namato, Y., Y. Asano, K. Dohi, M. Fujioka, H. Iida, Y. Kibe, N. Hattori, and J. Takeuchi: Primary IgA glomerulonephritis: Clinicopathological and immunohistological characteristics, *Q. J. Med.,* 47: 495, 1978.

387. Rodicio, J. L.: Idiopathic IgA nephropathy, *Kidney Int.,* 25:717, 1984.

388. Nicholls, K. M., K. F. Fairley, J. P. Dowling, and P. Kincaid-Smith: The clinical course of mesangial IgA associated nephropathy in adults, *Q. J. Med.,* 53:227, 1984.

389. Hyman, L. R., J. P. Wagnild, G. J. Beirne, and P. M. Burkholder: Immunoglobulin A distribution in glomerular disease: Analysis of immunofluorescence localization and pathogenetic significance, *Kidney Int.,* 3:397, 1973.

390. Hasbargen, J. A., and J. B. Copley: Utility of skin biopsy in the diagnosis of IgA nephropathy, *Am. J. Kid. Dis.,* 6:100, 1985.

391. Woodroffe, A. J., A. A. Gormly, P. E. McKenzie, A. M. Wootton, A. J. Thompson, A. E. Seymour, and A. R. Clarkson: Immunologic studies in IgA nephropathy, *Kidney Int.,* 18:366, 1980.

392. Czerkinsky, C., W. J. Koopman, S. Jackson, J. E. Collins, S. S. Crago, R. E. Schrohenloher, B. A. Julian, J. H. Galla, and J. Mestecky: Circulating immune complexes and immunoglobulin A rheumatoid factor in patients with mesangial immunoglobulin A nephropathies, *J. Clin. Invest.,* 77: 1931, 1986.

393. Waldo, F. B., L. Beischel, and C. D. West: IgA synthesis by lymphocytes from patients with IgA and their relatives, *Kidney Int.,* 29:1229, 1986.

394. Trascasa, M. L., J. Egido, J. Sancho, and L. Hernando: IgA glomerulonephritis (Berger's disease): Evidence of high serum levels of polymeric IgA, *Clin. Exp. Immunol.,* 42:247, 1980.

395. Valentijn, R. M., J. Radl, J. J. Haaijman, B. J. Vermeer, J. J. Weening, R. H. Kauffman, M. R. Daha, and L. A. van Es: Circulating and mesangial secretory component-binding IgA-1 in primary IgA nephropathy, *Kidney Int.,* 26:760, 1984.

396. Tomino, Y., H. Sakai, M. Miura, M. Endoh, and Y. Nomoto: Detection of polymeric IgA in glomeruli from patients with IgA nephropathy, *Clin. Exp. Immunol.,* 49:419, 1982.

397. Rifai, A., and K. Millard: Glomerular deposition of immune complexes prepared with monomeric

or polymeric IgA, *Clin. Exp. Immunol.,* 60:363, 1985.

398. Bene, M. C., G. Faure, B. Hurault de Ligny, M. Kessler, and J. Duheille: Immunoglobulin A nephropathy. Quantitative immunohisto-morphometry of the tonsillar plasma cells: Evidence of inversion of the immunoglobulin A versus immunoglobulin G secreting cell balance, *J. Clin. Invest.,* 71:1342, 1983.

399. Emancipator, S. N., G. R. Gallo, and M. E. Lamm: Experimental IgA nephropathy induced by oral immunization, *J. Exp. Med.,* 157:572, 1983.

400. Clarkson, A. R., A. J. Woodroffe, K. M. Bannister, J. D. Lomax-Smith, and I. Aarons: The syndrome of IgA nephropathy, *Clin. Nephrol.,* 21:7, 1984.

401. Rifai, A., and M. Mannik: Clearance of circulating IgA immune complexes is mediated by a specific receptor on Kupffer cells in mice, *J. Exp. Med.,* 160:125, 1984.

402. Gormly, A. A., P. S. Smith, A. E. Seymour, A. R. Clarkson, and A. J. Woodroffe: IgA glomerular deposits in experimental cirrhosis, *Am. J. Pathol.,* 104:50, 1981.

403. Callard, P., G. Feldman, D. Prandi, M. F. Belair, C. Mandet, Y. Weiss, P. Druet, J. P. Benhamou, and J. Bariety: Immune complex type glomerulonephritis in cirrhosis of the liver, *Am. J. Pathol.,* 80: 329, 1975.

404. Nochy, D., P. Callard, B. Bellon, J. Bariety, and P. Druet: Association of overt glomerulonephritis and liver disease: A study of 34 patients, *Clin. Nephrol.,* 6:422, 1976.

405. Kater, L., A. C. Jöbsis, E. H. Baart de la Faille-Kuyper, A. J. M. Vogten, and R. Grijm: Alcoholic hepatic disease. Specificity of IgA deposits in liver, *Am. J. Clin. Pathol.,* 71:51, 1979.

405a. Schifferli, J. A., Y. C. Ng, and D. K. Peters: The role of complement and its receptors in the elimination of immune complexes, *N. Engl. J. Med.,* 315:488, 1986.

406. Julian, B. A., P. A. Quiggins, J. S. Thompson, S. Y. Woodford, K. Gleason, and R. J. Wyatt: Familial IgA nephropathy. Evidence of an inherited mechanism of disease, *N. Engl. J. Med.,* 312:202, 1985.

407. Pape, J. F., O. J. Mellbye, B. Øystese, and E. K. Brodwall: Glomerulonephritis in dermatitis herpetiformis, *Acta Med. Scand.,* 203:445, 1978.

408. Helin, H., J. Mustonen, T. Revnala, and A. Pasternack: IgA nephropathy associated with celiac disease and dermatitis herpetiformis, *Arch. Pathol.,* 107:324, 1983.

409. Jennette, J. C., A. L. Ferguson, M. A. Moore, and D. G. Freeman: IgA nephropathy associated with

seronegative spondylarthropathies, *Arthr. Rheum.,* 25:144, 1982.

410. Shu, K-H., J-D. Liau, Y-F. Yang, Y-S. Lu, J-Y. Wang, J-L. Lau, and G. Chan: Glomerulonephritis in ankylosing spondylitis, *Clin. Nephrol.,* 25:169, 1986.

411. Ramirez, G., J. B. Stinson, E. T. Zaweada, and F. Moatamed: IgA nephritis associated with mycosis fungoides. Report of two cases. *Arch. Intern. Med.,* 141:1287, 1981.

412. Cohen, A. J., and E. D. Rosenstein: IgA nephropathy associated with disseminated tuberculosis, *Arch. Intern. Med.,* 145:554, 1985.

413. Endo, Y., and M. Hara: Glomerular IgA deposits in pulmonary diseases, *Kidney Int.,* 29:557, 1986.

414. Mustonen, J., H. Helin, and A. Pasternack: IgA nephropathy associated with bronchial small-cell carcinoma, *Am. J. Clin. Pathol.,* 76:652, 1981.

415. Kashiwabara, H., H. Shishido, S. Tomura, H. Tuchida, and T. Miyajima: Strong association between IgA nephropathy and HLA-DR4 antigen, *Kidney Int.,* 22:377, 1982.

416. Hiki, Y., Y. Kobayashi, S. Tateno, M. Sada, and N. Kashiwagi: Strong association of HLA-DR 4 with benign IgA nephropathy, *Nephron,* 32:222, 1982.

417. Praga, M., V. Gutierrez-Millet, J. J. Navas, L. M. Ruilope, J. M. Morales, J. M. Alcazar, I. Bello, and J. L. Rodicio: Acute worsening of renal function during episodes of macroscopic hematuria in IgA nephropathy, *Kidney Int.,* 28:69, 1985.

418. Lévy, M., G. Gonzalez-Burchard, M. Broyer, J-P. Dommergues, M. Foulard, J-P. Sorez, and R. Habib: Berger's disease in children. Natural history and outcome, *Medicine,* 64:157, 1985.

419. Abuelo, J. G., A. R. Esparza, R. A. Matarese, R. G. Endreny, J. S. Carvalho, and S. R. Allegra: Crescentic IgA nephropathy, *Medicine,* 63:396, 1984.

420. Mustonen, J., A. Pasternack, and I. Rantala: The nephrotic syndrome in IgA glomerulonephritis: Response to corticosteroid therapy, *Clin. Nephrol.,* 20:172, 1983.

421. Abreo, K., and S-F. Wen: A case of IgA nephropathy with an unusual response to corticosteroid and immunosuppressive therapy, *Am. J. Kid. Dis.,* 3:54, 1983.

422. Clarkson, A. R., A. E. Seymour, H. A. Thompson, W. D. G. Haynes, Y.-L. Chan, and B. Jackson: IgA nephropathy: A syndrome of uniform morphology, diverse clinical features, and uncertain prognosis, *Clin. Nephrol.,* 8:459, 1977.

423. Frascà, G. M., A. Vangelista, G. Biagini, and V. Bonomini: Immunological tubulo-interstitial deposits in IgA nephropathy, *Kidney Int.,* 22:184, 1982.

424. Hood, S. A., J. A. Velosa, K. E. Holley, and J. V. Donadio, Jr.: IgA-IgG nephropathy: Predictive indices of progressive disease, *Clin. Nephrol.,* 16:55, 1981.

425. Van de Putte, L. B. A., G. B. de la Riviere, and P. J. C. van Vriesman: Recurrent or persistent hematuria: Sign of mesangial immune-complex deposition, *N. Engl. J. Med.,* 290:1165, 1974.

426. Kupor, L. R., J. D. Mullins, and J. P. McPhaul, Jr: Immunopathologic findings in idiopathic renal hematuria, *Arch. Intern. Med.,* 135:1204, 1975.

427. Migone, L., G. Olivetti, L. Allegri, and P. Dall'Aglio: Mesangioproliferative glomerulonephritis, *Clin. Nephrol.,* 13:219, 1980.

428. Trachtman, H., R. A. Weiss, B. Bennett, and I. Greifer: Isolated hematuria in children: Indications for a renal biopsy, *Kidney Int.,* 25:94, 1984.

429. Berger, J., H. Yaneva, B. Nabarra, and C. Barbanel: Recurrence of mesangial deposition of IgA after renal transplantation, *Kidney Int.,* 7:232, 1975.

430. Clarkson, A. R., A. E. Seymour, A. J. Woodroffe, P. E. McKenzie, Y.-L. Chan, and A. M. Wootton: Controlled trial of phenytoin therapy in IgA nephropathy, *Clin. Nephrol.,* 13:215, 1980.

431. Egido, J., F. Rivera, J. Sancho, A. Barat, and L. Hernando: Phenytoin in IgA nephropathy: A long-term controlled trial, *Nephron,* 38:30, 1984.

432. McConville, J. M., C. D. West, and A. J. McAdams: Familial and non-familial benign haematuria, *J. Pediatr.,* 69:207, 1966.

433. Johnston, C., and S. Shuler: Recurrent haematuria in childhood: A five-year followup, *Arch. Dis. Child.,* 44:483, 1969.

434. Glasgow, E. F., M. W. Moncrieff, and R. H. R. White: Symptomless hematuria in childhood, *Br. Med. J.,* 2:687, 1970.

435. Labovitz, E. D., S. R. Steinmuller, L. W. Henderson, D. K. McCurdy, and M. Goldberg: "Benign" hematuria with focal glomerulonephritis in adults, *Ann. Intern. Med.,* 77:723, 1972.

436. Brown, E. A., K. Upadhyaya, J. P. Hayslett, M. Kashgarian, and N. J. Siegel: The clinical course of mesangial proliferative glomerulonephritis, *Medicine,* 58:295, 1979.

437. Pardo, V., G. Berian, D. F. Levi, and J. Strauss: Benign primary hematuria: Clinicopathologic study of 65 patients, *Am. J. Med.,* 67:817, 1979.

438. Tina, L., E. Jenis, P. Jose, C. Medani, Z. Papadopoulou, and P. Calcagno: The glomerular basement membrane in benign familial hematuria, *Clin. Nephrol.,* 17:1, 1982.

439. Rogers, P. W., N. A. Kurtzman, S. M. Bunn, and M. G. White: Familial benign essential hematuria, *Arch. Intern. Med.,* 131:257, 1973.

440. Grekas, D., A. R. Morley, R. Wilkinson, and D. N. S. Kerr: Isolated C3 deposition in patients without systemic disease, *Clin. Nephrol.,* 21:270, 1984.

441. Vehaskari, V. M., J. Rapola, O. Koskimies, E. Savilahti, J. Vilska, and N. Hallman: Microscopic hematuria in school children: Epidemiology and clinicopathologic evaluation, *J. Pediatr.,* 95:676, 1979.

442. Dische, F. E., M. J. Weston, and V. Parsons: Abnormally thin glomerular basement membranes associated with hematuria, proteinuria or renal failure in adults, *Am. J. Nephrol.,* 5:103, 1985.

443. Glassock, R. J., A. H. Cohen, S. G. Adler, and H. J. Ward: Secondary glomerular diseases in B. M. Brenner and F. C. Rector, Jr. (eds.), *The Kidney,* 3d ed., Saunders, Philadelphia, 1986, chap. 23.

444. O'Neil, W. M., C. L. Atkin, and H. A. Bloomer: Hereditary nephritis: A re-examination of its clinical and genetic features, *Ann. Intern. Med.,* 88:176, 1978.

445. Grünfeld, J.-P.: The clinical spectrum of hereditary nephritis, *Kidney Int.,* 27:83, 1985.

446. Habib, R., M-C. Gubler, N. Hinglais, L-H. Noël, D. Droz, M. Levy, P. Mathieu, J-M. Foidart, D. Perrin, E. Bois, and J-P. Grünfeld: Alport's syndrome: Experience at Hôpital Necker, *Kidney Int.,* 21(suppl. 11):S-20, 1982.

447. Yoshikawa, N., R. H. R. White, and A. H. Cameron: Familial hematuria: Clinico-pathologic correlations, *Clin. Nephrol.,* 17:172, 1982.

448. Krickstein, H. I., F. J. Gloor, and K. Balogh: Renal pathology in hereditary nephritis with nerve deafness, *Arch. Pathol.,* 82:506, 1966.

449. Churg, J., and R. L. Sherman: Pathologic characteristics of hereditary nephritis, *Arch. Pathol.,* 95:374, 1973.

450. Rumpelt, H.-J.: Hereditary nephropathy (Alport's syndrome): Correlation of clinical data with glomerular basement membrane alterations, *Clin. Nephrol.,* 13:203, 1980.

451. Feingold, J., E. Bois, A. Chompret, M. Broyer, M.-C. Gubler, and J-P. Grünfeld: Genetic heterogeneity of Alport's syndrome, *Kidney Int.,* 27:672, 1985.

452. Dibona, G. F.: Alport's syndrome: A genetic defect in biochemical composition of basement membrane of glomerulus, lens, and inner ear?, *J. Lab. Clin. Med.,* 101:817, 1983.

453. Olson, D. L., S. K. Anand, B. H. Landing, E. Heuser, C. M. Grushkin, and E. Lieberman: Diagnosis of hereditary nephritis by failure of glomeruli to bind anti-glomerular basement membrane antibodies, *J. Pediatr.,* 96:697, 1980.

454. McCoy, R. C., H. K. Johnson, W. J. Stone, and C. B. Wilson: Absence of nephritogenic GBM antigen(s) in some patients with hereditary nephritis, *Kidney Int.,* 21:642, 1982.

455. Jeraj, K., Y. Kim, R. L. Vernier, A. J. Fish, and A. F. Michael: Absence of Goodpasture's antigen in male patients with familial nephritis, *Am. J. Kid. Dis.,* 2:626, 1983.

456. Savage, C. O. S., C. D. Pusey, M. J. Kershaw, S. J. Cashman, P. Harrison, B. Hartley, D. R. Turner, J. S. Cameron, D. J. Evans, and C. M. Lockwood: The Goodpasture antigen in Alport's syndrome: Studies with a monoclonal antibody, *Kidney Int.,* 30:107, 1986.

457. Kashtan, C., A. J. Fish, M. Kleppel, K. Yoshioka, and A. F. Michael: Nephritogenic antigen determinance in epidermal and renal basement membranes of kindreds with Alport-type familial nephritis, *J. Clin. Invest.,* 78:1035, 1986.

458. Perrin, D., P. Jungers, J.-P. Grünfeld, S. Delons, L-H. Noël, and C. Zanati: Perimacular changes in Alport's syndrome, *Clin. Nephrol.,* 13:163, 1980.

459. Grünfeld, J-P., L-H. Noel, S. Hafez, and D. Droz: Renal prognosis in women with hereditary nephritis, *Clin. Nephrol.,* 23:267, 1985.

460. A report from the ASC/NIH Renal Transplant Registry: Renal transplantation in congenital and metabolic diseases, *J. Am. Med. Assoc.,* 232:148, 1975.

461. Wilson, C. B., and F. J. Dixon: Renal response to immunological injury, B. M. Brenner and F. C. Rector, Jr. (eds.), in *The Kidney,* 3d ed., Saunders, Philadelphia, 1986, pp. 840–843.

462. Sagel, I., G. Treser, A. Ty, N. Yoshizawa, H. Kleinberger, A. M. Yuceoglu, E. Wasserman, and K. Lange: Occurrence and nature of glomerular lesions after group A streptococci infections in children, *Ann. Intern. Med.,* 79:492, 1973.

463. Hyman, L. R., E. H. Jenis, G. S. Hill, S. W. Zimmerman, and P. M. Burkholder: Alternate C3 pathway activation in pneumococcal glomerulonephritis, *Am. J. Med.,* 58:810, 1975.

464. Sitprija, V., V. Pipatanagul, V. Boonpucknavig,

and S. Boonpucknavig: Glomerulonephritis in typhoid fever, *Ann. Intern. Med.*, 81:210, 1974.

465. Editorial: Nephritis in infectious mononucleosis, *Lancet*, 1:647, 1973.

466. Smith, M. C., J. H. Cooke, C. M. Zimmerman, J. J. Bird, B. L. Feaster, R. E. Morrison, and B. E. F. Reimann: Asymptomatic glomerulonephritis after nonstreptococcal upper respiratory infections, *Ann. Intern. Med.*, 91:967, 1979.

467. Lin, C-Y., and H-C. Hsu: Measles and acute glomerulonephritis, *Pediatrics*, 71:398, 1983.

468. Nagy, J., G. Bajtai, H. Brasch, T. Süle, M. Ambrus, G. Deák, and A. Hámori: The role of hepatitis B surface antigen in the pathogenesis of glomerulopathies, *Clin. Nephrol.*, 12:109, 1979.

469. Vitulb, B. B., S. O'Regan, J. P. de Chadarevian, and B. S. Kaplan: Mycoplasma pneumonia associated with acute glomerulonephritis, *Nephron*, 21:284, 1978.

470. Sitprija, V., M. Keoplung, V. Boonpucknavig, and S. Boonpucknavig: Renal involvement in human trichinosis, *Arch. Intern. Med.*, 140:544, 1980.

471. Jordan, S. C., B. Buckingham, R. Sakai, and D. Olson: Studies of immune-complex glomerulonephritis mediated by human thyroglobulin, *N. Engl. J. Med.*, 304:1212, 1981.

472. Ditlove, J., P. Weidmann, M. Bernstein, and S. G. Massry: Methicillin nephritis, *Medicine*, 56:483, 1977.

473. Beaufils, M., L. Morel-Maroger, J. D. Sraer, A. Kanfer, O. Kourilsky, and G. Richet: Acute renal failure of glomerular origin during visceral abscesses, *N. Engl. J. Med.*, 295:185, 1976.

474. Kaehny, W. D., T. Ozawa, M. I. Schwarz, R. E. Stanford, P. F. Kohler, and R. M. McIntosh: Acute nephritis and pulmonary alveolitis following pneumococcal pneumonia, *Arch. Intern. Med.*, 138:806, 1978.

475. Buka, I., and H. M. Coovadia: Typhoid glomerulonephritis, *Arch. Dis. Child.*, 55:305, 1980.

476. Dosik, G. M., J. U. Gutterman, E. M. Hersh, M. Akhtar, T. Sonada, and R. G. Horn: Nephrotoxicity from cancer immunotherapy, *Ann. Intern. Med.*, 89:41, 1978.

477. Lin, C.-Y., H.-C. Hsu, and H.-Y. Hung: Nephrotic syndrome associated with varicella infection, *Pediatrics*, 75:1127, 1985.

478. Rodriguez-Iturbe, B., R. Garcia, L. Rubio, J. Zabala, G. Moros, and R. Torres: Acute glomerulonephritis in the Guillain-Barré-Strohl syndrome: Report of nine cases, *Ann. Intern. Med.*, 78:391, 1973.

479. Jennings, R. B., and D. P. Earle: Poststreptococcal glomerulonephritis: Histopathologic and clinical studies of the acute, subsiding acute and early chronic latent phases, *J. Clin. Invest.*, 40:1525, 1961.

480. Hooke, D. H., W. W. Hancock, D. C. Gee, N. Kraft, and R. C. Atkins: Monoclonal antibody analysis of glomerular hypercellularity in human glomerulonephritis, *Clin. Nephrol.*, 22:163, 1984.

481. Dodge, W. F., B. H. Spargo, L. B. Travis, R. N. Srivastava, H. F. Carvajal, M. M. de Beukelaer, M. P. Longley, and J. A. Menchaca: Poststreptococcal glomerulonephritis: A prospective study in children, *N. Engl. J. Med.*, 286:273, 1972.

482. Villareal, H., Jr., V. A. Fischetti, I. van de Rijn, and J. B. Zabriskie: The occurrence of a protein in the extracellular products of streptococci isolated from patients with acute glomerulonephritis, *J. Exp. Med.*, 149:459, 1979.

483. Michael, A. F., Jr., K. N. Drummond, R. A. Good, and R. L. Vernier: Acute poststreptococcal glomerulonephritis: Immune deposit disease, *J. Clin. Invest.*, 45:237, 1966.

484. Tornroth, T.: The fate of subepithelial deposits in acute poststreptococcal glomerulonephritis, *Lab. Invest.*, 35:461, 1976.

485. Lewy, J. E., L. Salinas-Madrigal, P. B. Herdson, C. L. Pirani, and J. Metcoff: Clinico-pathologic correlations in acute poststreptococcal glomerulonephritis: A correlation between renal functions, morphologic damage, and clinical course of 46 children with acute poststreptococcal glomerulonephritis, *Medicine*, 50:453, 1971.

486. Dodge, W. F., B. H. Spargo, J. A. Bass, and L. B. Travis: The relationship between the clinical and pathologic features of poststreptococcal glomerulonephritis: A study of the early natural history, *Medicine*, 47:227, 1968.

487. Baldwin, D. S.: Chronic glomerulonephritis: Nonimmunologic mechanisms of progressive glomerular damage, *Kidney Int.*, 21:109, 1982.

488. Barnham, M., T. J. Thornton, and K. Lange: Nephritis caused by streptococcus zooepidemicus (Lancefield Group C), *Lancet*, 1:945, 1983.

489. Stetson, C. A., C. H. Rammelkamp, Jr., R. M. Krause, R. J. Kohen, and W. D. Perry: Epidemic acute nephritis: Studies on etiology, natural history, and prevention, *Medicine*, 34:431, 1955.

490. Freedman, P., H. P. Meester, H. J. Lee, E. C. Smith, B. S. Co, and B. D. Nidus: The renal response to streptococcal infection, *Medicine*, 49:433, 1970.

491. Anthony, B. F., E. L. Kaplan, L. W. Wannamaker, F. W. Briese, and S. S. Chapman: Attack rates of acute nephritis after type 49 streptococcal infec-

tion of the skin and of the respiratory tract, *J. Clin. Invest.,* 48:1697, 1969.

492. Nissenson, A. R., L. J. Baraff, R. N. Fine, and D. W. Knutson: Poststreptococcal acute glomerulonephritis: Fact and controversy, *Ann. Intern. Med.,* 91: 76, 1979.

493. Stollerman, G. H.: Rheumatogenic and nephritogenic streptococci, *Circulation,* 43:915, 1971.

494. Gibney, R., J. Reineck, G. A. Bannayan, and J. H. Stein: Renal lesions in acute rheumatic fever, *Ann. Intern. Med.,* 94:322, 1981.

495. Ben-Dov, I., E. M. Berry, and J. Kopolovic: Poststreptococcal nephritis and acute rheumatic fever in two adults, *Arch. Intern. Med.,* 145:338, 1985.

496. Friedman, J., I. van de Rijn, H. Ohkuni, V. A. Fischetti, and J. B. Zabriskie: Immunological studies of post-streptococcal sequelae. Evidence for presence of streptococcal antigens in circulating immune complexes, *J. Clin. Invest.,* 74:1027, 1984.

497. Lange, K., G. Seligson, and W. Cronin: Evidence for the in situ origin of poststreptococcal glomerulonephritis: Glomerular localization of endostreptosin and the clinical significance of the subsequent antibody response, *Clin. Nephrol.,* 19:3, 1983.

498. Vogt, A., S. Batsford, B. Rodriguez-Iturbe, and R. Garcia: Cationic antigens in poststreptococcal glomerulonephritis, *Clin. Nephrol.,* 20:271, 1983.

499. Yoshizawa, N., G. Treser, I. Sagel, A. Ty, U. Ahmed, and K. Lange: Demonstration of antigenic sites in glomeruli of patients with acute poststreptococcal glomerulonephritis by immunofluorescein and immunoferritin technics, *Am. J. Pathol.,* 70:131, 1973.

500. Fillit, H., S. P. Damle, J. D. Gregory, C. Violin, T. Poon-King, and J. B. Zabriskie: Sera from patients with poststreptococcal glomerulonephritis contain antibodies to glomerular heparan sulfate proteoglycan, *J. Exp. Med.,* 161:277, 1985.

501. McIntosh, R. M., R. Garcia, L. Rubio, D. Rabideau, J. E. Allen, R. I. Carr, and B. Rodriguez-Iturbe: Evidence for an autologous immune complex pathogenic mechanism in acute poststreptococcal glomerulonephritis, *Kidney Int.,* 14:501, 1978.

502. Rodriguez-Iturbe, B., V. N. Katiyar, and J. Coello: Neuraminidase activity and free sialic acid levels in the serum of patients with acute poststreptococcal glomerulonephritis, *N. Engl. J. Med.,* 304: 1506, 1981.

503. Griswold, W. R., J. R. McIntosh, R. Weil, III, and R. M. McIntosh: Neuraminidase treated homologous IgG and immune deposit renal disease in

504. inbred rats, *Proc. Soc. Exp. Biol. Med.,* 148:1018, 1975.

504. Rochlin, R. E., E. J. Lewis, and J. R. David: In vitro evidence for cellular hypersensitivity to glomerular-basement-membrane antigens in human glomerulonephritis, *N. Engl. J. Med.,* 283:497, 1970.

505. Filit, H. M., S. E. Read, R. L. Sherman, J. B. Zabriskie, and I. van de Rijn: Cellular reactivity to altered glomerular basement membrane in glomerulonephritis, *N. Engl. J. Med.,* 298:861, 1978.

506. Tipping, P. G., T. J. Neale, and S. R. Holdsworth: T lymphocyte participation in antibody-induced experimental glomerulonephritis, *Kidney Int.,* 27: 530, 1985.

507. Neild, G. H., K. Ivory, M. Hiramatsu, and D. G. Williams: Cyclosporin A inhibits acute serum sickness nephritis in rabbits, *Clin. Exp. Immunol.,* 52: 586, 1983.

508. Poon-King, T., I. Mohammed, R. Cox, E. V. Potter, N. M. Simon, A. C. Siegel, and D. P. Earle: Recurrent epidemic nephritis in south Trinidad, *N. Engl. J. Med.,* 277:728, 1967.

509. Kaplan, E. L., B. F. Anthony, S. S. Chapman, and L. W. Wannamaker: Epidemic acute glomerulonephritis associated with type 49 streptococcal pyoderma, I: Clinical and laboratory findings, *Am. J. Med.,* 48:9, 1970.

510. Rodriguez-Iturbe, B.: Epidemic poststreptococcal glomerulonephritis, *Kidney Int.,* 25:129, 1984.

511. Dillon, H. C., Jr., and M. S. A. Reeves: Streptococcal immune response in nephritis after skin infection, *Am. J. Med.,* 56:333, 1974.

512. Rodriguez-Iturbe, B., B. Baggio, J. Colina-Chourio, S. Favaro, R. Garcia, F. Sussana, L. Castillo, and A. Borsatti: Studies on the renin-aldosterone system in the acute nephritic syndrome, *Kidney Int.,* 19:445, 1981.

513. Powell, H. R., R. Rotenberg, A. L. Williams, and D. A. McCredie: Plasma renin activity in acute poststreptococcal glomerulonephritis and the hemolytic-uraemic syndrome, *Arch. Dis. Child.,* 49: 802, 1974.

514. Ferrario, F., O. Kourilsky, and L. Morel-Maroger: Acute endocapillary glomerulonephritis in adults: A histologic and clinical comparison between patients with and without initial acute renal failure, *Clin. Nephrol.,* 19:17, 1983.

515. Derrick, C. W., M. S. Reeves, and H. C. Dillon, Jr.: Complement and overt asymptomatic nephritis after skin infections, *J. Clin. Invest.,* 49:1178, 1970.

516. Lewis, E. J., C. B. Carpenter, and P. H. Schur: Serum complement levels in human glomerulonephritis, *Ann. Intern. Med.,* 75:555, 1971.

517. Williams, D. G., L. Morel-Maroger, O. Kourilsky, and D. K. Peters: C3 breakdown by serum from patients with acute poststreptococcal nephritis, *Lancet,* 2:360, 1972.

518. Halbwachs, L., M. Leveille, Ph. Lesavre, S. Wattel, and J. Leibowitch: Nephritic factor of the classical pathway of complement. Immunoglobulin G autoantibody directed against the classical pathway C3 convertase enzyme, *J. Clin. Invest.,* 65: 1249, 1980.

519. Meri, S.: Complement activation by circulating serum factors in human glomerulonephritis, *Clin. Exp. Immunol.,* 59:276, 1985.

520. McIntosh, R. M., W. R. Griswold, W. B. Chernack, G. Williams, J. Strauss, D. B. Kaufman, M. N. Koss, J. R. McIntosh, R. Cohen, and R. Weil, III: Cryoglobulins, III: Further studies of the nature, incidence, clinical diagnostic, prognostic and immunopathologic significance of cryoproteins in renal disease, *Q. J. Med.,* 44:285, 1975.

521. Rodríguez-Iturbe, B., L. Rubio, and R. Garcia: Attack rate of poststreptococcal nephritis in families, *Lancet,* 1:401, 1981.

522. Kaplan, E. L., and L. W. Wannamaker: Suppression of the antistreptolysin O response by cholesterol and by lipid extracts of rabbit skin, *J. Exp. Med.,* 144:754, 1976.

523. Weinstein, L., and J. LeFrock: Does antimicrobial therapy of streptococcal pharyngitis or pyoderma alter the risk of glomerulonephritis?, *J. Infect. Dis.,* 124:229, 1971.

524. McCrory, W. W., D. S. Fleisher, and W. B. Sohn: Effects of early ambulation on the course of nephritis in children, *Pediatrics,* 24:395, 1959.

525. Roy, S, III, W. M. Murphy, and B. S. Arant, Jr.: Poststreptococcal crescenteric glomerulonephritis in children: Comparison of quintuple therapy versus supportive care, *J. Pediatr.,* 98:403, 1981.

526. Leonard, C. D., R. B. Nagle, G. E. Striker, R. E. Cutler, and B. J. Scribner: Acute glomerulonephritis with prolonged oliguria: An analysis of 29 cases, *Ann. Intern. Med.,* 73:703, 1970.

527. Potter, E. V., S. Abidh, A. R. Sharrett, E. G. Burt, M. Svartman, J. F. Finklea, T. Poon-King, and D. P. Earle: Two- to six-year follow-up studies of nephritis in Trinidad, *N. Engl. J. Med.,* 298:767, 1978.

528. Potter, E. V., S. A. Lipschultz, S. Abidh, T. Poon-King, and D. P. Earle: Twelve to seventeen-year follow-up of patients with poststreptococcal acute glomerulonephritis in Trinidad, *N. Engl. J. Med.,* 307:725, 1982.

529. Garcia, R., L. Rubio, and B. Rodríguez-Iturbe: Long-term prognosis of epidemic poststreptococcal glomerulonephritis in Maracaibo: Follow-up studies 11–12 years after the acute episode, *Clin. Nephrol.,* 15:291, 1981.

530. Baldwin, D. S.: Poststreptococcal glomerulonephritis, *Am. J. Med.,* 62:1, 1977.

531. Schacht, R. G., M. C. Gluck, G. R. Gallo, and D. S. Baldwin: Progression to uremia after remission of acute streptococcal glomerulonephritis, *N. Engl. J. Med.,* 295:977, 1976.

532. Editorial: Is poststreptococcal glomerulonephritis progressive?, *Br. Med. J.,* 2:975, 1977.

533. Kurtzman, N. A.: Does acute poststreptococcal glomerulonephritis lead to chronic renal disease? *N. Engl. J. Med.,* 298:795, 1978.

534. Lien, J. W. K., T. H. Mathew, and R. Meadows: Acute poststreptococcal glomerulonephritis in adults: A long-term study, *Q. J. Med.,* 48:99, 1979.

535. Gutman, R. S., G. E. Striker, B. Gilliland, and R. E. Cutler: The immune complex glomerulonephritis of bacterial endocarditis, *Medicine,* 51:1, 1972.

536. Neugarten, J., and D. S. Baldwin: Glomerulonephritis in bacterial endocarditis, *Am. J. Med.,* 77: 297, 1984.

537. Neugarten, J., G. R. Gallo, and D. S. Baldwin: Glomerulonephritis in bacterial endocarditis, *Am. J. Kid. Dis.,* 3:371, 1983.

538. Arze, R. S., H. Rashid, R. Morley, M. K. Ward, and D. N. S. Kerr: Shunt nephritis: Report of two cases and review of the literature, *Clin. Nephrol.,* 19:48, 1983.

539. Morel-Maroger, L., J.-D. Sraer, G. Herreman, and P. Godeau: Kidney in subacute endocarditis: Pathological and immunofluorescence findings, *Arch. Pathol.,* 94:205, 1972.

540. Bayer, A. S., A. N. Theofilopoulos, D. B. Tillman, F. J. Dixon, and L. B. Guze: Use of circulating immune complex levels in the serodifferentiation of endocarditic and nonendocarditic septicemias, *Am. J. Med.,* 66:58, 1979.

541. Levy, R. L., and R. Hong: The immune nature of subacute bacterial endocarditis nephritis, *Am. J. Med.,* 54:645, 1973.

542. Perez, G. O., N. Rothfield, and R. C. Williams: Immune-complex nephritis in bacterial endocarditis, *Arch. Intern. Med.,* 136:334, 1976.

543. Kaufmann, D. B., and R. M. McIntosh: The pathogenesis of the renal lesion in a patient with streptococcal disease, infected ventriculoatrial shunt, cryoglobulinemia and nephritis, *Am. J. Med.,* 50: 262, 1971.

544. Strife, C. F., B. M. McDonald, E. J. Ruley, A. J. McAdams, and C. D. West: Shunt nephritis: The

nature of the serum cryoglobulins and their relation to the complement profile, *J. Pediatr.,* 88:403, 1976.

545. Stickler, G. B., M. H. Shin, E. C. Burke, K. E. Holley, R. H. Miller, and W. E. Segar: Diffuse glomerulonephritis associated with infected ventriculoatrial shunt, *N. Engl. J. Med.,* 279:1077, 1968.

546. Spain, D. M., and D. W. King: The effect of penicillin on the renal lesions of subacute bacterial endocarditis, *Ann. Intern. Med.,* 36:1086, 1952.

547. Nolan, C. M., and R. S. Abernathy: Nephropathy associated with methicillin therapy: prevalence and determinants in patients with staphylococcal bacteremia, *Arch. Intern. Med.,* 137:997, 1977.

548. Spitzer, R. E., A. E. Stitzel, and J. R. Urmson: Is glomerulonephritis after bacterial sepsis always benign?, *Lancet,* 1:871, 1978.

549. Schoeneman, M., B. Bennett, and I. Greifer: Shunt nephritis progressing to chronic renal failure, *Am. J. Kid. Dis.,* 2:375, 1982.

550. Herdman, R. C., R. J. Pickering, A. F. Michael, R. L. Vernier, A. J. Fish, H. Gerwurz, and R. A. Good: Chronic glomerulonephritis associated with low serum complement activity (chronic hypocomplementemic glomerulonephritis), *Medicine,* 49:207, 1970.

551. West, C. D., and A. J. McAdams: The chronic glomerulonephritides of childhood, *J. Pediatr.,* 93: 167, 1970.

552. Habib, R., C. Kleinknecht, M-C. Gubler, and M. Levy: Idiopathic membranoproliferative glomerulonephritis in children, *Clin. Nephrol.,* 1:194, 1973.

553. West, C. D.: Childhood membranoproliferative glomerulonephritis: An approach to management, *Kidney Int.,* 29:1077, 1986.

554. Cameron, J. S., D. R. Turner, J. Heaton, D. G. Williams, C. S. Ogg, C. Chantler, G. B. Haycock, and J. Hicks: Idiopathic mesangiocapillary glomerulonephritis and α_1-antitrypsin deficiency in children and adults and long-term prognosis, *Am. J. Med.,* 74:175, 1983.

555. Donadio, J. V., Jr., T. K. Slack, K. E. Holley, and D. M. Ilstrup: Idiopathic membranoproliferative (mesangiocapillary) glomerulonephritis: A clinicopathologic study, *Mayo Clin. Proc.,* 54:141, 1979.

556. Sissons, J. G. P., R. J. West, J. Fallows, D. C. Williams, B. J. Boucher, N. Amos, and D. K. Peters: The complement abnormalities of lipodystrophy, *N. Engl. J. Med.,* 294:461, 1976.

557. Coleman, T. H., J. Forristal, T. Kosaka, and C. D. West: Inherited complement component deficiencies in membranoproliferative glomerulonephritis, *Kidney Int.,* 24:681, 1983.

558. Berger, M., J. E. Balow, C. B. Wilson, and M. M. Frank: Circulating immune complexes and glomerulonephritis in a patient with congenital absence of the third component of complement, *N. Engl. J. Med.,* 308:1009, 1983.

559. Brzosko, W. J., K. Krawczynski, T. Nazarewicz, M. Morzycka, and A. Nowoslawski: Glomerulonephritis associated with hepatitis-B surface antigen immune complexes in children, *Lancet,* 2:477, 1974.

560. Kilcoyne, M. M., J. J. Daly, D. J. Gocke, G. E. Thomson, J. I. Meltzer, K. C. Hsu, and M. Tannenbaum: Nephrotic syndrome in heroin addicts, *Lancet,* 1:17, 1972.

561. Stachura, I., S. Jayakumar, and M. Pardo: Talwin addict nephropathy, *Clin. Nephrol.,* 19:147, 1982.

562. Morel-Maroger, L., and P. Verroust: Glomerular lesions in dysproteinemias, *Kidney Int.,* 5:249, 1974.

563. Cheigh, J. S., J. Mouradian, M. Susin, W. T. Stubenbord, L. Tapia, R. R. Riggio, K. H. Stenzel, and A. L. Rubin: Kidney transplant nephrotic syndrome: Relationship between allograft histopathology and natural course, *Kidney Int.,* 18:358, 1980.

564. Olson, J. L., T. M. Philips, M. G. Lewis, and K. Solez: Malignant melanoma with renal dense deposits containing tumor antigens, *Clin. Nephrol.,* 12:74, 1979.

565. Strife, C. F., G. Chuck, A. J. McAdams, C. A. Davis, and J. J. Kline: Membranoproliferative glomerulonephritis and α_1-antitrypsin deficiency in children, *Pediatrics,* 71:88, 1983.

566. Appel, G. B., V. D'Agati, M. Bergman, and C. L. Pirani: Nephrotic syndrome and immune complex glomerulonephritis associated with chlorpropamide therapy, *Am. J. Med.,* 74:337, 1983.

567. Ott, B. R., N. P. Libbey, R. J. Ryter, and W. M. Trebbin: Treatment of Schistosome-induced glomerulonephritis. A case report and review of the literature, *Arch. Intern. Med.,* 143:1477, 1983.

568. Strife, C. F., E. C. Jackson, and A. J. McAdams: Type III membranoproliferative glomerulonephritis: Long-term clinical and morphological evaluation, *Clin. Nephrol.,* 21:323, 1984.

569. Strife, C. F., A. J. McAdams, and C. D. West: Membranoproliferative glomerulonephritis characterized by focal, segmental proliferative lesions, *Clin. Nephrol.,* 18:9, 1982.

570. Sibley, R. K., and Y. Kim: Dense intramembranous deposit disease: New pathologic features, *Kidney Int.,* 25:660, 1984.

571. Galle, P., and P. Mahieu: Electron dense altera-

tion of kidney basement membranes: A renal lesion specific of a systemic disease, *Am. J. Med.,* 58:749, 1975.

572. Woodroffe, A. J., W. A. Border, A. N. Theofilopoulos, O. Gotze, R. J. Glassock, F. J. Dixon, and C. B. Wilson: Detection of circulating immune complexes in patients with glomerulonephritis, *Kidney Int.,* 12:268, 1977.

573. Ooi, Y. M., E. H. Vallota, and C. D. West: Serum immune complexes in membranoproliferative and other glomerulonephritides, *Kidney Int.,* 11:275, 1977.

574. Thompson, R. A.: IgG3 levels in patients with chronic membranoproliferative glomerulonephritis, *Br. Med. J.,* 1:282, 1972.

575. Bannister, K. M., G. S. Howarth, A. R. Clarkson, and A. J. Woodroffe: Glomerular IgG subclass distribution in human glomerulonephritis, *Clin. Nephrol.,* 19:161, 1982.

576. Lewis, E. J., G. J. Busch, and P. H. Schur: Gamma G globulin subgroup composition of the glomerular deposits in human renal diseases, *J. Clin. Invest.,* 49:1103, 1970.

577. Beck, O. G.: Distribution of virus antibody activity among human IgG subclasses, *Clin. Exp. Immunol.,* 43:626, 1981.

578. Nevins, T. E.: Lectin binding in membranoproliferative glomerulonephritis. Evidence for *N*-acetylglucosamine in dense intramembranous deposits, *Am. J. Pathol.,* 118:325, 1985.

579. George, C. R. P., S. J. Slichter, L. J. Quadrucci, G. E. Striker, and L. A. Harker: A kinetic evaluation of hemostasis in renal disease, *N. Engl. J. Med.,* 291:1111, 1974.

580. Donadio, J. V., Jr., C. F. Anderson, J. C. Mitchell, III, K. E. Holley, D. M. Ilstrup, V. Fuster, and J. H. Cheesebro: Membranoproliferative glomerulonephritis. A prospective clinical trial of platelet inhibitor therapy, *N. Engl. J. Med.,* 310:1421, 1984.

581. Zimmerman, S. W., A. V. Moorthy, W. H. Dreher, A. Friedman, and U. Varanasi: Prospective trial of warfarin and dipyridamole in patients with membranoproliferative glomerulonephritis, *Am. J. Med.,* 75:920, 1983.

582. West, C. D.: Pathogenesis and approaches to therapy of membranoproliferative glomerulonephritis, *Kidney Int.,* 9:1, 1976.

583. Vallota, E. H., J. Forristal, R. E. Spitzer, N. C. Davis, and C. D. West: Continuing C3 breakdown after bilateral nephrectomy in patients with membranoproliferative glomerulonephritis, *J. Clin. Invest.,* 50:552, 1971.

584. Daha, M. R., D. T. Fearon, and K. F. Austen: C3 nephritic factor (C3NeF): Stabilization of fluid phase and cell bound alternative pathway convertase, *J. Immunol.,* 116:1, 1976.

585. Daha, M. R., K. F. Austen, and D. T. Fearon: Heterogeneity, polypeptide chain composition, and antigenic reactivity of C3 nephritic factor, *J. Immunol.,* 120:1389, 1978.

586. Vallota, E. H., J. Forristal, N. C. Davis, and C. D. West: The C3 nephritic factor and membranoproliferative nephritis: Correlation of serum levels of the nephritic factor with C3 levels, with therapy and with progression of the disease, *J. Pediatr.,* 80:947, 1972.

587. West, C. D., and A. J. McAdams: Serum B_{1c} globulin levels in persistent glomerulonephritis with low serum complement: Variability unrelated to clinical course, *Nephron,* 7:193, 1970.

588. Magil, A. B., J. D. E. Price, G. Bower, C. P. Rance, J. Huber, and W. H. Chase: Membranoproliferative glomerulonephritis type I: Comparison of natural history in children and adults, *Clin. Nephrol.,* 11:239, 1979.

589. Watson, A. R., S. Poucell, P. Thorner, G. S. Arbus, C. P. Rance, and R. Baumal: Membranoproliferative glomerulonephritis type I in children: Correlation of clinical features with pathologic subtypes, *Am. J. Kid. Dis.,* 4:141, 1984.

590. Klein, M., S. Poucell, G. G. Arbus, M. McGraw, C. P. Rance, S-J. Yoon, and R. Baumal: Characteristics of a benign subtype of dense deposit disease: Comparison with the progressive form of this disease, *Clin. Nephrol.,* 20:163, 1983.

591. Strife, C. F., A. J. McAdams, and C. D. West: Membranoproliferative glomerulonephritis characterized by focal, segmental proliferative lesions, *Clin. Nephrol.,* 18:9, 1982.

592. Cameron, J. S., E. F. Glasgow, C. S. Ogg, and R. H. R. White: Membranoproliferative glomerulonephritis and persistent hypocomplementemia, *Br. Med. J.,* 4:7, 1970.

593. Donadio, J. V., Jr., T. K. Slack, K. E. Holley, and D. M. Ilstup: Idiopathic membranoproliferative (mesangiocapillary) glomerulonephritis: A clinicopathologic study, *Mayo Clin. Proc.,* 54:141, 1979.

594. McAdams, A. J., P. T. McEnery, and C. D. West: Mesangiocapillary glomerulonephritis: Changes in glomerular morphology with long-term alternate-day prednisone therapy, *J. Pediatr.,* 86:23, 1975.

595. A Report of the International Study of Kidney Disease in Children: Alternate day steroid therapy in membranoproliferative glomerulonephritis: A randomized controlled clinical trial (abstract), *Kidney Int.* 21:150, 1982.

596. Cattran, D. C., C. J. Cardella, J. M. Roscoe, R. C.

Charron, P. C. Rance, S. M. Ritchie, and P. N. Corey: Results of a controlled drug trial in membranoproliferative glomerulonephritis, *Kidney Int.*, 27:436, 1985.

597. Kincaid-Smith, P.: The natural history and treatment of mesangiocapillary glomerulonephritis, in P. Kincaid-Smith, T. H. Mathew, and E. L. Becker (eds.), *Glomerulonephritis: Morphology, Natural History, and Treatment,* Wiley, New York, 1973.

598. Cameron, J. S., C. Chantler, and D. Turner: Treatment of mesangiocapillary glomerulonephritis in children with combined immunosuppression and anti-coagulation, *Arch. Dis. Child.*, 55:446, 1980.

599. Curtis, J. J., R. J. Wyath, D. Bhathena, B. A. Lucas, N. H. Holland, and R. G. Luke: Renal transplantation for patients with type I and type II membranoproliferative glomerulonephritis: Serial complement and nephritic factor measurements and the problem of recurrence of disease, *Am. J. Med.*, 66:216, 1979.

600. Eddy, A., R. Sibley, S. M. Mauer, and Y. Kim: Renal allograft failure due to recurrent dense intramembranous deposit disease, *Clin. Nephrol.*, 21:305, 1984.

601. Merslin, A. G., and N. Rothfield: Systemic lupus erythematosus in childhood: Analysis of 42 cases, with comparative data on 200 adult cases, *Pediatrics,* 42:37, 1968.

602. Mahajan, S. K., N. G. Ordonez, P. J. Feitelson, V. S. Lim, B. H. Spargo, and A. I. Katz: Lupus nephropathy without clinical renal involvement, *Medicine,* 56:493, 1977.

603. Leehey, D. J., A. I. Katz, A. H. Azaran, A. J. Aronson, and B. H. Spargo: Silent diffuse lupus nephritis: Long-term follow-up, *Am. J. Kid. Dis.*, 2(suppl. 1):188, 1982.

604. Bennett, W. M., E. J. Boudana, D. J. Norman, and D. C. Houghton: Natural history of "silent" lupus nephritis, *Am. J. Kid. Dis.*, 1:359, 1982.

605. Brentjens, J. R., M. Sepulveda, T. Baliah, C. Bentzel, B. F. Erlanger, C. Elwood, M. Montes, K. C. Hus, and G. A. Andres: Interstitial immune complex nephritis in patients with systemic lupus erythematosus, *Kidney Int.*, 7:342, 1975.

606. Case Records of Massachusetts General Hospital (Case 2-1976), *N. Engl. J. Med.*, 294:100, 1976.

607. Tron, F., D. Ganeval, and D. Droz: Immunologically-mediated acute renal failure of nonglomerular origin in the course of systemic lupus erythematosus (SLE). Report of two cases., *Am. J. Med.*, 67:529, 1979.

608. Appel, G. B., F. G. Silva, C. L. Pirani, J. I. Meltzer, and D. Estes: Renal involvement in systemic lupus erythematosus: A study of 56 patients emphasizing histologic classification, *Medicine,* 57:371, 1978.

609. Hill, G. S.: Systemic lupus erythematosus and mixed connective tissue disease, in *Pathology of the Kidney,* 3d ed. R. H. Heptinstall, Little, Brown, Boston, 1983, chap. 17.

610. Lee, H. S., S. K. Mujais, B. S. Kasinath, B. H. Spargo, and A. I. Katz: Course of renal pathology in patients with systemic lupus erythematosus, *Am. J. Med.*, 77:612, 1984.

611. Tisher, C. C., H. B. Kelso, R. R. Robinson, J. C. Gunnells, and P. M. Burkholder: Intraendothelial inclusions in kidneys of patients with systemic lupus erythematosus, *Ann. Intern. Med.*, 75:537, 1971.

612. Grimley, P. M., G. L. Davis, Y-H. Kang, J. S. Dooley, J. Strohmaier, and J. H. Hoofnagle: Tuboloreticular inclusions in peripheral blood mononuclear cells related to systemic therapy with α-interferon, *Lab. Invest.*, 52:638, 1985.

613. Kim, Y. H., Y. J. Choi, and L. Reiner: Ultrastructural "fingerprint" in cryoprecipitate and glomerular deposits: A case report of systemic lupus erythematosus, *Hum. Pathol.*, 12:86, 1981.

614. Grishman, E., and J. Churg: Focal segmental lupus nephritis, *Clin. Nephrol.*, 17:5, 1982.

615. Bhuyan, U. N., A. N. Malaviya, S. C. Dash, and K. K. Malhotra: Prognostic significance of renal angiitis in systemic lupus erythematous (SLE), *Clin. Nephrol.*, 20:109, 1983.

616. Kant, K. S., V. E. Pollak, M. A. Weiss, H. I. Glueck, M. A. Miller, and E. V. Hess: Glomerular thrombosis in systemic lupus erythematosus: Prevalence and significance, *Medicine,* 60:71, 1981.

617. Austin, H. A., III, J. H. Klippel, J. E. Balow, N. G. H. le Riche, A. D. Steinberg, P. H. Plotz, and J. L. Decker: Therapy of lupus nephritis. Controlled trial of prednisone and cytotoxic drugs, *N. Engl. J. Med.*, 314:614, 1986.

618. Balow, J. E., H. A. Austin, III, L. R. Muenz, K. M. Joyce, T. T. Antonovych, J. H. Klippel, A. D. Steinberg, P. H. Plotz, and J. L. Decker: Effect of treatment on the evolution of renal abnormalities in lupus nephritis, *N. Engl. J. Med.*, 311:491, 1984.

619. Hughes, G. R. V.: Autoantibodies in lupus and its variants: Experience in 1000 patients, *Br. Med. J.*, 289:339, 1984.

620. Tan, E. M.: Antinuclear antibodies in diagnosis and management, *Hosp. Pract.*, 18(1):79, 1983.

621. Eisenberg, R. A., K. Dyer, S. Y. Craven, C. R. Fuller, and W. J. Yount: Subclass restriction and polyclonality of systemic lupus erythematosus marker antibody anti-Sm, *J. Clin. Invest.*, 75:1270, 1985.

622. Koffler, D., P. H. Schur, and H. G. Kunkel: Immunological studies concerning the nephritis of systemic lupus erythematosus, *J. Exp. Med.,* 126: 607, 1967.

623. Winfield, J. B., I. Faiferman, and D. Koffler: Avidity of anti-DNA antibodies in serum and IgG glomerular eluates from patients with systemic lupus erythematosus: Association of high avidity antinative DNA antibody with glomerulonephritis, *J. Clin. Invest.,* 59:90, 1977.

624. Koffler, D., V. Agnello, and H. G. Kunkel: Polynucleotide immune complexes in serum and glomeruli of patients with systemic lupus erythematosus, *Am. J. Pathol.,* 74:109, 1974.

625. Yamada, A., Y. Miyakawa, and K. Kosaka: Entrapment of anti-DNA antibodies in the kidney of patients with systemic lupus erythematosus, *Kidney Int.,* 22:671, 1982.

626. Diamond, B. A., D. E. Yelton, and M. D. Scharff: Monoclonal antibodies. A new technology for producing serologic reagents, *N. Engl. J. Med.,* 304: 1344, 1981.

627. Lafer, E. M., J. Rauch, C. Andrzewski, Jr., D. Mudd, B. Furie, B. Furie, R. S. Schwartz, and B. D. Stollar: Polyspecific monoclonal lupus autoantibodies reactive with both polynucleotides and phospholipids, *J. Exp. Med.,* 153:897, 1981.

628. Shoenfield, Y., J. Rauch, H. Massicotte, S. K. Datta, J. Andre-Schwartz, B. D. Stollar, and R. S. Schwartz: Polyspecificity of monoclonal lupus autoantibodies produced by human-human hybridomas, *N. Engl. J. Med.,* 308:414, 1983.

629. Cairns, E., J. Block, and D. A. Bell: Anti-DNA autoantibody-producing hybridomas of normal human lymphoid cell origin, *J. Clin. Invest.,* 74:880, 1984.

630. Schwartz, R. S., and B. D. Stollar: Origins of anti-DNA autoantibodies, *J. Clin. Invest.,* 75:321, 1985.

631. Atkinson, P. M., G. W. Lampman, B. C. Furie, Y. Naparstek, R. S. Schwartz, B. D. Stollar, and B. Furie: Homology of the NH_2-terminal amino acid sequences of the heavy and light chains of human monoclonal lupus autoantibodies containing the dominant 16/6 idiotype, *J. Clin. Invest.,* 75:1138, 1985.

631a. Naparstek, Y., J. Andre-Schwartz, T. Manser, L. J. Wysocki, L. Breitman, B. D. Stollar, M. Gefter, and R. S. Schwartz: A single germ-line V_H gene segment of normal A/J mice encodes autoantibodies characteristic of systemic lupus erythematosus, *J. Exp. Med.,* 164:614, 1986.

632. Steinberg, A. D., E. S. Raveche, C. A. Laskin, H. R. Smith, T. Santoro, M. L. Miller, and P. H. Plotz: Systemic lupus erythematosus: Insights from animal models, *Ann. Intern. Med.,* 100:714, 1984.

633. Smoler, J. S., T. M. Chused, W. M. Leiserson, J. P. Reeves, D. Alling, and A. D. Steinberg: Heterogeneity of immunoregulatory T-cell subsets in systemic lupus erythematosus. Correlation with clinical features, *Am. J. Med.* 72:783, 1982.

634. Morimoto, C., E. L. Reinherz, S. F. Schlossman, P. H. Schur, J. A. Mills, and A. D. Steinberg: Alterations in immunoregulatory T cell subsets in active systemic lupus erythematosus, *J. Clin. Invest.,* 66:1171, 1980.

635. Morimoto, C., T. Abe, and M. Homma: Altered function of suppressor T lymphocytes in patients with active systemic lupus erythematosus—In vitro immune response to autoantigen, *Clin. Immunol. Immunopathol.,* 13:161, 1979.

636. Miller, K. B., and R. S. Schwartz: Familial abnormalities of suppressor-cell function in systemic lupus erythematosus, *N. Engl. J. Med.,* 301:803, 1979.

637. Sakane, T., A. D. Steinberg, J. P. Reeves, and I. Green: Studies of immune functions of patients with systemic lupus erythematosus: Complement-dependent immunoglobulin M anti-thymus-derived cell antibodies preferentially inactivate suppressor cells, *J. Clin. Invest.,* 63:954, 1979.

638. Morimoto, C., E. L. Reinherz, J. A. Distaso, A. D. Steinberg, and S. F. Schlossman: Relationship between systemic lupus erythematosus, T cell subsets, anti-T cell antibodies, and T cell functions, *J. Clin. Invest.,* 73:689, 1984.

639. Neilson, E. G., and B. Zakheim: T cell regulation, anti-idiotypic immunity, and the nephritogenic immune response, *Kidney Int.,* 24:289, 1983.

640. Abdou, N. I., H. Wall, H. B. Lindsley, J. F. Halsey, and T. Suzuki: Network theory in autoimmunity. In vitro suppression of serum anti-DNA antibody binding to DNA by anti-idiotypic antibody in systemic lupus erythematosus, *J. Clin. Invest.,* 67:1297, 1981.

641. Frank, M. M., M. I. Hamburger, T. J. Lawley, R. P. Kimberly, and P. H. Plotz: Defective reticuloendothelial system Fc-receptor function in systemic lupus erythematosus, *N. Engl. J. Med.,* 300:518, 1979.

642. Hamburger, M. I., T. J. Lawley, R. P. Kimberly, P. H. Plotz, and M. M. Frank: A serial study of splenic reticuloendothelial system Fc receptor functional activity in systemic lupus erythematosus, *Arth. Rheum.,* 25:48, 1982.

643. Wilson, J. G., W. W. Wong, P. H. Schur, and D. T. Fearon: Mode of inheritance of decreased C3b

receptors on erythrocytes of patients with systemic lupus erythematosus, *N. Engl. J. Med.*, 307: 981, 1982.

644. Agnello, V.: Complement deficiency states, *Medicine*, 57:1, 1978.

645. Provost, T. T., F. C. Arnett, and M. Reichlin: Homozygous C2 deficiency, lupus erythematosus, and anti-Ro (SSA) antibodies, *Arth. Rheum.*, 26: 1279, 1983.

646. Fielder, A. H. L., M. J. Walport, J. R. Batchelor, R. I. Rynes, C. M. Black, I. A. Dodi, and G. R. V. Hughes: Family study of the major histocompatibility complex in patients with systemic lupus erythematosus: Importance of null alleles of C4A and C4B in determining disease susceptibility, *Br. Med. J.*, 286:425, 1983.

647. Schifferli, J. A., Y. C. Ng, and D. K. Peters: The role of complement and its receptors in the elimination of immune complexes, *N. Engl. J. Med.*, 315:488, 1986.

648. Schifferli, J. A., G. Steiger, G. Hauptmann, P. J. Spaeth, and A. G. Sjoholm: Formation of soluble immune complexes in sera of patients with various hypocomplementemic states. Difference between inhibition of immune precipitation and solubilization, *J. Clin. Invest.*, 76:2127, 1985.

649. McDevitt, H. O.: The HLA system and its relation to disease, *Hosp. Pract.*, 20(7):57, 1985.

650. Schwartz, R. S.: Immunologic and genetic aspects of systemic lupus erythematosus, *Kidney Int.*, 19: 474, 1981.

651. Reinersten, J. L., J. H. Klippel, A. H. Johnson, A. D. Steinberg, J. L. Decker, and D. L. Mann: B-lymphocyte alloantigens associated with systemic lupus erythematosus, *N. Engl. J. Med.*, 299: 515, 1978.

652. Reveille, J. D., W. B. Bias, J. A. Winkelstein, T. T. Provost, C. A. Dorsch, and F. C. Arnett: Familial systemic lupus erythematosus: Immunogenetic studies in eight families, *Medicine*, 62:21, 1983.

653. Roubinian, J. R., N. Talal, J. S. Greenspan, J. R. Goodman, and P. K. Siiteri: Effect of castration and sex hormone treatment on survival, antinucleic acid antibodies, and glomerulonephritis in NZB/NZW F_1 mice, *J. Exp. Med.*, 147:1568, 1978.

654. Roubininan, J. R., R. Papoian, and N. Talal: Androgenic hormones modulate antibody responses and improve survival in murine lupus, *J. Clin. Invest.*, 59:1066, 1977.

655. Miller, M. H., M. B. Urowitz, D. D. Gladman, and D. W. Killinger: Systemic lupus erythematosus in males, *Medicine*, 62:327, 1983.

656. Inman, R. D., L. Jovanovic, J. A. Markenson, C. Longcope, M. Y. Dawood, and M. D. Lockshin: Systemic lupus erythematosus in men. Genetic and endocrine features, *Arch. Intern. Med.*, 142: 1813, 1982.

657. Lahita, R. G., H. L. Bradlow, H. G. Kunkel, and J. Fishman: Increased 16α-hydroxylation of estradiol in systemic lupus erythematosus, *J. Clin. Endocrinol. Metab.*, 53:174, 1981.

658. Dixon, F. J.: Murine SLE models and autoimmune disease, *Hosp. Pract.*, 17(3):63, 1982.

659. Lahita, R. G., N. Chiorazzi, A. Gibofsky, R. I. Winchester, and H. G. Kunkel: Familial systemic lupus erythematosus in males, *Arth. Rheum.*, 26:39, 1983.

660. Emlen, W., R. Ansari, and G. Burdick: DNA–anti-DNA immune complexes. Antibody protection of a discrete DNA fragment from DNAase digestion in vitro, *J. Clin. Invest.*, 74:185, 1984.

661. Reichlin, M., and M. Mattoli: Correlation of a precipitin reaction to an RNA protein antigen and a low prevalence of nephritis in patients with systemic lupus erythematosus, *N. Engl. J. Med.*, 286:908, 1972.

662. Izui, S., P. H. Lambert, and P. A. Miescher: In vitro demonstration of a particular affinity of glomerular basement membrane and collagen for DNA: A possible basis for a local formation of DNA–anti-DNA complexes in systemic lupus erythematosus, *J. Exp. Med.*, 144:428, 1976.

663. Tan, E. M., P. H. Schur, R. I. Carr, and H. G. Kunkel: Deoxyribonucleic acid (DNA) and antibodies to DNA in the serum of patients with systemic lupus erythematosus, *J. Clin. Invest.*, 45:1732, 1966.

664. Raptis, L., and H. A. Menard: Quantitation and characterization of plasma DNA in normals and patients with systemic lupus erythematosus, *J. Clin. Invest.*, 66:1391, 1980.

665. Biesecker, G., S. Katz, and D. Koffler: Renal localization of the membrane attack complex in systemic lupus erythematosus nephritis, *J. Exp. Med.*, 154:1779, 1981.

666. Biesecker, G., L. Lavin, M. Ziskind, and D. Koffler: Cutaneous localization of the membrane attack complex in discoid and systemic lupus erythematosus, *N. Engl. J. Med.*, 306:264, 1982.

667. Falk, R. J., A. P. Dalmasso, Y. Kim, S. Lam, and A. Michael: Radioimmunoassay of the attack complex of complement in serum from patients with systemic lupus erythematosus, *N. Engl. J. Med.*, 312:1594, 1985.

668. Donadio, J. V., Jr., J. H. Burgess, and K. E. Holley: Membranous lupus nephropathy: A clinicopathologic study, *Medicine*, 56:527, 1977.

669. Friend, P. S., Y. Kim, A. F. Michael, and J. V. Donadio: Pathogenesis of membranous nephropathy in systemic lupus erythematosus: Possible role of nonprecipitating DNA antibody, *Br. Med. J.*, 1:25, 1977.

670. Asano, Y., and Y. Nakamoto: Avidity of anti-native DNA antibody and glomerular immune complex localization in lupus nephritis, *Clin. Nephrol.*, 10: 134, 1978.

671. Hoyer, J. R., A. F. Michael, and L. W. Hoyer: Immunofluorescent localization of antihemophilic factor antigen and fibrinogen in human renal disease, *J. Clin. Invest.*, 53:1375, 1974.

672. Cole, E. H., J. Schulman, M. Urowitz, E. Keystone, C. Williams, and G. A. Levy: Monocyte procoagulant activity in glomerulonephritis associated with systemic lupus erythematosus, *J. Clin. Invest.*, 75:861, 1985.

673. Perry, H. M., Jr.: Late toxicity to hydralazine resembling systemic lupus erythematosus or rheumatoid arthritis, *Am. J. Med.*, 54:58, 1973.

674. Perry, H. M., Jr.: Possible mechanisms of the hydralazine-related lupus-like syndrome, *Arth. Rheum.*, 24:1093, 1981.

675. Blomgren, S. E., J. J. Condemi, and J. H. Vaughan: Procainamide-induced lupus erythematosus: Clinical and laboratory observations, *Am. J. Med.*, 52: 338, 1972.

676. Lahita, J. R., J. Kluger, D. E. Drayer, D. Koffler, and M. M. Reidenberg: Antibodies to nuclear antigens in patients treated with procainamide or acetylprocainamide, *N. Engl. J. Med.*, 301:1382, 1979.

677. Lavie, C. J., J. Biundo, R. J. Quinet, and J. Waxman: Systemic lupus erythematosus (SLE) induced by quinidine, *Arch. Intern. Med.*, 145:446, 1985.

678. West, S. G., M. McMahon, and J. P. Portanova: Quinidine-induced lupus erythematosus, *Ann. Intern. Med.*, 100:840, 1984.

679. Chalmers, A., D. Thompson, H. E. Stein, G. Reid, and A. C. Patterson: Systemic lupus erythematosus during penicillamine therapy for rheumatoid arthritis, *Ann. Intern. Med.*, 97:659, 1982.

680. Record, N. B., Jr.: Acebutolol-induced pleuropulmonary lupus syndrome, *Ann. Intern. Med.*, 95:326, 1981.

681. Dupont, A., and R. Six: Lupus-like syndrome induced by methlydopa, *Br. Med. J.*, 285:693, 1982.

682. Fritzler, M. J., and E. M. Tan: Antibodies to histones in drug-induced and idiopathic lupus erythematosus, *J. Clin. Invest.*, 62:560, 1978.

683. Hahn, B. H., G. C. Sharp, W. S. Irvin, O. S. Kantor, C. A. Gardner, M. K. Bagby, H. M. Perry, Jr., and C. K. Osterland: Immune responses to hydralazine and nuclear antigens in hydralazine-induced lupus erythematosus, *Ann. Intern. Med.*, 76:365, 1972.

684. Tan, E. M., and J. P. Portanova: The role of histones as nuclear-autoantigens in drug-related lupus erythematosus, *Arth. Rheum.*, 24:1064, 1981.

685. Perry, H. M., Jr., E. M. Tan, S. Carmody, and A. Sakamoto: Relationship of acetyl transferase activity to antinuclear antibodies and toxic symptoms in hypertensive patients treated with hydralazine, *J. Lab. Clin. Med.*, 76:114, 1970.

686. Woosley, R. L., D. E. Drayer, M. M. Reidenberg, A. S. Nies, K. Carr, and J. A. Oates: Effect of acetylator phenotype on the rate at which procainamide induces antinuclear antibodies and the lupus syndrome, *N. Engl. J. Med.*, 298:1157, 1978.

687. Mansilla-Tinoco, R., S. J. Harland, P. J. Ryan, R. M. Bernstein, C. T. Dollery, G. R. V. Hughes, C. J. Bulpitt, A. Morgan, and J. M. Jones: Hydralazine, antinuclear antibodies, and the lupus syndrome, *Br. Med. J.*, 284:936, 1982.

688. Cameron, H. A., and L. E. Ramsay: The lupus syndrome induced by hydralazine: A common complication with low dose treatment, *Br. Med. J.*, 289:410, 1984.

689. Batchelor, J. R., K. I. Welsh, R. M. Tinoco, C. T. Dollery, G. R. V. Hughes, R. Bernstein, P. Ryan, P. F. Naish, G. M. Aber, R. F. Bing, and G. I. Russell: Hydralazine-induced systemic lupus erythematosus: Influence of HLA-DR and sex on susceptibility, *Lancet*, 1:1107, 1980.

690. Magil, A. B., H. S. Ballon, and A. Rae: Focal proliferative lupus nephritis. A clinicopathologic study using the W. H. O. classification, *Am. J. Med.*, 72:620, 1982.

691. DeFronzo, R. A., C. R. Cooke, M. Goldberg, M. Cox, A. R. Myers, and Z. S. Agus: Impaired renal tubular potassium secretion in systemic lupus erythematosus, *Ann. Intern. Med.*, 86:268, 1977.

692. Lloyd, W., and P. H. Schur: Immune complexes, complement, and anti-DNA antibodies in exacerbations of systemic lupus erythematosus, *Medicine*, 60:208, 1981.

693. Gilliam, J. N., D. E. Cheatum, E. R. Hurd, P. Stastny, and M. Ziff: Immunologlobulin in clinically uninvolved skin in systemic lupus erythematosus: Association with renal disease, *J. Clin. Invest.*, 53:1434, 1974.

694. Pennebaker, J. S., J. N. Gilliam and M. Ziff: Immunoglobulin classes of DNA binding activity in serum and skin in systemic lupus erythematosus, *J. Clin. Invest.*, 60:1331, 1977.

695. Ahmed, A. R., and T. T. Provost: Incidence of a positive lupus band test using sun-exposed and unexposed skin, *Arch. Dermatol.,* 115:228, 1979.

696. Weinstein, J: Hypocomplementemia in hydralazine-associated systemic lupus erythematosus, *Am. J. Med.,* 65:553, 1978.

697. Clinicopathologic Conference: Renal failure, dyspnea and anemia in a 57 year-old woman, *Am. J. Med.,* 71:876, 1981.

698. Bjorck, S., C. Svalander, and G. Westberg: Hydralazine-associated glomerulonephritis, *Acta Med. Scand.,* 218:261, 1985.

699. Shapiro, K. S., V. W. Pinn, J. T. Harrington, and A. S. Levey: Immune complex glomerulonephritis in hydralazine-induced SLE, *Am. J. Kid. Dis.,* 3:270, 1984.

700. Zech, P., S. Colon, M. Labeeuw, J. Bernheim, and N. Blanc-Brunat: Nephrotic syndrome in procainamide induced lupus nephritis, *Clin. Nephrol.,* 11:218, 1979.

701. Sharp, G. C., W. S. Irvin, C. M. May, H. R. Holman, F. C. McDuffie, E. V. Hess, and F. R. Schmid: Association of antibodies to ribonucleoprotein and Sm antigens with mixed connective-tissue disease, systemic lupus erythematosus and other rheumatic disease, *N. Engl. J. Med.,* 295:1149, 1976.

702. Sharp, G. C.: Subsets of SLE and mixed connective tissue disease, *Am. J. Kid. Dis.,* 2(suppl. 1):201, 1982.

703. Zwelman, B., J. Kornblum, J. Cornog, and E. A. Hildreth: The prognosis of lupus nephritis: A role of clinical-pathologic correlations, *Ann. Intern. Med.,* 69:441, 1968.

704. Cameron, J. S.: Diseases of the urinary system: Treatment of glomerulonephritis by drugs, *Br. Med. J.,* 1:1520, 1977.

705. Hughes, G. R. V.: Systemic lupus erythematosus: Treatment and prognosis, *Br. Med. J.,* 2:1019, 1979.

706. Urowitz, M. B., A. A. M. Bookman, B. E. Koehler, D. A. Gordon, H. A. Smythe, and M. A. Ogryzlo: The bimodal mortality pattern of systemic lupus erythematosus, *Am. J. Med.,* 60:221, 1976.

707. Pollak, V. E., C. L. Pirani, and F. D. Schwartz: The natural history of the renal manifestations of systemic lupus erythematosus, *J. Lab. Clin. Med.,* 63: 537, 1964.

708. Cameron, J. S., D. R. Turner, C. S. Ogg, D. G. Williams, M. H. Lessof, C. Chantler, and S. Leibowitz: Systemic lupus with nephritis: A long-term study, *Q. J. Med.,* 48:1, 1979.

709. Finlander, P., M. Koss, R. Kitridou, and W. A. Border: Glomerulonephritis in systemic lupus erythematosus, *Am. J. Nephrol.,* 1:53, 1981.

710. Donadio, J. V., Jr., K. E. Holley, R. H. Ferguson, and D. M. Ilstrup: Treatment of lupus nephritis with prednisone and combined prednisone and cyclophosphamide, *N. Engl. J. Med.,* 299:1151, 1978.

711. Hecht, B., N. Siegel, M. Adler, M. Kashgarian, and J. P. Hayslett: Prognostic indices in lupus nephritis, *Medicine,* 55:163, 1976.

712. Hayslett, J. P., M. Kashgarian, C. D. Cook, and B. H. Spargo: The effect of azathioprine on lupus glomerulonephritis, *Medicine,* 51:393, 1972.

713. Shelp, W. D., J. M. B. Bloodworth, Jr., and R. E. Rieselbach: Effect of azathioprine on renal histology and function in lupus nephritis, *Arch. Intern. Med.,* 128:566, 1971.

714. Donadio, J. V., Jr., K. E. Holley, R. D. Wagoner, R. H. Ferguson, and F. C. McDuffie: Treatment of lupus nephritis with prednisone and combined prednisone and azathioprine, *Ann. Intern. Med.,* 77:829, 1972.

715. Decker, J. L., J. H. Klippel, P. H. Plotz, and A. D. Steinberg: Cyclophosphamide or azathioprine in lupus glomerulonephritis. A controlled trial: Results at 28 months, *Ann. Intern. Med.,* 83:606, 1975.

716. Donadio, J. V., Jr., K. E. Holley, and D. M. Ilstrup: Cytotoxic drug treatment of lupus nephritis, *Am. J. Kid. Dis.,* 2(suppl. 1):178, 1982.

717. Steinberg, E. B., H. R. Smith, and A. D. Steinberg: Cyclophosphamide therapy in murine lupus: effect of combining multiple subsets into a single randomized study (letter), *Arth. Rheum.,* 26:1293, 1983.

718. Felson, D. T., and J. Anderson: Evidence for the superiority of immunosuppressive drugs and prednisone over prednisone alone in lupus nephritis. Results of a pooled analysis, *N. Engl. J. Med.,* 311:1528, 1984.

719. Austin, H. A., III, L. R. Muenz, K. M. Joyce, T. T. Antonovych, and J. E. Balow: Diffuse proliferative lupus nephritis: Identification of specific pathologic features affecting renal outcome, *Kidney Int.,* 25:689, 1984.

720. Garcia, D. L., S. Anderson, H. G. Rennke, and B. M. Brenner: Chronic steroid therapy amplifies glomerular injury in rats with reduced renal mass (abstract), *Clin. Res.,* 34(2):697a, 1986.

721. Austin, H., J. Klippel, N. leRiche, J. L. Decker, and J. E. Balow: Immunosuppressive therapy of lupus nephritis (abstract), *Kidney Int.,* 27:204, 1985.

722. Plotz, P. H., J. H. Klippel, J. L. Decker, D. Grauman, B. Wolff, B. C. Brown, and G. Rutt: Bladder

complications in patients receiving cyclophosphamide for systemic lupus erythematosus or rheumatoid arthritis, *Ann. Intern. Med.,* 91:221, 1979.

723. Elliott, R. W., D. M. Essenhigh, and A. R. Morley:
Cyclophosphamide treatment of systemic lupus
erythematosus: Risk of bladder cancer exceeds
benefit, *Br. Med. J.,* 284:1160, 1982.

724. Steinberg, A. D.: Cyclophosphamide. Should it be
used daily, monthly, or never?, *N. Engl. J. Med.,*
310:458, 1984.

725. Zizic, T. M., C. Marcoux, D. S. Hungerford, J-V.
Dansereau, and M. B. Stevens: Corticosteroid
therapy associated with ischemic necrosis of bone
in systemic lupus erythematosus, *Am. J. Med.,* 79:
596, 1985.

726. Pinching, A. J., C. M. Lockwood, B. A. Pussell,
A. J. Rees, P. Sweny, D. J. Evans, N. Bowley, and
D. K. Peters: Wegener's granulomatosis: Obser-
vations on 18 patients with severe renal disease,
Q. J. Med., 52:435, 1983.

727. Raij, L., S. Azar, and W. Keane: Role of hypertension in progressive glomerular immune injury,
Hypertension, 7:398, 1985.

728. Neugarten, J., H. D. Feiner, R. G. Schacht, G. R.
Gallo, and D. S. Baldwin: Aggravation of experimental glomerulonephritis by superimposed clip
hypertension, *Kidney Int.,* 22:257, 1982.

729. Levinsky, R. J., J. S. Cameron, and J. F. Soothill:
Serum immune complexes and disease activity in
lupus nephritis, *Lancet,* 1:564, 1977.

730. Kimberly, R. P., M. D. Lockshin, R. L. Sherman,
J. S. McDougal, R. D. Inman, and C. L. Christian:
High-dose intravenous methylprednisolone pulse
therapy in systemic lupus erythematosus, *Am. J.
Med.,* 70:817, 1981.

731. Cathcart, E. S., M. A. Scheinberg, B. A. Idelson,
and W. G. Couser: Beneficial effects on methylprednisolone "pulse" therapy in diffuse proliferative lupus nephritis, *Lancet,* 1:163, 1976.

732. Ponticelli, C., P. Zucchielli, G. Banfi, L. Cagnoli, P.
Scalia, S. Pasquali, and G. Imbasciati: Treatment
of diffuse proliferative lupus nephritis by intravenous high-dose methylprednisolone, *Q. J. Med.,*
51:17, 1982.

733. Jacob, H. S.: Pulse steroids in hematologic diseases, *Hosp. Pract.,* 20 (8):87, 1985.

734. Weiler, J. M., and B. D. Packard: Methylprednisolone inhibits the alternative and amplification pathways of complement, *Infect. Immun.,* 38:
122, 1982.

735. Warren, D. J., and R. S. Smith: High-dose prednisolone, *Lancet,* 1:594, 1983.

736. Bocanegra, T. S., M. O. Castaneda, L. R. Espinoza,

F. B. Vasey, and B. F. Germain: Sudden death
after methylprednisolone pulse therapy, *Ann. Intern. Med.,* 95:122, 1981.

737. Moses, R. E., A. McCormick, and W. Nickey:
Fatal arrhythmia after pulse methylprednisolone
therapy (letter), *Ann. Intern. Med.,* 95:781, 1981.

738. Otra-Sibu, N., C. Chantler, M. Bewick, and G.
Haycock: Comparison of high-dose intravenous
methylprednisolone with low-dose oral prednisolone in acute renal allograft rejection in children,
Br. Med. J., 285:258, 1982.

739. Barry, J. M., D. H. Craig, S. M. Fischer, G. M.
Fuchs, R. K. Lawson, and W. M. Bennett: An
analysis of 100 primary cadaver kidney transplants,
J. Urol, 124:783, 1980.

740. Bach, M. C., A. Sahyoun, J. L. Adler, R. M. Schles-
inger, J. Breman, P. Madras, F.-K. P'eng, and
A. P. Monaco: Influence of rejection therapy on
fungal and nocardial infections in renal-transplant
recipients, *Lancet,* 1:180, 1973.

741. Verrier Jones, J., R. H. Cumming, P. A. Bacon, J.
Evers, I. D. Fraser, J. Bothamley, C. R. Tribe, P.
David, and G. R. V. Hughes: Evidence for a therapeutic effect of plasmaphersis in patients with
systemic lupus erythematosus, *Q. J. Med.,* 48:555,
1979.

742. Lewis, E. J.: Plasmapheresis for the treatment of
severe lupus nephritis: Uncontrolled observations,
Am. J. Kid. Dis., 2(suppl. 1):182, 1982.

743. Editorial: Hazards of apheresis, *Lancet,* 2:1025,
1982.

744. Prickett, J. D., D. R. Robinson, and A. D. Steinberg: Dietary enrichment with the polyunsaturated fatty acid eicosapentaenoic acid prevents
proteinuria and prolongs survival in NZB×NZW
F_1 mice, *J. Clin. Invest.,* 68:556, 1981.

745. Kant, K. S., V. E. Pollak, A. Dosekun, P. Glas-
Greenwalt, M. Weiss, and H. I. Glueck: Lupus
nephritis with thrombosis and abnormal fibrinolysis: Effect of ancrod, *J. Lab. Clin. Med.,* 105:77,
1985.

746. Jarrett, M. P., L. B. Sablay, L. Walter, P. Barland,
and A. I. Grayzel: The effect of continuous normalization of serum hemolytic complement on
the course of lupus nephritis. A five year prospective study, *Am. J. Med.,* 70:1067, 1981.

747. Schur, P. H., and J. Sanderson: Immunologic factors and clinical activity in systemic lupus erythematosus, *N. Engl. J. Med.,* 278:533, 1968.

748. Epstein, W. V.: Immunologic events preceding
clinical exacerbation of systemic lupus erythematosus, *Am. J. Med.,* 54:631, 1973.

749. Singsen, B. H., B. H. Bernstein, K. K. King, and V.

Hansen: Systemic lupus erythematosus in childhood: Correlations between changes in disease activity and serum complement levels, *J. Pediatr.*, 89:358, 1976.

750. Gladman, D. D., M. B. Urowitz, and E. C. Keystone: Serologically active, clinically quiescent systemic lupus erythematosus: A discordance between clinical and serologic features, *Am. J. Med.*, 66:210, 1979.

751. Sharon, E., D. Kaplan, and H. S. Diamond: Exacerbation of systemic lupus erythematosus after withdrawal of azathioprine therapy, *N. Engl. J. Med.*, 288:122, 1973.

752. Wallace, D. J., T. E. Podell, J. M. Weiner, M. B. Cox, J. R. Klinenberg, S. Forouzesh, and E. L. Dubois: Lupus nephritis. Experience with 230 patients in a private practice from 1950 to 1980, *Am. J. Med.*, 72:209, 1982.

753. Austin, H. A., III, L. B. Muenz, K. A. Joyce, T. A. Antonovych, M. E. Kullick, J. H. Klippel, J. L. Decker, and J. E. Balow: Prognostic factors in lupus nephritis. Contribution of renal histologic data, *Am. J. Med.*, 75:382, 1983.

754. Tejani, A., A. D. Nicastri, C-K. Chen, S. Fikrig, and K. Gurumurthy: Lupus nephritis in black and Hispanic children, *Am. J. Dis. Child.*, 137:481, 1983.

755. Wilson, H. A., M. E. Hamilton, D. A. Spyker, C. M. Brunner, W. M. O'Brien, J. S. Davis, III, and J. B. Winfield: Age influences the clinical and serologic expression of systemic lupus erythematosus, *Arth. Rheum.*, 24:1230, 1981.

756. Coplon, N. S., C. J. Diskin, J. Petersen, and R. S. Swenson: The long-term clinical course of systemic lupus erythematosus in end-stage renal disease, *N. Engl. J. Med.*, 308:186, 1983.

757. Austin, H. A., III, L. B. Muenz, K. A. Joyce, T. A. Antonovych, M. E. Kullick, J. Klippel, J. L. Decker, and J. E. Balow: Prognostic factors in lupus nephritis. Contribution of renal histologic data, *Am. J. Med.*, 75:382, 1983.

758. Kimberly, R. P., M. D. Lockshin, R. L. Sherman, J. F. Beary, J. Mouradian, and J. S. Cheigh: "End-stage" lupus nephritis: Clinical course to and outcome on dialysis. Experience with 39 patients, *Medicine*, 60:277, 1981.

759. Correia, P., J. S. Cameron, C. S. Ogg, D. G. Williams, M. Bewick, and J. A. Hicks: End-stage renal failure in systemic lupus erythematosus with nephritis, *Clin. Nephrol.*, 22:293, 1984.

760. Amend, W. J. C. Jr., F. Vincenti, N. J. Feduska, O. Salvatierra, Jr., W. H. Johnston, J. Jackson, N. Tilney, M. Garovoy, and E. L. Burwell: Recurrent

systemic lupus erythematosus involving renal allografts, *Ann. Intern. Med.*, 94:444, 1981.

761. Ziff, M., and J. H. Helderman: Dialysis and transplantation in end-stage lupus nephritis, *N. Engl. J. Med.*, 308:218, 1983.

762. Kimberly, R. P., M. D. Lockshin, R. L. Sherman, J. Mouradian, and S. Saal: Reversible "end-stage" lupus nephritis. Analysis of patients able to discontinue dialysis, *Am. J. Med.*, 74:361, 1983.

763. Ginzler, E. M., A. D. Nicastri, C.-K. Chen, E. A. Friedman, H. S. Diamond, and D. Kaplan: Progression of mesangial and focal to diffuse lupus nephritis, *N. Engl. J. Med.*, 291:693, 1974.

764. Kimberly, R. P., J. R. Gill, R. E. Bowden, H. R. Keiser, and P. H. Plotz: Elevated urinary prostaglandins and the effects of aspirin on renal function in lupus erythematosus, *Ann. Intern. Med.*, 89:336, 1978.

765. Kimberly, R. P., and P. H. Plotz: Aspirin-induced depression of renal function, *N. Engl. J. Med.*, 296:418, 1977.

766. Hayslett, J. P.: Effect of pregnancy in patients with SLE, *Am. J. Kid. Dis.*, 2(suppl. 1):223, 1982.

767. Fine, L. G., E. V. Barnett, G. M. Danovitch, A. R. Nissenson, M. E. Conolly, S. M. Lieb, and C. T. Barrett: Systemic lupus erythematosus in pregnancy, *Ann. Intern. Med.*, 94:667, 1981.

768. Imbasciati, E., M. Surian, S. Bottino, P. Cosci, G. Colussi, G. C. Ambroso, E. Massa, L. Minetti, G. Pardi, and C. Ponticelli: Lupus nephropathy and pregnancy. A study of 26 pregnancies in patients with systemic lupus erythematosus and nephritis, *Nephron*, 36:46, 1984.

769. Jungers, P., M. Dougados, C. Pelissier, F. Kuttenn, F. Tron, P. Lesaure, and J-F. Bach: Lupus nephropathy and pregnancy. Report of 104 cases in 36 patients, *Arch. Intern. Med.*, 142:771, 1982.

770. Spargo, B. H., N. G. Ordonez, and J. C. Ringus: The differential diagnosis of crescentic glomerulonephritis: The pathology of specific lesions with prognostic implications, *Hum. Pathol.*, 8:187, 1977.

771. Beirne, G. J., J. P. Wagnild, S. W. Zimmerman, P. D. Macken, and P. M. Burkholder: Idiopathic crescentic glomerulonephritis, *Medicine*, 56:349, 1977.

772. Wilson, C. B., and F. J. Dixon: Antiglomerular basement membrane antibody induced glomerulonephritis, *Kidney Int.*, 3:74, 1973.

773. Stilmant, M. M., W. K. Bolton, B. C. Sturgill, G. W. Schmitt, and W. G. Couser: Crescentic glomerulonephritis without immune deposits: Clinicopathologic features, *Kidney Int.*, 15:184, 1979.

774. Couser, W. G.: Idiopathic rapidly progressive glomerulonephritis, *Am. J. Nephrol.,* 2:57, 1982.

775. Bacani, R. A., F. Velasquez, A. Kanter, C. L. Pirani, and V. E. Pollak: Rapidly progressive (non-streptococcal) glomerulonephritis, *Ann. Intern. Med.,* 69:463, 1968.

776. Magil, A. B.: Histogenesis of glomerular crescents. Immunohistochemical demonstration of cytokeratin in crescent cells, *Am. J. Pathol.,* 120:222, 1985.

777. Thomson, N. M., S. R. Holdsworth, E. F. Glasgow, and R. C. Atkins: The macrophage in the development of experimental crescentic glomerulonephritis, *Am. J. Pathol.,* 94:223, 1979.

778. Atkins, R. C., E. F. Glasgow, S. R. Holdsworth, and F. E. Matthews: The macrophage in human rapidly progressive glomerulonephritis, *Lancet,* 1: 830, 1976.

779. Hooke, D. H., W. W. Hancock, D. C. Gee, N. Kraft, and R. C. Atkins: Monoclonal antibody analysis of glomerular hypercellularity in human glomerulonephritis, *Clin. Nephrol.,* 22:163, 1984.

780. Schreiner, G. F., R. S. Cotran, V. Pardo, and E. R. Unanue: A mononuclear cell component in experimental immunological glomerulonephritis, *J. Exp. Med.,* 147:369, 1978.

781. Andres, G., J. Brentjens, R. Kohli, R. Anthone, S. Anthone, T. Baliah, M. Montes, B. K. Mookerjee, A. Prezyna, M. Sepulveda, R. Venuto, and C. Elwood: Histology of human tubulo-interstitial nephritis associated with antibodies to renal basement membranes, *Kidney Int.,* 13:480, 1978.

782. Beirne, G. J., G. N. Octaviano, W. L. Kopp, and R. O. Burns: Immunohistology of the lung in Goodpasture's syndrome, *Ann. Intern. Med.,* 69: 1207, 1968.

783. McCluskey, R. T., P. Vassalli, G. Gallo, and D. S. Baldwin: An immunofluorescent study of pathogenic mechanisms in glomerular diseases, *N. Engl. J. Med.,* 274:695, 1966.

784. Hoyer, J. R., A. F. Michael, and L. W. Hoyer: Immunofluorescent localization of antihemophilic factor antigen and fibrinogen in human renal disease, *J. Clin. Invest.,* 53:1375, 1974.

785. Min, K. W., F. Gyorkey, P. Gyorkey, J. Y. Yium, and G. Eknoyan: The morphogenesis of glomerular crescents in rapidly progressive glomerulonephritis, *Kidney Int.,* 5:47, 1974.

786. Bonsib, S. M.: Glomerular basement membrane discontinuities. Scanning electron microscopic study of acellular glomeruli, *Am. J. Pathol.,* 119: 357, 1985.

787. Serra, A., J. S. Cameron, D. R. Turner, B. Hartley, C. S. Ogg, G. H. Neild, D. G. Williams, D. Taube, C. B. Brown, and J. A. Hicks: Vasculitis affecting the kidney: Presentation, histopathology, and long-term outcome, *Q. J. Med.,* 53:181, 1984.

788. Vassalli, P., and R. T. McCluskey: The pathogenic role of the coagulation process in rabbit Masugi nephritis, *Am. J. Pathol.,* 45:653, 1964.

789. Thomson, N. M., J. Moran, I. J. Simpson, and D. K. Peters: Defibrination with ancrod in nephrotoxic nephritis in rabbits, *Kidney Int.,* 10:343, 1976.

790. Thomson, N. M., I. J. Simpson, D. J. Evans, and D. K. Peters: Defibrination with ancrod in experimental chronic immune complex nephritis, *Clin. Exp. Immunol.,* 20:527, 1975.

791. Cole, E. H., J. Schulman, M. Urowitz, E. Keystone, C. Williams, and G. A. Levy: Monocyte procoagulant activity in glomerulonephritis associated with systemic lupus erythematosus, *J. Clin. Invest.,* 75:861, 1985.

792. Wiggins, R. C., A. Glatfelter, and J. Brukman: Procoagulant activity in glomeruli and urine of rabbits with nephrotoxic nephritis, *Lab. Invest.,* 53:156, 1985.

793. Steblay, R. W.: Glomerulonephritis induced in sheep by injections of heterologous glomerular basement membrane and Freund's complete ad-'juvant, *J. Exp. Med.,* 116:253, 1962.

794. Lerner, R. A., and F. J. Dixon: Transfer of ovine experimental allergic glomerulonephritis (EAG) with serum, *J. Exp. Med.,* 124:431, 1966.

795. Lerner, R. A., R. J. Glassock, and F. J. Dixon: The role of anti-glomerular basement membrane antibody in the pathogenesis of human glomerulonephritis, *J. Exp. Med.,* 126:989, 1967.

796. Koffler, D., J. Sanderson, R. Carr, and H. G. Kunkel: Immunologic studies concerning the pulmonary lesions in Goodpasture's syndrome, *Am. J. Pathol.,* 54:293, 1969.

797. McPhaul, J. J., Jr., and F. J. Dixon: Characterization of human antiglomerular basement membrane antibodies eluted from glomerulonephritic kidneys, *J. Clin. Invest.,* 49:308, 1970.

798. Wilson, C. B., and F. J. Dixon: Renal response to immunologic injury, in B. M. Brenner and F. C. Rector, Jr. (eds.), *The Kidney,* 3d ed., Saunders, Philadelphia, 1986, pp. 817–825.

799. Rees, A. J., D. K. Peters, D. A. S. Compston, and J. R. Batchelor: Strong association between HLA-DRW2 and antibody-mediated Goodpasture's syndrome, *Lancet,* 1:966, 1978.

800. Rees, A. J., D. K. Peters, N. Amos, K. I. Welsh, and J. R. Batchelor: The influence of HLA-linked genes on the severity of anti-GBM antibody-mediated nephritis, *Kidney Int.,* 26:444, 1984.

801. Willoughby, W. F., and F. J. Dixon: Experimental hemorrhagic pneumonitis produced by heterologous anti-lung antibody, *J. Immunol.,* 104:28, 1970.

802. Steblay, R. W.: Autoimmune glomerulonephritis induced in sheep by injections of human lung and Freund's adjuvant, *Science,* 160:204, 1968.

803. Wilson, C. B., and R. C. Smith: Goodpasture's syndrome associated with influenza A2 virus infection, *Ann. Intern. Med.,* 76:91, 1972.

804. Abboud, R. T., W. H. Chase, H. S. Ballon, and S. Grzyboswki: Goodpasture's syndrome: Diagnosis by transbronchial lung biopsy, *Ann. Intern. Med.,* 89:635, 1978.

805. Kleinknecht, D., L. Morel-Maroger, P. Callard, J.-P. Adhemar, and P. Mahieu: Antiglomerular basement membrane nephritis after solvent exposure, *Arch. Intern. Med.,* 140:230, 1980.

806. Yoshioaka, K., A. F. Michael, J. Velosa, and A. J. Fish: Detection of hidden nephritogenic antigen determinants in human renal and nonrenal basement membranes, *Am. J. Pathol.,* 121:156, 1985.

807. McPhaul, J. J., and J. D. Mullens: Glomerulonephritis mediated by antibody to glomerular basement membrane: Immunological clinical and histological characteristics, *J. Clin. Invest.,* 57:351, 1976.

808. Donaghy, M., and A. J. Rees: Cigarette smoking and lung hemorrhage in glomerulonephritis caused by antibodies to glomerular basement membrane, *Lancet,* 2:1390, 1983.

809. Lockwood, C. M., A. J. Pinching, P. Sweny, A. J. Rees, B. Pussell, J. Uff, and D. K. Peters: Plasma-exchange and immunosuppression in the treatment of fulminating immune-complex crescentic nephritis, *Lancet,* 1:63, 1977.

810. Adu Ntoso, K., J. E. Tomaszewski, S. A. Jimenez, and E. G. Neilson: Penicillamine-induced rapidly progressive glomerulonephritis in patients with progressive systemic sclerosis, *Am. J. Kid. Dis.,* 8: 159, 1986.

811. Walker, P. D., E. C. Deeves, G. Sahba, J. D. Wallin, and W. M. O'Neill, Jr.: Rapidly progressive glomerulonephritis in a patient with syphilis. Identification of antitreponemal antibody and treponemal antigen in renal tissue, *Am. J. Med.,* 76:1106, 1984.

812. Bolton, W. K., F. L. Tucker, and B. C. Sturgill: New avian model of experimental glomerulonephritis consistent with mediation by cellular immunity, *J. Clin. Invest.,* 73:1263, 1984.

813. Tipping, P. G., T. J. Neale, and S. R. Holdsworth: T lymphocyte participation in antibody-induced experimental glomerulonephritis, *Kidney Int.,* 27: 530, 1985.

814. A Report of the Southwest Pediatric Nephrology Study Group: A clinico-pathologic study of crescentic glomerulonephritis in 50 children, *Kidney Int.,* 27:450, 1985.

815. Boyce, N. W., and S. R. Holdsworth: Pulmonary manifestations of the clinical syndrome of acute glomerulonephritis and lung hemorrhage, *Am. J. Kid. Dis.,* 8:31, 1986.

816. Heaf, J. G., F. Jorgensen, and L. P. Nielsen: Treatment and prognosis of extracapillary glomerulonephritis, *Nephron,* 35:217, 1983.

817. Bolton, W. K., and W. G. Couser: Intravenous pulse methylprednisolone therapy of acute crescentic rapidly progressive glomerulonephritis, *Am. J. Med.,* 66:495, 1979.

818. Hind, C. R. K., C. M. Lockwood, D. K. Peters, H. Paraskevakou, D. J. Evans, and A. J. Rees: Prognosis after immunosuppression of patients with crescentic nephritis requiring dialysis, *Lancet,* 1: 263, 1983.

819. Neild, G. H., J. S. Cameron, C. S. Ogg, D. R. Turner, D. G. Williams, C. Chantler, and J. Hicks: Rapidly progressive glomerulonephritis with extensive glomerular crescent formation, *Q. J. Med.,* 52:395, 1983.

820. Booth, L. J., and G. M. Aber: Immunosuppressive therapy in adults with proliferative glomerulonephritis: Controlled trial, *Lancet,* 2:1010, 1970.

821. Report by the Medical Research Council Working Party: Controlled trial of azathioprine and prednisone in chronic renal disease, *Br. Med. J.,* 2:239, 1971.

822. Brown, C. B., D. Turner, C. S. Ogg, D. Wilson, J. S. Cameron, and C. Chantler: Combined immunosuppression and anticoagulation in rapidly progressive glomerulonephritis, *Lancet,* 2:1166, 1974.

823. Kincaid-Smith, P: Anticoagulants are of value in the treatment of renal disease, *Am. J. Kid. Dis.,* 3:299, 1984.

824. Frye, K. H., D. Hancock, H. Moutsopoulos, H. D. Humes, and A. I. Arieff: Low-dosage heparin in rapidly progressive glomerulonephritis, *Arch. Intern. Med.,* 136:995, 1976.

825. Border, W. A.: Anticoagulants are of little value in the treatment of renal disease, *Am. J. Kid. Dis.,* 3:308, 1984.

826. O'Neil, W. M., W. B. Etheridge, and H. A. Bloomer: High-dose corticosteroids, *Arch. Intern. Med.,* 139:514, 1979.

827. Cole, B. R., J. T. Brockelback, R. A. Kienstra, J. M. Kissane, and A. M. Robson: "Pulse" methypred-

nisolone therapy in the treatment of severe glomerulonephritis, *J. Pediatr.,* 88:307, 1976.

828. Oredugba, O., D. C. Mazumdar, J. S. Meyer, and H. Lubowitz: Pulse methylprednisolone therapy in idiopathic rapidly progressive glomerulonephritis, *Ann. Intern. Med.,* 92:504, 1980.

829. Balow, J. E.: Renal vasculitis, *Kidney Int.,* 27:954, 1985.

830. Rosenblatt, S. G., W. Knight, G. A. Bannayan, C. B. Wilson, and J. H. Stein: Treatment of Goodpasture's syndrome with plasmapheresis: A case report and review of the literature, *Am. J. Med.,* 66:689, 1979.

831. Kincaid-Smith, P., and A. J. F. D'Apice: Plasmapheresis in rapidly progressive glomerulonephritis, *Am. J. Med.,* 65:564, 1978.

832. Lockwood, C. M., S. Worlledge, A. Nicholas, C. Cotton, and D. K. Peters: Reversal of impaired splenic function in patients with nephritis or vasculitis (or both) by plasma exchange, *N. Engl. J. Med.,* 300:524, 1979.

833. Rosen, R. D., E. M. Hersh, J. T. Sharp, K. B. McCredie, F. Gyorkey, W. N. Suki, G. Eknoyan, and M. A. Reisberg: Effect of plasma exchange on circulating immune complexes and antibody formation in patients treated with cyclophosphamide and prednisone, *Am. J. Med.,* 63:674, 1977.

834. Bystryn, J.-C., M. W. Graf, and J. W. Uhr: Regulation of antibody formation by serum antibody, II: Removal of specific antibody by means of exchange transfusion, *J. Exp. Med.,* 132:1279, 1970.

835. Bruns, F. J., S. Adler, D. P. Segel, and D. S. Fraley: Long-term follow-up of aggressively treated rapidly progressive glomerulonephritis (abstract), *Kidney Int.,* 29:181, 1986.

836. Savage, C. O. S., C. D. Pusey, C. Bowman, and A. J. Rees: Antiglomerular basement membrane antibody mediated disease in the British Isles 1980–4, *Br. Med., J.,* 292:301, 1986.

837. Briggs, W. A., J. P. Johnson, S. Teichman, H. C. Yeager, and C. B. Wilson: Antiglomerular basement membrane antibody-mediated glomerulonephritis and Goodpasture's syndrome, *Medicine,* 58:348, 1979.

838. De Torrente, A., M. M. Popovtzer, S. J. Guggenheim, and R. W. Schrier: Serious pulmonary hemorrhage, glomerulonephritis, and massive steroid therapy, *Ann. Intern. Med.,* 83:218, 1975.

839. Rees, A. J., C. M. Lockwood, and D. K. Peters: Enhanced allergic tissue injury in Goodpasture's syndrome by intercurrent bacterial infection, *Br. Med. J.,* 2:723, 1977.

840. Peters, D. K.: The major glomerulopathies, *Hosp. Pract.,* 16(10):117, 1981.

841. Bailey, R. R., I. J. Simpson, K. L. Lynn, T. J. Neale, P. B. Doak, and A. R. McGiven: Goodpasture's syndrome with normal renal function, *Clin. Nephrol.,* 15:211, 1981.

842. Teague, C. A., P. B. Doak, I. J. Simpson, S. P. Rainer, and P. B. Herdson: Goodpasture's syndrome: An analysis of 29 cases, *Kidney Int.,* 13:492, 1978.

843. Maddock, R. K., Jr., L. E. Stevens, K. Reemtsma, and H. A. Bloomer: Goodpasture's syndrome: Cessation of pulmonary hemorrhage after bilateral nephrectomy, *Ann. Intern. Med.,* 67:1258, 1967.

844. Nowakowski, A., R. B. Grove, L. H. King, Jr., T. T. Antonovych, R. W. Fortner, M. R. Knieser, B. C. Carter, and J. H. Knepshield: Goodpasture's syndrome: Recovery from severe pulmonary hemorrhage after bilateral nephrectomy, *Ann. Intern. Med.,* 75:243, 1971.

845. Eisinger, A. J.: Goodpasture's syndrome: Failure of nephrectomy to cure pulmonary hemorrhage, *Am. J. Med.,* 55:565, 1973.

846. Bergren, H., J. Jervell, E. K. Brodwall, A. Flatmark, and O. Mellbye: Goodpasture's syndrome. A report of seven patients including long-term follow-up of three who received a kidney transplant, *Am. J. Med.,* 68:54, 1980.

847. Dahlberg, P. J., S. B. Kurtz, J. V. Donadio, Jr., K. E. Holley, J. A. Velosa, D. E. Williams, and C. B. Wilson: Recurrent Goodpasture's syndrome, *Mayo Clin. Proc.,* 53:533, 1978.

848. Heptinstall, R. H.: Pathology of end-stage kidney disease, *Am. J. Med.,* 44:656, 1968.

849. Velosa, J., K. Miller, and A. F. Michael: Immunopathology of the end-stage kidney: Immunoglobulin and complement component deposition in nonimmune disease, *Am. J. Pathol.,* 84:149, 1976.

850. Baker, P. J., S. Adler, Y. Yang, and W. G. Couser: Complement activation by heat-killed human kidney cells: Formation, activity and stabilization of cell-bound C3 convertases, *J. Immunol.,* 133:877, 1984.

851. Murphy, F. D., and E. G. Schultz: Natural history of glomerular nephritis: report of patients treated ten to twenty-five years after acute stage, *Arch. Intern. Med.,* 97:783, 1956.

852. Levitt, J. I.: Deterioration of renal function after discontinuation of long-term prednisone-azathioprine therapy in primary renal disease, *N. Engl. J. Med.,* 282:1125, 1970.

7

VASCULAR DISEASES OF THE KIDNEY

Robert M. Black

Vascular diseases of the kidney impair renal function by reducing renal blood flow (Table 7–1). This may result from partial or complete occlusion of large, medium, or small vessels and may have an immunologic (e.g., vasculitis) or nonimmunologic (e.g., thromboembolism) pathogenesis. Furthermore, the clinical manifestations of these disorders are highly variable. Consequently, the diagnosis of vascular diseases of the kidney must be made by correlating the history, physical examination, and other laboratory data with the renal abnormalities.

SYSTEMIC VASCULITIS

CLASSIFICATION AND PATHOGENESIS

The classification of systemic vasculitis has been difficult in part because the etiologies and pathogeneses of the various disorders

TABLE 7-1. Vascular Diseases of the Kidney

Systemic vasculitis
   Polyarteritis
   Wegener's granulomatosis
   Hypersensitivity vasculitis
   Miscellaneous renal vasculitis
Progressive systemic sclerosis (scleroderma)
Hemolytic-uremic syndromes
   Thrombotic thrombocytopenic purpura
   Childhood hemolytic-uremic syndrome
   Adult hemolytic-uremic syndrome
Preeclampsia
Renal cortical necrosis
Thromboembolic diseases
   Blood clot
   Atheroma
Sickle cell nephropathy
Radiation nephritis

are undefined. Table 7-2 outlines a scheme which differentiates the vasculitides according to the size and site of vascular involvement.

Despite the variability in clinicopathologic changes, the different types of vasculitis are generally thought to be the result of immunologic mechanisms, particularly immune complex deposition in the blood vessel wall. Favoring this hypothesis is the presence of circulating immune complexes (CIC) in many patients, especially those with active vasculitis.[1-4] Although immunoglobulin deposition is rarely found at the tissue site of disease activity,[5,6] this could reflect rapid removal of complexes from the vascular wall in lesions over 24 to 48 h old.[7]

In some cases, an inciting antigen has been identified in the vascular lesions, offering further support for the immune complex hypothesis. Hepatitis B surface antigen (HbsAg) is the most common example of this phenomenon.[8] However, the observations that HbsAg is not associated with clinical vasculitis in most carriers and that its presence has been reported in several clinically different vasculitic syndromes (including polyarteritis and cryoglobulinemia) indicate that *host factors* must also be important.

Potential host factors include the type and quantity of antibody produced and the ability of the reticuloendothelial system to clear CIC, thereby minimizing tissue deposition.[4] Decreased clearance, for example, may predispose patients with hairy cell leukemia and splenic disease to the development of polyarteritis nodosa.[9,10]

Factors in addition to complex formation may also play an important role in tissue deposition. These include high blood flow and pressure in the microcirculation (in the

TABLE 7-2. Major Causes of Renal Vasculitis

Disorder	Vessels Primarily Affected

Polyarteritis
   Classsic polyarteritis nodosa
   Microscopic polyarteritis
   Churg-Strauss syndrome
   "Overlap" syndrome
	Small- and medium-sized muscular arteries (occasionally arterioles)

Wegener's granulomatosis	Granulomatous vasculitis of small- and medium-sized arteries (respiratory tract and kidneys)

Hypersensitivity vasculitis
   Henoch-Schönlein purpura
   Essential mixed cryoglobulinemia
   Serum sickness
	Small blood vessels particularly postcapillary venules

kidney and lung, for example) and the release of soluble mediators from activated basophils, mast cells, or platelets which increase vascular permeability.

The following sequence has been proposed to explain the pathogenesis of tissue injury in acute immune complex vasculitis (Fig. 7–1).[1,5,11] The deposition of immune complexes in the vascular wall (either as intact complexes or by in situ complex formation; see p. 149) initiates an inflammatory reaction that is both complement- and neutrophil-dependent. Complement can directly damage the vascular wall via formation of the membrane attack complex (C5b-C9) and can act indirectly by increasing vascular permeability (anaphylatoxin activity) and by promoting the accumulation of neutrophils (chemotactic activity) (see p. 153). The neutrophils can then perpetuate vascular injury by the release of oxygen free radicals, collagenase, elastase, prostaglandins, and macrophage chemotactic factors.

While this hypothesis is supported by some experimental data, the pathogenesis of chronic, granulomatous vasculitis (e.g., Wegener's granulomatosis) is poorly understood. Recently, anticytoplasmic antibodies have been detected in Wegener's granulomatosis, again supporting, but not proving, an im-

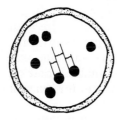

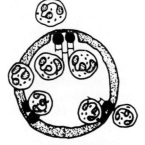

1) Circulating soluble immune complexes in antigen excess

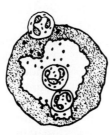

2) Increased permeability via platelet derived vasoactive amines and IgE mediated reactions

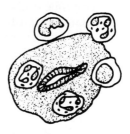

3) Trapping of immune complexes along basement membrane of vessel wall and activation of complement components (C)

4) Complement derived chemotactic factors (C3a, C5a, C567) cause accumulation of neutrophils

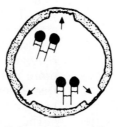

5) Neutrophils release lysosomal enzymes (collagenase, elastase); activation of C5b–C9 (membrane attack complex) directly injures vessel wall

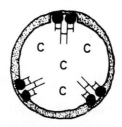

6) Damage and necrosis of vessel wall, thrombosis occlusion, hemorrhage

FIG. 7–1. Mechanism of immune complex vasculitis (see text). (*Adapted from A. S. Fauci, B. F. Haynes, and P. Katz, Ann. Intern. Med., 89:660, 1978.*)

mune complex pathogenesis.[12] Alternatively, the presence of granulomas could indicate involvement of cell-mediated immunity.

POLYARTERITIS

Polyarteritis nodosa (PAN) typically affects the small- and medium-sized muscular arteries. It tends to spare smaller vessels and is usually not associated with eosinophilia or significant pulmonary involvement. However, lung disease, allergic manifestations, and small vessel vasculitis, all may be seen in patients who otherwise appear to have classic PAN. As a result, three subdivisions of polyarteritis have evolved with different pathologic and clinical characteristics (Table 7–2).[1]

CLASSIC POLYARTERITIS NODOSA

Classic PAN primarily affects the small- and medium-sized muscular arteries.[13] The lesions tend to be segmental and commonly are found at bifurcations or branchings of arteries, with distal spread occasionally involving the arterioles. Early lesions are characterized by neutrophilic infiltration of all layers of the vascular wall with subsequent fibrinoid necrosis, disruption of the elastic lamina, and thrombosis, ischemia, and infarction of varying severity. (Fig. 7–2a). Mononuclear cell infiltration is then seen as the lesion becomes subacute. Aneurysm formation appears to follow this sequence, with inflammation of the intima and adventitia and weakening of the arterial wall ultimately causing incomplete arterial rupture.[14] Typically, lesions of all ages are found, suggesting that continuous immune complex deposition is occurring.

The phase of active injury is followed by healing. This is characterized by resolution of inflammation and subsequent fibrous thickening of the vascular wall, occasionally

causing further narrowing or obliteration of the vascular lumen (Fig. 7–2b).

Renal involvement may be associated with both arterial and glomerular changes.[13,15-17] The arterial lesions are similar to those in other vessels and, in classic PAN, predominantly affect the arcuate and interlobular arteries (Fig. 7–2). In the variants of PAN (see below), the distal interlobular arteries and afferent glomerular arterioles also may be affected, and eosinophils as well as neutrophils may be present in the inflammatory lesions. Thrombosis can result in partial or total occlusion of the vessel, with infarction of the surrounding parenchyma. Immunofluorescent microscopy may show deposition of IgG and complement in the involved vessels. However, negative findings do not necessarily exclude an immune complex pathogenesis since complexes may be rapidly removed from the vascular wall.[7] Furthermore, relatively small complexes can cause tissue damage without complex deposition being detectable histologically.[18]

The resolution of inflammation and thickening of the vascular wall seen in the healing phase results in a histologic picture in the kidney similar to that induced by chronic hypertension. These disorders can be differentiated by examining the elastic lamina, which is extensively disrupted by vasculitis but only reduplicated in hypertension.[13,15]

The glomerular lesions of classic PAN are induced primarily by ischemia and include segmental areas of fibrinoid necrosis and sclerosis with minimal cell proliferation.[13,16] Immunofluorescent and electron microscopy usually do not demonstrate evidence of immunoglobulin deposition in the glomeruli,[16,17] a pattern which is consistent with the ischemic nature of the lesion.

The glomerular changes may be particularly important from a diagnostic viewpoint, since vascular involvement is focal. Thus, a percutaneous renal biopsy may not demonstrate abnormal vessels, particularly if the disease is limited to the larger arteries. How-

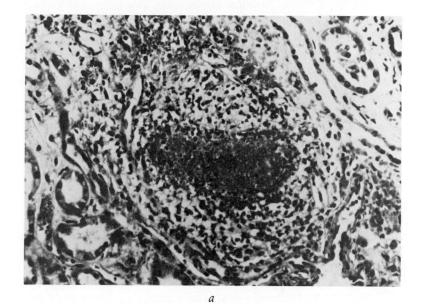

a

FIG. 7-2. Pathologic arterial changes in renal vasculitis. (*a*) Active lesion in a medium-sized artery reveals neutrophilic and mononuclear cell infiltration of the vascular wall with disruption of the elastic lamina and thrombus formation. (*b*) Healing is characterized by fibrous thickening of the damaged vascular wall, frequently resulting in further narrowing of the vascular lumen.

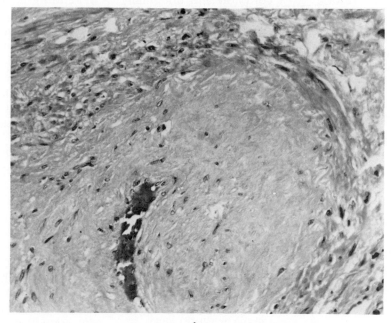

b

ever, the triad of necrotizing glomerular lesions, negative immunofluorescence, and systemic symptoms is strongly suggestive of systemic vasculitis.[16,19]

Clinical Manifestations. Polyarteritis nodosa is most common in middle-aged men, but can affect any age group.[16] Patients typically present with nonspecific symptoms such as fever, weight loss, and arthralgias. Other findings in the history and physical examination are dependent upon the extent of clinically significant organ involvement (Table 7–3).

Hypertension is ultimately present in over 50 percent of patients with classic PAN.[20] The elevation in blood pressure may be severe, and hypertensive crisis may rarely be the presenting sign of systemic vasculitis.[21] The mechanism primarily involves stimulation of the renin-angiotensin system by glomerular ischemia.[22,23]

Polyneuropathy, due to involvement of vasa vasora,[24] is a common and potentially disabling complication of PAN. Although the neurologic examination may be normal in the early stages of neural involvement, the typical clinical findings are those of a mononeuritis multiplex. This finding is diagnostically important because vasculitis is, with the exception of diabetes mellitus, the primary cause of an asymmetric polyneuropathy in the United States.

Central nervous system involvement also may occur in about 40 percent of patients.[24] Diffuse disturbances in cerebral, cerebellar, or brainstem function are frequently present, leading to headache or altered mental status. Other patients, however, may have more focal lesions causing a cerebrovascular accident or seizures.

Cardiac involvement is less common, occurring in approximately 30 percent of patients.[1,20] This is usually manifested as congestive heart failure, but myocardial infarction or pericarditis may also occur.

Renal involvement is seen in most patients at some time during the course of their disease.[16,25,26] The urinary findings are variable, depending in part upon the site of vascular involvement. Dysmorphic red blood cells, red cell casts, and mild proteinuria are commonly found, particularly if the small glomerular vessels are directly involved.[25] In comparison, hematuria may be absent with little or no casts or proteinuria if only the larger vessels are diseased, since, in this setting, there may be glomerular ischemia but no necrosis.[25]

Azotemia is common in untreated patients, occurring in up to 85 percent of cases.[16,27] The nephrotic syndrome is unusual (reflecting the secondary nature of glomerular involvement), and plasma complement levels are typically normal.[20]

Diagnosis. The diagnosis of PAN is often suggested by the clinical and laboratory evidence of multisystem involvement. In some patients, associated conditions may increase the statistical likelihood of PAN. These include HbsAg (40 percent in inner city pa-

TABLE 7–3. Major Clinical Features of Classic Polyarteritis Nodosa

Organ System	Typical Features
General	Fever, weakness, weight loss
Musculoskeletal	Arthralgias, myalgias, rare arthritis
Kidney	Abnormal sediment, renal insufficiency, hypertension, flank pain if infarction
Nervous system	Mononeuritis multiplex, cranial neuropathy
Heart	Angina, infarction, congestive heart failure
Liver	Subclinical disease to chronic active hepatitis—latter only with hepatitis B infection
Gastrointestinal tract	Infarction of viscera
Uncommon	Skin (subcutaneous nodules, livedo reticularis), lungs, spleen, genitourinary tract

tients),[22] intravenous drug abuse,[22] and hairy cell leukemia.[9,10]

Although the history and physical examination may be suggestive, a definitive diagnosis can be made only by demonstrating characteristic vascular changes either by biopsy or angiography. A biopsy should be obtained from a *clinically involved organ* such as a peripheral nerve, testis (if there is testicular pain), or the kidney.[1] For example, sural nerve biopsy is a procedure that can diagnose PAN if there is evidence of neural involvement by neurologic examination or by nerve conduction studies.[28] This test has the advantage of low morbidity (in possible contrast to renal biopsy), with most patients experiencing only mild numbness in the distribution of the sural nerve.

If no easily biopsied tissue appears to be involved, angiography of the celiac and renal vessels will often be diagnostic, demonstrating microaneurysms and irregular, segmental constrictions in the larger vessels with occlusion of smaller penetrating arteries (Fig. 7–3). These findings are virtually pathognomonic of systemic vasculitis although they may rarely be found in other disorders including fibromuscular dysplasia,[29] systemic lupus erythematosus,[30] Wegener's granulomatosis,[31] Henoch-Schönlein purpura,[32] or chronic ergot use.[33]

Renal biopsy, which carries a theoretically increased risk of bleeding, should be done only if the arteriogram is negative (or cannot be performed) or if no other easily accessible tissue seems to be involved. In some patients, however, renal biopsy is performed initially because of the lack of systemic symptoms that would suggest the possible presence of PAN.

Since PAN is a necrotizing disease, any delay in the onset of therapy may lead to potentially disabling and irreversible organ damage or death.[1,24] Consequently, *rapid evaluation is essential* in these patients. Once the vascular injury is sufficiently severe, control

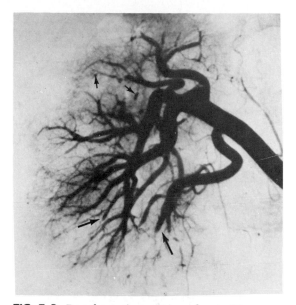

FIG. 7–3. Renal arteriogram in polyarteritis nodosa. Both microaneurysms (small arrows) and abrupt cutoff of medium-sized arteries (large arrows) can be seen, changes which are virtually pathognomonic of large-vessel vasculitis.

of the inflammatory process may be ineffective, since scarring during the healing phase can lead to progressive narrowing of the vascular lumen (Fig. 7–2b).

MICROSCOPIC POLYARTERITIS

This variant of classic PAN is associated with a similar pathologic lesion, but smaller vessels are affected. In the kidney, distal interlobular arteries and afferent glomerular arterioles are typically involved.[13,25,34] Eosinophils as well as neutrophils may be seen in the inflammatory lesions.

Glomerular damage is usually more prominent than in classic PAN since there is direct involvement of the glomerular capillaries by the inflammatory process. This is manifested by areas of fibrinoid necrosis with collapse of surrounding capillaries (Fig. 7-4), thickening of the glomerular basement membrane,

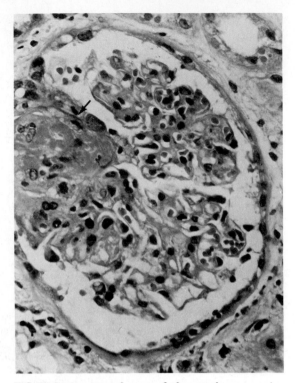

FIG. 7-4. Segmental area of glomerular necrosis in a patient with systemic vasculitis.

variable degrees of mesangial and endothelial cell proliferation, and, in severe cases, crescent formation similar to that found in rapidly progressive glomerulonephritis.[13,17,34] Since the vascular disease tends to involve some but not all vessels, the glomerular disease may be focal (affecting some but not all glomeruli) and segmental (affecting part of but not the entire glomerular tuft) with the severity of damage varying between affected glomeruli.

Immunofluorescent and electron microscopy usually does not demonstrate evidence of immune complex deposition in the glomeruli,[17] and a percutaneous renal biopsy may not demonstrate abnormal vessels. In this setting, the combination of a *focal, necrotizing glomerulonephritis without evidence of immune complex deposition* is highly suggestive of vasculitis.[16,19,25] The other disorders that are associated with focal and segmental lesions [lupus nephropathy, IgA nephropathy, anti-GBM (glomerular basement membrane) antibody disease, Henoch-Schönlein purpura] also have characteristic positive findings on immunofluorescent and electron microscopy (see Chap. 6 and "Hypersensitivity Vasculitis," below).

As in classic PAN, other major visceral organs may be involved.[34] As a result, differentiation between these disorders may be difficult. However, hypertension is unusual in the microscopic form, and the urinary sediment is more likely to be active due in part to the direct involvement of the glomerular capillaries.[25]

CHURG-STRAUSS SYNDROME (ALLERGIC GRANULOMATOSIS)

The Churg-Strauss syndrome is characterized by systemic involvement in which there is usually prominent extravascular granuloma formation, with eosinophilic infiltration involving arterioles and venules.[35] The kidneys may show a focal, segmental necrotizing glomerulonephritis (occasionally with crescents) as well as a focal or diffuse interstitial nephritis with eosinophilic infiltrates and granulomas.[35]

Clinical Manifestations. The clinical findings in this disorder are somewhat different from those in classic PAN. The typical picture can be divided into three phases.[35] Allergic symptoms are frequently the first finding in a patient who is between 20 and 30 years old and who may have no prior atopic history. Subsequently, asthmatic symptoms begin (second phase) with an increase in peripheral eosinophils and with eosinophilic tissue infiltration. The third phase is heralded by the onset of systemic vasculitis, usually several years after the onset of asthma.

This sequence is variable and, although asthma usually precedes the onset of vasculitis, the two processes can on occasion occur simultaneously. A short interval between the onset of asthma and the start of vasculitis carries a poorer prognosis.[36] Often, asthmatic and allergic symptoms improve as systemic vasculitis develops. Why this occurs is unclear.

When compared to PAN, renal involvement is mild, with renal failure occurring in fewer than 10 percent of patients.[35] Hypertension is common (75 percent), however, despite the relatively minor renal damage. Skin rash (usually purpuric), mononeuritis multiplex, cerebrovascular involvement (psychosis, stroke), and cardiac disease may also occur. Involvement of the heart is frequently the most serious site of disease activity. In one large series, for example, almost half the deaths were secondary to cardiac vasculitis.[35]

Laboratory findings are similar to those in classic PAN with the additional evidence of an allergic component, including eosinophilia and, frequently, an elevated plasma IgE concentration. Plasma complement levels are normal, and HbsAg is usually absent.

Diagnosis. The clinical findings of asthma, eosinophilia, and multisystem disease suggest the possible presence of the Churg-Strauss syndrome. The correct diagnosis may be overlooked, however, since all manifestations of the disease may not be present simultaneously.

The chest x-ray may be suggestive, typically revealing patchy or nodular infiltrates or diffuse interstitial disease. The infiltrates in this disorder do not cavitate, unlike those in Wegener's granulomatosis, but can be confused with the lung involvement in several other disorders including sarcoidosis (which can occasionally be associated with glomerulonephritis; see Chap. 8) and allergic bronchopulmonary aspergillosis. Consequently, a definitive diagnosis can be made only by biopsy of an involved organ, such as the lung or kidney.

OVERLAP SYNDROME

In some patients, both small- and medium-sized vessels are involved, leading to additional findings atypical of classic PAN such as purpuric skin lesions (similar to those in hypersensitivity vasculitis), eosinophilia, and pulmonary involvement. Patients in this category are considered to have an "overlap" syndrome[1,37,38] but appear to have a course similar to that of classic PAN.[37]

COURSE AND TREATMENT

The prognosis in patients with untreated classic PAN is poor with the survival rate being only 50 percent at 3 months, 35 percent at 6 months, and 10 to 15 percent at 5 years (Fig. 7–5).[20,25] The overall prognosis in patients with microscopic PAN may be somewhat better, but this is still a serious disease.[25,32]

Treatment has substantially improved the outcome in this disorder. Corticosteroids alone (1 mg/kg per day of prednisone) can increase the 5-year survival to about 50 percent.[20,26] Improvement can be expected in up to two-thirds of patients within the first 6 months of therapy.[26] Nevertheless, the mortality rate in these patients remains unacceptably high due primarily to renal failure (particularly in microscopic PAN), cerebral or mesenteric infarction, and cardiac failure.[25] Furthermore, some survivors have persistent symptoms due either to the underlying disease or to corticosteroid toxicity.

Dramatic, *long-term remissions* have been induced with cytotoxic agents, such as cyclophosphamide, even in patients who are corticosteroid-resistant.[20,22,39] The dosage schedule is similar to that used for Wegener's granulomatosis (see below). Clinical improvement in classic PAN is manifested by ameli-

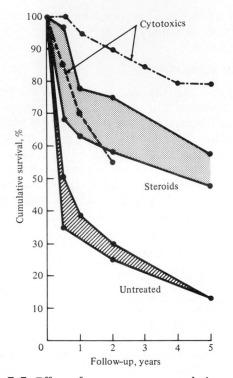

FIG. 7–5. Effect of treatment on cumulative survival of patients with polyarteritis nodosa. Shaded areas represent the range of survival in untreated patients and in those treated with steroids. Separate slopes (dotted lines) are shown for two series reporting the effects of cytotoxic agents. (*From J. E. Balow and H. A. Austin: Vasculitic diseases of the kidney, in W. N. Suki and S. G. Massry (eds.), Therapy of Renal Diseases and Related Disorders, Martinus Nijhoff, Boston, 1984.*)

oration of symptoms, normalization of the erythrocyte sedimentation rate, reduction of the plasma creatinine concentration, a less active urine sediment, and even resolution of aneurysms on arteriography.[39] Azathioprine may be less toxic but is also frequently less effective, particularly in patients with advanced disease.[22,40] The role, if any, for plasma exchange is unclear,[25] although there

is some evidence that patients with aggressive disease may benefit.[4,41]

In summary, oral corticosteroids alone can be used in patients with classic PAN who have relatively *stable* disease.[25,34,42] Most of these patients should be started on 1 mg/kg per day of prednisone in divided doses. Patients with more aggressive disease should receive immunosuppressive agents (e.g., cyclophosphamide) concurrently, especially when there is involvement of viscera with low tolerance to a vascular insult (such as heart, nervous system, or gastrointestinal tract) or when there is progressive renal failure.[25,39] Intravenous pulse therapy with either methylprednisolone or cyclophosphamide (see "Wegener's Granulomatosis: Course and Treatment," below) may also be necessary as initial therapy in patients with fulminant disease. It is important to emphasize that even patients who acutely require dialysis may, with aggressive therapy, recover enough renal function to allow dialysis to be discontinued.[41] Thus, the severity of renal dysfunction should not preclude an attempt at therapy. Similarly, recent evidence suggests that patients with PAN associated with HbsAg or intravenous drug abuse may also respond favorably to immunosuppressive therapy.[22]

Once the symptoms and disease activity are controlled, the doses of corticosteroids and immunosuppressive agents should be reduced. Corticosteroids can be slowly converted to an alternate-day schedule after a remission has been induced.[25] At this time, it may also be possible to switch from cyclophosphamide (if this has been used) to azathioprine, which is usually better tolerated.[16,25] However, it is imperative to continue therapy for *1 to 2 years* after disease activity has been controlled to minimize the risk of relapse.[1]

Most patients with the Churg-Strauss syndrome, in comparison, respond to corticosteroids alone, although azathioprine, cyclophosphamide, and chlorambucil have been successfully used in severe cases.[35] The vasculitic phase lasts less than 12 months in most patients with late relapses in the minority. Therefore, therapy can be stopped in most patients with this variant of PAN after 1 year in remission.

Dialysis can be instituted in patients who progress to end-stage renal failure. Renal transplantation has also been successfully performed,[43] but it may be necessary to substitute cyclophosphamide for azathioprine (which is frequently used to prevent graft rejection) if the disease recurs.

WEGENER'S GRANULOMATOSIS

Wegener's granulomatosis (WG) is another distinctive vasculitic syndrome. The classic triad in this disorder, each component of which occurs in 85 to 95 percent of patients, consists of a necrotizing granulomatous vasculitis of the upper (nasopharynx, paranasal sinuses) and lower (lungs) respiratory tract, and a necrotizing glomerulonephritis. A disseminated medium- and small-vessel vasculitis affecting virtually any organ also may be present (Table 7-4).

PATHOLOGY

The histologic changes in the respiratory tract consist of necrotizing vasculitis involving the small- and medium-sized vessels with granuloma formation. However, granulomas and evidence of vascular involvement are infrequently found on renal biopsy, where the major changes are similar to those in microscopic PAN: focal, segmental areas of fibrinoid necrosis and sclerosis of the glomerular tufts, varying degrees of hypercellularity, and in severe cases, crescent formation (Fig. 7-4).[17,44-46] Immunofluorescent studies may be negative or may show irregular granular deposits of IgG, IgM, and C3.[44] Electron microscopy may also show scattered deposits, although not in amounts sufficient to account for the degree of glomerular injury.

CLINICAL PRESENTATION

Wegener's granulomatosis usually occurs in middle-aged adults, without a predilection

TABLE 7-4. Characteristic Clinical Findings in Wegener's Granulomatosis

Organ System	Approximate Frequency, percent	Typical Features
Nasopharynx	75	Necrotizing granuloma with mucosal ulceration; saddle nose deformity
Paranasal sinuses	90	Pansinusitis; necrotizing granuloma; secondary bacterial infection
Eyes	60	Keratoconjunctivitis; granulomatous sclerouveitis
Ears	35	Serous otitis media; secondary bacterial infection
Lungs	95	Multiple nodular cavitary infiltrates; necrotizing granulomatous vasculitis
Kidneys	85	Focal and segmental glomerulitis; necrotizing glomerulonephritis later in course
Heart	15	Coronary vasculitis; pericarditis
Nervous system	20	Mononeuritis multiplex; cranial neuritis
Skin	40	Dermal vasculitis with secondary ulcerations
Joints	50	Polyarthralgias

SOURCE: A. S. Fauci, B. R. Haynes, and P. Katz, *Ann. Intern. Med.,* 89:660, 1978.

for either sex.[11,44] Extrarenal manifestations *almost always* precede clinical renal involvement.

The presenting symptoms in WG are usually nonspecific, such as fever, arthralgias, weight loss, and weakness. Symptoms that are more suggestive of WG include rhinorrhea, sinus pain, dyspnea, chest pain, cough and hemoptysis (Table 7–4).[44,47]

The findings on physical examination vary with the pattern of organ involvement. A careful examination of the mouth and nasopharynx is essential since lesions in this area are easy to biopsy and allow the diagnosis to be made with minimal risk.

The GFR may be normal in patients with little or no renal involvement, but varying degrees of renal insufficiency are seen with more advanced disease. The urinalysis is often abnormal with mild proteinuria, red blood cells, and frequently, red cell casts.

Laboratory findings are nondiagnostic. Anemia, leukocytosis, and an elevated erythrocyte sedimentation rate are common. Eosinophilia, rheumatoid factor, and circulating immune complexes may be present in some patients, but plasma complement levels are usually normal.[44,48]

Radiographic evidence of respiratory tract involvement is common. The chest x-ray typically reveals solitary or multiple pulmonary nodules in the middle and lower lung fields. The nodules tend to be poorly defined and may undergo central necrosis, leading to a cavitary appearance. Less commonly, only a solitary pulmonary infiltrate is seen. Sinus films may be abnormal in the presence of sinusitis, an important finding since this area can be easily and safety biopsied.

DIAGNOSIS

Although the diagnosis may seem apparent in patients presenting with the classic triad, a biopsy of affected tissue is essential since other disorders, which may require markedly different therapy, can have identical clinical manifestations. Nasal involvement in WG, for example, may be confused with midline granuloma or a neoplasm.[48]

Diagnostic problems may also occur in patients with the "limited" form of WG, which is characterized by respiratory, but not clinically evident, renal involvement.[11,49,50] In this setting, the differential diagnosis may include such diverse disorders as metastatic tumor, sarcoidosis, tuberculosis, or lymphomatoid granulomatosis.[44,51]

Renal biopsy in WG is often similar to that in polyarteritis (see above).[44] Consequently, the finding of a segmental necrotizing glomerulonephritis with minimal immunofluorescent staining in a patient with concomitant pulmonary involvement should raise the possibility of WG.

COURSE AND TREATMENT

The prognosis for patients with untreated WG is extremely poor. Mean survival is 5 months[52] with only 10 percent alive at 2 years.[25] Renal and respiratory failure are the major causes of death. While spontaneous remissions may occur, they appear to be temporary,[44] and patients with the "limited" form of WG without renal involvement and a more benign course are rare.[49,50,53] Most, if not all, of these patients probably have an earlier form of the disease, where renal involvement has not occurred or is not yet detectable.[54]

The use of corticosteroids leads to a remission in some patients.[44] However, these remissions are typically temporary, as the mean survival rate is only increased to about 12 months.[55]

The addition of cytotoxic agents, particularly cyclophosphamide, has dramatically altered the course of the disease, as *complete and long-lasting remissions* can be induced in as many as 90 percent of patients.[1,46-48] These remissions frequently persist long after active therapy has been discontinued.[48]

Early institution of therapy is extremely important since tissue necrosis cannot be reversed. As a result, end-stage renal disease may ensue in severely affected patients even if the inflammatory process can subsequently be controlled.[56] However, the requirement for dialysis during the *acute phase* does not preclude the institution of aggressive therapy, since sufficient functional recovery may occur to allow dialysis to be discontinued.[41]

Oral cyclophosphamide (1 to 2 mg/kg per day) can be initiated in patients with active but relatively stable disease. The dose is increased by 25 mg every 2 weeks until a response is seen or leukopenia occurs. In patients with fulminant renal or respiratory failure, however, cyclophosphamide should be administered in higher doses (4 mg/kg per day) for the first 3 days. An alternative to oral therapy in these patients is intermittent intravenous pulse cyclophosphamide (0.5 to 1.0 g/m^2 every month) as has been used in lupus nephritis (see p. 250).[57] Although this regimen may be as or more effective and less toxic than daily cyclophosphamide,[57] there is little experience at present with this form of therapy in Wegener's granulomatosis.[25]

Risks of cyclophosphamide therapy include marrow suppression, infection, hemorrhagic cystitis, bladder fibrosis and carcinoma, the late development of malignancy, and gonadal fibrosis with infertility (see p. 192).[58] Intravenous pulse cyclophosphamide has not, as yet, been associated with hemorrhagic cystitis (because of the short exposure), and late malignancy may be less common;[25,57] however, herpes zoster seems to occur as frequently as it does with oral cyclophosphamide.[57,59]

Conventional doses of prednisone (1 mg/kg per day in divided doses) are also given initially. Corticosteroids may be useful in diminishing the acute inflammatory reaction (particularly with pericardial, eye, or skin involvement) until the effects of cyclophosphamide become apparent, usually within 14 days. Pulse methyprednisolone (250 to 1000 mg daily for 3 days) given intravenously may be used in severe disease,[56,60] although this regimen has additional acute risks (arrhythmias, hypertension) in some patients.[61-63]

Daily corticosteroids (in divided doses) are continued until the disease is brought under control by cyclophosphamide. At this time, a single daily dose can be started and ultimately changed to an alternate-day schedule. The prednisone dose can be reduced to 10 to 15 mg every other day after remission has been induced.[25] Corticosteroids can then be slowly discontinued if the patient remains well.

Cyclophosphamide is continued until there is no evidence of disease activity or toxicity develops. Patients in remission may then be switched from cyclophosphamide to azathioprine to reduce the risk of toxicity.[44] Immunosuppressive therapy should be continued for *at least* 1 year after remission is induced.

Systemic symptoms may rapidly resolve in patients who respond to treatment. This early clinical response is presumably secondary to corticosteroid therapy. In contrast, the chest x-ray, urinalysis, and glomerular filtration rate (GFR) typically improve over 10 days to 2 months after cyclophosphamide has been started.[44,60]

Patients who achieve a clinical and laboratory remission may relapse. As a result, careful, long-term follow-up is imperative since relapses may occur after as late as 1 year or more after therapy has been discontinued.[64]

Most relapses are associated with treatment using corticosteroids alone, reductions in cyclophosphamide dosage, the use of azathioprine in place of cyclophosphamide, or superimposed infection.[46,65,66] When relapse follows infection, treatment of the infection with conventional antimicrobials (but without a change in immunosuppressive therapy) does not usually induce remission.[66] However, recent studies suggest that the use of trimethoprim-sulfamethoxazole (in contrast to other antimicrobials) in this setting may be associated with clinical and laboratory improvement. This finding suggests a possible immunosuppressive action of this antimicrobial combination.[67]

Patients who do not respond to therapy or who begin treatment after sufficient renal damage has already occurred may develop irreversible end-stage renal disease. In this setting, either dialysis[68,69] or renal transplantation may be successful.[56,65] The disease can, on occasion, recur in the transplanted kidney even though the recipient is frequently treated with azathioprine and prednisone to prevent rejection.[65,68] In this setting, switching from azathioprine to cyclophosphamide usually leads to remission.[65,70]

HYPERSENSITIVITY VASCULITIS

Hypersensitivity vasculitis (HV) refers to a heterogeneous group of diseases characterized by vasculitis of the small vessels (arterioles, capillaries, and especially venules), in contrast to the small- and medium-sized arteries affected in classic PAN. There is prominent involvement of the skin (occasionally without evidence of other systemic abnormalities), and an inciting agent can often be identified.[71-73] Drugs are commonly implicated with a penicillin, sulfonamide, thiazide, or allopurinol being most often found.

Dermal vessels from involved skin are surrounded by an intense inflammatory infiltrate. There is a characteristic fragmentation and destruction of neutrophils and other inflammatory cells, resulting in a histopathologic picture which is termed a leukocytoclastic (nuclear dust) vasculitis.

In the kidney, vascular involvement is found primarily in the distal interlobular arteries and glomerular arterioles. The ensuing glomerular ischemia may cause a segmental, necrotizing glomerulonephritis, with variable cell proliferation and crescent formation similar to that seen in PAN (Fig. 7–4). In contrast to PAN, focal or diffuse glomerular deposition of immunoglobulin and complement is common. The class of antibody deposited can help distinguish among the variants of HV. For example, prominent IgA deposition is, in a patient with HV, diagnostic of Henoch-Schönlein purpura (see below).

CLINICAL PRESENTATION

Skin lesions are the *most prominent abnormality* in HV. This may be manifested by the acute onset of maculopapular, vesicular, urticarial, or most often, *palpable* purpuric lesions, which are most prominent over the lower extremities.[71-73] The lesions may vary from the size of a pinpoint to several centimeters in diameter, and, in more severe cases, may develop bullae or ulcerate. Typically, these changes begin 7 to 10 days after antigen exposure.

In some patients, skin involvement may be the only manifestation of HV.[71-74] However, many patients have systemic involvement. When the kidney is affected, one of three variants of HV is usually present: Henoch-Schönlein purpura, essential mixed cryoglobulinemia, or serum sickness. Much less commonly, vasculitic skin lesions and kidney disease are seen as part of the overlap syndrome[37] or with urticarial (hypocomplementemic) vasculitis.[75-77]

HENOCH-SCHÖNLEIN PURPURA

Henoch-Schönlein purpura (HSP) most commonly affects young children but can also occur in adults.[78-82] Most cases occur in late winter or early spring, seasons associated with frequent upper respiratory tract infections. This finding suggests that the precipitating antigen is commonly infectious.[83]

Pathology. The most distinctive pathologic changes in HSP are found in the skin and on renal biopsy. Immune complexes containing IgA (as demonstrated by immunofluorescent microscopy) are present in the affected dermal vessels in up to 75 percent of patients, if early lesions are biopsied.[84-87] Clinically uninvolved skin may also show similar vascular IgA deposition, but a negative test does not exclude the diagnosis of HSP.[85,88,89]

The pathologic changes in the kidney are identical to those in IgA nephropathy (see p. 215).[90] The most common lesion is a mild glomerulonephritis with focal and segmental mesangial cell proliferation. In severe cases, however, areas of fibrinoid necrosis and crescent formation are frequently found. The characteristic immunofluorescent change in HSP is prominent mesangial IgA deposition*; IgG and C3 may also be seen, but there is less intense deposition of these inflammatory components. Electron microscopy reveals dense deposits in the mesangium and, occasionally, in the capillary loops.

Clinical Manifestations. A classic tetrad of palpable purpura, arthralgias or arthritis, abdominal pain, and hematuria is present in most, but not all, patients. Skin involvement is ultimately present in 100 percent, but may not be evident at onset. Lesions are most prominent over the extensor surfaces of the distal arms and legs and buttocks (Fig. 7–6). In children, lesions may begin as a maculopapular or urticarial eruption with progression to a more typical, hemorrhagic lesion.

Renal involvement is common in HSP. It usually occurs within 3 months of the onset

---

*Although other diseases may be associated with mesangial IgA deposition (such as chronic liver disease[91] and lupus nephritis[92]), the clinical picture, normal liver functions, and negative serologies will tend to exclude these disorders.

of skin or visceral symptoms but may, in some patients, occur before or years after the extrarenal changes.[80] Most patients present with microscopic hematuria and mild proteinuria.[81] However, more severe involvement can occur, characterized by an acute nephritic syndrome with oliguria, hypertension, proteinuria, hematuria (which may be macroscopic), and an active urinary sediment containing red cell and granular casts. Glomerular crescents are commonly seen in these patients, and nephrotic range proteinuria (>3.5 g/day) may be present.[79]

Diagnosis. The diagnosis of HSP may be strongly suspected if the classic tetrad is present. Biopsy of early skin lesions or uninvolved skin can establish the diagnosis if IgA is seen in the dermal vessels. Renal biopsy is indicated (once the diagnosis is established) only in patients with progressive renal insufficiency or persistent nephrotic syndrome, since the necessity for therapy may be dependent upon the severity of the changes that are found. Laboratory studies in HSP are nonspecific, and plasma complement levels are usually normal despite C3 deposition on renal biopsy.

Course and Therapy. The usual course of HSP is self-limited, even when glomerulonephritis is present. Episodic purpura may recur over several months with transient hematuria or, at times, renal insufficiency.[81] There is, however, no uniform relationship between recurrent disease and prognosis. There is also no consistent correlation between the severity of nephritis and the severity of the extrarenal manifestations.[81]

The extent of renal involvement is typically the most important indicator of long-term prognosis.[25] The ultimate outlook for most patients with renal involvement is good, even when hematuria persists.[79,80,93] Some patients may, however, develop acute renal failure with oliguria. The percentage of these

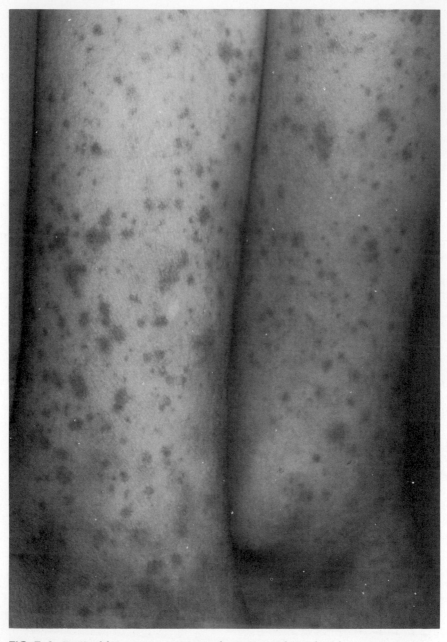

FIG. 7–6. Typical lower extremity involvement with "palpable purpura" in a patient with Henoch-Schönlein purpura. Immunofluorescent staining of dermal vessels may reveal IgA deposition. (*Courtesy of Dr. Gregory F. Bishop.*)

patients who will have an improvement in renal function after resolution of the acute episode correlates inversely with the presence and extent of glomerular crescents (Table 7–5).[83,94] Patients with marked proteinuria are also less likely to completely recover normal renal function.[83]

Guidelines for therapy in HSP are limited by the benign course in most patients and by a lack of controlled studies when therapy has been attempted. Consequently, specific treatment should be *initiated only in those patients with unusually debilitating or progressive disease.*[81]

There has been anecdotal improvement in arthritic and gastrointestinal symptoms in HSP patients treated with corticosteroids. Intussusception may be prevented, but it is not reversed.[81] However, neither the skin lesions nor renal involvement appear to respond to conventional corticosteroid therapy alone,[83,95] and these drugs do not alter the duration of the illness or the frequency of relapse.

Intravenous pulse methylprednisolone (see "Wegener's Granulomatosis: Course and Therapy," above) may have some use in patients with rapidly progressive (crescentic) glomerulonephritis.[96] Immunosuppressive agents (such as cyclophosphamide[25]) and plasmapheresis[97,98] may be considered in patients with progressive renal failure unresponsive to corticosteroids, although there is no definitive proof of efficacy in this setting.

In patients who recover from the acute episode(s), persistent proteinuria or renal insufficiency may be associated with late progression to renal failure due both to activity of the underlying disease and to hemodynamic mechanisms initiated by nephron loss (see Chap. 4).[99] The unusual patient who develops end-stage renal disease requiring dialysis may undergo successful renal transplantation. Despite the administration of prednisone and azathioprine, recurrent disease is not uncommon (especially in patients with continued skin or gastrointestinal symptoms) and can lead to loss of the renal allograft.[99,100]

ESSENTIAL MIXED CRYOGLOBULINEMIA

Most cryoproteins are immunoglobulins which precipitate in the cold and dissociate upon rewarming. Three types of cryoglobulins have been identified[101]:

1. A monoclonal immunoglobulin, most often seen in multiple myeloma or Waldenström's macroglobulinemia.
2. A mixed cryoglobulin with a monoclonal component, which represents autoantibody, and an IgG immunoglobulin, which acts as antigen.

TABLE 7–5. Henoch-Schönlein Purpura: Glomerular Crescents and Prognosis

Percent Glomeruli Affected by Crescents	No. of Patients	Recovery	Minimal Renal Abnormality	Persisting Nephropathy	Terminal Failure
>80	19	2	4	1	12 (60%)
50–80	20	4	5	5	6 (30%)
<50	42	22	11	7	2 (5%)
Total	81	28	20	13	20

SOURCE: From J. S. Cameron, Henoch-Schönlein purpura nephritis, in S. G. Massry and R. J. Glassock (eds.), *Textbook of Nephrology,* Williams and Wilkins, Baltimore, 1983.

3. A mixed cryoglobulin in which both the immunoglobulin and antiimmunoglobulin components are polyclonal, most commonly found in chronic inflammatory disorders.

Cryoglobulins, which are part of an antigen-antibody complex, may contribute to the development of glomerulonephritis in a variety of disorders including SLE (systemic lupus erythematosus, in which the cryoglobulin may contain anti-DNA antibodies) and poststreptococcal glomerulonephritis.[102,103]

In essential mixed cryoglobulinemia (EMC), there are circulating immune complexes that usually have three components: an antigen, an immunoglobulin directed against the antigen, and a monoclonal IgM rheumatoid factor directed against the immunoglobulin.[104,105] The inciting antigen cannot generally be identified. However, hepatitis B virus, DNA, and *Coccidioides immitis* antigens have, in isolated cases, been found in the cryoprecipitates (and in some cases the glomeruli).[102,106,107]

The biochemical characteristics of cryoglobulins are incompletely understood. It is possible that a lack of carbohydrate groups may be responsible in some way for cryoprecipitation, since cryoimmunoglobulins lack certain carbohydrate groups present in noncryoimmunoglobulins.[105] It has been hypothesized that there may be a presecretory defect of B-cell antibody secretion with defective glycosylation. An alternative possibility is a postsecretory defect caused by cleavage of the carbohydrate moiety from the circulating antibody (perhaps by a microorganism).[108]

Pathology. The predominant pathologic changes in EMC are found in the skin and on renal biopsy. Skin biopsy reveals the typical changes of hypersensitivity vasculitis. In contrast to HSP, IgA deposition is not prominent in this disorder.

The pathologic findings in the kidney may be highly suggestive of EMC. Light microscopy typically reveals diffuse mesangial and endothelial cell proliferation, which may in some patients lead to a lobular appearance similar to that in membranoproliferative glomerulonephritis (see Chap. 6). Of particular importance, many patients have numerous intraluminal thrombi composed of precipitated cryoglobulins (Fig. 7–7*a* and *b*).[108] Generalized crescent formation[108] may be present in patients with more severe disease, while only focal proliferative changes may be seen in patients with mild involvement. Immunofluorescent microscopy demonstrates granular deposition of IgG, IgM, C3, and less often C4 (Fig. 7–7*c*). Mesangial and subendothelial deposits and cellular proliferation are found on elecron microscopy, changes similar to those in type I membranoproliferative glomerulonephritis. However, the presence of intraluminal thrombi points to the diagnosis of EMC.

Clinical Manifestations. Patients usually present with recurrent episodes of palpable purpura, invariably involving the lower extremities, which may progress to ulceration.[108] Arthralgias, lymphadenopathy, hepatosplenomegaly, Raynaud's phenomenon, and neuropathy may also be present.

When renal involvement occurs (in over 50 percent of patients), it *always* follows the skin lesions and may have a latent period of four or more years.[108] The clinical findings are variable and range from asymptomatic hematuria and proteinuria to acute renal failure with oliguria, edema, and hypertension.[101,109] The urinalysis may contain red and white cells, cellular casts, and protein, depending upon the degree of renal involvement. Azotemia is present at onset in fewer than 50 percent of patients.[104]

Diagnosis. Essential mixed cryoglobulinemia should be suspected in patients with the skin lesions of a hypersensitivity vasculitis, who also have renal involvement. The demonstration of a high mixed IgM-IgG (or sometimes IgA) cryoglobulin titer with a monoclonal component by immunoelectrophoresis is diagnostic.[101,110] Abnormal liver function tests are frequently present* and may reflect underlying hepatitis B infection in some patients[101,110] Low C4 levels are also commonly found, but C3 may be normal.[†,108] Renal biopsy should be reserved for patients with progressive renal disease or for those in whom the diagnosis is in doubt.

Course and Therapy. In most patients, the renal disease is slowly progressive, leading to renal failure over a period of months to years.[101,108] Hypertension and renal insufficiency are poor prognostic signs. While complement levels alone do not predict renal involvement or prognosis, the presence of hypocomplementemia in the presence of azotemia is associated with a very poor outcome.[104,108]

Treatment should be limited to patients with disabling or progressive disease, since the effectiveness of therapy is uncertain. Oral corticosteroids alone and pulse methylprednisolone have been used with limited success.[104,108,111] Consequently, in patients with *acute, severe disease* (progressive renal failure, distal necroses requiring amputation, or advanced neuropathy), corticosteroids should be used in conjunction with plasmapheresis‡

(to remove the circulating cryoglobulins and to desaturate reticuloendothelial receptors, thereby enhancing the clearance of immune complexes)[112,113] and with cytotoxic agents. This regimen has been effective in inducing remission in many patients with acute, severe disease.* Optimal therapy is less clear in patients with chronic, slowly progressive disease, but prednisone and cyclophosphamide (or chlorambucil) have been used in this setting.

Those who progress to terminal renal failure can be successfully dialyzed. Renal transplantation should be postponed, however, until the disease is clinically inactive to prevent recurrence in the transplanted kidney.

SERUM SICKNESS

Serum sickness (SS) was formerly caused primarily by the administration of heterologous antisera, which are now rarely used.[114] At the present time, serum sickness-like illnesses are usually caused by medications which probably act as haptens.[115] Most cases are caused by penicillins[116] and phenytoin,[117-119] but many other drugs have been implicated.[113] Certain viral infections (particularly acute type B hepatitis) can also be associated with a syndrome clinically identical with SS.[120]

The clinical picture is a systemic one with fever, urticaria, arthralgias, lymphadenopathy, and sometimes edema. In most patients, the onset of symptoms is 7 to 10 days after antigen exposure, the time required to produce a sufficient amount of antibody, and, subsequently, antigen-antibody complexes (see Fig. 5–7). This time course may be altered with a secondary antigen exposure (symptoms beginning within 2 to 7 days

---

*Liver disease may contribute to the development or persistence of EMC since the liver is the primary site of removal of cryoglobulins from the plasma.[108]

†The reduction in early complement components may be the result of decreased synthesis of C1, C2, or C4 with normal production of C3. Alternatively, it is possible that cryoprecipitates may have the ability to fix the early complement components (C1, C2, and C4) in the cold only after being drawn, but cannot activate C3 in vivo or in the cold.[109]

‡Acute renal failure due to precipitation of cryoglobulins in the glomerular capillaries can occur in EMC during plasmapheresis if the reinfused plasma is not sufficiently warmed.[112]

*Plasmapheresis alone or combined with corticosteroid therapy may effectively induce a sustained remission in some patients with EMC and acute renal failure *without* the addition of cytotoxic therapy.[113]

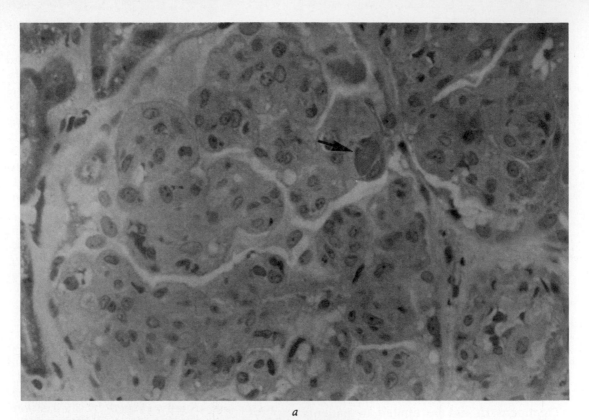

a

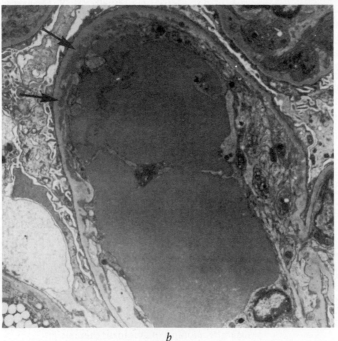

b

FIG. 7–7. Pathologic changes in essential mixed cryoglobulinemia. (*a*) Diffuse proliferative glomerulonephritis with intracapillary thrombus formation (arrow). (*b*) Electron microscopy of the intracapillary thrombus, composed of precipitated cryoglobulins. Characteristic subendothelial dense deposits are also present (arrows).

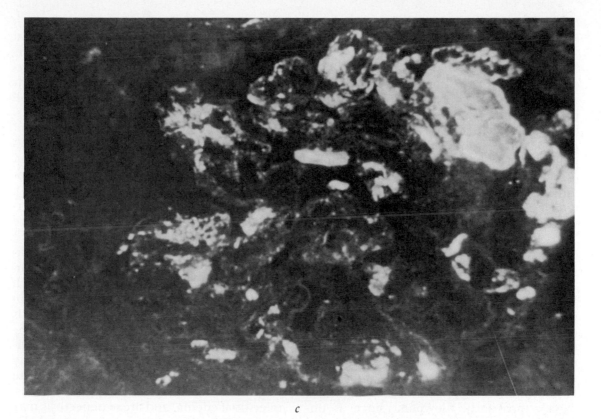

FIG. 7–7 (Continued).   (*c*) Immunofluorescent staining with anti-IgM antiserum. (*Courtesy of Dr. Jerome B. Jacobs.*)

after exposure due to the accelerated antibody response) or with the use of a long-acting drug such as benzathine penicillin (in which the onset of the disease is delayed and the duration of symptoms prolonged).[121]

The urinalysis in patients with renal involvement typically reveals red cells with cellular casts and protein. Acute renal failure is uncommon but may occur with heavy or prolonged antigen exposure.[122] In this setting, renal biopsy reveals an immune complex glomerulonephritis with segmental or diffuse endothelial cell proliferation, and deposition of immunoglobulin (mainly IgG) and C3 in the glomerular capillary walls.[122]

The diagnosis of SS is usually apparent from the history and physical examination. Recent antigen exposure (usually a medication) can be elicited from most patients. Hypocomplementemia may be present, and patients with a prodrome of acute hepatitis may be HbsAg or antibody-positive.[120,123]

Treatment of SS should be directed toward identifying and removing the inciting drug or antigen. This should lead to resolution of the disease within a period of days to a few weeks.[121] Immunosuppressive therapy with corticosteroids or cytotoxic agents should be reserved for the infrequent patient with fulminant or progressive disease.

MISCELLANEOUS CAUSES OF RENAL VASCULITIS

There are several other uncommon vasculitic disorders that are infrequently associated with major renal involvement. These include urticarial (hypocomplementemic) vasculitis,[75-77] rheumatoid vasculitis,[124,125] and an arteritic process in SLE[124] or in relapsing polychondritis.[126-128] Large vessel vasculitides (such as temporal arteritis and Takayasu's arteritis) may involve the main renal arteries, but usually spare the smaller intrarenal vessels.[129-131]

PROGRESSIVE SYSTEMIC SCLEROSIS

Progressive systemic sclerosis (PSS) is an uncommon disease characterized by prominent changes in the skin and frequent evidence of multisystem involvement, most often affecting the lungs, gastrointestinal tract, kidneys, and heart.[132-134] Renal involvement (scleroderma renal crisis) is particularly important from a prognostic viewpoint since, if untreated, it is usually associated with rapid progression to end-stage renal failure, which is a major cause of death in this disorder.

PATHOLOGY

Obliterative vascular lesions and increased collagen accumulation are the major pathologic changes in PSS. In the kidney, the primary abnormalities are in the vessels. In patients with acute disease, the interlobular (but not the larger arcuate or interlobar) arteries reveal concentric, onionskin thickening, a change that appears to be produced by proliferation of the smooth muscle cells of the media, when then migrate into the intima. There is also a marked increase in intimal mucoid or collagenous ground substance (Fig. 7-8a).[133-146] These changes result in narrowing of the vascular lumen, which may become obliterated, leading to cortical microinfarcts. Extensive fibrosis is characteristically found in the adventitia and interstitium around the affected vessels. Similar vascular lesions may be present in the small arteries of other organs.[133,136]

The distal interlobular arteries and afferent glomerular arterioles are also involved, although the histologic changes are different. In these vessels, fibrinoid necrosis and occasionally fibrin thrombi are found (Fig. 7-8b).

A variety of glomerular and tubulointersitial changes also may be seen and are thought to be primarily due to ischemia.[133,134] The glomerular lesions include focal thickening of the glomerular basement membrane, mild mesangial hypercellularity which may induce a lobular appearance of the glomerular tuft, and areas of fibrinoid necrosis or, with healing, sclerosis.[136,137]

The tubulointerstitial changes are dependent upon the rapidity of onset and severity of the vascular involvement. In the acute stage, swelling of the tubular epithelial cells, interstitial edema, and areas of necrosis may be seen. With more chronic lesions, tubular atrophy and interstitial fibrosis with mononuclear cell infiltration are usually present.

The immunofluorescent findings are variable. IgM and C3 are frequently found in the vessels (even in patients without clinical evidence of renal disease), and fibrin may be seen in vessels undergoing fibrinoid necrosis.[138,139] Glomerular deposition of immunoglobulins or complement is unusual, except as a nonspecific finding in sclerotic areas. Electron microscopy reveals wrinkling of the glomerular basement membrane and sclerosis in the mesangial areas. In addition, fibrinlike material may be deposited between the endothelial cells and the basement membrane in the acute phase of the disease (similar to Fig. 7-9c below).[140]

Similar histopathologic changes may be seen with polyarteritis nodosa, malignant

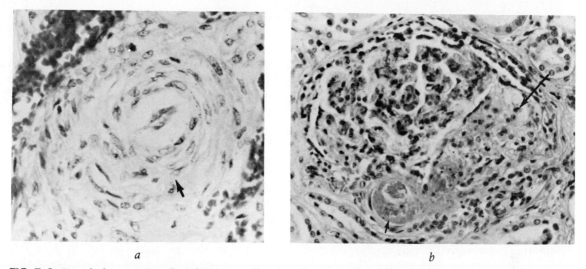

a　　　　　　　　　　　　　*b*

FIG. 7–8. Renal changes in scleroderma. (*a*) Interlobular artery reveals concentric, onionskin thickening (arrow), with marked narrowing of the vascular lumen. (*b*) Fibrinoid necrosis and fibrin thrombus are seen in afferent glomerular arteriole (small arrow) associated with fibrinoid necrosis of a segment of the glomerular tuft (large arrow). These changes are not specific for scleroderma since they may also be found in malignant hypertension and the hemolytic-uremic syndromes.

nephrosclerosis, the hemolytic-uremic syndromes, and chronic transplant rejection.[136] In contrast to polyarteritis, there is no inflammatory infiltrate in the vessel wall in PSS, and the elastic membrane is intact, not disrupted. However, differentiation between PSS and either malignant nephrosclerosis or the hemolytic-uremic syndromes may not be possible on the basis of the histologic examination.[136] Thus, the characteristic extrarenal findings of PSS are essential in establishing the diagnosis of this disorder.

The preceding discussion refers to the pathologic changes in acute scleroderma renal disease. Less commonly, a chronic form of renal involvement is seen, characterized by intimal thickening of the arcuate and larger interlobular arteries without changes in the smaller vessels.[138] The significance of these findings is uncertain, however, since there is little or no clinical evidence of renal disease (with at most mild proteinuria being present) in these patients. Furthermore, these changes are similar to those that may accompany atherosclerosis, aging, and hypertension. Consequently, one should be reluctant to ascribe renal involvement to PSS in patients with fibrous intimal thickening of the renal arterial system and chronic renal failure but without a history of acute scleroderma renal disease.[135,136]

PATHOGENESIS

The pathogenesis of PSS is unknown. Nevertheless, a great deal of information has been obtained which sheds light on the possible mechanisms that may be involved. Based on these data, three theories have been proposed: impaired control of the vascular microcirculation, abnormal collagen metabolism, and autoimmune vascular damage.[141]

The vascular theory proposes that *vasoregu-*

latory failure in the microcirculation, resulting in intracapillary hypertension, is the primary change in PSS.[142] In normal subjects, the mean capillary hydrostatic pressure is much less than that in the major arteries due to the resistance at the precapillary arteriole.[143] However, dilation of this arteriole would raise the intracapillary pressure, since more of the systemic pressure would be transmitted to the capillary. This could cause edema (due to increased movement of fluid from the vascular space into the interstitium) as well as capillary dilation and the development of telangiectases. If this high microvascular pressure persisted, arteriolar hyperplasia and eventually fibrosis might ensue, a sequence similar to that induced by severe hypertension, except that systemic hypertension is not required. These secondary arteriolar changes could then result in narrowing of the vascular lumen, increased tendency to vasospasm, and ischemic scarring in the skin and internal organs. The deposition of fibrin also may contribute to the vascular lesions, since endothelial damage can activate the coagulation pathway.[144]

This hypothesis is, as yet, unproved, and the cause of the arteriolar dilation is unknown. However, the observation that control of hypertension in scleroderma renal crisis (see "Course and Treatment," below) can, in some patients, lead to an improvement in renal function and, less often, regression of the dermal changes[145-149] is consistent with a central role for microvascular hypertension.

In addition to these structural changes in the vessels, patients with PSS also have evidence of increased vasospasm.[134] This most often is manifested clinically by Raynaud's phenomenon, resulting from a marked reduction in digital blood flow upon exposure to the cold.[150,151] Furthermore, immersing the hands in cold water may cause a reversible decrease in *renal* blood flow to the outer renal cortex (the site of 85 percent of glomeruli), a finding not seen in normal subjects.[134] This effect may be mediated in part by hyperactivity of the renin-angiotensin system since patients with PSS (even without clinically evident renal disease) frequently have an elevated plasma renin activity[139] and may demonstrate an exaggerated release of renin after standing or cold exposure.[152] However, baseline plasma renin activity is elevated mainly in those patients with histologic evidence of renal arterial involvement, suggesting that the enhanced renin response is secondary to renal ischemia produced by previous vascular injury.[139]

The hypothesis that *abnormal collagen metabolism* is the primary defect in PSS has come primarily from the observations that collagen accumulation in the skin is increased in this disorder and that dermal fibroblasts from patients with PSS synthesize more collagen than normal fibroblasts when incubated in vitro.[141,151,153,154] Furthermore, lymphocytes from these patients show increased blastogenic reactivity when incubated with skin extracts or pure collagen, a finding that may be important since activated lymphocytes can release soluble mediators (lymphokines) that both attract fibroblasts and enhance their collagen production.[155,156] Thus, sensitization of lymphocytes to collagen could be the primary abnormality in PSS. The subsequent release of lymphokines could then result in enhanced collagen synthesis and the characteristic vascular and dermal lesions.

It seems likely, however, that these alterations in lymphocyte and fibroblast function represent *secondary* phenomena. For example, a primary increase in collagen production cannot explain many of the common features of PSS, particularly the development of telangiectases, the frequent occurrence of Raynaud's phenomenon, edema of the skin, and the development of arterial lesions before the onset of fibrosis.[137,142] In contrast, primary vascular injury can account for all the changes in this disorder. Also consistent with the vascular hypothesis is the similarity of the renal changes in scleroderma to those in malignant nephrosclerosis and the hemolytic-uremic syndromes,[136] disorders in which endothelial damage appears to be an early finding (see "Hemolytic-Uremic Syndromes," below).

Since PSS is often associated with a variety of immunologic abnormalities, a third theory suggests that the vascular lesions reflect *immunologic injury*.[141,157,158] Autoantibodies are frequently present (see below[159]) as, occasionally, are autoimmune diseases such as Hashimoto's thyroiditis, Sjögren's syndrome, systemic lupus erythematosus, dermatomyositis, and primary biliary cirrhosis. However, these immune phenomena do not correlate well with the duration or severity of the disease.[141]

Recently, however, high titers of a PSS-specific autoantibody (anti-Scl-70) have been detected in the serum of severely affected patients. The antigen (Scl-70) against which this antibody is directed appears to be identical with the abundant nuclear enzyme DNA topoisomerase I.[160] Thus, anti-Scl-70 could be involved in the pathogenesis of PSS. Conversely, cell damage, especially in PSS patients with severe, progressive disease, could cause release of Scl-70 with secondary antibody formation.

In addition to autoantibody formation in PSS, abnormalities in T-cell activity are also present. The total circulating T-cell number is reduced, a change that is associated with an increase in the normal helper-to-suppressor T-cell ratio. It has been suggested that an inherited or acquired defect in suppressor T cells (or enhanced helper-inducer cell activity) could allow proliferation of a clone of cells reactive against collagen. These cells could then release lymphokines that could injure the vascular endothelium and promote fibroblast accumulation and activation.[151]

In summary, none of the three theories alone seems to explain all the abnormalities found in PSS. Most data favor the vascular hypothesis, but the event which triggers vessel damage remains unknown.

CLINICAL PRESENTATION

Progressive systemic sclerosis is most often a disease of females in the 20 to 50 year-old group, although almost any age and either sex may be affected. The signs and symptoms are due to the obliterative arterial lesions, the increase in collagen deposition (fibrosis), and secondary smooth muscle atrophy.

The earliest manifestations of PSS are usually nonspecific and include weakness, early fatigability, and diffuse musculoskeletal aching and stiffness. Raynaud's phenomenon or signs of skin involvement are also generally present, occurring in over 90 percent of patients. The initial skin changes may be local or diffuse, producing swelling which most prominently affects the distal extremities and face. This is followed by progressive induration, resulting in tight, thickened skin and a boardlike facial appearance. Ischemic ulcers and calcinosis may occur in severe cases. These cutaneous changes usually precede clinically evident visceral involvement (which does not occur in all patients) by a variable period. However, one or several organ systems may occasionally be affected prior to the onset of sclerodermatous alterations in the skin.

The clinical signs of visceral involvement reflect the pattern of organ damage (Table 7–6).[134,161] In the gastrointestinal tract and lungs, for example, these changes can lead, respectively, to ulceration, perforation, infarction, or hemorrhage anywhere in the gut or to pulmonary hypertension. Fibrosis and smooth muscle atrophy in these organs may cause dysphagia, constipation (both due to

TABLE 7-6. Major Clinical Signs of Progressive Systemic Sclerosis

Organ System	Approximate Frequency, percent	Typical Features
Skin	>90	Edema or thickening of skin; telangiectases; calcinosis; Raynaud's phenomenon (95 percent)
Gastrointestinal tract	50–70	Dysphagia; malabsorption; ulceration, infarction, perforation, or hemorrhage
Lungs	50	Dyspnea; restrictive lung disease; cor pulmonale
Heart	50	Pericarditis; heart failure (due to cor pulmonale, hypertension, or myocardial ischemia or fibrosis); conduction abnormalities
Kidneys	40–50	Hypertension (often malignant); acute renal failure
Joints and muscles	20–50	Arthralgias; arthritis; muscle weakness and stiffness

SOURCE: Data from Refs. 132, 134, and 161.

decreased motility), or dyspnea (due to diffusion defects).

SCLERODERMA RENAL CRISIS

The classic form of renal involvement in PSS, scleroderma renal crisis (SRC), is characterized by abrupt onset and rapid progression to renal failure within 1 to 2 months (if untreated), with a relatively benign urinary sediment.[133,134,162] Severe hypertension is commonly, but not always, present.[136] There is no prior evidence of renal disease in most patients; isolated mild, hypertension alone does not predict which patients will ultimately develop this complication.[163]

The frequency of SRC is estimated to be as high as 20 to 25 percent.[134] However, the actual frequency may be lower since most series are from referral centers, which may preferentially see more severe disease. Patients with SRC seem to present more frequently in the fall and winter[137] (perhaps reflecting a role for cold-induced vasospasm)

and almost always present early in the course of their disease (within 4 years after onset).[163] While most patients with SRC have elevated plasma renin activity, a mild increase in this parameter is not necessarily predictive of future disease.[163-165]

It has been proposed that the abrupt onset of the renal failure may result from the superimposition of a stimulus which leads to renal vasoconstriction (such as hypovolemia, heart failure, or, perhaps, cold exposure) upon the preexisting renal vascular disease.[134] The net effect is a critical narrowing of the interlobular arteries, leading to renal ischemia, necrosis, and increased activation of the renin-angiotensin system which can produce both hypertension and more intense renal ischemia. The development of hypertension can then promote further renal damage, as evidenced by the partial improvement in renal function, which may follow strict control of the blood pressure.[145,147,149] However, systemic hypertension is clearly a secondary factor in SRC, since some patients develop acute renal failure *without* an elevation of blood pressure.[133,134,136]

DIAGNOSIS

The diagnosis of PSS is usually suggested by the characteristic clinical findings of the disease, particularly the dermal changes, Raynaud's phenomenon, dysphagia with decreased esophageal motility, and evidence of decreased diffusing capacity on pulmonary function testing. Although the diagnosis can usually be confirmed by skin biopsy, this is not necessary in most patients.

The urinalysis is usually normal or only mildly abnormal (mild proteinuria with few cells or casts), even in patients with advanced renal disease.[134] This combination of acute renal failure with a benign urinalysis may be of some diagnostic importance, since it is found in only a few other conditions, which usually can be easily differentiated from PSS. Included in this group are prerenal disease, urinary tract obstruction, atheroembolic disease, hypercalcemia, multiple myeloma, and some cases of acute tubular necrosis.

Serologic testing for autoantibodies directed against the cell nucleus [antinuclear antibodies (ANA)] is useful in equivocal cases of PSS. Over 90 percent of PSS patients have antinuclear antibodies in their serum.[166] A speckled pattern on immunofluorescent staining is most common, frequently being seen in patients early in the course of their disease. This pattern correlates well with the presence of extractable nuclear antigen (ENA), which contains several antigens including the Sm antigen and RNP (ribonuclear protein).[167]

The presence of other antinuclear antibodies in PSS may vary with the severity of the disease. Anticentromere antibodies, for example, may be found in the sera of patients who have the CREST syndrome (calcinosis, Raynaud's phenomenon, esophageal motility abnormalities, sclerodactyly, and telangiectasia), or other limited forms of PSS.[168-170] In contrast, patients with severe, diffuse PSS are more likely to have anti-Scl-70 antibody (approximately 20 percent of patients with PSS) in their serum.[160,170,171] These last two autoantibodies are highly specific for PSS.

COURSE AND TREATMENT

The course of PSS is variable, being dependent upon the pattern of organ involvement. In some patients, the disease remains mild and prognosis for long-term survival is good. As an example, patients with the CREST syndrome may follow a relatively benign course for 10 years or more, although late deterioration can occur.[172] On the other hand, patients with early visceral involvement tend to have slowly progressive disease which may terminate abruptly in acute renal failure. Pregnancy should probably be avoided in patients with systemic involvement, since it may be associated with exacerbation of PSS and an increased incidence of toxemia, premature births and perinatal mortality.[173]

The overall mortality rate in PSS is approximately 65 percent at 7 years.[134] Renal failure accounts for about 40 percent of these deaths, with respiratory and cardiac failure or gastrointestinal complications (such as intestinal infarction or perforation) being responsible for most of the remaining mortality. The average survival time after the onset of azotemia and malignant hypertension may be as short as 1 month if antihypertensive therapy or dialysis are not instituted.[134] However, aggressive therapy of SRC has reduced the prominence of renal failure as a cause of death.[174]

No form of treatment has been shown to definitely alter the course of the extrarenal disease.[167,175] Thus, supportive measures aimed at specific symptoms constitute the therapeutic regimen for most patients. These include adequate nutrition, the avoidance of cold exposure, lubricating oils and physical therapy for the digital changes, antibiotics for malabsorption, and calcium blocking agents (particularly nifedipine)[176] or less often other vasodilators (such as reserpine)[177] for severe Raynaud's phenomenon.

There is, however, one setting in which therapy is extremely important: control of the blood pressure may lead to improved renal and patient survival in *scleroderma renal crisis.* In the past, standard oral antihypertensive agents were frequently ineffective, and nephrectomy was occasionally required to remove the source of renin secretion, thereby decreasing both the blood pressure and systemic angiotensin II-mediated vasoconstriction. In one early study of patients on hemodialysis, for example, only 1 of 8 patients who had not had bilateral nephrectomy survived 6 months, in contrast to 3 of 7 patients who had undergone surgery.[162]

The availability of more potent and specific oral antihypertensive agents has dramatically altered the course of SRC, since effective treatment of hypertension can stabilize or improve renal function in many patients.[145,147,149] Although the use of β-blockers and potent vasodilators (such as minoxidil) can allow control of blood pressure without nephrectomy,[145,178,179] the antihypertensive agent of choice for SRC is a converting enzyme inhibitor, since this group of drugs specifically reverses the angiotensin II-mediated hypertension.[147-149,174,180] With captopril, for example, up to 90 percent of patients have a significant reduction in blood pressure, 70 to 80 percent may have an improvement in GFR (if therapy is begun before the onset of advanced renal failure), and approximately 50 percent have a sustained long-term (over 2 years) response.[149,174]

Successful treatment of SRC may also be associated with rapid and persistent improvement in cutaneous sclerodermatous changes, Raynaud's phenomenon, and the microangiopathic hemolytic anemia.[145-147] These findings suggest that hypertension, although not a primary event, may exacerbate and perpetuate the vascular disease.

The optimal treatment of chronic progressive renal failure in PSS is uncertain, aside from strict control of hypertension and possibly protein restriction (to reduce intraglomerular hypertension; see Chap. 4).[181] Hemodialysis, continuous ambulatory peritoneal dialysis (CAPD), and transplantation have all effectively prolonged life, although each modality has some problems with its use. Reductions in peripheral blood flow can lead to difficulties in vascular access and fistula flow in patients being hemodialyzed. If these problems limit the effectiveness of this procedure, peritoneal dialysis can be used. CAPD is usually successful even though the peritoneal clearances of urea and creatinine are often decreased in PSS, possibly due to local vascular disease.[182] Clearances may change from summer to winter, however, with changes in ambient temperature.[182]

Renal transplantation is an acceptable alternative to dialysis[183-185] and may be associated with a reduction in symptoms (especially Raynaud's phenomenon).[185] However, a relatively frequent problem in the small number of patients who have received transplants is recurrence of PSS in the graft, leading to progressive renal failure.[185] This is most likely to occur in patients in whom end-stage renal disease developed within 1 year of the clinical onset of PSS. The frequency of this problem may be overestimated, however, since chronic transplant rejection can cause a similar pathologic picture.[136,184]

HEMOLYTIC-UREMIC SYNDROMES

The hemolytic-uremic syndromes are typically characterized by acute renal failure of varying severity, a microangiopathic hemolytic anemia, and thrombocytopenia. The classic histologic lesions, which appear to cause most of the symptoms, are micro-thrombi consisting primarily of platelets and, to a lesser degree, fibrin. Three distinct disorders with different clinical features, but apparently similar pathologic changes and pathogenetic mechanisms, are included under the term hemolytic-uremic syndrome (HUS): thrombotic thrombocytopenic purpura (TTP), childhood HUS, and adult HUS (Table 7–7). Although other diseases such as malignant nephrosclerosis, progressive systemic sclerosis, and systemic vasculitis may be associated with acute renal failure and a microangiographic hemolytic anemia, small vessel platelet thrombi are not pathogenetically important in these disorders.

PATHOLOGY

The histologic findings in the kidney are similar in each of the forms of HUS.[186-189] The acute stage is characterized by platelet and fibrin thrombi occluding the glomerular capillaries, arterioles, and small interlobular arteries (Fig. 7–9a). The interlobular arteries also may show mucoid intimal thickening, similar to that seen in progressive systemic

sclerosis (see Fig. 7–8a). These vascular changes can lead to marked ischemia, resulting in areas of arteriolar, glomerular, and, in severe cases, cortical necrosis. Later changes include narrowing of the glomerular capillaries by endothelial cell swelling and increased masangial matrix and cellularity. Fibrin thrombi may be relatively sparse at this stage, presumably due to local fibrinolysis.

The site of major pathologic change (glomeruli versus arterioles) appears to be of prognostic importance. Glomerular involvement (consisting of intracapillary thrombi) predominates in young children who have a high rate of spontaneous recovery. In comparison, older children and adults develop prominent mucoid arterial lesions, a finding that is associated with a more marked elevation in blood pressure and less frequent recovery of renal function.[187,190]

Immunofluorescent studies demonstrate extensive fibrin deposition in the arterial and glomerular lesions (Fig. 7–9b).[187,191] Immunoglobulins and complement are usually absent, although IgM and C3 have occasionally been found.[192,193] The significance of the latter findings is uncertain since typical dense deposits thought to represent immune com-

TABLE 7–7. Clinical Characteristics of the Hemolytic-Uremic Syndromes

Disorder	Clinical Setting	Clinical Features
TTP	Most often affects females between the ages of 10 and 50. Usually idiopathic.	Characteristic pentad: fever, microangiopathic hemolytic anemia, thrombocytopenic purpura, renal failure (usually slowly progressive), and neurologic abnormalities.
Childhood HUS	Primarily affects children under the age of 4 following an episode of gastroenteritis or, less often, an upper respiratory infection.	Acute renal failure, microangiopathic hemolytic anemia, and thrombocytopenia.
Adult HUS	May rarely follow gastroenteritis as in children, but most common in women who are postpartum or taking oral contraceptives, in cancer patients (if treated with mitomycin C or the combination of cisplatin and bleomycin), or in transplant patients taking cyclosporine.	Acute renal failure, microangiopathic hemolytic anemia, and thrombocytopenia, but fever, neurologic abnormalities, and a cardiomyopathy may also be present.

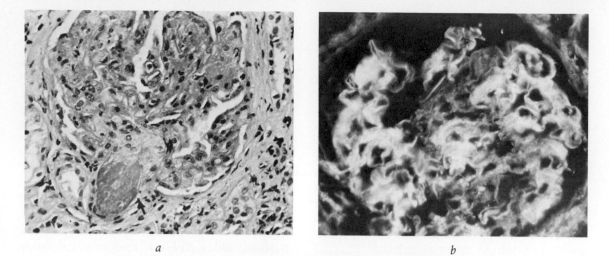

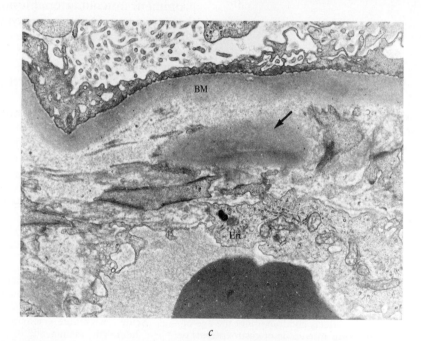

FIG. 7–9. Glomerular changes in the hemolytic-uremic syndrome. (*a*) Large thrombus occluding the afferent arteriole (arrow). Although there is no hypercellularity, capillary loops are mostly closed due to both fibrin deposition and swelling of the endothelial cells. (*b*) Immunofluorescent microscopy demonstrates extensive glomerular fibrin deposition. (*Courtesy of Dr. Robert Colvin.*) (*c*) Electron microscopy reveals widening of the subendothelial region [between the basement membrane (BM) and endothelial cell (En)] by both electron-lucent and electron-dense, fibrillar material (arrow), which may represent incompletely polymerized fibrin. A red cell is seen in the capillary lumen.

TABLE 7-8. Typical Hematologic Findings in HUS and DIC

Finding	HUS	DIC
Composition of thrombi	Platelets with a thin rim of fibrin	Platelets and fibrin
Platelet turnover	Increased	Increased
Fibrinogen turnover	Normal	Increased
Platelet count	Decreased	Decreased
Plasma levels of fibrinogen and clotting factors V, VIII	Usually normal or increased	Usually decreased
Prothrombin and partial thromboplastin times	Normal or slightly increased	Increased
Fibrin degradation products	Increased	Increased

plex deposition are not seen on electron microscopy in HUS. It is possible, however, that activation of the alternate complement pathway may occur as a secondary event, being initiated by ischemic damage to the glomerular or vascular cells.[194]

The major glomerular change observed on electron microscopy is thickening of the capillary wall. This is due to widening of the subendothelial space by both electron-lucent material of uncertain composition and electron-dense granular or fibrillar material which may represent incompletely polymerized fibrin. (Fig. 7-9c).[186,195] Swelling of the endothelial cells and intracapillary thrombi composed, in part, of platelets also may be seen. Similar ultrastructural changes are present in the arterioles, including thrombi, endothelial cell swelling, and the deposition of fibrin-like material.[195]

The vascular lesions frequently are not limited to the kidney. This is particularly true in TTP and, to a lesser degree, in HUS in which arteriolar and capillary thrombi may be found in the brain, heart, adrenal gland, pancreas, and other organs.[189,195,196]

PATHOGENESIS

The presence of intravascular thrombi raises the possibility that HUS represents a localized form of disseminated intravascular coagulation (DIC). However, there are several major differences between these two disorders which suggest that they are probably not related (Table 7-8). The characteristic laboratory findings in DIC—thrombocytopenia, hypofibrinogenemia, reduced plasma levels of factors V and VIII, prolonged prothrombin and partial thromboplastin times, and elevated fibrin degradation products—are produced by intravascular activation of the coagulation system.[197-199] For example, thromboplastins may be released into the circulation in obstetric complications or with certain tumors.[197-200] This results sequentially in the formation of fibrin thrombi, consumption of clotting factors and platelets (Fig. 7-10), and secondary fibrinolysis. In this setting, heparin, but not inhibitors of platelet function such as dipyridamole, may return fibrinogen and platelet turnover to normal (Fig. 7-11).[201]

In contrast, HUS appears to represent relatively *isolated platelet consumption* and not generalized activation of the coagulation pathway. This is manifested by thrombi that frequently contain platelets with only a thin rim of fibrin,[188] and by an increase in platelet, but not fibrinogen turnover (Fig. 7-10).[188,201] As a result, thrombocytopenia is typically present, but the prothrombin and partial thromboplastin times as well as the plasma levels of fibrinogen and factors V and VIII are usually, but not always, normal.[187,188,202-204] Elevated levels of fibrin degradation products may be present in HUS and are presumably

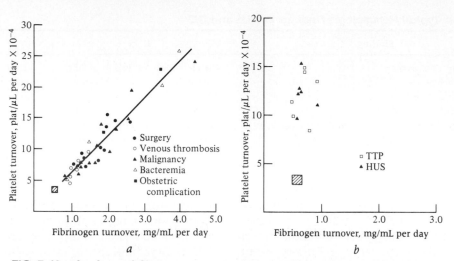

FIG. 7-10. Platelet and fibrin turnover in thrombotic disorders. (*a*) Platelet and fibrinogen consumption are directly related in venous thrombosis and disorders associated with DIC. (*b*) In contrast, TTP and the HUS are associated with selective platelet consumption. Normal values are shown by the shaded areas. (*Adapted from L. A. Harker and S. J. Slichter, N. Engl. J. Med., 287:999, 1972. Reprinted by permission from the New England Journal of Medicine.*)

due to the effect of the fibrinolytic system on the fibrin present in the thrombi. Since platelet consumption is primary, platelet turnover is normalized by dipyridamole and aspirin but not by heparin (Fig. 7-11).*

The factors responsible for the platelet consumption in HUS are unknown. Two theories, which are not necessarily mutually exclusive, have been proposed. In the first, it is postulated that some insult (such as a virus, endotoxin, some chemotherapeutic agents, or immune complex formation) *injures the vascular endothelium.* This results in the exposure of collagen, which then leads to platelet aggregation and a platelet thrombus.[201,205,206] Support for this hypothesis has

*In addition to these pathogenetic differences, DIC and HUS have somewhat different clinical manifestations. In particular, renal failure is characteristically found in the HUS but is unusual in DIC unless produced by some underlying abnormality such as septicemia or shock.[198,199]

been demonstrated experimentally using the chemotherapeutic agent, mitomycin C, which can cause HUS in humans (see "Adult Hemolytic-Uremic Syndrome," below). Mitomycin C infusion into the renal artery of the rat results in the formation of renal lesions indistinguishable from those in human HUS.[207] The earliest detectable abnormality seen in this setting is glomerular endothelial damage, which occurs *prior* to platelet accumulation.

The second hypothesis proposes that HUS is caused by *primary intravascular platelet aggregation.* This could be due either to the *presence* of a substance that promotes the formation of platelet thrombi or to a *deficiency* of an inhibitor of platelet aggregation.

The presence of a circulating *platelet aggregating factor* (PAF) in TTP is suggested by the observation that normal platelets tend to aggregate when incubated in plasma from patients with TTP.[208] This pro-aggregating activity is not present in normal plasma. The nature of the PAF is not well understood, but one possibility has come from the demonstration of unusually large factor VIII—von Willebrand factor (FVIII/vWF) multimers in patients with chronic relapsing TTP.[209] These platelet-aggregating multimers are similar to those synthesized by normal human endothelial cells. However, the FVIII/vWF depolymerase that decreases the size of these very large multimers in normal plasma may be deficient in patients with TTP. The favorable response to plasma exchange in many patients with this disorder (see "Thrombotic Thrombocytopenic Purpura: Course and Treatment," below)[210] may be due to the removal of these multimers (or of some other PAF).[211]

Alternatively, *deficiency of a normal circulating inhibitor of platelet aggregation* could be of primary importance in some patients. This hypothesis is supported by the reduction in platelet aggregation and the dramatic reversal of symptoms that can follow the infusion of normal plasma in some patients with active TTP.[212,213] It is possible in this setting that fresh frozen plasma supplies a factor that normally inhibits platelet aggregation by, for example, promoting the catabolism of the large FVIII/vWF multimers described above, by correcting an absolute or relative decrease in prostacyclin action (due to reduced production or increased degradation),[210,214-218] or by neutralizing an, as yet, unidentified PAF.

While the mechanism of action of this inhibitor of platelet aggregation remains unknown, recent evidence strongly suggests that it is an *immunoglobulin of the IgG class.*[219-222] IgG from patients with active HUS appears to lack this platelet inhibitory activity, as does IgG from normal infants and children under the age of 4 (the group most likely to develop childhood HUS).[219]

In addition to the uncertainty about the mechanisms responsible for the platelet aggregation and consumption in the hemolytic-uremic syndrome, the triggering factors are also incompletely understood and appear to vary with age. In young children (and less commonly in adults), the development of HUS is frequently preceded by an infection, most often viral or bacterial gastroenteritis.[206] It has been proposed that the common denominator in these conditions is injury to the intestinal mucosa, which might allow a toxin (such as verotoxin from *Escherichia coli*)

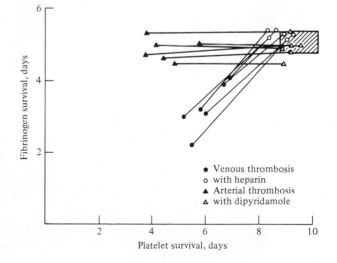

FIG. 7-11. Effects of heparin and dipyridamole treatment on thrombotic disorders. Heparin interrupts the platelet and fibrinogen consumption of venous thrombosis and DIC, whereas dipyridamole (but not heparin) prevents the selective platelet consumption associated with arterial thrombosis as in TTP or HUS. The shaded area represents the normal range for platelet and fibrinogen survival. (*From L. A. Harker and S. J. Slichter, N. Engl. J. Med., 287:999, 1972. Reprinted by permission from the New England Journal of Medicine.*)

• Venous thrombosis
○ with heparin
▲ Arterial thrombosis
△ with dipyridamole

Fibrinogen survival, days

Platelet survival, days

to enter the bloodstream and produce HUS either by damaging the arterial endothelium or by causing primary platelet aggregation.[206,223-225] HUS has also followed other infectious causes of gastroenteritis such as *Shigella*,[225] *Salmonella*,[226] *Yersinia*,[227] *Campylobacter*,[228,229] and enteroviruses.[230]

In comparison, the hemolytic-uremic syndrome in adults is most often idiopathic[187,189] or associated with pregnancy (particularly in the postpartum period),[187,231-234] the use of oral contraceptives,[235-237] or cancer chemotherapy with mitomycin C[238-240] or the combination of bleomycin and cisplatin.[241] Although pregnancy and its complications may predispose to the development of DIC, it is not known how they might lead to the selective platelet consumption characteristic of HUS. With chemotherapy, it is possible that direct vascular toxicity may occur.[207,217,241]

In addition to impairing organ function, arterial thrombi also appear to be responsible for the characteristic red cell abnormalities seen in HUS (Fig. 7–12). The erythrocytes undergo traumatic fragmentation as they move through the partially occluding fibrin stands.[242] A primary role for *intrarenal hemolysis* is suggested by resolution of the microangiopathic changes that has occurred in several adults with HUS in whom nephrectomy was performed for severe hypertension and end-stage renal failure.[232,243] However, hemolysis does not necessarily occur only in the kidney.[244]

THROMBOTIC THROMBOCYTOPENIC PURPURA

TTP is a rare disorder which may occur at any age, but primarily affects females between the ages of 10 and 50. It is characterized by five prominent findings, each of which is found in more than 90 percent of patients:[189] fever, thrombocytopenia, which is usually accompanied by purpura; neurologic abnormalities; renal disease; and a microangiopathic hemolytic anemia.

CLINICAL PRESENTATION

Most patients with TTP begin with a flu-like prodrome (fever, malaise, fatigue, nausea,

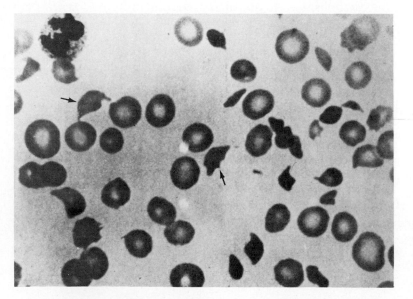

FIG. 7–12. Peripheral blood smear in microangiopathic hemolytic anemia revealing helmet cells (arrows) and other fragmented red cells.

vomiting), which then progresses to purpuric skin lesions, pallor, and neurologic symptoms that may fluctuate in severity.[189] The neurologic manifestations that may occur include headache, abnormal mental status, paresthesias, seizures, and coma. Focal findings, such as aphasia or hemiparesis, are less commonly seen.[188,189] In some patients, clinically important thrombi may also develop in other organs, resulting, for example, in intestinal or myocardial infarction.

The laboratory findings typically include thrombocytopenia, anemia with a microangiopathic blood smear, and findings characteristic of intravascular hemolysis: indirect hyperbilirubinemia, low haptoglobin, high plasma lactate dehydrogenase, and a moderate reticulocytosis (unless there is severe renal failure). The urinalysis may be normal, but usually contains red cells, mild proteinuria, and, in rare cases, red cell casts.[245] Renal insufficiency is generally of mild to moderate severity, although acute anuric renal failure may occur.[246] Hypocomplementemia may be found, but appears to reflect activation of complement by viral products, proteolytic enzymes, or damaged renal tissue, rather than by immune complex deposition.[247]

DIAGNOSIS

The diagnosis of this rare syndrome is usually suggested by the characteristic clinical and laboratory findings. The demonstration of hyaline thrombi in the small arteries and capillaries on gingival or bone marrow biopsy has been used to confirm the diagnosis, but false-negative results are common.[189,248] Consequently, a renal biopsy may be required if the diagnosis is uncertain or if less invasive biopsies are negative.

Other disorders which can present with similar findings to TTP are disseminated intravascular coagulation, systemic vasculitis, and adult HUS. In contrast to DIC, which is usually associated with sepsis, shock, or an obstetrical complication, a precipitating disorder cannot usually be identified in TTP. Furthermore, most coagulation tests other than the platelet count and fibrin degradation products are usually normal or only slightly abnormal in TTP (Table 7–8).[188,204] Although systemic vasculitis can present with fever, renal insufficiency, purpura, and a microangiopathic hemolytic anemia, thrombocytopenia is uncommon and the primary neurologic abnormalities are more often in the peripheral (mononeuritis multiplex), not the central, nervous system (see "Systemic Vasculitis," above).

The differentiation between TTP and adult HUS is made primarily on clinical grounds. In TTP, for example, neurologic symptoms are prominent, while renal insufficiency is typically mild. In contrast, acute renal failure is the major visceral abnormality in adult HUS. This distinction may be arbitrary, however, since a common event can lead to both clinical disorders.* Therefore, a search for the causes of adult HUS (see below) should be made in all patients who present with TTP.

COURSE AND TREATMENT

Thrombotic thrombocytopenic purpura can present as an acute fulminant illness or as a chronic, slowly progressive disease. If untreated, it is almost uniformly fatal with about three-fourths of patients dying within 3 months of presentation.[189] Therefore, *prompt diagnosis and initiation of therapy are imperative* to prevent both severe bleeding from thrombocytopenia and necrosis with potentially irreversible loss of organ function from thrombotic lesions.

A variety of therapies have been tried in

---

*A strong association between adult HUS and chemotherapy with cisplatin and bleomycin has been suggested. In one study of five patients, however, two developed a syndrome typical of TTP, while the remainder presented with the usual features of HUS.[241]

an attempt to improve the grim prognosis in TTP. Heparin generally has been ineffective, a finding that is not surprising since heparin does not reverse the platelet consumption characteristic of this disorder.[201] Corticosteroids,[248,249] splenectomy,[248,250,251] and antiplatelet agents alone have also had limited benefit in most patients.[252-255] Prostacyclin infusions have had some success, but are not available at this time for routine use.[216]

The treatment of TTP has been revolutionized by protocols using fresh frozen plasma infusions alone[212,213,256] *or combined with plasma exchange.*[254,257,258] These therapies, which are usually given in conjunction with antiplatelet agents, have led to remission of the disease in up to 80 to 90 percent of patients.[254] Fresh frozen plasma may replace the missing inhibitor of platelet aggregation (possibly an IgG),[219,220] while plasmapheresis presumably removes platelet aggregating factors or toxins.

A reasonable approach to therapy for TTP patients with relatively *stable,* and not life-threatening, disease is to begin with fresh frozen plasma infusions (3 units/day) and antiplatelet agents (aspirin and dipyridamole). If no response, as evidenced by an increased platelet count, is seen within 48 h, plasmapheresis should be performed with plasma replacement. In patients who still do not respond, gamma globulin infusion[220,221] or vincristine[214,215] should be considered. The beneficial effect of vincristine, which occurs by an unknown mechanism, is delayed for 2 to 10 days. Corticosteroids and splenectomy should probably be reserved for patients who fail these other modalities.[248-250]

These recommendations should be modified in the face of *fulminant* disease. In this setting, plasmapheresis with fresh frozen plasma replacement should be started immediately, since time is not available to see if fresh frozen plasma alone will be effective.

It is important to be aware of two potentially adverse effects of therapy in patients with TTP. Some patients may have a bleeding episode after antiplatelet agents,[255] and

focal central nervous system deficits have been reported after platelet transfusions.[259] The latter problem is presumably related to consumption of the infused platelets by the formation of new thrombi. Consequently, platelet infusions should be used only in patients with marked bleeding due to thrombocytopenia.

Patients who respond to therapy typically show an improvement in their platelet count and neurologic symptoms within hours to days after therapy is started. However, the anemia and microangiopathy persist for weeks to months in most patients.[254] Those who progress to end-stage renal failure may be successfully dialyzed or transplanted, although TTP may recur in the renal allograft.[260]

CHILDHOOD HEMOLYTIC-UREMIC SYNDROME

The childhood hemolytic-uremic syndrome is a relatively common cause of acute renal failure in children under 4 years of age.[206,261] The disease may occur in older children as well. Both sporadic cases and miniepidemics are seen,[206,225] and the disease appears to be endemic in some areas, such as Argentina.[262] There is also an increased incidence within certain families, which may reflect exposure to a common environmental agent as well as increased genetic susceptibility.[263]

CLINICAL PRESENTATION

The most common predisposing factor for the development of HUS in children is an episode of gastroenteritis (primarily viral or bacterial), frequently with bloody diarrhea, and, in some patients, melena or hematemesis.[206,225,261,264,265] In one study, gastroenteritis occurred in 34 of 39 children, with the other five having had prior upper respiratory infections.[261] Infections in other organ systems can also precipitate the HUS in isolated cases.[266]

The initial illness is followed within 3 days to 3 weeks by the sudden onset of pallor, oliguria or anuria, and frequently manifestations of a bleeding tendency such as petechiae or purpura. Less common complaints include abdominal pain, fever, and neurologic changes such as altered mental status and seizures.[261,267] The last symptoms may be in part due to uremic encephalopathy and usually do not reflect cerebrovascular thrombi as in TTP. However, hemorrhagic cerebral infarcts have occurred in childhood HUS, leading to a syndrome that fulfills the criteria for TTP.[268,269]

In addition to pallor and purpura, the physical examination reveals hypertension and hepatomegaly in approximately one-half of patients and, less often, jaundice and neurologic changes.[261,269] Activation of the renin-angiotensin system by glomerular ischemia appears to be responsible for the elevation in blood pressure.[270]

The laboratory findings in childhood HUS are similar to those in TTP (see above), except that the renal disease tends to be more severe. Acute, anuric renal failure occurs in over 50 percent of patients with concomitant moderate to marked elevations in the BUN (blood urea nitrogen) and plasma creatinine concentration.[271] The urinalysis is often relatively benign, revealing mild proteinuria with few cells or casts.

DIAGNOSIS

The diagnosis of childhood HUS is generally made on the basis of the characteristic clinical and laboratory findings. There is no specific test that can be used to confirm the diagnosis other than renal biopsy, which is not only unnecessary but usually contraindicated because of thrombocytopenia. Although the presence of hypocomplementemia in some patients[193,247] may suggest poststreptococcal or membranoproliferative glomerulonephritis (see Chap. 6), these disorders are not associated with the hematologic abnormalities of HUS.

COURSE AND TREATMENT

Early studies found a mortality rate of 60 to 80 percent in childhood HUS[272] with heart or renal failure, bleeding, and sepsis being the major causes of death.[261] However, the mortality rate has been reduced to under 5 percent in the last 15 years.[261,267,273,274]

The major factors responsible for the improved prognosis in this disorder appear to be better supportive care (treatment of anemia, infection, and hypertension) and early peritoneal dialysis.[272] Consequently, it is recommended that peritoneal dialysis be instituted if anuria persists for more than 48 h, regardless of the BUN, plasma creatinine concentration, or fluid and electrolyte status.

Most children with HUS recover with supportive care alone,[261,267,272,275] with the hematologic and renal abnormalities improving within 1 to 2 weeks.[261,267] There are, however, several settings in which children with HUS are at greater risk of persistent renal failure (due to diffuse cortical necrosis) or death. These include a lack of improvement by 2 weeks, no antecedent gastroenteritis, and recurrent or familial disease.[261,263,267,274] The increased severity in familial HUS is seen primarily if the episodes are widely spaced (more than 9 to 12 months apart), suggesting some genetic predisposition rather than exposure to a common agent as with closely spaced cases.[263] In addition, the prognosis appears to be worse in Argentina, where up to 20 percent of children develop chronic renal failure and 33 percent become hypertensive.[262] These late complications are uncommon in the United States,[273] where the mortality rate is under 3 percent and the incidence of chronic renal failure is less than 5 percent.[275] The reason for this difference is not known.

Considering the clinical and pathogenetic similarities between HUS and TTP, anecdotal reports suggest that children with more severe disease can be treated with the regimen outlined above for TTP.[222,276-278] This includes children who do not show an improvement in renal function within 7 days, who have hemorrhage due to severe thrombocytopenia, or who have severe multisystem disease (especially with otherwise unexplained central nervous system involvement).[279] Fresh frozen plasma and antiplatelet agents[278,280,281] can be used initially, with plasmapheresis added in children who do not respond within 48 h or who have fulminant disease.

A variety of other modalities have been tried in selected patients. Included in this group are experimental infusions of prostacyclin, which has shown some success,[282] and corticosteroids, heparin, and urokinase, which generally have been without benefit.[261,272,273] Platelet transfusions should be avoided if possible, since the infused platelets, if consumed in the ongoing thrombus formation, may be associated with the rapid appearance of focal neurologic symptoms.[259,280]

Children who develop chronic progressive renal failure may be successfully transplanted, but the disease not infrequently recurs.[283,284] Prophylactic administration of antiplatelet agents posttransplantation as well as the avoidance of cyclosporine, which can cause the HUS (see "Adult Hemolytic Uremic Syndrome," below), may minimize the incidence of recurrent disease in this setting.[283]

ADULT HEMOLYTIC-UREMIC SYNDROME

The adult form of the hemolytic-uremic syndrome is another uncommon disorder.[187,196] This condition is frequently idiopathic,[187] although its occasional occurrence within families suggests a genetic or environmental predisposition.[285] In some patients, however, an underlying disorder can be identified (see Table 7-7). In women, for example, the onset of the disease often occurs in the postpartum period[231-234] or in patients taking oral contraceptives.[235-237] How these conditions might produce HUS is not known.

Adult hemolytic-uremic syndrome has also been described with certain malignancies (usually mucinous adenocarcinomas of the gastrointestinal tract, pancreas, or prostate)[286] and with chemotherapy using mitomycin C[238-240] or the combination of cisplatin and bleomycin.[241] The pathogenesis of chemotherapy-induced HUS is uncertain. However, the possibility that primary vascular damage may be the initiating event is supported by the association of Raynaud's phenomenon, lung fibrosis, and skin fibrosis with bleomycin therapy,[241] by the development of acute vascular ischemic events after combination therapy with cisplatin and bleomycin,[287] and by the observation that mitomycin C can directly injure the vascular endothelium.[207]

Cyclosporine, an immunosuppressive agent used primarily to prevent organ rejection, has also been associated with adult HUS.[288-291] This complication was initially observed in bone marrow transplant recipients.[289-291] Its recent description in patients with renal allografts[288] has probably been delayed because of the clinical and histopathologic similarities between the HUS and hyperacute transplant rejection.[292] Pathologically, the lack of inflammatory changes in the vascular wall and the absence of vascular IgG and C3 deposition (by immunofluorescent microscopy) favor the diagnosis of the HUS.[288] Furthermore, better cross-matching techniques have made hyperacute rejection rare.

Other uncommon causes of adult HUS have also been described. These include infectious gastroenteritis (as commonly occurs in children)[223,226] and after a snakebite.[293]

CLINICAL PRESENTATION

The mode of presentation in adult HUS is similar to that in children. Many patients have prodromal, viral-like symptoms followed by the onset of pallor, oliguria or anuria, and frequently bleeding manifestations such as purpura or, in women, vaginal bleeding.[187,196,237] Fever and neurologic involvement (such as seizures) may also occur, resulting in a clinical syndrome that is indistinguishable from TTP.[196] Furthermore, signs or symptoms of congestive heart failure are found at some time in the course of many patients with postpartum HUS, and appear to result from a cardiomyopathy (the etiology of which is uncertain), rather than from fluid overload secondary to acute renal failure.[231,232]

The onset of the disease varies with the setting in which it occurs. For example, postpartum HUS usually occurs 1 day to 10 weeks after an *uncomplicated* pregnancy and delivery.[232,234] Chemotherapy-induced HUS may appear shortly after chemotherapy or many months after treatment has been discontinued,[239-241] suggesting that long-term followup is required in patients receiving the implicated agents.

The physical examination typically reveals pallor and, in over 80 percent of patients, hypertension which may be severe.[187,232] Pulmonary rales and a gallop rhythm may be heard if congestive heart failure is present. The laboratory findings are similar to those described above for TTP. The urinalysis may contain red blood cells and, rarely, red cell casts, but is frequently benign, showing only mild proteinuria.

DIAGNOSIS

The diagnosis of adult HUS can be easily missed unless the triad of acute renal failure, a microangiopathic hemolytic anemia, and thrombocytopenia is present. A history of recent pregnancy, oral contraceptive use, malignancy, especially if treated with mitomycin C or the combination of bleomycin and cisplatin, or cyclosporine therapy should suggest the hemolytic-uremic syndrome. The differential diagnosis is similar to that in TTP

(see above), which has many features in common with adult HUS. If the diagnosis is in doubt, a renal biopsy can be performed unless contraindicated by severe thrombocytopenia.

COURSE AND TREATMENT

Adult hemolytic-uremic syndrome generally has a poor prognosis, particularly when compared with childhood HUS (where the mortality rate is under 5 percent with spontaneous recovery the rule). In addition to the different settings in which these syndromes develop, the vessels involved by the pathologic changes appear to be important determinants of the ultimate outcome.[187] For example, glomerular involvement is most prominent in childhood HUS, a change that is typically reversible. In contrast, larger arterial lesions predominate in adult HUS, causing a greater degree of persistent ischemia and necrosis.

Recovery, when it occurs, is typically seen within the first few weeks after presentation, but may be delayed and may be incomplete.[241,294] However, only 20 to 30 percent of patients with adult HUS survive without the need for dialysis or transplantation.[187,232-234] Patient survival appears to be particularly poor in postpartum HUS, where congestive heart failure due to the associated cardiomyopathy is a major cause of death.[232] The outcome may be better in patients with a diarrheal prodrome (as in childhood HUS)[294] and in patients taking cyclosporine.[288,290]

The effectiveness of therapy in adult HUS is uncertain. In view of the poor prognosis in the untreated patient, however, it is reasonable to attempt any form of therapy that might be of benefit without posing undue risk. Considering the pathogenetic, clinical, and prognostic similarities between adult HUS and TTP, and the apparent responsiveness of TTP to treatment, it may be efficacious to use a similar regimen in the two disorders. Thus, antiplatelet agents and fresh frozen plasma infusion should be used in patients with indolent disease, and plasma exchange with plasma replacement should be added in patients without evidence of improvement in 48 to 72 h or used initially in patients with acute renal failure or more aggressive disease. Anecdotal reports suggest that such a regimen may be effective in at least some patients.[295-297] Other modalities that have been used with apparent success in selected patients include vincristine[298-300] and antiplatelet agents alone.[285,301] Heparin appears to be of little benefit as it does not prevent disease progression.[232,302,303]

In contrast to the poor prognosis in most forms of untreated adult HUS, spontaneous recovery has been observed in over 50 percent of patients who developed HUS while taking cyclosporine.[288,290] Substitution of azathioprine for cyclosporine, or a reduction in cyclosporine dose, appears to improve the clinical and laboratory status of transplant recipients in this setting.[284,288]

Those patients with adult hemolytic-uremic syndrome who progress to end-stage renal disease may be successfully transplanted. Oral contraceptives should be avoided, since estrogen therapy has been associated with recurrent disease, even after renal transplantation.[231,304] The safety of cyclosporine in patients with a history of HUS is unknown.[283,284,305]

THE KIDNEY IN PREGNANCY

NORMAL PHYSIOLOGY

Major changes in systemic hemodynamics and renal function occur during normal pregnancy (Table 7-9). The cardiac output, for example, increases by 30 to 40 percent during the first trimester.[306,307] This change, which is maintained throughout the pregnancy, is associated with the retention of approximately 900 to 1000 meq of sodium and 6 to 8 L of water.[308] To some degree, these

TABLE 7-9. Hemodynamic Alterations in Normal Pregnancy

Increased cardiac output
Sodium and water retention
Reduced systemic blood pressure
Increased plasma renin activity
Increased renal blood flow and GFR

elevations in output and volume are required to meet the needs of the fetus and placenta. However, true volume expansion is also present as evidenced by a 30 to 40 percent rise in plasma volume, by enhanced perfusion of other organs such as the kidney, and by the development of mild peripheral edema (to which partial obstruction of the inferior vena cava by the enlarged uterus also contributes) in up to 80 percent of pregnant women.[308]

The factors responsible for this volume expansion are incompletely understood. Enhanced secretion of aldosterone and estrogens probably plays an important role by promoting tubular sodium reabsorption.[308,309] These humoral changes are, however, partially antagonized by an elevation in GFR and by increased production of prostaglandins and progesterone, both of which tend to augment sodium and water excretion.[308,309]

Despite the multiple influences on renal sodium handling, the degree of sodium retention is independent of alterations in sodium intake, suggesting that *sodium balance is being strictly regulated.*[308] It is possible that sodium retention reflects an *appropriate response* to systemic vasodilatation and relative hypotension.* The systemic blood pressure falls early

---

*Several other observations also suggest a hypovolemia-induced resetting of volume regulation in normal pregnancy. For example, the plasma sodium concentration falls by about 5 meq/L and remains at that level despite variations in fluid intake. This response is presumably mediated by a volume depletion-induced lowering of the osmotic threshold for the release of antidiuretic hormone.[310] Similarly, preliminary studies suggest that atrial natriuretic peptide levels are normal, not elevated as might be expected if plasma volume expansion reflected true hypervolemia.[311]

in pregnancy and, during the second trimester, is often 10 mmHg below baseline, declining to a mean of 105/60.[309] This reduction in blood pressure is induced by a marked decline in peripheral vascular resistance, due both to the uterine vasculature acting as a "low-resistance" shunt and to impaired vascular responsiveness to the pressor action of angiotensin II,[312,313] norepinephrine,[314,315] and possibly vasopressin.[315] Increased production of vasodilator prostaglandins by the uterus (a response that helps to maintain uterine perfusion)[316] and by arterial endothelium appears to play an important role in the resistance to vasopressors.[317,318] These changes become attenuated near term, as both vascular resistance and systemic blood pressure rise toward normal.[309]

A dramatic rise in plasma renin activity accompanies the reduction in peripheral vascular resistance. This response is due to an estrogen-mediated increase in hepatic production of renin substrate[319] and to enhanced *renal and uterine* secretion of renin.[320,321] The net effect is a three- to fivefold elevation in the plasma concentration of angiotensin II. The rise in renal renin production probably represents (at least in part) an appropriate attempt to maintain the systemic and renal perfusion pressure, since the administration of an angiotensin II inhibitor results in a further decline in the already reduced blood pressure.[322] In comparison, uterine renin (at least as studied in pregnant rabbits) may have a predominantly local effect as the generation of angiotensin II acts to enhance uterine perfusion by promoting uterine prostaglandin synthesis.[323]

Renal function also changes during pregnancy as the elevation in cardiac output leads to a rise in both renal plasma flow and GFR. The increase in GFR is apparent within 1 month of conception and reaches a peak approximately 40 to 50 percent above nonpregnant levels by the end of the first trimester (Fig. 7–13).[324,325] This glomerular hyperfiltration lowers the P_{cr} to about 0.4 to

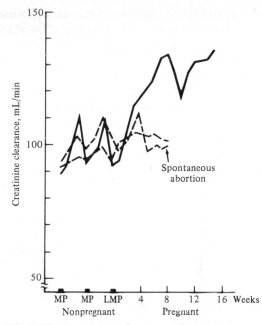

FIG. 7–13. Creatinine clearance data on nine women, measured before pregnancy and through the end of the first trimester. The solid line represents the mean GFR, and the broken lines represent two women who aborted spontaneously during the first trimester. MP = menstrual period; LMP = last menstrual period. (*From J. M. Davidson and M. C. B. Noble, Br. J. Obstet. Gynaecol., 88:10, 1980, and M. D. Lindheimer and A. Katz, in B. M. Brenner and F. C. Rector (eds.), The Kidney, 3d ed., Saunders, Philadelphia, 1986.*)

0.5 mg/dL.[309] As a result, a relatively "normal" P_{cr} of 0.7 to 0.8 mg/dL in pregnancy may be indicative of some impairment in renal function. The GFR normally decreases by about 20 percent during the last month of pregnancy, but is still well above nonpregnant levels.[326,327] These changes in renal function return to pre-pregnancy values within 3 months after delivery.[326]

Acid-base and electrolyte changes also occur during normal pregnancy. The most common are (1) chronic respiratory alkalosis, resulting from direct stimulation of the medullary respiratory center by progesterone[328];

and (2) mild hyponatremia, due to resetting of the hypothalamic osmoreceptors.[310]

PREECLAMPSIA

Preeclampsia is usually characterized by the gradual onset of hypertension, proteinuria, and edema, beginning after 20 weeks of gestation. It is most common during the last trimester of a first pregnancy and develops in 5 to 10 percent of all pregnancies. This disorder may progress to a convulsive phase termed *eclampsia*.[329]

It is important to emphasize that none of these findings alone is diagnostic of preeclampsia. Edema, for example, is common in normal pregnancy, proteinuria can reflect preexistent renal disease, and hypertension can occur as a late transient event.[329]

PATHOLOGY

Renal involvement in preeclampsia is primarily limited to the glomeruli.[330-332] The major change on light microscopy is swelling of the endothelial and mesangial cells, resulting in narrowing or obliteration of the capillary lumens (Fig. 7–14a). This characteristic morphological alteration is called *glomerula endotheliosis*.[333] Glomerular cellularity is typically normal or only mildly increased.

Electron microscopy reveals occlusion of the capillary lumens by the swollen endothelial cells and deposition of granular or fibrillar material both within the endothelial cells and on the endothelial side of the basement membrane (Fig. 7–14b).

Immunofluorescence studies have been of major importance in this disorder, demonstrating that the intracellular and subendothelial deposits are composed at least in part of fibrin-like material (see Fig. 7–9c).[332] The absence of the characteristic fibrillar pattern of fibrin on electron microscopy has led to the suggestion that this material may represent incompletely polymerized fibrin. Immunoglobulins and complement usually are not found on immunofluorescent staining of the glomeruli or vessels, although focal, nonspecific deposition of IgM, IgG, and C3 occasionally may be seen.[333,334]

The renal lesion typically reverses soon after delivery, and the glomeruli revert to a normal appearance in 2 to 3 weeks.[335] In contrast, the renal abnormalities are frequently more severe in those patients with severe preeclampsia. In this setting, extensive platelet and fibrin thrombi may be found, occasionally resulting in renal cortical necrosis or delayed functional recovery.[336]

Similar pathologic changes may be seen in other organs. Fibrin deposition has been demonstrated both in the placental vessels[337] and outlining the hepatic sinusoids in preeclampsia.[338] In those patients who progress to eclampsia, fibrin thrombi with focal areas of necrosis and hemorrhage may be found in the brain, liver, and adrenal and pituitary glands.[336]

PATHOGENESIS

The pathogenesis of preeclampsia remains incompletely understood.[309,329] The placenta is thought to play a central role, since delivery results in rapid resolution of the disease. The nature of this relationship, however, is unclear. Four etiologic factors have been proposed, each of which may play a contributory role: uterine ischemia, decreased production of vasodilator prostaglandins, activation of the coagulation system, and immunologic factors (Fig. 7–15).

Uterine Ischemia. The possible role of uterine ischemia in the pathogenesis of preeclampsia has been suggested by the following experimental and clinical observations:

1. Chronically decreasing uterine blood flow (by partially clamping the uterine artery) in pregnant animals can induce renal le-

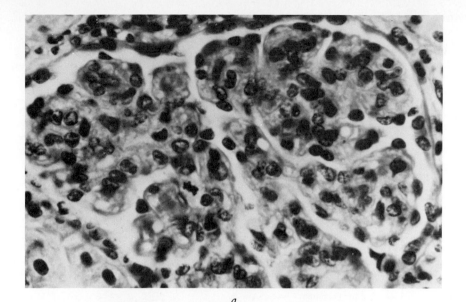

a

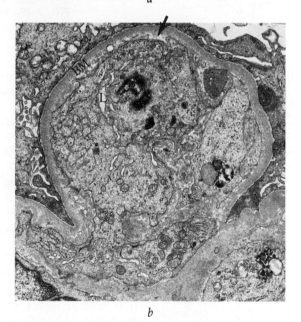

b

FIG. 7–14. Histologic changes in the glomeruli in preeclampsia. (*a*) Light microscopy reveals narrowing or obliteration of the capillary lumens due to swelling of endothelial and mesangial cells (*glomerular endotheliosis*). Glomerular cellularity is relatively normal. (*b*) Electron microscopy shows virtual obliteration of the capillary lumen (L) due to swelling of the endothelial cell. Widening of the subendothelial area of the glomerular basement membrane (BM) by both electron-lucent and electron-dense material also can be seen (arrow). The latter change is similar to that in HUS (see Fig. 7–9*c*).

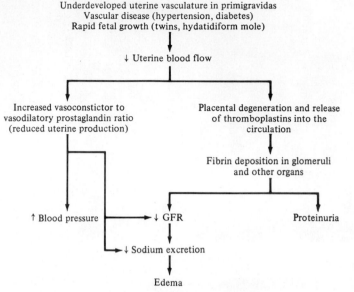

FIG. 7-15. Proposed model for the development of preeclampsia.

sions indistinguishable from those in preeclampsia.[339,340] This finding, however, has not been reproducible in all animal models.

2. Prospective studies have shown that the metabolic clearance rate of dehydroisoandrosterone sulfate, thought to be a possible measure of uteroplacental blood flow, is reduced in patients who subsequently develop preeclampsia, 3 to 4 weeks before the onset of clinically evident disease.[341,342] Furthermore, other markers of blood flow to the placenta have detected a 50 percent reduction in preeclamptic women compared to normal pregnant controls, with the degree of ischemia paralleling the severity of the disease.[343]

3. Preeclampsia occurs primarily in patients in whom decreased placental perfusion would be more likely to occur. Included in this group are patients with underlying vascular diseases such as hypertension or diabetes mellitus, patients with a hydatidiform mole or multiple births in whom the increased metabolic needs may exceed the placental blood supply, and primigravidas who may have a "less-developed" uterine

vasculature than multiparous women.*[344] This proposed imbalance between supply and demand may also explain why preeclampsia occurs in the third trimester (except in patients with hydatidiform mole), which is the time of rapid fetal growth.

Abnormal Prostaglandin Metabolism. Prostaglandin metabolism during normal and preeclamptic pregnancies appears to be different. In normal women, both uteroplacental and renal synthesis of the vasodilators prostaglandin E_2 (PGE_2) and prostacyclin are increased,[316,345,346] an effect that may be mediated in part by enhanced prolactin production.[347] If, however, prostaglandin synthesis is inhibited by indomethacin during normal pregnancy, there is a concomitant reduction in uterine blood flow, suggesting that at least

*The increased risk of preeclampsia in primigravidas may be related to factors other than a hypothetically immature vasculature. There is evidence, for example, that it is the first pregnancy with a given father, rather than the first pregnancy itself, that predisposes toward preeclampsia (see "Immunologic Factors," below).

one of the functions of increased uteroplacental prostaglandin production is the maintenance of local perfusion.[348] Thus, diminished PGE_2 or prostacyclin synthesis could promote the development of uterine ischemia and preeclampsia.[316,349-351] A reduction in vasodilator prostaglandin production also could explain the observation that, as early as the 24th week of pregnancy, patients who are destined to develop preeclampsia display a progressive increase in sensitivity to the pressor effect of infused angiotensin II (Fig. 7–16).[312,352]

Alternatively, a change in the *relative, rather than the absolute, production* of prostacyclin (a vasodilator and platelet deaggregator) and thromboxane B_2 (a vasoconstrictor and promoter of platelet aggregation) may be important in preeclampsia. Uteroplacental synthesis of these two compounds is relatively similar in normal pregnancy[316]; in comparison, there appears to be an increase in the production of thromboxane B_2 and a decrease in that of prostacyclin in preeclampsia.[316,353] The admin-

istration of a prostaglandin synthesis inhibitor in this setting can preferentially reduce thromboxane synthesis.[316] This finding may explain the apparent ability of low-dose aspirin (with or without dipyridamole) to prevent preeclampsia in high-risk pregnancies (see "Prevention," below).[354,355] This beneficial effect could result from an improvement in uterine blood flow and/or from diminished platelet aggregation.

These humoral abnormalities—high level of vasoconstrictors; low level of vasodilators—also may play an important role in the hypertension that accompanies preeclampsia. Although the plasma renin activity and angiotensin II concentration are somewhat lower than in normal pregnancy,[322] this may well be counteracted by the increase in vascular reactivity (Fig. 7–16).[309,312,313]

Activation of the Coagulation System. The fibrin deposition that occurs in the kidney and other organs in preeclampsia suggests an im-

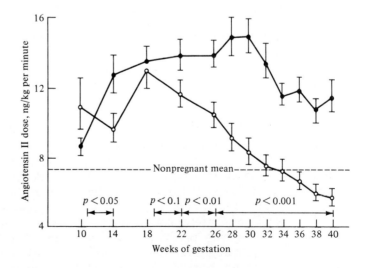

FIG. 7–16. Comparison of the mean angiotensin II dose (nanograms per kilogram per minute) required to raise the diastolic blood pressure 20 mmHg in 120 primigravidas who remained normotensive (filled circles) and 72 who ultimately developed preeclampsia (open circles). A higher dose is required in normotensive pregnancies than in nonpregnant females (broken line), suggesting resistance to the effect of angiotensin II. However, women who developed toxemia showed a progressive fall in angiotensin II resistance (which was significant after the 23rd week), eventually becoming more sensitive to angiotensin II than normal women. (*From N. F. Gant, G. I. Daley, S. Chand, P. J. Whalley, and P. C. MacDonald, J. Clin. Invest., 52:2682, 1973, by copyright permission of the American Society for Clinical Investigation.*)

portant role for the coagulation system.[332,337,338] This hypothesis is supported by the demonstration that lesions similar to those in preeclampsia can be produced in experimental animals by the infusion of thromboplastin.[356] Furthermore, the early findings of increased platelet and factor VIII consumption in women with preeclampsia[357-359] suggest that mild intravascular coagulation may be present. It is possible that the increase in thromboxane B_2 production could contribute to these changes, since this substance is a potent stimulator of platelet aggregation.[316]

Reduced fibrin removal also may promote thrombus formation in preeclampsia. The normal glomerulus contains a plasminogen activator which, by initiating fibrinolysis, plays an important role in the removal of fibrin.[360] However, glomerular plasminogen activity appears to be diminished in pregnancy,[361] a change that would tend to facilitate glomerular fibrin deposition.

Immunologic Factors. The immune system also may contribute to the uteroplacental abnormalities of preeclampsia. It has been observed, for example, that multiparous women who have a new baby with a different father have an increased risk of preeclampsia, similar to that in a true primigravida.[362] The mechanism by which this might occur is not known. One possibility that has been proposed is that the quantity of blocking antibodies, which "block" an immune response directed against paternal antigens in placental tissue, would be expected to be low during a first pregnancy with a given father. These "protective" antibodies should then increase with subsequent pregnancies, thereby decreasing the risk of preeclampsia (unless there is some underlying vascular disease).[362] Further support for an immune basis has come from the observation that placental deposition of complement components is greater in patients with preeclampsia, with the most prominent deposition seen in severe cases.[363] However, it is possible that this finding is the result, rather than the primary cause, of placental damage in this setting.

In summary, placental vascular insufficiency with a subsequent disruption of placental metabolism may be central to the development of preeclampsia. The initiating event that triggers this disorder (an abnormality of prostaglandin metabolism, of the coagulation system, or of the immune system) remains unknown.

CLINICAL PRESENTATION

Preeclampsia usually develops in primigravidas or in women with preexistent vascular disease (most often due to hypertension, diabetes mellitus, or primary renal disease). The physical examination is characterized by the gradual onset of high blood pressure (which may be labile), beginning after the 20th week of pregnancy and most commonly in the third trimester. However, a significantly higher baseline blood pressure (that is still within the normal range) may be observed from as early as 9 to 12 weeks of gestation in women who subsequently become preeclamptic.[364]

The severity of the hypertension often increases with the duration of the disease. Initially, the blood pressure may be 140/90 or less. If, however, the delivery of the fetus is delayed, the blood pressure may eventually exceed 180/120. These more severely affected women also may have headaches, abdominal pain, visual disturbances, hyperactive deep tendon reflexes, hemolysis (with a microangiopathic blood smear), elevated plasma levels of hepatic enzymes (transaminases and lactate dehydrogenase), and a low platelet count (the last three findings have been called the HELLP syndrome).[365] Seizures are considered to be indicative of eclampsia.

Peripheral edema occurs in most patients with preeclampsia (but is also often part of normal pregnancy). The edema is frequently generalized, with the most prominent involvement occurring in the face and hands. It appears to result from the combination of a mild reduction in GFR and the presence of intact tubular function, thereby allowing enhanced sodium reabsorption. (A similar sequence occurs in acute glomerulonephritis.)[366] Prostaglandin deficiency in preeclampsia may also be important, since prostaglandins can decrease renal tubular sodium reabsorption.[367]

In the early phase of preeclampsia, urinary protein excretion may remain within the normal range (at which time only pregnancy-induced hypertension can be diagnosed). However, proteinuria gradually increases with time and can reach nephrotic levels (>3.5 g/day) if delivery is delayed.[320,330] The urine sediment is typically benign, containing only a few red and white cells,[330] and renal function is usually well maintained with only minor elevations in the P_{cr} (0.2 to 0.3 mg/dL) occurring in most patients.[330] An exception may be seen in severe preeclampsia, in which disseminated intravascular coagulation, renal cortical necrosis, and renal failure may occur.[336]

The plasma uric acid concentration is elevated in almost all patients with preeclampsia, due to diminished uric acid excretion.[330,368] The enhanced sodium reabsorption in preeclampsia may be responsible for this effect, since tubular urate reabsorption varies with that of sodium.[369] As a result, the plasma uric acid concentration, which is usually under 4.5 mg/dL in normal pregnancy, is generally greater than 5.5 mg/dL in mild preeclampsia and may exceed 7.5 mg/dL in more severe cases.[330]

A common hematologic abnormality in preeclampsia is mild thrombocytopenia, which is thought to reflect platelet consumption as the coagulation system is activated (see "Pathogenesis," above).[358,370] This change may be detected as early as the 28th week, indicating that coagulation abnormalities begin well before the onset of clinical symptoms.[359] However, the other hematologic findings of disseminated intravascular coagulation—prolonged prothrombin time, hypofibrinogenemia, reduced factor VIII level, and increased fibrin degradation products—usually are not found[370,371] unless there is severe preeclampsia or eclampsia.[372,373]

DIAGNOSIS

The clinical diagnosis of preeclampsia is based on the development of hypertension and proteinuria.[329,330] Edema is also common but is hard to distinguish from the fluid retention that is seen in normal pregnancy. These problems usually begin in the third trimester; an earlier onset suggests an underlying disorder such as essential hypertension, diabetes mellitus, kidney disease, or the presence of a hydatidiform mole.[320]

The diagnosis is not always easy to establish, however, since proteinuria and edema may be either absent[330] or due to some underlying renal disease. In one large series, for example, the clinical diagnosis of preeclampsia could be confirmed histologically on renal biopsy in 85 percent of primiparas, but in only 38 percent of multiparas, most of whom had either benign nephrosclerosis or underlying primary renal disease.[374] These findings support the notion that preeclampsia in the absence of a predisposing disease is primarily a disorder of first pregnancies.[309]

The new onset of hypertension during pregnancy is most commonly due to preeclampsia, but may also be caused by preexistent renal disease or an underlying tendency to essential hypertension. Consequently, there are three issues that need to be addressed in the evaluation and appropriate management of preeclampsia: early diagnosis, distinguishing preeclampsia or pregnancy-induced hypertension from essential hypertension, and distinguishing preeclampsia from other causes of renal disease.

Early Diagnosis of Preeclampsia. The optimal initial step in the diagnosis of preeclampsia is to identify early in pregnancy those patients who are at greatest risk. One such group is patients with underlying vascular disease. This probably explains the higher frequency of preeclampsia (or pregnancy-induced hypertension) in patients with diabetes mellitus or chronic hypertension.

In addition to identifying patients with preexistent vascular disease, several tests have been described that attempt to detect patients likely to develop preeclampsia. Perhaps the most predictive has been the measurement of hemodynamic sensitivity to an infusion of angiotensin II (Fig. 7–16). Patients prone to develop preeclampsia demonstrate increased responsiveness as early as the 24th week of pregnancy. In one large study, 26 of 58 patients with a positive test subsequently developed preeclampsia or pregnancy-induced hypertension, in comparison to only 8 of 173 patients with a negative test.[375]

Blood pressure measurements in the second trimester may also be useful in determining which women are more likely to develop preeclampsia. An apparently normal mid-trimester blood pressure above 125/80 (mean arterial pressure > 90 to 95 mmHg) is associated with an increased risk of later preeclampsia.[376]

A third predictive test is the "roll-over" test, which assesses the blood pressure response to changes in position. This procedure is performed at 28 weeks by measuring the blood pressure every 5 min until stable in the left lateral recumbent and then the supine position.[377,378] An increase in diastolic pressure, when supine, of greater than 20 mmHg is considered to be a positive test (even in patients with a normally low resting pressure) and is associated with a 75 to 80 percent incidence of preeclampsia or pregnancy-induced hypertension. This is in contrast to a less than 10 percent incidence in patients with a smaller rise in blood pressure. The exaggerated response to changes in posture may reflect increased sensitivity to or increased activity of vasoconstrictive factors, since positive responders also demonstrate an enhanced blood pressure response to infused angiotensin II (Fig. 7–16).[377] The roll-

over test has the advantage of being easier to perform than serial angiotensin II infusions.

Until the present time, early identification* of patients at risk has not been widely pursued, in part due to the absence of any definitive therapy other than close monitoring and the institution of bed rest if progressive hypertension occurs. However, the recent suggestion that low-dose aspirin may be beneficial in high-risk patients[354,355] may, if shown to be true, make these predictive tests more valuable (see "Prevention," below).

Pregnancy-Induced Hypertension. The development of hypertension during pregnancy is not always indicative of preeclampsia.[329] Hypertension is considered to be present when the blood pressure exceeds 140/90 mmHg or there is an increase in systolic pressure of 30 mmHg or in diastolic pressure of 15 mmHg over baseline values.[378] This elevation in blood pressure may reflect preeclampsia, an underlying hypertensive tendency, or late or transient hypertension (which resolves after delivery).[329,383]

Differentiating between preeclampsia and underlying essential hypertension is important from a therapeutic and prognostic viewpoint (see "Prognosis," below). Unless there is a documented past history of hypertension, however, this distinction may be difficult because the systemic blood pressure commonly falls in the second trimester, occasionally reaching the normal range in patients with previously elevated levels. Consequently, the presence of a diastolic blood pressure below 90 mmHg during early pregnancy does

---

*Several other laboratory abnormalities have been used experimentally to detect patients likely to develop preeclampsia including: a reduced metabolic clearance of dehydroisoandrosterone, thought to be a reflection of uterine ischemia or dysfunction[341]; an increased fibronectin concentration, thought to be a marker of endothelial damage[379,380]; and an altered plasma phospholipid ratio.[381,382] These tests are limited, however, since their sensitivities and specificities are uncertain, and since they are not routinely available.

not exclude the presence of underlying hypertension.[335] In contrast, *the appearance of proven, de novo, third trimester hypertension in a primipara is sufficient reason to proceed with therapy (see "Treatment," below) as though the patient has preeclampsia.*[329]

The patient's age, gravid status, degree of proteinuria, and plasma uric acid concentration can also be used to attempt to distinguish preeclampsia from essential hypertension (Table 7-10). For example, the plasma uric acid concentration generally increases in preeclampsia but is unaffected by essential hypertension. However, hyperuricemia typically is a relatively late finding in preeclampsia, occurring at a time when more specific manifestations are also present. In isolation, therefore, the plasma uric acid concentration is of little use in making a definitive diagnosis of preeclampsia or in predicting who will subsequently develop this disorder.[384] The hematologic abnormalities of preeclampsia (thrombocytopenia, hemolysis, disseminated intravascular coagulation) also tend to be late findings[365] and are not helpful for early diagnosis.

Transient hypertension of pregnancy is characterized by hypertension, usually developing in the last trimester, but without other signs and symptoms of preeclampsia (such as proteinuria) or a history of chronic hypertension. The prognosis in terms of fetal and maternal outcome is good, although some of these women will develop essential hypertension later in life.[329] The probability of developing chronic hypertension in this setting is greater in those patients who are still hypertensive by the tenth postpartum day.[385]

Distinguishing Underlying Renal Disease from Preeclampsia. The major causes of renal disease developing during pregnancy are listed in Table 7-11.[386,387] Preeclampsia is the most common disorder occurring in the last half of pregnancy and is characterized by proteinuria and by relatively normal renal function. In contrast, postpartum hemolytic-uremic syndrome (see p. 334), acute tubular necrosis (see Chap. 3), and renal cortical necrosis (see "Renal Cortical Necrosis," below), are associated with acute renal failure, but little or no proteinuria.

The distinction between severe preeclampsia (which can cause acute renal failure due to the formation of intravascular thrombi)[336] and the postpartum hemolytic-uremic syndrome may be somewhat more difficult. The former usually occurs in patients with preceding evidence of mild preeclampsia, who also have neurologic dysfunction (including seizures) and the laboratory findings of disseminated intravascular coagulation. In comparison, the hemolytic-uremic syndrome typically occurs in patients who have had an uncomplicated pregnancy and who have thrombocytopenia, but usually a normal pro-

TABLE 7-10. Characteristics of Hypertension due to Preeclampsia and Underlying Essential Hypertension

Finding	Preeclampsia	Essential Hypertension
Age	Frequently less than 20	Often greater than 30
Gravida	Primarily primigravida	Primigravida or multigravida
Hypertension before pregnancy	No	May be present
Proteinuria	Present	Absent or trace
Plasma uric acid concentration	>5.5 mg/dL	<5.5 mg/dL
Blood pressure after delivery	Normal by 6 to 12 weeks	Hypertension may persist
Future development of hypertension	Similar to control population	Common

TABLE 7-11. Major Causes of Renal Disease in Pregnancy

First half
 Acute tubular necrosis resulting from septic abortion
 Prerenal disease due to hyperemesis gravidarum
Second half
 Preeclampsia
 Renal cortical necrosis or acute tubular necrosis due to abruptio placentae or placenta previa
 Postpartum hemolytic-uremic syndrome
 Urinary tract obstruction

thrombin time, partial thromboplastin time, and plasma fibrinogen concentration.[187,234] This differentiation is important for therapeutic and prognostic reasons: severe preeclampsia tends to resolve spontaneously within 1 to 2 weeks of delivery, whereas spontaneous recovery is unusual in the hemolytic-uremic syndrome and plasma exchange may be tried (see "Adult Hemolytic-Uremic Syndrome," above).

It may also be difficult to diagnose urinary tract obstruction during pregnancy. Renal ultrasonography usually reveals some degree of dilatation of the renal collecting system and ureters in normal pregnancy, resulting from smooth muscle relaxation (caused in part by prostaglandins) as well as from pressure by the enlarged uterus.[388] Consequently, hydronephrosis on ultrasonography is not necessarily diagnostic of obstruction; this may make it difficult to diagnose the rare case in which the pregnant uterus occludes both ureters, causing acute renal failure.[388,389] This possibility can be confirmed in some patients by the resolution of renal insufficiency when the patient is in the lateral recumbent position.[389]

In summary, the diagnosis of preeclampsia is frequently difficult to establish. A classic case would be a primagravida under the age of 25, who has a negative history of hypertension and renal disease, and who develops slowly increasing hypertension and proteinuria during the third trimester.[390] Such a pa-

tient would also be likely to have had increased sensitivity to angiotensin II (Fig. 7-16) or a positive roll-over test[377,378] if studied at the end of the second trimester.

TREATMENT

Untreated preeclampsia is associated with an increased incidence of stillbirths, neonatal deaths, and, in patients who progress to severe preeclampsia or eclampsia, maternal mortality due primarily to intracerebral hemorrhage.[330] The definitive therapy consists of delivery of the fetus and placenta, which results in rapid and usually complete resolution of the clinical abnormalities, even in severely affected patients.[330,372] Magnesium sulfate may be required in some patients for control of marked neuromuscular irritability or frank seizures.[329]

The only reason to delay delivery is evidence of fetal immaturity (and subsequently a high risk of respiratory distress syndrome).[391,392] In this setting, several options are available, depending upon the severity of the disease:

1. Bed rest, preferably in the lateral recumbent position, can be used if maternal involvement is relatively mild and the fetus is not near term. Antihypertensive agents are not usually added unless the diastolic blood pressure is above 100 to 105 mmHg.[329]
2. Delivery is indicated, regardless of the status of the fetus, if there are signs of severe disease that pose direct risk to the mother. These include uncontrollable hypertension, symptoms such as headache, visual disturbances, or seizures, and the presence of the HELLP syndrome or disseminated intravascular coagulation.[309,365] It has been suggested that the prophylactic administration of glucocorticoids (12 mg of dexamethasone intramuscularly on two consecutive days) may decrease the risk of respiratory distress syndrome and overall mortality in the infant if delivery is required before 34 weeks gestation.[393]

Hypertension during Pregnancy. The minimum level of *chronic hypertension* (due to underlying hypertension or renal disease) that will adversely affect the fetus is unknown.[394] Prospective studies have shown an increased fetal mortality when maternal diastolic blood pressure is persistently greater than 95 mmHg.[395,396] These findings, however, do not necessarily indicate that antihypertensive treatment will be beneficial. Some studies, for example, have observed an increased fetal and maternal morbidity only in those hypertensive patients who later developed preeclampsia.[397,398]

The conclusions from studies comparing the risks and benefits of antihypertensive treatment in pregnancy have been inconsistent.[394] These trials have been criticized since none is optimally designed. Furthermore, limited data suggest that an acute, marked reduction in maternal blood pressure decreases ureteroplacental perfusion, which can cause fetal compromise.[329] Thus, there are no data presently available that clearly indicate the minimum level of blood pressure elevation that should be treated in the pregnant woman.

A reasonable approach, therefore, should strongly consider the potential benefits as well as possible adverse effects of antihypertensive therapy on the mother and fetus. Most physicians choose to institute antihypertensive therapy for chronic hypertension if the diastolic blood pressure is above 90 to 95 mmHg in the first or second trimester or above 100 mmHg in the third trimester.[329,399,400]

Once a decision to treat the hypertensive pregnant woman has been made, there are three drugs that, when given orally, do not appear to have significant adverse effects on the mother or fetus: *methyldopa, β-adrenergic blockers, and hydralazine.* The major fetal side-effect of methyldopa is the development of minor and reversible neonatal tremors; in comparison, another centrally acting α_2-recep-

tor agonist, clonidine, has been associated with an embryopathy in animals, and its use is contraindicated in pregnancy.[329] Several β-adrenergic blockers have been found to be as safe as methyldopa,[329,400] but neonatal bradycardia and hypoglycemia have been observed in selected cases. Hydralazine should probably be used as a second-line drug in pregnancy since, when given alone, it has limited efficacy and can cause reflex tachycardia (which can be prevented with methyldopa or a β-blocker).

Diuretic use in the management of hypertension in pregnancy is generally felt to be of more risk than benefit, since preeclamptic patients have a low plasma volume,[401,402] which, if reduced further, may aggravate placental ischemia.[403,404] Consequently, diuretics or marked sodium restriction should probably be avoided in the absence of left ventricular failure. In comparison, volume expansion has been suggested as a treatment for preeclampsia based on the low intravascular volume. Additional data are required before this type of therapy can be routinely recommended, since most studies have not convincingly shown benefit.[309]

More potent and more rapidly acting agents may be necessary in patients with severe blood pressure elevations (diastolic pressure > 110 mmHg), in patients with evidence of central nervous system involvement, or in patients refractory to or intolerant of methyldopa, β-blockade, and oral hydralazine. Parenteral hydralazine is the antihypertensive medication used most commonly in this setting. Patients who do not respond can be treated with a calcium channel blocker[405] or diazoxide. Intravenous diazoxide may cause uterine atony with arrest of labor and a rapid drop in blood pressure (which could jeopardize the fetus) if conventional doses are given. However, mini-infusions (beginning with a 30-mg bolus) appear to avoid these problems.[406] *Nitroprusside and converting enzyme inhibitors should not be used,* since the former has caused cyanide poisoning[397] and since both have caused fetal death in animals.[323,400,407] Converting enzyme inhibitors act by reducing the formation of angiotensin II which, in the pregnant uterus, promotes the production of vasodilator prostaglandins.[323] Interfering with this process leads to uterine ischemia, which could account for the marked fetal wastage.[323]

PREVENTION

The optimal medical care of preeclampsia would be to prevent its development. Preliminary reports suggest that antiplatelet agents (low-dose aspirin with or without dipyridamole) may *prevent* the development of preeclampsia in susceptible patients, presumably by inhibition of excess thromboxane synthesis and/or platelet aggregation.[354,355] In one study, for example, 46 primigravidas likely to develop preeclampsia (as detected by increased sensitivity to infused angiotensin II; see Fig. 7–16) were treated with low-dose aspirin (60 mg/day) or placebo.[355] Preeclampsia, eclampsia, or pregnancy-induced hypertension developed in 12 of 23 placebo-treated patients but in only 2 of 23 (both of whom had only mild hyptertension) treated with aspirin. However, further clinical trials are necessary before the place of aspirin in the prevention of preeclampsia is defined, since increased fetal mortality may occur in patients treated with higher doses of this drug.[408]

PROGNOSIS

The long-term prognosis of preeclampsia is variable. When toxemia occurs in primigravidas, there does not appear to be an increased risk of eventually developing either chronic hypertension or renal disease.[374,383,409,410] Recurrent hypertension and proteinuria in a second pregnancy are also unusual in women who have had preeclampsia during their first pregnancy, occurring in fewer than 4 percent of cases.[411] These data suggest that preeclampsia in primigravidas is primarily a self-limited disease.

In comparison, preeclampsia occurring in multigravidas is more likely to be associated with underlying renal disease or a tendency toward hypertension.[374] It is not surprising, therefore, that these women have a twofold increase in the incidence of late hypertension (when compared to the general population).[374,409,410]

Isolated hypertension (without proteinuria) during pregnancy generally has little effect on fetal outcome unless preeclampsia develops, there is significant end-organ damage (such as renal failure), or the hypertension is secondary to a pheochromocytoma. For reasons that are poorly understood, fetal and maternal mortality is high in pregnant women with this rare endocrine form of hypertension.[329,412] Women with transient hypertension of pregnancy should receive long-term blood pressure follow-up, since the risk of developing subsequent chronic hypertension may be increased.[329]

COURSE OF UNDERLYING KIDNEY DISEASE

There are two important questions that need to be addressed when women with underlying renal disease become pregnant:

1. What is the effect of pregnancy on the kidney disease?
2. What is the effect of kidney disease on the pregnancy?

When evaluating the effect of pregnancy on preexistent renal disease, it is important to distinguish between changes in clinical manifestations and possible changes in the rate of deterioration of renal function. In women with relatively normal baseline renal function ($P_{cr} < 1.5$ mg/dL), for example, proteinuria increases in about 50 percent and hypertension can develop or worsen in about 20 to 25 percent of cases.[413-416] Marked worsening of edema also may occur in women with underlying nephrotic syndrome. These findings, however, tend to resolve after delivery. Furthermore, there is usually no evidence of an accelerated deterioration of renal function as long as adequate blood pressure control has been maintained.[413,416]

The course may be somewhat different in patients with mild chronic renal insufficiency (P_{cr} between 1.5 and 2.9 mg/dL). The P_{cr} in this setting tends to decrease during the first half of pregnancy (as it does in women without renal disease), but often rises above baseline as the pregnancy progresses.[417] Several small studies have also suggested that about one-third of such women have an *irreversible* decline in GFR that is greater than would have been predicted from previous observation of the patient.[417,418]

This possible adverse effect of pregnancy on underlying renal disease may be related to the associated renal hyperperfusion. As described in Chap. 4, intraglomerular hypertension may be a common denominator in the progressive nature of many kidney diseases. Thus, the elevated intraglomerular hydrostatic pressure that drives the hyperfiltration of pregnancy could be responsible for exacerbating the preexistent disease. There is as yet no confirmatory evidence in support of this hypothesis. Repetitive pregnancy in normal rats does not lead to glomerular sclerosis, probably because the intraglomerular hypertension is not sustained.[419] It is possible, however, that the outcome would be different if superimposed on an already present rise in intraglomerular pressure that has been induced by previous loss of functioning nephrons.

The histopathologic type of kidney disease may also be important in predicting progression of renal insufficiency after pregnancy. Data in this area are limited, but it appears that accelerated progression is most likely in active lupus nephritis, membranoproliferative glomerulonephritis, and, possibly, focal glomerulosclerosis (see the individual disorders in Chap. 6).[415,420–422]

The effect of preexistent renal disease on the course of pregnancy is somewhat better established. The rate of live births and fetal survival are above 90 percent in women with normal renal function, with the latter possibly declining slightly with moderate renal insufficiency (P_{cr} between 1.5 and 2.9 mg/dL).[418,422] In comparison, women with more severe baseline renal dysfunction ($P_{cr} \geq 3.0$ mg/dL) frequently have amenorrhea or anovulatory menstrual cycles. In this setting, the likelihood of conception and then carrying the baby to term is very low.[418,422]

The outcome of pregnancy and its effect on renal function in patients with renal transplants has become an important area of interest as the number of premenopausal women who have received allografts has increased. The majority of these patients have been treated with prednisone and azathioprine.* Many have had successful pregnancies with normal fetal development and delivery, although the incidence of prematurity appears to be increased.[423] It may be difficult to determine whether preeclampsia or rejection is present when renal function changes in this setting.[424] Consequently, renal transplant biopsy should be considered during pregnancy in all patients in whom renal function deteriorates without an identified cause so that antirejection therapy can be started or the fetus can be delivered.

RENAL CORTICAL NECROSIS

Renal cortical necrosis (RCN) refers to a clinicopathologic entity that is characterized by acute, frequently anuric renal failure and varying degrees of necrosis (or infarction) of all the cortical components (tubules as well as glomeruli). This disorder most often occurs with abruptio placentae (or another complication of late pregnancy such as placenta previa), septic shock, or any cause of severe hypovolemia such as burns or acute hemor-

---

*The safety of cyclosporine in pregnancy is not known.

rhagic pancreatitis.[425-427] Cortical necrosis may also be found in other conditions such as systemic vasculitis, scleroderma, and the hemolytic-uremic syndromes. The necrosis in these disorders, however, is usually limited to the glomeruli and arterioles, although true RCN may occur.[428] In addition, medullary as well as cortical necrosis may result from occlusion of the renal vessels by thromboemboli or a dissecting aneurysm.

PATHOLOGY

The major pathologic change in RCN is necrosis of all elements in the renal cortex (Fig. 7–17).[426,429] The degree to which this occurs is variable. In the patchy forms, only focal areas of the cortex are affected, with the proximal tubules frequently more severely necrosed than the glomeruli and distal tubules. The vessels also may become necrotic, and scattered thrombi may be found in the interlobular arteries, arterioles, and glomeruli. Furthermore, proximal tubular necrosis may be observed in nonnecrotic areas, resulting in a histologic appearance similar to acute tubular necrosis.[429]

In more advanced cases, virtually the entire cortex may be destroyed with the arteries showing a greater degree of necrosis and thrombosis. However, even in this setting, renal tissue is usually preserved just under the capsule (these nephrons, however, are not functional since their inner cortical segments are necrotic), in the juxtamedullary region, and in the medulla.[427,429] The last two effects may be due to perfusion of the juxtamedullary and medullary areas by the arcuate arteries rather than the thrombosed interlobular arteries. Preservation of the juxtamedullary nephrons may be physiologically important since it may account for the partial recovery of renal function that occurs in some patients (see "Treatment and Prognosis," below). In contrast, sparing of the sub-

capsular cortex is not seen when RCN develops in the recently transplanted kidney. This finding is probably due to the destruction of capsular collateral vessels at the time of donor nephrectomy.[429]

In severe cases of RCN, areas of necrosis also may be found in organs other than the kidney including the adrenal gland, spleen, lung, pancreas, anterior pituitary gland, and gastrointestinal tract.[426]

PATHOGENESIS

The pathogenesis of renal cortical necrosis is incompletely understood, as both disseminated intravascular coagulation (DIC) and severe renal ischemia have been postulated to be important. The presence of fibrin thrombi, the histologic similarity to the generalized Shwartzman reaction, and, in many patients with abruptio placentae, laboratory evidence of DIC[427,430] suggest that activation of the coagulation system with subsequent intravascular fibrin deposition could be of primary importance in RCN. In patients with abruptio placentae, for example, the release of thromboplastins from the damaged placenta could initiate fibrin formation which then persists because fibrinolysis is impared in late pregnancy.[361] Of interest in this regard is the observation that the Shwartzman reaction can be more readily produced in pregnant animals than in nongravid controls.[431]

However, the relationship between RCN and DIC is uncertain. Most patients with RCN (other than those with an obstetrical complication) have neither extensive fibrin thrombus formation nor the laboratory findings of DIC.[429] Furthermore, RCN is an unusual occurrence in patients with established DIC.[429]

Alternatively, severe renal ischemia may be the primary event in RCN. The observation that all the disorders that can produce RCN also may be associated with postischemic acute tubular necrosis (ATN) (see Chap. 3)

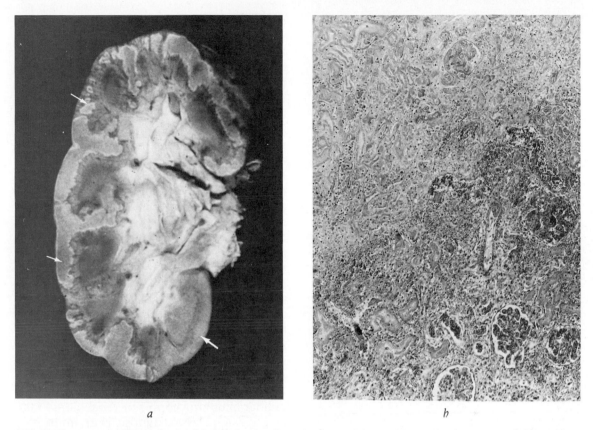

a   *b*

FIG. 7-17. Gross and histologic changes in renal cortical necrosis. (*a*) Gross specimen reveals extensive cortical necrosis (small arrows) and congestion of the medulla. The only normal area of cortex is at the lower pole (large arrow). (*b*) Histologic examination shows infarction involving all constituents of the outer cortex. Relatively normal cortical tissue can be seen in the lower part of the diagram.

suggests that ATN and RCN may represent different ends of a spectrum of renal damage induced by a marked reduction in renal perfusion. Also consistent with this hypothesis is the frequent presence of areas of proximal tubular necrosis in patients with patchy RCN.[429]

Furthermore, the following experiment indicates that the fibrin thrombi found in RCN could be the *result* rather than the cause of the renal ischemia. If the renal artery is clamped for 2 to 3 h, release of the clamp does not then result in the reestablishment

of flow through the kidney, presumably due to swelling or sloughing of the endothelial cells, leading to obliteration of the vascular lumen.[432] In this setting, the kidney initially becomes congested (as blood enters but cannot leave) with stasis of blood leading to the late formation of fibrin thrombi.

In summary, most of the evidence favors severe renal ischemia as the major pathogenetic event in the majority of patients who develop RCN. In addition, a hypercoagulable state induced by release of thromboplastins into the circulation can, in some patients, lead to intravascular fibrin deposition and a further reduction in renal perfusion.

CLINICAL PRESENTATION

RCN is characterized by the abrupt onset of oliguria or anuria, frequently accompanied by gross hematuria, flank pain, and hypotension.[425,426,433] These findings occur in any of the clinical settings described above, with abruptio placentae or another third-trimester complication such as placenta previa accounting for more than 50 percent of cases.[427]

The laboratory findings in RCN are nonspecific. The BUN and plasma creatinine concentration increase daily, reflecting the acute reduction in renal perfusion. In addition to hematuria and mild proteinuria, the urinalysis may reveal white cells, tubular epithelial cells, and granular casts. The hematologic abnormalities associated with DIC are usually absent, except in patients with an underlying obstetrical complication.

DIAGNOSIS

The differential diagnosis of RCN includes ATN, other causes of acute renal failure in late pregnancy (see Table 7–11), and other causes of anuria. Several clinical clues may suggest RCN rather than ATN. For example, flank pain, gross hematuria, and anuria are common in RCN, but are rare in ATN. Furthermore, renal function usually begins to improve within 7 to 21 days in ATN with virtually complete recovery eventually occurring in most patients. In contrast, prolonged anuria or oliguria is characteristic of RCN, with either no or only partial late improvement in renal function.[426]

The major causes of renal disease in late pregnancy (in addition to RCN and ATN) are preeclampsia and postpartum hemolytic-uremic syndrome (HUS) (see "The Kidney in Pregnancy," above). Although preeclampsia may precede the development of abruptio placentae and RCN, preeclampsia alone is not associated with the acute renal failure or the active urinary sediment characteristic of RCN. The diagnosis of postpartum HUS is suggested by the onset of acute renal failure, a microangiopathic hemolytic anemia, and thrombocytopenia 1 day to 8 weeks after delivery. In contrast to RCN, the pregnancy and delivery are usually uncomplicated in this disorder.

Although there are many causes of acute renal failure (see Chap. 3), only a few other than RCN are associated with *anuria*. These include shock, complete urinary tract obstruction (which can usually be excluded by ultrasonography), one of the hemolytic-uremic syndromes, and rarely, severe glomerulonephritis, vasculitis, or complete bilateral vascular occlusion. The typical settings in which RCN occurs usually allow it to be differentiated from these disorders. However, radiographic procedures or renal biopsy may be indicated if the diagnosis is in doubt.

Noninvasive studies, such as ultrasonography[434] or CT scanning[435] are generally the initial radiologic procedures of choice in this setting. Using these tests, the diagnosis of RCN can often be made rapidly and usually with little discomfort or risk to the patient. For example, most other causes of acute renal failure are associated with an increase in echogenicity of the renal cortex on ultrasonography. Thus, the characteristic finding of a hypoechoic zone adjacent to the renal capsule is highly suggestive of RCN. However, only patchy cortical ischemia is present in relatively mild cases, producing an echographic pattern similar to that seen in ATN.[426] Consequently, it may be necessary in some patients to perform a renal biopsy (although focal lesions may be missed) or preferably a renal arteriogram, which demonstrates an absent cortical nephrogram in severe cases.[426] Although the finding of renal parenchymal calcifications on a plain film of the abdomen also suggests the presence of RCN, calcium deposition occurs during the healing phase and cannot usually be visualized radiologically for 1 to 2 months.[427,436] Therefore, a plain film of the abdomen is not likely to be helpful during the acute phase of the illness.

TREATMENT AND PROGNOSIS

No specific therapy has been shown to affect the course of RCN. Thus, treatment must be aimed at reversing the underlying predisposing condition (such as delivery of the fetus and placenta in abruptio placentae) and at preventing the complications of renal failure with control of fluid and electrolyte intake and, if necessary, dialysis.

Prior to the availability of dialysis, the prognosis in RCN was extremely poor, with the mortality rate approaching 95 percent.[426] However, chronic dialysis has led to improved survival rates in this disorder. In addition, approximately 20 to 40 percent of patients will begin to show increases in urine output and renal function within 2 to 4 months, with the creatinine clearance eventually stabilizing between 15 and 50 mL/min.[426,427] This partial recovery, which is sufficient to allow dialysis to be discontinued, is presumed to occur at least in part in the juxtamedullary nephrons, which are usually spared from irreversible ischemic necrosis (see "Pathogenesis," above).[427,429] The recovery phase may, however, be followed by a gradual deterioration in renal function over a period of years, a change that may reflect hemodynamically mediated injury involving the surviving glomeruli (see Chap. 4).[426]

Either dialysis or renal transplantation can be used in those patients with end-stage renal disease. Transplantation has been successfully performed in a small number of patients.[426] Rapid loss of the graft has occurred in some cases,[437] with necrosis of the renal cortical parenchyma but little cellular infiltrate on pathologic examination. The pathogenesis of these changes is unclear, however, since cortical necrosis in the early posttransplant period may reflect hyperacute rejection or arterial or venous thrombosis of the allograft rather than recurrent RCN.[429] Consequently, the frequency of recurrence of RCN in the renal transplant is unknown; concern about this complication should not preclude transplantation in appropriate cases.

ARTERIAL THROMBOEMBOLIC DISEASES

Thrombus formation or embolization can involve either the arterial or venous circulation in the kidney. Depending upon the rapidity with which this occurs and the degree of vascular occlusion, one of three effects may be seen: ischemic infarction, ischemic atrophy, or, with some cases of renal vein thrombosis, no change in renal function. In the last setting, the main clinical concerns are the development of pulmonary emboli or extension of the thrombus into the inferior vena cava. Renal vein thrombosis most often occurs in patients with the nephrotic syndrome and is reviewed in Chap. 5.

Appropriate preventive and therapeutic measures can minimize both the incidence and the complications of renal thromboemboli. Therefore, it is important to be aware of the predisposing conditions and presenting signs associated with these relatively uncommon disorders. Since acute nonatheromatous occlusion of the renal arteries and atheroemboli tend to have somewhat different clinical characteristics, these disorders will be discussed separately.

ACUTE NONATHEROMATOUS OCCLUSION OF THE RENAL ARTERIES

The renal arteries may be occluded by emboli, by thrombi, or by a dissecting aortic aneurysm. Emboli from the left atrium, left ventricle, or ulcerated atheromatous lesions in the aorta are likely to involve the kidney, which normally receives approximately 20 percent of the cardiac output. The major nonatheromatous causes of renal *emboli* are blood clots originating in the heart in patients with atrial arrhythmias or mural thrombi, and vegetations in patients with bacterial endocarditis.[438-440] Less often, tumor or fat emboli may be found. In addition, intentional embolization by an injection of gelatin sponge material (Gelfoam) into the renal vessels supplying the tumor has been used in the management of renal malignancies.[441]

Renal artery *thrombosis* is usually superimposed upon an underlying atheromatous lesion or follows an episode of trauma in which an intimal tear promotes thrombus formation.[442] It may also be seen with renal artery aneurysms, following inflammation of the renal artery (e.g., vasculitis) and, rarely, as a spontaneous finding.[438,443]

PATHOLOGY AND PATHOGENESIS

The major pathologic change is infarction of the renal parenchyma, generally involving both the cortex and the medulla. The infarcts are typically wedge-shaped, radiating outward from the occluded vessel. On light microscopy, a central area of necrosis with hemorrhage and loss of cellular detail is seen. This is surrounded by a hyperemic rim with neutrophilic infiltration. With time, scarring occurs resulting in contraction of the necrotic areas and a decrease in renal mass.

The magnitude of these changes is dependent upon the size and number of vessels involved and the degree and duration of occlusion. If the main renal artery is totally occluded, virtually the entire kidney may become infarcted, although a thin rim of outer cortex is frequently spared due to collateral blood flow from capsular vessels.[444] Irreversible necrosis occurs if the renal artery is totally occluded for more than 2 to 3 h,[445] although collateral flow may preserve some renal tissue for a more prolonged period.[442] In comparison, a shorter duration of ischemia can cause acute tubular necrosis without permanent injury.[446]

If vascular occlusion is not complete, however, longer periods of renal ischemia can be tolerated without irreversible damage.[447] This is in part due to the fact that the major portion of renal oxygen consumption is utilized for active tubular reabsortion. Since the GFR ceases when the mean arterial pressure falls below 40 to 50 mmHg, there is no tubular reabsorption, and therefore the renal oxygen requirement falls dramatically.[448] In this setting, the small amount of persistent renal perfusion provides both oxygen and enough substrates to allow anaerobic metabolism to maintain renal viability.[448,449] Thus, ischemic atrophy rather than infarction may be seen, a pattern similar to that usually found with atheroemboli.

CLINICAL PRESENTATION AND DIAGNOSIS

The clinical manifestations of renal arterial occlusion are extremely varied. The typical presenting symptoms are nonspecific and include abdominal or flank pain, nausea, and vomiting.[438-440,444] However, some patients are asymptomatic, particularly if there is only a segmental infarct or incomplete vascular occlusion. In symptomatic patients, abdominal or flank tenderness and fever are usually found on physical examination. In addition, the history and physical examination may reveal evidence of an underlying predisposition to systemic embolization (such as atrial fibrillation, myocardial infarction, or bacterial endocarditis) or of extrarenal embolization (such as skin lesions or the acute onset of focal neurologic deficits).

The routine laboratory tests are nondiagnostic.[440,444] Leukocytosis is common, the plasma creatinine concentration (P_{cr}) may be elevated (particularly if both kidneys are involved), and the urinalysis usually reveals mild proteinuria and, in approximately one-third of patients, microscopic hematuria.[439,440,444] The lack of hematuria in many patients with this disorder is caused in part by a marked reduction of the blood supply to the infarcted area, resulting in loss of glomerular filtration and urine flow from the involved nephrons.

There is, however, one laboratory finding that, in the appropriate clinical setting, strongly suggests the presence of renal infarction: a markedly elevated plasma lactate dehydrogenase (LDH) level (usually greater than 5 times the upper limit of normal) with no or only minimal elevation in plasma transaminase levels.[440,450,451] The only other disorders that are commonly associated with a similar pattern are myocardial infarction (at 3 to 14 days), hemolysis (particularly with a megaloblastic anemia), and transplant rejection.[451,452] These conditions can be differentiated from one another on clinical grounds and, if necessary, by measuring the urinary excretion of LDH. The latter is normal in extrarenal disorders since the enzyme is too large to be filtered, but is elevated with renal infarction or transplant rejection since the excreted LDH is derived from the kidney.[450]

Once the diagnosis is suspected, radiologic studies can be used to confirm the diagnosis. The procedures of choice to demonstrate a segmental or generalized decrease in renal perfusion are a radioisotope renogram or a renal arteriogram[440] (Fig. 7–18). The former procedure has the advantage of being noninvasive and, if positive, may obviate the need for arteriography. An IVP is less sensitive; it typically demonstrates partial or complete nonvisualization of the affected kidney, but may appear normal with segmental lesions. The kidney size is initially unchanged, since scarring of the necrotic areas and a reduction in size does not occur for several weeks.[453] Calcification of the infarcted region is also a late finding.

COURSE AND TREATMENT

As described above, complete occlusion results in irreversible infarction unless blood flow is restored within 2 to 3 h. Collateral flow, however, may preserve enough renal tissue so that revascularization may be beneficial as late as 24 to 48 h after injury or even later with incomplete occlusion.[442] Treatment must also be aimed at preventing further embolization.

Surgical embolectomy can result in improved renal function in some patients.[439,454] However, surgery is associated with a higher mortality rate and with no apparent increase in the rate of functional recovery when compared to the use of anticoagulation therapy alone.[455] This is true even in patients with bilateral embolization and advanced renal failure, most of whom will regain a significant amount of renal function if treated medically with anticoagulants.[440] As a result, persistent dialysis is rarely necessary, even for patients requiring dialysis during the acute stage of the disease.[440] The efficacy of anticoagulation is due to a decrease both in the incidence of further embolization and in the degree of renal infarction since extension of the clot to complete occlusion may be prevented.

Standard anticoagulation therapy for renal emboli consists of intravenous heparin followed by oral warfarin. It may be proved desirable, however, to initiate therapy with a thrombolytic agent (such as streptokinase) in an attempt to lyse the occluding blood

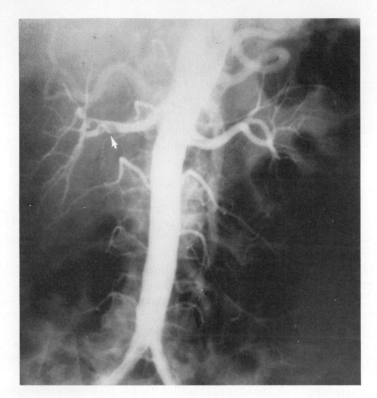

FIG. 7-18. Renal arteriogram in renal embolization demonstrates filling defects due to emboli in the right renal artery (arrow).

clot.[456-460] The risks of systemic bleeding and of possibly decreasing adherence of the intracardiac thrombus to the endocardium (a change that could promote further embolization) can be minimized by low-dose, local intraarterial infusion at the site of occlusion.

The likelihood of a successful result is related in part to the rapidity with which therapy is instituted. Unfortunately, recognition of the presence of renal infarction is often delayed. In one study of 17 patients with renal emboli, the diagnosis was most often made on the third to sixth day with only five patients being diagnosed on the first day.[440] It is important to be aware, therefore, that the triad of abdominal or flank pain, acute renal insufficiency, and a marked elevation in the plasma LDH level (without an equivalent change in the transaminases) strongly suggests the presence of renal in-farction, particularly in a patient with underlying cardiac disease.

Although generally not indicated as initial therapy, there may be a role for surgery in the treatment of this disorder. In patients with incomplete renal infarction (as evidenced by a continued urine output), embolectomy can lead to improved renal function even if performed as late as 6 weeks after the acute event, indicating that ischemic atrophy can still be reversed.[439,461] Therefore, surgery might be considered in stable patients with severe renal failure who have shown no improvement after 4 to 6 weeks of anticoagulation therapy.

Although surgery is not indicated for other causes of renal emboli (such as bacterial endocarditis in which appropriate antimicrobials are the treatment of choice), it may be effective in patients with renal artery thrombosis. In this setting, insertion of a bypass graft or thrombectomy should be considered if the patient has developed either severe hypertension or advanced renal failure, particularly if surgery can be performed within 24 h of injury.[442,462,463]

Although the renal prognosis is usually relatively good in patients with renal emboli, the early and late mortality rate remain high. This is due both to extrarenal embolization (particularly to the brain and intestine) and to the underlying disease (such as atherosclerotic heart disease or endocarditis).[139,440] In contrast, patients with traumatic renal artery thrombosis are frequently young and have a survival rate similar to the general population, unless uncorrectible hypertension or renal failure is present.

The late management of renal infarction involves treatment of hypertension. The elevation in blood pressure commonly develops in the first week after infarction but usually subsides after a period of 2 to 3 weeks.[464] Persistent hypertension, however, may occur and may be severe. It is usually mediated by the renin-angiotensin system and, therefore, responds to therapy with converting enzyme inhibitors and diuretics.

RENAL ATHEROEMBOLI

Atheroemboli to the kidneys and other organs occur in patients with advanced, erosive atheromatous disease. Although they may occur spontaneously, clinically important renal atheroemboli more often result from manipulation of the aorta during arteriography, angioplasty, or aortic aneurysm surgery.[465-468] In addition, spontaneous renal atheroemboli can be demonstrated on postmortem examination in up to 12 percent of patients over the age of 80.[469] These patients, however, tend to have a relatively small number of emboli, and the presence of renal insufficiency due to embolic disease is unusual.

PATHOLOGY

The pathognomonic pathologic change in this disorder is the demonstration of atheroemboli, usually in the medium-sized and small renal arteries (Fig. 7-19). The emboli consist of fragments of acellular or hyaline material with biconcave, parallel slits representing dissolved cholesterol crystals.[443,444,465,470] They can be identified only by viewing a frozen section under polarized light, since the crystals are dissolved by paraffin processing. With time, the atheroembolus appears to act as a foreign body resulting in intimal proliferation, macrophage infiltration, giant cell formation, and fibrosis, which may further narrow the vascular lumen.[443,444] Similar emboli are commonly found in other organs as well, particularly the pancreas, spleen, and lower extremities.[466,467,470]

In contrast to other forms of renal embolization, atheroemboli tend to lodge in the smaller vessels and most often cause incomplete vascular occlusion, probably because of their irregular shape and nondistensibility. As a result, ischemic atrophy (tubular atrophy with dilatation and interstitial fibrosis) rather than infarction is usually seen.[443,465,470] This difference is clinically important since the symptoms (abdominal or flank pain) and signs (high plasma LDH level) associated with renal infarction are typically absent in patients with atheroembolic disease.

CLINICAL PRESENTATION

Atheroembolism is primarily a disease of men over the age of 50, the group in which atheromatous disease is generally most prevalent. In patients who develop renal infarction, the signs and symptoms are similar to those described above for other causes of renal arterial occlusion. More often, however, ischemic atrophy occurs and no symptoms referable to the kidney are present. In this setting, the patient is usually found to have acute or subacute renal failure as an

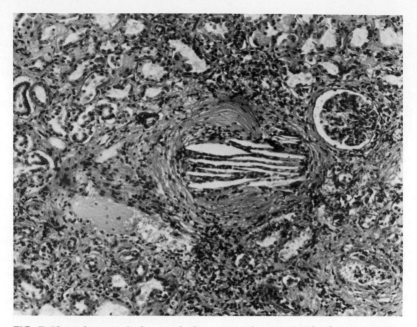

FIG. 7-19. Atheroembolus occluding a renal artery with characteristic slits representing dissolved cholesterol crystals.

incidental finding, frequently following abdominal aortic surgery or arteriography (such as a transfemoral carotid arteriogram for cerebrovascular disease). Symptoms, if present, are due to extrarenal emboli resulting in visual defects, acute pancreatitis, myalgias, or splenic infarction.[471]

The physical examination may reveal findings suggestive of systemic atheroembolism. These include bright orange plaques in the retinal arterioles,[472] subcutaneous nodules, livido reticularis,[473,474] or areas of mottling or gangrene in the toes despite palpable pedal pulses.[465,471] Furthermore, a variable increase in blood pressure may occur, presumably due to activation of the renin-angiotensin system by renal ischemia.[470,475]

The laboratory findings are nonspecific. The BUN and P_{cr} usually begin to rise on the first day following an arteriogram or aortic surgery. The urinalysis may be normal or may reveal mild proteinuria with few cells or casts.

In some patients, however, findings are present which suggest immunologic activation, probably in response to the exposed surface of the atheroembolus. These include hypocomplementemia,[476,477] peripheral eosinophilia,[476,478,479] and rarely, eosinophiluria.[479] Furthermore, the urine sediment may occasionally be more active with hematuria and cellular (including red cell) or granular casts.[480] As a result of these serologic and urinary findings, a systemic vasculitis, glomerulonephritis, or acute interstitial nephritis may be suspected.[479-482]

DIAGNOSIS

In the absence of symptoms or specific laboratory tests, the diagnosis of atheroemboli as the cause for acute renal failure is frequently difficult. The history and the course of the disease may provide suggestive clues. For example, atheroemboli should be considered in any patient developing renal failure after catheterization of the aorta or aortic aneurysm surgery. Although acute tubular necrosis (ATN) due to radiocontrast media or hypotension is much more common in this setting, ATN tends to follow a different course from atheroembolic disease (Fig. 7–20). With ATN, the P_{cr} rises progressively, and dialysis may be required until renal function begins to improve spontaneously, generally within 4 to 21 days. In comparison, atheroembolic disease is usually characterized by an *acute, self-limited, and irreversible* decline in renal function, since emboli typically lodge in the kidney at the time of or shortly after aortic manipulation but not on subsequent days. For example, atheroembolism is more likely than ATN if the P_{cr} increases from 1.2 to 5.0 mg/dL in the first 4 days after a transfemoral carotid arteriogram and then remains at approximately the same level indefinitely. It is important to remember, however, that occasional patients with biopsy-proven atheroembolic disease may show some improvement in renal function with time.[473,482]

The history and course of the disease are not helpful in all cases. An inciting event, for example, cannot be identified in patients with spontaneous atheroemboli. Furthermore, slowly progressive rather than acute, self-limited renal failure occurs in some patients.[444,465] This may be due to new emboli (particularly in patients with spontaneous atheroemboli) or to progressive narrowing of the vascular lumen by the fibrotic reaction that eventually ensues.[444,468,473] In these settings, the only clue to the diagnosis may be evidence of extrarenal embolization, particularly to the retina or toes.

In those patients in whom no clinical clues are present, the differential diagnosis includes other causes of acute renal failure with a benign urinalysis: prerenal disease, obstruction, and a variety of tubulointerstitial disorders (see Chap. 8). If appropriate diagnostic tests rule out prerenal disease and obstruction, biopsy of the kidney (or a subcutaneous nodule or skin lesion,[473] if present) may be required to establish the diagnosis. However, percutaneous biopsy may miss the affected vessels, since atheroembolism is a focal disease.

In some patients, widespread atheroembolization can result in a picture similar to

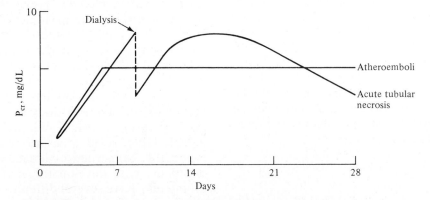

FIG. 7–20. Comparison of the typical courses of acute tubular necrosis and atheroembolic disease of the kidney. See text for details.

that in systemic vasculitis: abdominal pain, myalgias, and acute renal failure.[479-482] The frequent presence of eosinophilia, hypocomplementemia, and rarely hematuria with cellular casts may not allow these disorders to be distinguished without a biopsy of the kidney or other affected organ.

TREATMENT AND COURSE

No treatment is effective in atheroembolic disease, other than preventing further manipulation of the aorta by avoiding aortic catheterization. As described above, renal function tends to stabilize at a reduced level shortly after the inciting episode. In those patients who develop advanced renal insufficiency, dialysis may be required to prolong life. In some patients, a significant improvement in GFR may occur with time, but long-term survival is usually limited because of the presence of severe, generalized atherosclerotic vascular disease.

SICKLE CELL NEPHROPATHY

It is estimated that 8 percent of American blacks have sickle hemoglobin (sickle cell trait, hemoglobin SA), and that one in 625 has sickle cell disease (hemoglobin SS).[483] Renal involvement is common. The principal renal manifestation in sickle cell trait is recurrent hematuria, but a variety of other pathologic and functional alterations are typically present in sickle cell disease (Table 7–12). Thus, sickle cell disease should be considered in the differential diagnosis of black patients with such problems as hematuria and papillary necrosis.

PATHOLOGY

The medulla is the portion of the kidney most severely affected in sickle cell nephrop-

TABLE 7-12. Renal Manifestations of Sickle Cell Anemia

Hematuria

Renal infarction and papillary necrosis, which may predispose to urinary tract infection

Abnormal tubular function
  Reduced concentrating ability
  Reduced acid and potassium secretion
  Increased uric acid and creatinine secretion
  Increased phosphate reabsorption

Nephrotic syndrome which may progress to renal failure

athy. The primary changes are congestion and stasis of the vasa recta capillaries by sickled erythrocytes with focal areas of hemorrhage or necrosis, ultimately leading to interstitial inflammation, tubular atrophy, and fibrosis.[484,485] Microangiographic studies (Fig. 7–21) have demonstrated that the vasa recta are almost completely absent in older patients with hemoglobin SS. The remaining few vessels are spiraled and dilated, and end blindly.[486] Both hematuria and papillary necrosis are logical consequences of these vascular abnormalities as are disturbances in renal concentrating ability and acidification (see below).[487]

Glomerular lesions are also common in patients with sickle cell disease. Glomerular size, especially in the juxtamedullary population, is markedly increased early in the course of the disease, perhaps reflecting the substantial rise in GFR that frequently occurs (see "Pathogenesis," below).[488,489] Furthermore, the glomerular capillaries may be congested by sickled erythrocytes. With time, light microscopy reveals mild mesangial hypercellularity, focal areas of sclerosis, and eventually, glomerular hyalinization.[490]

Patients who develop the nephrotic syndrome may have several different patterns of glomerular disease, with focal glomerulosclerosis being most common.[490] In some patients, however, the light microscopic ap-

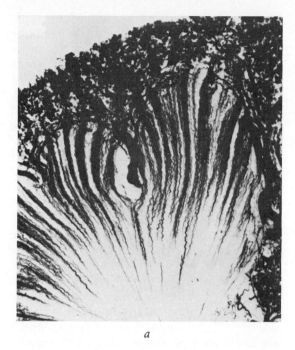

a

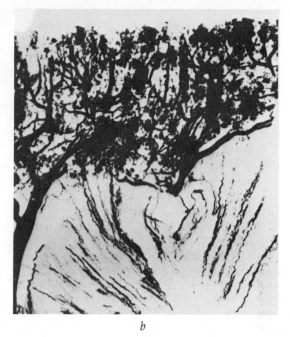

b

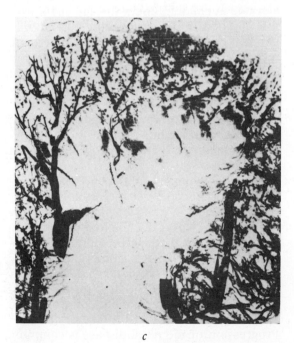

c

FIG. 7–21. Injection microangiographs of kidneys from an individual with no hemoglobinopathy (*a*), a patient with sickle cell trait (*b*), and a patient with sickle cell disease (*c*). The renal cortical surface is at the top of the figure, and the medullary pyramid is at the bottom. In the normal kidney, vasa recta are visible radiating into the renal papilla, and the cortical vasculature is dense and uniform. In sickle trait, the cortical vasculature is somewhat decreased, and the vasa recta are attenuated and distorted. In sickle cell disease, there is a considerable decrease in the cortical vasculature, and the vasa recta are virtually absent. [*From L. W. Statius van Eps and L. E. Earley, The Kidney in Sickle Cell Disease, in L. E. Earley and C. W. Gottschalk (eds.), Strauss and Welt's Diseases of the Kidney, 3d ed., Little, Brown, Boston, 1979.*]

pearance resembles that of membranoproliferative glomerulonephritis (see Fig. 6-16), in which lobulation with mesangial hypercellularity and thickening and splitting of the glomerular basement membrane (GBM) are prominent.[491,492] Immunofluorescence studies in these patients reveal granular deposition of IgG and C3 along the GBM, a finding similar to that in other immune complex disorders. Electron microscopy usually demonstrates increased mesangial cellularity and matrix, basement membrane thickening with interposition of mesangial cytoplasm into the capillary walls, and electron-dense deposits in the mesangium and along the subendothelial surface of the GBM.[488,491,492] Few, if any, glomerular changes are present in patients with sickle trait, and glomerular size is normal.[488]

PATHOGENESIS

The primary event in sickle cell nephropathy appears to be *sickling of erythrocytes in the medullary capillaries*. The result is sludging of blood in the inner medulla, causing ischemia. An important factor in the initiation of sickling is the combination of medullary hypoxia (due to countercurrent exchange of oxygen; see Fig. 3–11) and interstitial hypertonicity, which removes water from the erythrocyte, thereby concentrating the hemoglobin S. Increased acidity of the renal medullary blood may also enhance sickling.[493]

The net effect is increased viscosity and a reduction in flow in the vasa recta capillaries, the severity of which is proportional to the quantity of hemoglobin S that is present. Consequently, lesions are most marked in patients with homozygous sickle cell anemia (hemoglobin SS), but less severe with heterozygous sickle cell trait (hemoglobin AS) or a combined hemoglobinopathy (such as hemoglobin SC disease) (Fig. 7-21).[486]

The resultant medullary stasis and ische-

mia can lead to loss of function of the papillary (inner medullary) structures, resulting in tubular abnormalities similar to those observed in experimental animals in whom the papilla has been removed surgically. These include decreased concentrating ability,[486,494,495] impaired urinary acidification,[496] and reduced excretion of potassium[497] (see below).

The hematuria frequently found in patients with sickle cell disease may be due to one or both of two factors: engorgement and subsequent rupture of vessels proximal to the obstructed vasa recta;[485] and the development of papillary necrosis, which may be detectable by intravenous pyelography (see Fig. 8–2).[498]

In addition to the medullary changes, cortical abnormalities also may occur in sickle cell disease, particularly glomerulosclerosis.[488,490] These glomerular changes, which are not seen with sickle cell trait,[488] may be related to hyperperfusion of the kidney.[487] The GFR and renal blood flow are markedly elevated in children under the age of 10, with the GFR occasionally exceeding 200 mL/min per $1.73 \, m^2$ (Fig. 7–22).[499-501] This hyperemic response appears to be mediated at least in part by vasodilator prostaglandins, released in an attempt to counteract the medullary ischemia described above.[487] Anemia alone does not seem to play an important role in the renal vasodilatation, since the hemodynamic changes are not reversed by blood transfusions.

The GFR typically falls to normal by the end of the second decade, and is usually reduced below normal in patients over the age of 30.[499,502] This decline in renal function is associated with the development of glomerulosclerosis.[490] This glomerular scarring may reflect *hemodynamically mediated injury* that was initiated by the high intraglomerular pressure that presumably contributed to the early elevation in GFR (see Chap. 4).[503] Progression of the renal disease is common,

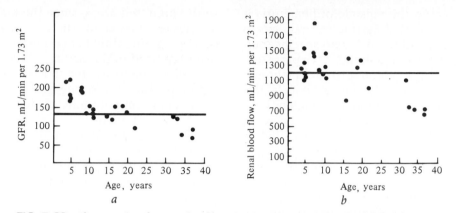

FIG. 7–22. Changes in glomerular filtration rate (*a*) and renal blood flow (*b*) with increasing age in patients with sickle cell disease. Both parameters are above normal in young children, decrease to normal between the ages of 10 to 20, and are ultimately reduced over the age of 30. The circles represent average values in individual patients; and the solid line is equal to the mean normal values in children and adults (corrected for body surface area). (*From J. N. Ettledorf, J. D. Smith, A. H. Tuttle, and L. W. Diggs, Am. J. Med., 18:243, 1955.*)

and renal failure is one of the major causes of death in adults with sickle cell disease.[504]

In selected patients, the nephrotic syndrome has also been caused by membranoproliferative glomerulonephritis[487,491,505] or, rarely, by membranous nephropathy, disorders which are associated with immune complex deposition.[487,506] IgG and IgM antibodies eluted from the glomerular basement membrane can, in at least some of these patients, bind to a renal tubular cell antigen.[507] It has been suggested that the development of glomerulonephritis in this setting may be related to initial ischemic tubular damage, leading to exposure or entry into the systemic circulation of these previously "unseen" antigens.[491,505,507]

CLINICAL PRESENTATION, DIAGNOSIS, AND TREATMENT

The clinical manifestations of sickle cell nephropathy are variable, ranging from subclinical disturbances in water or potassium excretion to gross hematuria or the nephrotic syndrome (Table 7–12). The diagnosis of any of these abnormalities is based upon confirming the presence of hemoglobin S by appropriate studies such as hemoglobin electrophoresis.

HEMATURIA

Painless gross hematuria is one of the most common renal complaints in patients with sickle cell *trait*.[508] Furthermore, it is a major cause of urinary bleeding in blacks, accounting for as many as one-third of cases.[509] It is unclear why hematuria is more common in sickle trait than in sickle cell disease, but it may be related to the much greater prevalence of the former disorder.[493]

Hematuria can occur spontaneously or follow mild trauma, is frequently recurrent,[509] may be microscopic or macroscopic, and is usually unilateral.[484,510] Although it had been suggested that hematuria more commonly arose from the left kidney,[511] this has not been confirmed in later studies.[512,513]

In most cases, the episode of hematuria is mild and self-limited, lasting several days to several weeks and requiring no specific therapy. However, some patients have persistent gross hematuria which produces enough blood loss to lower the hematocrit. In this setting a variety of therapeutic regimens have been tried, each of which aims to decrease vascular engorgement by reducing medullary sickling. For example, diminishing medullary interstitial osmolality can decrease the intracellular hemoglobin S concentration and therefore sickling by preventing osmotic water loss from the erythrocyte.[514] This can be achieved by the combination of a high fluid intake and low doses of a loop diuretic, which act by diminishing the release of antidiuretic hormone and by reducing sodium chloride reabsorption in the loop of Henle, respectively. The administration of sodium bicarbonate, which may retard sickling by its ability to alkalinize hemoglobin S, and correction of the anemia with blood transfusions, thereby reducing the concentration of hemoglobin S, may also be useful.[514]

Diminishing fibrinolysis with ε-aminocaproic acid has also been used.[515] However, the efficacy of this agent has not been proved, and its use can lead to increased clot formation in the renal pelvis. In rare cases of severe hemorrhage, unilateral nephrectomy has been performed.[511] Although it will control bleeding, hematuria may recur in the remaining kidney. The latter two forms of therapy, therefore, should be reserved for the rare patient with severe bleeding refractory to other forms of management.

RENAL INFARCTION AND PAPILLARY NECROSIS

Renal infarcts can occur in patients with either sickle cell disease[516] or sickle cell trait.[517] Despite the local vascular occlusion, however, blood may continue to be supplied to the infarcted areas, since the major renal arteries remain patent. This may be the cause of large, perinephric hematomas which have been reported in this setting.[518,519]

Papillary necrosis, due to vasa recta sludging or thrombosis, is one of the most common renal complications of sickle cell anemia.[520] Most patients are asymptomatic, and the GFR is usually unaffected. However, scar formation may predispose to urinary tract infections,[521] and radiographic findings on pyelography may show central cavities in the papillae.

REDUCED CONCENTRATING ABILITY

Diminished concentrating ability is an early and universal finding in sickle cell disease.[486,494,495] Sickling in the vasa recta capillaries presumably interferes with countercurrent exchange, causing inefficient trapping of solute in the inner medulla.[487] As a result, the maximum urine osmolality that can be achieved by 10-year-old children is only 400 to 450 mosmol/kg (the normal maximum urinary osmolality is 900 to 1400 mosmol/kg).[494,522-525] This concentrating defect is reversible after multiple blood transfusions in homozygous patients less than 10 to 15 years old, but is irreversible in patients who are older.[495,522] These findings suggest that sickling in the vasa recta produces at first a functional, reversible alteration in the countercurrent mechanism that ultimately cannot be corrected because of the development of pathologic changes in the inner medulla such as microinfarcts, tubular atrophy, and interstitial fibrosis. These changes are less severe and occur later in patients with sickle cell trait or hemoglobin SC disease.[525]

In most patients, intermittent nocturia is the major symptom, since maximum concentrating ability is most important overnight when there is little or no fluid intake. Water balance is generally maintained as long as fluid intake is adequate. However, negative fluid balance may occur if intake is reduced or extrarenal losses are enhanced.

REDUCED RENAL HYDROGEN AND POTASSIUM EXCRETION

An *incomplete* form of distal renal tubular acidosis may be seen in patients with sickle cell anemia. This is characterized by an inability to lower the urine pH below 5.3 even though the net urinary acid excretion, the plasma bicarbonate concentration, and the arterial pH remain normal.[496,526,527] Urinary acidification remains intact in patients with sickle trait.[527,528]

Potassium excretion also may be impaired in sickle cell disease, occasionally causing hyperkalemia.[497,529] This is probably a result of ischemic injury to the distal nephron (the site of potassium secretion) since the plasma aldosterone concentration is generally normal.[497] Potassium handling is unimpaired in patients with sickle trait.[530]

ABNORMAL PROXIMAL TUBULAR FUNCTION

As discussed above, sickle cell nephropathy is associated with disturbances in function related to impaired medullary transport. Proximal tubular function (both secretion and reabsorption), however, is supernormal.[487] The mechanism by which this occurs is not known. It is possible, for example, that enhanced proximal function is required because of the high GFR and the need to compensate for sodium wasting in the more distal medullary segments (Fig. 7-23).

The increase in proximal tubular function

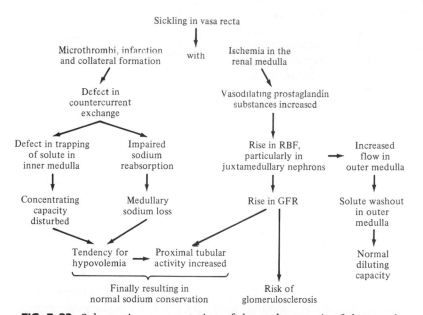

FIG. 7-23. Schematic representation of the pathogenesis of the renal abnormalities in sickle cell anemia. (*From P. E. de Jong and L. W. Statius van Eps: Kidney Int., 27:711, 1985. Reprinted by permission from Kidney International.*)

is not limited to the reabsorption of sodium, as uric acid, creatinine, and phosphate handling are also affected. Increased uric acid secretion helps maintain normal plasma uric acid levels in sickle cell anemia, even though uric acid turnover is increased (as a result of red cell breakdown).[531,532] Creatinine secretion is also increased by 20 to 25 percent above normal.[487] Thus, the creatinine clearance can significantly overestimate the GFR (see p. 4). By comparison, the plasma phosphorus levels may be higher than normal because there is enhanced proximal phosphate reabsorption in this setting.[533,534]

NEPHROTIC SYNDROME

Heavy proteinuria, which may be associated with progressive renal failure, is an unusual complication of sickle cell anemia that does not occur with sickle cell trait or hemoglobin SC disease.[491,492,535] As described above, the most common glomerular lesion is focal glomerulosclerosis,[490] probably induced by the initially high glomerular flow rates and intraglomerular hypertension. Membranoproliferative glomerulonephritis without hypocomplementemia[491] and membranous nephropathy have also been described.[487,506] Patients with these disorders tend to present with edema, proteinuria, and frequently hypertension with renal insufficiency. (In comparison, the prevalence of hypertension in patients with sickle cell disease and normal renal function appears to be lower than in the general population, possibly reflecting higher vasodilator prostaglandin production or a tendency to sodium wasting.)[536-538]

No therapy has been shown to alter the course of these glomerular diseases. Thus, treatment is largely supportive, aiming to minimize hemodynamically mediated injury with blood pressure control (preferentially with a converting enzyme inhibitor if there are no contraindications such as hyperkalemia) and dietary protein restriction (see

Chap. 4). Chronic dialysis has been effective in patients who progress to end-stage renal failure.[539]

RADIATION NEPHRITIS

As with other organs, the kidneys are sensitive to radiation damage, particularly when exposed to a cumulative dose of more than 2300 rads.[540] Radiation nephritis, which was a relatively common disorder in the past,[541,542] is almost never seen today. The disappearance of this form of renal disease has followed improved techniques for localized radiation therapy, a reduction in the use of radiation for nonmalignant diseases, and the widespread use of chemotherapy rather than whole abdominal radiation for intraabdominal malignancies. As a result of these changes, the major current setting in which this disorder may occur is in the radiation treatment of disseminated retroperitoneal malignancies.

PATHOLOGY

Vascular, glomerular, and tubulointerstitial changes of varying severity are found in radiation nephritis.[542-544] The arterial lumina are frequently narrowed due to extensive fibrous intimal thickening, a change similar to that in progressive systemic sclerosis or the hemolytic-uremic syndrome (see Figs. 7–8 and 7–9). Fibrinoid necrosis and intravascular thrombi may also be seen, particularly in the smaller arteries.

The glomerular damage, which may in part be secondary to ischemia, is initially manifested by endothelial cell swelling, increased mesangial matrix, splitting of the GBM, and, in some patients, areas of fibrinoid necrosis. With time, these lesions progress to focal or diffuse glomerulosclerosis.

Immunofluorescence studies are negative for immunoglobulins and complement,[544] a finding consistent with the nonimmunologic nature of the disease. Electron microscopy reveals expansion of the subendothelial region of the basement membrane due to deposition of electron-lucent material (similar to that in Fig. 7-9c).[544] The origin of this material and its significance are not known.

Tubulointerstitial disease is typically prominent in radiation nephritis and may be more severe than the vascular or glomerular lesions. Interstitial edema and tubular necrosis are seen in the early stages, followed by the development of interstitial fibrosis, mononuclear cell infiltration, and tubular atrophy.

PATHOGENESIS

Experimental and human studies have revealed that the extent of radiation-induced injury is dependent upon several factors, including the dose of radiation, the interval from the time of exposure, and individual susceptibility. In general, clinically important renal changes are not seen unless the total radiation dose exceeds 2300 rads.[540] In addition, there is a variable interval before renal dysfunction becomes apparent, ranging from 6 months to 12 or more years.[541] Neither the factors responsible for this latent period nor the primary site of damage within the kidney are known. The observation that renal blood flow begins to fall after as few as 400 rads suggests that the earliest changes may be in the vessels.[545] However, there frequently is no correlation between the severity of the vascular changes and those in the glomeruli, tubules, or interstitium,[541,546] indicating that the sensitivity of the different renal components to radiation may vary from patient to patient.

The elevation in blood pressure commonly seen in radiation nephritis appears to be mediated primarily by the renin-angiotensin system.[547] A vicious cycle may be involved, since vessels exposed to radiation are more sensitive to the effects of hypertension; this is manifested by the development of fibrinoid necrosis at a lower blood pressure than required in normal vessels.[546,548] Thus, hypertension in radiation nephritis could produce further vascular disease, resulting in increased renal ischemia, renin secretion, hypertension, and renal insufficiency. This effect of vascular injury is important clinically since 25 to 30 percent of patients with radiation nephritis ultimately develop malignant hypertension, which is a major cause of morbidity and mortality in this disorder.

CLINICAL PRESENTATION AND COURSE

The course of radiation nephritis is variable, as both acute and more chronic syndromes may occur.[541] Patients with *acute radiation nephritis* usually present within 6 to 12 months after exposure with nonspecific symptoms such as headache, lassitude, nausea, vomiting, and dyspnea. Hypertension, congestive heart failure, anemia, proteinuria, and renal insufficiency are frequently found at this time. If the hypertension is not adequately treated, progression to malignant hypertension commonly occurs.

Thrombocytopenia and a microangiopathic hemolytic anemia also can occur in this setting, leading to a clinical picture that is suggestive of the hemolytic-uremic syndrome.[549] This similarity is not surprising, since vascular damage can initiate the hemolytic-uremic syndrome[206,207] and the vascular lesions in the two disorders are similar histologically.

The prognosis of acute radiation nephritis is variable. Patients who develop malignant hypertension have an appreciable rate of mortality or progression to end-stage renal failure. However, patients who survive the acute episode without severe hypertension may undergo partial resolution of the disease with gradual improvement both in the GFR and in the degree of hypertension.

Chronic radiation nephritis may follow an episode of acute radiation nephritis or occur de novo after a latent period of as long as 12 years. The primary changes in this disorder are a variable degree of renal insufficiency and an abnormal urinalysis characterized by mild proteinuria and granular cysts. Patients with mild disease may remain asymptomatic. However, progression to renal failure or malignant hypertension eventually occurs in approximately one-third to one-half of patients.

Late malignant hypertension may develop in some patients without prior evidence of nephritis. The latent period in this condition ranges from 1.5 to 11 years and tends to be somewhat shorter in patients with bilateral disease. Others may present with a moderate elevation in blood pressure and normal renal function. Most of these patients tend to follow a course similar to that in essential hypertension, although progression to malignant hypertension is somewhat more common.

Patients who develop *intermittent isolated proteinuria* following radiation therapy generally have an excellent prognosis. This disorder tends not to be associated with an increased incidence of hypertension or renal insufficiency.

DIAGNOSIS AND TREATMENT

The diagnosis of radiation nephritis is made by inference from the history of radiation to the kidneys and the development of one of the characteristic clinical syndromes associated with this disorder. Since there is no specific therapy, prevention by limiting exposure of the kidneys is of primary importance. Once radiation nephritis has developed, treatment is largely supportive. Control of hypertension is particularly important in view of the relatively poor prognosis associated with the development of malignant hypertension.

REFERENCES

1. Fauci, A. S., B. F. Haynes, and P. Katz: The spectrum of vasculitis: Clinical, pathologic, immunologic, and therapeutic considerations, *Ann. Intern. Med.,* 89:660, 1978.
2. Howell, S. B., and W. V. Epstein: Circulating immunoglobulin complexes in Wegener's granulomatosis, *Am. J. Med.,* 60:259, 1976.
3. Woodroffe, A. J., W. A. Border, O. Theofilopoulos, O. Gotze, R. J. Glassock, F. J. Dixon, and C. B. Wilson: Detection of circulating immune complexes in patients with glomerulonephritis, *Kidney Int.,* 12:268, 1977.
4. Lockwood, C. M., S. Worlledge, A. Nicholas, C. Cotton, and D. K. Peters: Reversal of impaired splenic function by plasma exchange, *N. Engl. J. Med.,* 300:254, 1979.
5. Cochran, C. G.: Mechanisms involved in the deposition of immune complexes in tissue, *J. Exp. Med.,* 134(suppl):75s, 1971.
6. McCluskey, R. T., and R. Feinberg: Vasculitis in primary vasculidities, granulomatoses, and connective tissue diseases, *Hum. Pathol.,* 14:305, 1983.
7. Braverman, I. M., and A. Yen: Demonstration of immune complexes in spontaneous and histamine-induced lesions in normal skin of patients with leukocytoclastic angiitis, *J. Invest. Dermatol.,* 64:105, 1975.
8. Shusterman, N., and W. T. London: Hepatitis B and immune-complex disease, *N. Engl. J. Med.,* 310:43, 1984.
9. Elkon, K. B., G. R. Hughes, and V. Catovsky: Hairy cell leukemia with polyarteritis nodosa, *Lancet,* 2:280, 1979.
10. Goedert, J. J., J. R. Neefe, F. S. Smith, N. I. Stahl, E. S. Jaffee, and A. S. Fauci: Polyarteritis nodosa, hairy cell leukemia and splenosis, *Am. J. Med.,* 71:323, 1981.

11. Fulmer, J. D., and H. B. Kaltreider: The pulmonary vasculidities, *Chest*, 82:615, 1982.
12. van der Wande, F. J.: Anticytoplasmic antibodies in Wegener's granulomatosis, *Lancet*, 2:48, 1985.
13. Heptinstall, R. H.: *Pathology of the Kidney*, 3d ed., Little, Brown, Boston, 1983, chap. 16.
14. Fisher, R. G.: Renal artery aneurysms in polyarteritis nodosa: A multiepisodic phenomenon, *Am. J. Radiol.*, 136:983, 1981.
15. Davson, J., J. Ball, and R. Platt: The kidney in periarteritis nodosa, *Q. J. Med.*, 17:178, 1948.
16. Serra, A., J. S. Cameron, D. R. Turner, B. Hartley, C. S. Ogg, G. H. Neild, D. G. Williams, D. Taube, C. B. Brown, and J. A. Hicks: Vasculitis affecting the kidney: Presentation, histopathology, and long-term outcome, *Q. J. Med.*, 53:181, 1984.
17. Spargo, B. H., N. G. Ordonez, and J. C. Ringus: The differential diagnosis of crescentic glomerulonephritis. The pathology of specific lesions with prognostic implications. *Hum. Pathol.*, 8:187, 1977.
18. Germuth, F. G., Jr., A. J. Valdes, J. J. Taylor, O. L. Wise, and F. Rodriguez: Fatal immune complex glomerulonephritis without deposits, *Johns Hopkins Med. J.*, 136:189, 1975.
19. Weiss, M. A., and J. D. Crissman: Segmental necrotizing glomerulonephritis: Diagnostic, prognostic, and therapeutic significance., *Am. J. Kid. Dis.*, 6:199, 1985.
20. Leib, E. S., C. Restivo, and H. E. Paulus: Immunosuppressive and corticosteroid therapy of polyarteritis nodosa, *Am. J. Med.*, 67:941, 1979.
21. O'Connell, M. T., D. B. Kubrusly, and A. M. Fournier: Systemic necrotizing vasculitis seen initially as hypertensive crisis, *Arch. Intern. Med.*, 145:265, 1985.
22. Case Records of the Massachusetts General Hospital (Case 36-1985), *N. Engl. J. Med.*, 313:622, 1985.
23. Stockigt, J. R., D. J. Topliss, and M. J. Hewett: High-renin hypertension in necrotizing vasculitis, *N. Engl. J. Med.*, 300:1218, 1979.
24. Moore, P. M., and A. S. Fauci: Neurologic manifestations of systemic vasculitis, *Am. J. Med.*, 71:517, 1981.
25. Balow, J. E.: Renal vasculitis, *Kidney Int.*, 27:954, 1985.
26. Frohnert, P. P., and S. G. Sheps: Long-term follow-up study of peri-arteritis nodosa, *Am. J. Med.*, 43:8, 1967.
27. Scott, D. G., P. A. Bacon, P. J. Elliott, C. R. Tribe, and T. B. Wallington: Systemic vasculitis in a district general hospital 1972–1980. Clinical and laboratory features, classification, and prognosis of 80 cases, *Q. J. Med.*, 51:292, 1982.
28. Wees, S. J., I. N. Sunwoo, and S. J. Oh: Sural nerve biopsy in systemic necrotizing vasculitis, *Am. J. Med.*, 71:525, 1981.
29. Meyers, D. S., C. E. Grim, and W. F. Keitzer: Fibromuscular dysplasia of the renal artery with medial dissection: A case simulating polyarteritis nodosa, *Am. J. Med.*, 56:412, 1974.
30. Longstreth, P. L., M. Korobkin, and A. J. Palumbinskas: Renal microaneurysms in a patient with systemic lupus erythematosus, *Radiology*, 113:65, 1974.
31. Baker, S. B., and D. R. Robinson: Unusual renal manifestations of Wegener's granulomatosis. Report of two cases, *Am. J. Med.*, 64:883, 1978.
32. De Shazo, R. D., A. I. Levinson, O. J. Lawless, and G. Weisbaum: Systemic vasculitis with coexistent large and small vessel involvement. A classification dilemma, *J. Am. Med. Assoc.*, 238:1940, 1977.
33. Corrocher, R., C. Brugnara, R. Mason, G. Taddei, P. Mexxalani, and G. De Sandre: Multiple arterial stenoses in chronic ergot toxicity (letter), *N. Engl. J. Med.*, 310:261, 1984.
34. Savage, C. O. S., C. G. Winearls, D. J. Evans, A. J. Rees, and C. M. Lockwood: Microscopic polyarteritis: Presentation, pathology, and prognosis, *Q. J. Med.*, 56:467, 1985.
35. Lanham, J. G., K. B. Elkon, C. D. Pusey, and G. R. Hughes: Systemic vasculitis with asthma and eosinophilia: A clinical approach to the Churg-Strauss syndrome, *Medicine*, 63:65, 1984.
36. Chumbley, L. C., F. G. Harrison, Jr., and R. A. DeRemee: Allergic granulomatosis and angiitis (Churg-Strauss syndrome), *Mayo Clin. Proc.*, 52:477, 1977.
37. Leavitt, R. Y., and A. S. Fauci: Polyangiitis overlap syndrome, *Am. J. Med.*, 81:79, 1986.
38. Cupps, T. R., and A. S. Fauci: *The Vasculidities*, Philadelphia, Saunders, 1981.
39. Fauci, A. S., J. L. Doppman, and S. M. Wolff: Cyclophosphamide-induced remissions in advanced polyarteritis nodosa, *Am. J. Med.*, 64:890, 1978.
40. Garges, L., R. Beaulieu, E. Bardana, and B. Pirofsky: Combined azathioprine-steroid therapy in periarteritis nodosa, *Clin. Res.*, 21:268, 1973.
41. Hind, C. R. K., H. Paraskevakov, C. M. Lockwood, D. J. Evans, D. K. Peters, and A. J. Rees: Prognosis after immunosuppression of patients with crescentic nephritis requiring dialysis, *Lancet*, 1:263, 1983.
42. Cohen, R. D., D. L. Conn, and D. M. Ilstrup: Clinical features, prognosis, and response to treatment in polyarteritis, *Mayo Clin. Proc.*, 55:146, 1980.
43. Montalbert, C., A. Corvallo, B. Broumand, D. Noble, L. A. Austine, and C. B. Currier, Jr.: Suc-

cessful renal transplantation in polyarteritis nodosa, *Clin. Nephrol.,* 14:206, 1980.

44. Pinching, A. J., C. M. Lockwood, B. A. Pussell, A. J. Rees, P. Sweeny, D. J. Evans, N. Bowley, and D. K. Peters: Wegener's granulomatosis: Observations on 18 patients with severe renal disease, *Q. J. Med.,* 52:435, 1983.

45. Horn, R. G., A. S. Fauci, A. S. Rosenthal, and S. M. Wolff: Renal biopsy pathology in Wegener's granulomatosis, *Am. J. Pathol.,* 74:423, 1974.

46. Wolff, S. M., A. S. Fauci, R. G. Horn, and D. C. Dale: Wegener's granulomatosis, *Ann. Intern. Med.,* 81:513, 1974.

47. Wolff, S. M., and A. S. Fauci: Wegener's granulomatosis: Studies in eighteen patients and a review of the literature, *Medicine,* 52:535, 1973.

48. Fauci, A. S., B. F. Haynes, P. Katz, and S. M. Wolff: Wegener's granulomatosis: Prospective clinical trial and therapeutic experience with eighty-five patients for 21 years, *Ann. Intern. Med.,* 98:76, 1983.

49. Carrington, C. B., and A. A. Liebow: Limited forms of angiitis and granulomatosis of Wegener's type, *Am. J. Med.,* 41:497, 1966.

50. Israel, H. L., and A. S. Patchefsky: Treatment of Wegener's granulomatosis of the lung, *Am. J. Med.,* 58:617, 1975.

51. Israel, H. L., A. S. Patchefsky, and M. J. Saldena: Wegener's granulomatosis, lymphomatoid granulomatosis, and benign lymphocytic angiitis and granulomatosis of the lung. Recognition and treatment, *Ann. Intern. Med.,* 87:691, 1977.

52. Walton, E. W.: Giant cell granuloma of the respiratory tract (Wegener's granulomatosis), *Br. Med. J.,* 2:265, 1958.

53. Case Records of the Massachusetts General Hospital (Case 26-1985), *N. Engl. J. Med.,* 312:1695, 1985.

54. Case Records of the Massachusetts General Hospital (Case 17-1986), *N. Engl. J. Med.,* 314:1170, 1986.

55. Hollander, D., and R. T. Manning: The use of alkylating agents in the treatment of Wegener's granulomatosis, *Ann. Intern. Med.,* 67:393, 1967.

56. Kjellstrand, C. M., R. L. Simmons, J. M. Uranga, T. J. Buselmeier, and J. S. Najarian: Acute fulminant Wegener's granulomatosis: Therapy with immunosuppression, hemodialysis, and renal transplantation, *Arch. Intern. Med.,* 134:40 1974.

57. Austin, H. A., J. H. Klippel, J. E. Balow, N. G. H. le Riche, A. D. Steinberg, P. H. Plotz, and J. L. Decker: Therapy of lupus nephritis, *N. Engl. J. Med.,* 314:614, 1986.

58. Ambrus, J. L., and A. S. Fauci: Diffuse histiocytic lymphoma in a patient treated with cyclophosphamide for Wegener's granulomatosis, *Am. J. Med.,* 76:745, 1984.

59. Cupps, T. R., G. J. Silverman, and A. S. Fauci: Herpes zoster in patients with treated Wegener's granulomatosis: A possible role for cyclophosphamide, *Am. J. Med.,* 69:881, 1980.

60. Harrison, H. L., M. A. Linshaw, C. B. Lindsley, and F. E. Cuppage: Bolus corticosteroids and cyclophosphamide for initial treatment of Wegener's granulomatosis, *J. Am. Med. Assoc.,* 244:1599, 1980.

61. Bocanegra, T. S., M. O. Kastaneda, L. R. Espinoza, F. B. Vasey, and B. F. Germain: Sudden death after methylprednisolone pulse therapy, *Ann. Intern. Med.,* 95:122, 1981.

62. Mose, R. E. A. McCormick, and W. Nickey: Fatal arrhythmia after pulse methylprednisolone therapy (letter), *Ann. Intern. Med.,* 95:781, 1981.

63. Warren, D. J., and R. S. Smith: High dose prednisolone, *Lancet,* 1:594, 1983.

64. Thomson, M., D. Gee, C. Wood, S. R. Holdsworth and R. C. Alkins: Wegener's granulomatosis with renal involvement: Is it ever cured? (abstract), *Kidney Int.,* 26:241, 1984.

65. Steinman, T. I., B. F. Jaffe, A. P. Monaco, S. M. Wolff, and A. S. Fauci: Recurrence of Wegener's granulomatosis after kidney transplantation, *Am. J. Med.,* 68:458, 1980.

66. Pinching, A. J., A. J. Rees, B. A. Pussell, C. M. Lockwood, R. J. Mitchison, and D. K. Peters: Relapses in Wegener's granulomatosis: The role of infection, *Br. Med. J.,* 281:836, 1980.

67. De Remee, R. A., T. J. McDonald, and L. H. Weiland: Wegener's granulomatosis: Observations on treatment with antimicrobial agents, *Mayo Clin. Proc.,* 60:27, 1985.

68. Kuross, S., T. Davin, and C. M. Kjellstrand: Wegener's granulomatosis with severe renal failure: Clinical course and results of dialysis and transplantation, *Clin. Nephrol.,* 16:172, 1981.

69. Cuevas, J., A. Pelegri, M. Morlans, J. Fort, J. Bonal, and L. Piera: Wegener's granulomatosis and hemodialysis (letter), *Clin. Nephrol.,* 18:109, 1981.

70. Curtis, J. J., A. G. Diethelm, G. A. Herrera, W. T. Crowell, and J. D. Whelchel: Recurrence of Wegener's granulomatosis in a cadaver renal allograft, *Transplantation,* 36:452, 1983.

71. Sams, W. M., Jr., E. G. Thorne, P. Small, M. F. Maso, R. M. McIntosh, and R. E. Stanford: Leukocytoclastic vasculitis, *Arch. Dermatol.,* 112:219, 1976.

72. Winkelmann, R. K., and W. B. Ditto: Cutaneous and visceral syndromes of necrotizing or "allergic angiitis": A study of 38 cases, *Medicine,* 43:59, 1964.

73. Mullick, F. G., H. A. McAllister, Jr., B. M. Wagner, and J. J. Fenoglio, Jr.: Drug-related vasculitis: Clinicopathologic correlations in 30 patients, *Hum. Pathol.,* 10:313, 1979.

74. Cupps, T. R., R. M. Springer, and A. S. Fauci: Chronic, recurrent small-vessel cutaneous vasculitis, *J. Am. Med. Assoc.,* 247:1994, 1982.

75. Sanchez, N. P., R. K. Winkelman, A. L. Schroeter, and C. H. Dicken: The clinical and histopathologic spectrum of urticarial vasculitis: Study of forty cases, *J. Am. Acad. Dermatol.,* 7:599, 1982.

76. Shultz, D. R., G. O. Perez, J. E. Volanakis, V. Pardo, and S. H. Moss: Glomerular disease in two patients with urticarial-cutaneous vasculitis and hypocomplementemia, *Am. J. Kid. Dis.,* 1:257, 1981.

77. Gammon, W. R.: Urticarial vasculitis, *Dermatol. Clinics,* 3:97, 1985.

78. Cream, J. J., J. M. Grumpel, and R. D. G. Peachey: Schönlein-Henoch purpura in adults: A study of 77 adults with anaphylactoid or Schönlein-Henoch purpura, *Q. J. Med.,* 39:461, 1970.

79. Roth, D. A., D. R. Wilz, and G. B. Theil: Schönlein-Henoch syndrome in adults, *Q. J. Med.,* 55:145, 1985.

80. Koskimies, O., S. Mir, J. Rapola, and J. Vilska: Henoch-Schönlein nephritis: Long-term prognosis of unselected patients, *Arch. Dis. Child.,* 56:482, 1981.

81. Austin, H. A., III, and J. E. Balow: Henoch-Schönlein nephritis: Prognostic features and the challenge of therapy, *Am. J. Kid. Dis.,* 2:512, 1983.

82. Cameron, J. S.: Henoch-Schönlein purpura: Clinical presentation, *Contrib. Nephrol.,* 40:246, 1984.

83. Meadow, S. R., R. F. Glasgow, R. H. R. White, M. W. Moncrieff, J. S. Cameron, and C. S. Ogg: Schönlein-Henoch nephritis, *Q. J. Med.,* 41:241, 1972.

84. Crumb, C. K.: Renal involvement in Schönlein-Henoch syndrome, in W. N. Suki (ed.), *The Kidney in Systemic Disease,* Wiley, New York, 1976, p. 43.

85. Cameron, J. S.: The nephritis of Schönlein-Henoch purpura: Current problems, in P. Kincaid-Smith, A. J. D'Apice, and R. C. Atkins (eds.), *Progress in Glomerulonephritis,* Wiley, New York, 1979, p. 283.

86. Kauffman, R. H., W. A. Herrmann, C. J. L. M. Meyers, M. R. Dana, and L. A. van Es: Circulating IgA-immune complexes in Henoch-Schönlein purpura. A longitudinal study of their relationship to disease activity and vascular deposition of IgA, *Am. J. Med.,* 69:859, 1980.

87. Levinsky, R. J., and T. M. Barratt: IgA immune complexes in Henoch-Schönlein purpura, *Lancet* 2:1100, 1979.

88. Baart de la Faille-Kuyper, E. H., L. Kater, and R. H. Kuyten: Occurrence of vascular IgA deposits in clinically normal skin in patients with renal disease, *Kidney Int.,* 9:424, 1976.

89. Hene, R. J., P. Velthuis, A. van de Wiel, D. Klepper, E. J. Dorhout Mees, and L. Kater: The revelance of IgA deposits in vessel walls of clinically normal skin, *Arch. Intern. Med.,* 146:745, 1986.

90. Namato, Y., Y. Asano, K. Dohi, M. Fukioka, H. Iida, Y. Kibe, N. Hattori, and J. Takeuchi: Primary IgA glomerulonephritis: Clinicopathological and immuno-histological characteristics, *Q. J. Med.,* 47:495, 1978.

91. Nochy, D., P. Druet, and J. Bariety: IgA nephropathy in alcoholic liver disease, *Contrib. Nephrol.,* 40:268, 1984.

92. Makdassy, R., M. Beaufils, A. Meyrier, F. Mignon, L. Moulonguet-Doleris, and G. Richet: Pathologic conditions associated with IgA mesangial nephropathy: Preliminary results, *Contrib. Nephrol.,* 40:292, 1984.

93. Balow, J. E., and H. Austin: Vasculitic diseases of the kidney, in W. N. Suki, and S. G. Massry (eds.), *Therapy of Renal Diseases and Related Disorders,* Martinus Nijhoff, Boston, 1984, pp. 273–282.

94. Cameron, JS: The nephritis of Henoch-Schönlein purpura: Current problems, in P. Kincaid-Smith, A. J. D'Apice, and R. C. Atkins (eds.), *Glomerulonephritis. Recent Advances,* Wiley, New York, 1979.

95. Counan, R., M. H. Winterborn, R. H. R. White, J. M. Heaton, S. R. Meadow, N. H. Bluet, H. Swetschin, J. S. Cameron, and C. Chantler: Prognosis of Henoch-Schönlein nephritis in children, *Br. Med. J.,* 2:11, 1977.

96. Bolton, W. K., and W. G. Couser: Intravenous pulse methylprednisolone therapy of acute crescentic rapidly progressive glomerulonephritis, *Am. J. Med.,* 66:495, 1979.

97. Kauffmann, R. H., and D. A. Houwert: Plasmapheresis in rapidly progressive Henoch-Schönlein glomerulonephritis and the effect on circulating IgA immune complexes, *Clin. Nephrol.,* 16:155, 1981.

98. Ito, K., F. Narumi, and M. Ono: The evaluation of the clinical effect of plasma exchange therapy on purpura nephritis in childhood (abstract), *Int. Cong. Nephrol.,* 8:259A, 1981.

99. Meadow, S. R.: The prognosis of Henoch-Schönlein nephritis, *Clin. Nephrol.,* 9:87, 1978.

100. Baliah, T., K. H. Kim, S. Anthone, M. Montes, and G. A. Andres: Recurrence of Henoch-Schönlein purpura in transplanted kidneys, *Transplantation,* 18:343, 1974.

101. Brouet, J. C., J. P. Clauvel, F. Danon, M. Klein, and M. Seligmann: Biologic and clinical significance of cryoglobulins: A report of 86 cases, *Am. J. Med.,* 57:775, 1974.

102. Roberts, J. L., and E. J. Lewis: Identification of

antinative DNA antibodies in cryoglobulinemic states, *Am. J. Med.,* 65:437, 1978.

103. McIntosh, R. M., W. R. Griswold, W. B. Chernack, G. Williams, J. Strauss, D. B. Kaufman, M. N. Koss, J. R. McIntosh, R. Cohen, and R. Weil III: Cryoglobulins, III: Further studies of the nature, incidence, clinical diagnostic, prognostic, and immunopathologic significance of cryoproteins in renal disease, *Q. J. Med.,* 44:285, 1975.

104. Lockwood, C. M.: Lymphoma, cryoglobulinemia, and renal disease, *Kidney Int.,* 16:522, 1979.

105. Levo, Y.: Nature of cryoglobulinemia, *Lancet,* 1:285, 1984.

106. Levo, Y., P. D. Gorevic, H. J. Kassab, H. Tobias, and E. C. Franklin: Liver involvement in the syndrome of mixed cryoglobulinemia, *Ann. Intern. Med.,* 87:287, 1977.

107. Gambles, C. N., and S. W. Rugles: The immunopathogenesis of glomerulonephritis associated with mixed cryoglobulinemia, *N. Engl. J. Med.,* 299:81, 1978.

108. Gorevic, P. D., H. J. Kassab, Y. Levo, R. Kohn, M. Meltzer, P. Prose, and E. C. Franklin: Mixed cryoglobulinemia: Clinical aspects and long term follow-up of 40 patients, *Am. J. Med.,* 69:287, 1980.

109. Clinicopathologic Conference: Pain, purpura and death in an elderly woman, *Am. J. Med.,* 78:839, 1985.

110. Case records of the Massachusetts General Hospital (Case 2-1985), *N. Engl. J. Med.,* 312:103, 1985.

111. De Vecchi, A., G. Montagnino, C. Possi, F. Tarantino, F. Locatelli, and C. Ponticelli: Intravenous methylprednisolone pulse therapy in essential mixed cryoglobulinemia nephropathy, *Clin. Nephrol.,* 19:221, 1983.

112. Evan, T. W., A. J. Nicholls, J. R. Shortland, A. M. Ward, and C. B. Brown: Acute renal failure in essential mixed cryoglobulinemia: Prescription and reversal by plasma exchange, *Clin. Nephrol.,* 21:287, 1984.

113. Ferri, C., L. Moriconi, G. Gremignai, P. Migliorini, G. Paleologo, P. V. Fossella, and S. Bombardieri: Treatment of the renal involvement in mixed cryoglobulinemia with prolonged plasma exchange, *Nephron,* 43:246, 1986.

114. Van Pirquet, C. F., and B. Schick: *Serum Sickness,* Williams and Wilkins, Baltimore, 1951.

115. Parker, C. W.: Allergic reactions in man, *Pharmacol. Rev.,* 34:85, 1982.

116. Reynolds, J. S.: Serum sickness: An old problem with new implications, *Allergy,* 24:337, 1966.

117. Haruda, F.: Phenytoin hypersensitivity: 38 cases, *Neurology,* 29:1480, 1979.

118. Josephs, S. H., S. F. Rothman, and R. H. Buckley: Phenytoin hypersensitivity, *J. Allergy Clin. Immunol.,* 66:166, 1980.

119. Tomsick, R. S.: The phenytoin syndrome, *Cutis,* 32:535, 1983.

120. McElgunn, P. S. J.: Dermatologic manifestations of hepatitis B virus infection, *J. Am. Acad. Dermatol.,* 8:539, 1983.

121. Parker, C. W.: Drug allergy, *N. Engl. J. Med.,* 292:511, 1975.

122. De la Pava, S., G. Nigogosyan, and J. W. Pickren: Fatal glomerulonephritis after receiving horse antihuman cancer serum, *Arch. Intern. Med.,* 109:391, 1962.

123. Eknoyan, G., F. Gyorkey, C. Dickson, M. Martinez-Maldonado, W. N. Suki, and P. Gyorkey: Renal, morphological, and immunological changes associated with acute viral hepatitis, *Kidney Int.,* 1:413, 1972.

124. Lakhanpal, S., D. L. Conn, and J. T. Lie: Clinical and prognostic significance of vasculitis as a manifestation of connective tissue disease syndrome, *Ann. Intern. Med.,* 101:743, 1984.

125. Scott, D. G. I., P. A. Bacon, and C. R. Tribe: Systemic rheumatoid vasculitis: A clinical and laboratory study of 50 cases, *Medicine,* 60:288, 1981.

126. Firestein, G. S., H. E. Gruber, M. N. Weisman, N. J. Zvaifler, J. Barker, and J. D. O'Duffy: Mouth and genital ulcers with inflamed cartilage. MAGIC syndrome, *Am. J. Med.,* 79:65, 1985.

127. Espinoza, L. R., A. Richman, T. Bocanegra, I. Pina, F. B. Vasey, S. I. Rifkin, and B. F. Germaine: Immune complex-mediated renal involvement in relapsing polychondritis, *Am. J. Med.,* 71:181, 1981.

128. Michet, C. J., C. H. McKenna, H. S. Luthra, and W. M. O'Fallon: Relapsing polychondritis, *Ann. Intern. Med.,* 104:74, 1986.

129. Truong, L., R. G. Kopelman, G. S. Williams, and C. L. Pirani: Temporal arteritis and renal disease, *Am. J. Med.,* 78:171, 1985.

130. Lagneau, P., and J. B. Michel: Renovascular hypertension and Takayasu's disease, *J. Urol.,* 134:876, 1985.

131. Lai, K. N., K. W. Chan, and C. P. Ho: Glomerulonephritis associated with Takayasu's arteritis: Report of three cases and review of literature, *Am. J. Kid. Dis.,* 7:197, 1986.

132. Medsger, T. A., Jr., A. T. Masi, G. P. Rodnan, T. G. Benedek, and H. Robinson: Survival with systemic sclerosis (scleroderma): A life-table analysis of clinical and demographic factors in 309 patients, *Ann. Intern. Med.,* 75:369, 1971.

133. D'Angelo, W. A., J. F. Fries, A. T. Masi, and L. E.

Shulman: Pathologic observations in systemic scle- rosis (scleroderma): A study of fifty-eight autopsy cases and fifty- eight matched controls, *Am. J. Med.,* 46:428, 1969.

134. Cannon, P. J., M. Hassar, D. B. Chase, W. J. Casa- rella, S. C. Sommers, and E. C. LeRoy: The relation- ship of hypertension and renal failure in sclero- derma (progressive systemic sclerosis) to structural and functional abnormalities of the renal cortical circulation, *Medicine,* 53:1, 1974.

135. Traub, R. M., A. P. Shapiro, G. P. Rodnan, T. A. Medsger, R. H. McDonald, V. D. Steen, T. A. Osial, and S. F. Tolchin: Hypertension and renal failure (scleroderma renal crisis) in progressive sysemic sclerosis. *Medicine,* 62:335, 1983.

136. Heptinstall, R.H.: *Pathology of the Kidney,* 3d ed., Lit- tle, Brown, Boston, 1983, chap. 18.

137. Norton, W. L., and J. M. Nardo: Vascular disease in progressive systemic sclerosis (scleroderma), *Ann. Intern. Med.,* 73:317, 1970.

138. McCoy, R. C., C. C. Tisher, P. F. Pepe, and L. A. Cleveland: The kidney in progressive systemic scle- rosis: Immunohistochemical and antibody elution studies, *Lab. Invest.,* 35:124, 1976.

139. Kovalchik, M. R., S. J. Guggenheim, J. H. Silver- man, J. S. Robertson, and J. C. Steigerwald: The kidney in progressive systemic sclerosis: A pro- spective study, *Ann. Intern. Med.,* 89:881, 1978.

140. Kincaid-Smith, P.: The role of coagulation in the obliteration of glomerular capillaries, in P. Kincaid- Smith, T. H. Mathew, and E. L. Becker (eds.), *Glomerulonephritis: Morphology, Natural History, and Treatment,* Wiley, New York, 1972.

141. Lee, E. B., G. J. Anhalt, J. J. Voorhees, and L. A. Diaz: Pathogenesis of scleroderma, *Int. J. Dermatol.,* 23:85, 1984.

142. Fries, J. F.: The microvascular pathogenesis of scle- roderma: An hypothesis, *Ann. Intern. Med.,* 91:788, 1979.

143. Rose, B. D.: *Clinical Physiology of Acid-Base and Elec- trolyte Disorders,* 2d ed., McGraw-Hill, New York, 1984, chap 1.

144. Gratwick, G. M., R. Klein, J. S. Sergent, and C. L. Christian: Fibrinogen turnover in progressive sys- temic sclerosis, *Arth. Rheum.,* 21:343, 1978.

145. Wasner, C., C. R. Cooke, and J. F. Fries: Successful medical treatment of scleroderma renal crisis, *N. Engl. J. Med.,* 299:873, 1978.

146. Barker, D. J., and M. J. Farr: Resolution of cuta- neous manifestations of systemic sclerosis after haemodialysis, *Br. Med. J.,* 1:501, 1976.

147. Lopez-Overjero, J. S., S. D. Sall, W. A. D'Angelo, J. S. Cheigh, K. H. Stenzel, and J. H. Laragh: Reversal of vascular and renal crisis of scleroderma by oral angiotensin converting enzyme blockade, *N. Engl. J. Med.,* 300:1417, 1979.

148. Fries, J. F., C. Wasner, J. Brown, and P. Feigen- baum: A controlled trial of antihypertensive ther- apy in systemic sclerosis (scleroderma), *Ann. Rheum. Dis.,* 43:407, 1984.

149. Beckett, V. L., J. V. Donadio, L. A. Brennan, Jr., D. L. Conn, E. Y. S. Chao, and K. E. Holley: Use of captopril as early therapy for renal scleroderma: A prospective study, *Mayo Clin. Proc.,* 60:763, 1985.

150. LeRoy, E.C., J. A. Downey, and P. J. Cannon: Skin capillary blood flow in scleroderma, *J. Clin. Invest.,* 50:930, 1971.

151. Postlethwaite, A. E., and A. E. Kang: Pathogenesis of progressive systemic sclerosis, *J. Lab. Clin. Med.,* 103:506, 1984.

152. Cannon, P. J.: Medical management of renal scle- roderma, *N. Engl. J. Med.,* 299:886, 1978.

153. LeRoy, E. C.: Increased collagen synthesis by scle- roderma skin fibroblasts in vitro: A possible defect in the regulation or activation of the scleroderma fibroblast, *J. Clin. Invest.,* 54:880, 1974.

154. Buckingham, R. B., R. K. Prince, G. P. Rodnan, and F. Taylor: Increased collagen accumulation in der- mal fibroblast cultures from patients with progres- sive systemic sclerosis (scleroderma). *J. Lab. Clin. Med.,* 92:5, 1978.

155. Kondo, H., B. S. Robin, and G. P. Rodnan: Cutane- ous antigen-stimulating lymphokine production by lymphocytes of patients with progressive systemic sclerosis, *J. Clin. Invest.,* 58:1388, 1976.

156. Kang, A. H.: Fibroblast activation, *J. Lab. Clin. Med.,* 92:1, 1978.

157. Dubois, E. L., S. Chandor, G. J. Fliou, and M. Bischel: Progressive systemic sclerosis and localized scleroderma (morphea) with positive LE cell test and unusual systemic manifestations compatible with lupus erythematosus: Presentation of 14 cases including one set of identical twins, one with scle- roderma and the other with SLE: Review of the literature, *Medicine,* 50:199, 1971.

158. Sharp, G. C., W. S. Irvin, E. M. Tan, R. Gould, and H. R. Holman: Mixed connective tissue disease— An apparently distinct rheumatic disease syndrome associated with a specific antibody to an extract- able nuclear antigen (ENA), *Am. J. Med.,* 52:148, 1972.

159. Rothfield, N. F., and G. P. Rodnan: Serum antinu- clear antibodies in progressive systemic sclerosis (scleroderma), *Arth. Rheum.,* 11:607, 1968.

160. Shero, J. H., B. Bordwell, N. F. Rothfield, and W. C. Earnshaw: High titers of autoantibodies to topoiso-

merase I (Scl-70) in sera from scleroderma patients, *Science,* 231:737, 1986.

161. Tumulty, P. A.: Clinical synopsis of scleroderma, simulator of other diseases, *Johns Hopkins Med. Bull.,* 122:236, 1968.

162. LeRoy, E. C., and R. M. Fleischmann: The management of renal scleroderma: Experience with dialysis, nephrectomy and transplantation, *Am. J. Med.,* 64:974, 1978.

163. Steen V. D., T. A. Medsger, T. A. Osial, G. L. Ziegler, A. P. Shapiro, and G. P. Rodnan: Factors predicting development of renal involvement in progressive systemic sclerosis, *Am. J. Med.,* 76:779, 1984.

164. Beckett, V. L., D. L. Conn, V. Fuster, P. J. Osmundson, C. G. Strong, E. Y. S. Chao, J. H. Chesebro, and W. M. O'Fallon: Trial of platelet-inhibiting drugs in scleroderma, *Arth. Rheum.,* 27:1137, 1984.

165. Wynn, J., N. Fineberg, L. Matzer, X. Cortada, W. Armstrong, J. C. Dillon, and E. L. Kinney: Prediction of survival in progressive systemic sclerosis by multivariate analysis of clinical features, *Am. Ht. J.,* 110:123, 1985.

166. Bernstein, R. M., J. C. Steigerwald, and E. M. Tan: Association of antinuclear and antinucleolar antibodies in progressive systemic sclerosis, *Clin. Exp. Immunol.,* 48:43, 1982.

167. LeRoy, E. C.: Scleroderma (systemic sclerosis), in W. N. Kelly, E. D. Harris, S. Ruddy, and C. B. Sledge (eds.), *Textbook of Rheumatology,* Saunders, Philadelphia, 1985.

168. Moroi, Y., C. Peebles, M. J. Fritzler, J. Steigerwald, and E. M. Tan: Autoantibodies to centromere (kinetochore) in scleroderma sera, *Proc. Natl. Acad. Sci. USA,* 77:1627, 1980.

169. Kleinsmith, D. M., R. H. Heinzerling, and T. K. Burnham: Antinuclear antibodies as immunologic markers for a benign subset and different characteristics of scleroderma, *Arch. Dermatol.,* 118:882, 1982.

170. Tan, E. M., G. P. Rodman, I. Garcia, Y. Moroi, M. J. Fritzler, and C. Peebles: Diversity of antinuclear antibodies in progressive systemic sclerosis: Anticentromere antibody and its relationship to CREST syndrome, *Arth. Rheum.,* 23:617, 1980.

171. Douvas, A. S., M. Achten, and E. M. Tan: Identification of a nuclear protein (Scl-70) as a unique target of human antinuclear antibodies in scleroderma, *J. Biol. Chem.,* 254:10514, 1979.

172. Salerni, R., G. P. Rodnan, D. F. Leon, and J. S. Shaver: Pulmonary hypertension in the CREST syndrome variant of progressive systemic sclerosis (scleroderma), *Ann. Intern. Med.,* 86:394, 1977.

173. Larlen, J. R., and W. A. Cook: Renal scleroderma and pregnancy, *Obstet. Gynecol.,* 44:349, 1974.

174. Thurm, R. H., and J. C. Alexander: Captopril in the treatment of scleroderma renal crisis, *Arch. Intern. Med.,* 144:733, 1984.

175. Follansbee, W. P.: The cardiovascular manifestations of systemic sclerosis (scleroderma), *Clin. Prob. Cardiol.,* 11:245, 1986.

176. Rodeheffer, R. J., J. A. Rommer, F. Wigley, and C. R. Smith: Controlled double blind trial of nifedipine in the treatment of Raynaud's phenomenon, *N. Engl. J. Med.,* 308:880, 1983.

177. Winkelmann, R. K., R. R. Kierland, H. O. Perry, S. A. Muller, and W. M. Sams, Jr: Management of scleroderma, *Mayo Clin. Proc.,* 46:128, 1971.

178. Lam, M., E. S. Ricanti, M. A. Khan, and I. Kushner: Reversal of severe renal failure in systemic sclerosis, *Ann. Intern. Med.,* 89:642, 1978.

179. Mitnick, P.D., and P. U. Feig: Control of hypertension and reversal of renal failure in scleroderma, *N. Engl. J. Med.,* 299:871, 1978.

180. Smith, C. D., R. D. Smith, and J. H. Korn: Hypertensive crisis in systemic sclerosis: Treatment with the new oral angiotensin converting enzyme inhibitor MK 421 (enalapril) in captopril intolerant patients, *Arth. Rheum.,* 27:826, 1984.

181. Brenner, B. M.: Nephron adaptation to renal injury or ablation, *Am. J. Physiol.,* 249:F324, 1985.

182. Copley, J. B., and B. J. Smith: Continuous ambulatory peritoneal dialysis in scleroderma, *Nephron,* 40:353, 1985.

183. Keane, W. F., B. Danielson, and L. Raij: Successful renal transplantation in progressive systemic sclerosis, *Ann. Intern. Med.,* 85:199, 1976.

184. Merino, G. E., D. E. R. Sutherland, C. M. Kjellstrand, R. L. Simmons, and J. S. Najarian: Renal transplantation for progressive systemic sclerosis with renal failure: Case report and review of previous experience, *Am. J. Surg.,* 133:745, 1977.

185. Paul, M., R. A. Bear, and L. Sugar: Renal transplantation in scleroderma, *J. Rheumatol.,* 11:406, 1984.

186. Vitsky, B. H., Y. Suzuki, L. Strauss, and J. Churg: The hemolytic-uremic syndrome: A study of renal pathologic alterations, *Am. J. Pathol.,* 57:627, 1969.

187. Morel-Maroger, L., A. Kanfer, K. Solez, J. D. Sraer, and G. Richet: Prognostic importance of vascular lesions in acute renal failure with microangiopathic hemolytic anemia (hemolytic-uremic syndrome): Clinicopathologic study in 20 adults, *Kidney Int.,* 15:548, 1979.

188. Neame, P. B., J. Hirsh, G. Browman, J. Denburg, T. J. D'Souza, A. Gallus, and M. C. Brian: Thrombotic thrombocytopenic purpura: A syndrome of

intravascular platelet consumption, *Can. Med. Assoc. J.*, 144:1108, 1976.

189. Amorosi, E. L., and J. E. Ultmann: Thrombotic thrombocytopenic purpura: Report of 16 cases and review of the literature, *Medicine*, 45:139, 1966.

190. Habib, R., M. Levy, M.-F. Gagnadoux, and M. Broyer: Prognosis of the hemolytic uremic syndrome in children, *Adv. Nephrol.*, 11:99, 1982.

191. Hoyer, J. R., A. F. Michael, and L. W. Hoyer: Immunofluorescent localization of antihemophilic factor antigen and fibrinogen in human renal diseases. *J. Clin. Invest.*, 53:1375, 1974.

192. McCoy, R. C., C. R. Abramowsky, and R. Kreuger: The hemolytic uremic syndrome with positive immunofluorescence studies, *J. Pediatr.*, 85:170, 1974.

193. Monnens, L., J. Molenaar, P. H. Lambert, W. Proesmans, and P. Van Munster: The complement system in hemolytic-uremic syndrome in childhood, *Clin. Nephrol.*, 13:168, 1980.

194. Baker, P. J., and S. G. Osofsky: Activation of human complement by heat-killed, human kidney cells grown in cell culture, *J. Immunol.*, 124:81, 1980.

195. Heptinstall, R. H.: *Pathology of the Kidney*, 3d ed., Little, Brown, Boston, 1983, chap. 18.

196. Clarkson, A. R., J. R. Lawrence, R. Meadows, and A. H. Seymour: The haemolytic uremic syndrome in adults, *Q. J. Med.*, 39:227, 1970.

197. Marder, V. J.: Consumptive thrombohemorrhagic disorders, in W. J. Williams, E. Beutler, A. J. Erslev, and M. A. Lichtman (eds.), 3d ed., *Hematology*, McGraw-Hill, New York, 1983, chap. 158.

198. Coleman, R. W., S. J. Robboy, and J. D. Minna: Disseminated intravascular coagulation (DIC): An approach, *Am. J. Med.*, 52:679, 1972.

199. Deykin, D.: The clinical challenge of disseminated intravascular coagulation, *N. Engl. J. Med.*, 283:636, 1970.

200. Talbert, L. M., and P. M. Blatt: Disseminated intravascular coagulation in obstetrics, *Clin. Obstet. Gynecol.*, 2:889, 1979.

201. Harker, L. A., and S. J. Slichter: Platelet and fibrinogen consumption in man, *N. Engl. J. Med.*, 287:999, 1972.

202. Avalos, J. S., M. Vitacco, F. Molinas, J. Penalver, and C. Gianantonio: Coagulation studies in the hemolytic-uremic syndrome, *J. Pediatr.*, 76:538, 1970.

203. Katz, J., A. Luris, F. F. Path, B. S. Kaplan, D. Paed, S. Krawitz, and J. Metz: Coagulation findings in the hemolytic-uremic syndrome of infancy: Similarity to hyperacute renal allograft rejection, *J. Pediatr.*, 78:426, 1971.

204. Jaffee, E. A., R. L. Nachman, and C. Merskey: Thrombotic thrombocytopenic purpura—Coagulation parameters in twelve patients, *Blood*, 42:499, 1973.

205. Gore, I.: Disseminated arteriolar and capillary platelet thrombosis: A morphologic study of its histogenesis, *Am. J. Pathol.*, 26:155, 1950.

206. Drummond, K. N.: Hemolytic-uremic syndrome—then and now, *N. Engl. J. Med.*, 312:116, 1985.

207. Cattell, V.: Mitomycin-induced hemolytic uremic kidney, *Am. J. Pathol.*, 121:88, 1985.

208. Lian, E. C.-Y.: The role of increased platelet aggregation in thrombotic thrombocytopenic purpura, *Sem. Thromb. Hemostasis*, 6:401, 1980.

209. Moake, J. L., C. K. Rudy, J. H. Troll, M. J. Weinstein, N. M. Colannino, J. Azocar, R. H. Seder, S. L. Hong, and D. Deykin: Unusually large plasma factor VIII: von Willebrand factor multimers in chronic relapsing thrombotic thrombocytopenic purpura, *N. Engl. J. Med.*, 307:1432, 1982.

210. Myers, T. J., C. J. Wakem, E. D. Ball, and S. J. Tremont: Thrombotic thrombocytopenic purpura: Combined treatment with plasmapheresis and antiplatelet agents, *Ann. Intern. Med.*, 92:149, 1980.

211. Brandt, J. T., M. S. Kennedy, and D. A. Senhauser: Platelet aggregating factor in TTP (letter), *Lancet*, 2:463, 1979.

212. Byrnes, J. J., and M. Khurana: Treatment of thrombotic thrombocytopenic purpura with plasma, *N. Engl. J. Med.*, 297:1386, 1977.

213. Lian, E. C.-Y., D. R. Harkness, J. J. Byrnes, H. Wallach, and R. Nunez: Presence of a platelet aggregating factor in the plasma of patients with thrombocytopenic purpura (TTP) and its inhibition by normal plasma, *Blood*, 53:333, 1979.

214. Sennett, M. L., and M. E. Conrad: Treatment of thrombotic thrombocytopenic purpura, *Arch. Intern. Med.*, 146:266, 1986.

215. Gutterman, L. A., and T. D. Stevenson: Treatment of thrombotic thrombocytopenic purpura with vincristine, *J. Am. Med. Assoc.*, 247:1433, 1982.

216. Fitzgerald, G. A., R. I. Mass, R. Stein, J. R. Oates, and L. J. Roberts: Intravenous prostacyclin in thrombotic thrombocytopenic purpura, *Ann. Intern. Med.*, 95:319, 1981.

217. Dupperay, A., L. Tranqui, J. L. Alix, M. Manoeurier, and D. Cardonnier: Effect of mitomycin C on the biosynthesis of prostacyclin by primary cultures of human umbilical cord vein endothelial cells (abstract), *Kidney Int.*, 25:730, 1984.

218. Chen, Y. C., E. R. Hall, B. McLeod, and K. K. Wu: Accelerated prostacyclin degradation in thrombotic thrombocytopenic purpura, *Lancet*, 2:267, 1981.

219. Lian, E. C.-Y., P. T. K. Mui, F. A. Siddiqui, A. Chiu, and L. L. S. Chiu: Inhibition of platelet-aggregating activity in thrombotic thrombocytopenic plasma by normal adult immunoglobulin G, *J. Clin. Invest.,* 73:548, 1984.

220. Wong, P., K. Itoh, and S. Yoshida: Treatment of thrombotic thrombocytopenic purpura with intravenous gamma globulin, *N. Engl. J. Med.,* 314:385, 1986.

221. Viero, P., S. Cortelazzo, M. Buelli, B. Comotti, B. Minetti, R. Bassan, and T. Barbui: Thrombotic thrombocytopenic purpura and high-dose immunoglobulin treatment, *Ann. Intern. Med.,* 104:282, 1986.

222. Monnens, L., W. van de Meer, C. Langenhuysen, P. van Munster, and C. van Oostrom: Platelet aggregating factor in the epidemic form of HUS in childhood, *Clin. Nephrol.,* 24:135, 1985.

223. Neill, M. A., J. Agosti, and H. Rosen: Hemorrhagic colitis with *Escherichia coli* 0157:H7 preceding adult HUS, *Arch. Intern. Med.,* 145:2215, 1985.

224. Karmali, M. A., M. Petric, C. Lim, and P. C. Flemming: *Escherichia coli* cytotoxin, haemolytic-uraemic syndrome, and haemorrhagic colitis (letter), *Lancet,* 2:1299, 1983.

225. Koster, F., J. Levin, L. Walker, K. S. K. Tung, R. H. Gilman, M. M. Rahaman, M. A. Majid, S. Islam, and R. C. Williams, Jr.: Hemolytic-uremic syndrome after shigellosis, *N. Engl. J. Med.,* 298:927, 1978.

226. Baker, N. M. A., E. Mills, I. Rachman, and J. E. P. Thomas: Haemolytic-uraemic syndrome in typhoid fever, *Br. Med. J.,* 2:84, 1974.

227. Prober, C. G., B. Tune, and L. Hoder: Yersenia pseudotuberculosis septicemia, *Am. J. Dis. Child,* 133:623, 1979.

228. Chamovitz, B. N., A. Hartstein, S. R. Alexander, A. B. Terry, P. Short, and R. Katon: Campylobacter jejuni-associated hemolytic uremic syndrome in a mother and daughter, *Pediatrics,* 71:253, 1983.

229. Delans, R. J., J. D. Biuso, S. R. Saba, and G. Ramirez: Hemolytic-uremic syndrome after Campylobacter-induced diarrhea in an adult, *Arch. Intern. Med.,* 144:1074, 1984.

230. Austin, T. W., and C. G. Ray: Coxsackie virus group B infection and the hemolytic uremic syndrome, *J. Infect. Dis.,* 127:678, 1973.

231. Robson, J. S., A. M. Martin, V. A. Ruckley, and M. K. MacDonald: Irreversible post-partum renal failure, *Q. J. Med.,* 37:423, 1968.

232. Strauss, R. G., and R. W. Alexander: Post-partum hemolytic uremic syndrome, *Obstet. Gynecol.,* 47:169, 1976.

233. Finkelstein, F. O., M. Kashgarian, and J. P. Hay-slett: Clinical spectrum of postpartum renal failure, *Am. J. Med.,* 57:649, 1974.

234. Hayslett, J. P.: Postpartum renal failure, *N. Engl. J. Med.,* 312:1556, 1985.

235. Brown, C. B., J. S. Robson, D. Thomson, A. R. Clarkson, J. S. Cameron, and C. S. Ogg: Haemolytic uremic syndrome in women taking oral contraceptives, *Lancet,* 1:1479, 1973.

236. Ashouri, O. S., T. C. Marbury, T. J. Fuller, E. Gaffney, W. G. Grubb, and J. R. Cade: Hemolytic-uremic syndrome in two postmenopausal females taking a conjugated estrogen preparation, *Clin. Nephrol.,* 17:212, 1982.

237. Hauglustaine, D., B. van Damme, Y. van Renterghem, and P. Michielsen: Recurrent hemolytic uremic syndrome during oral contraception, *Clin. Nephrol.,* 15:148, 1981.

238. Winn, R., S. Mulgoakar, and M. G. Jacobs: Mitomycin-induced hemolytic-uremic syndrome: Successful treatment with corticosteroids and plasma exchange, *Arch. Intern. Med.,* 143:1617, 1983.

239. Hanner, R. W., R. Verani, and E. J. Weinman: Mitomycin-associated acute renal failure, *Arch. Intern. Med.,* 143:803, 1983.

240. Valavaara, R., and E. Nordman: Renal complications of mitomycin C therapy with special reference to the total dose, *Cancer,* 55:47, 1985.

241. Jackson, A. M., B. D. Rose, L. G. Graff, J. B. Jacobs, J. H. Schwartz, G. M. Strauss, J. P. S. Yang, M. R. Rudnick, I. B. Elfenbein, and R. G. Narins: Thrombotic microangiopathy and renal dysfunction associated with antineoplastic chemotherapy, *Ann. Intern. Med.,* 104:41, 1984.

242. Bull, B. S., and I. N. Kuhn: The production of schistocytes by fibrin strands (a scanning electron microscope study), *Blood,* 35:104, 1970.

243. Giromini, M., and C. Laperrouze: Prolonged survival after bilateral nephrectomy in an adult with hemolytic uraemic syndrome, *Lancet,* 2:169, 1969.

244. Bohle, A., B. Grabensee, R. Fischer, E. Berg, and H. Klust: On 4 cases of HUS without microangiopathy, *Clin. Nephrol.,* 24:88, 1985.

245. Eknoyan, G., and S. A. Riggs: Renal involvement in patients with thrombotic thrombocytopenic purpura, *Am. J. Nephrol.,* 6:117, 1986.

246. Dunea, G., R. C. Muehrcke, S. Nakamoto, and F. D. Schwartz: Thrombotic thrombocytopenic purpura, with acute anuric renal failure, *Am. J. Med.,* 41:1000, 1966.

247. Cameron, J. S., and R. Vick: Plasma C3 in haemolytic-uraemic syndrome and thrombotic thrombocytopenic purpura, *Lancet,* 2:975, 1973.

248. Goldenfarb, P. B., and S. C. Finch: Thrombotic

thrombocytopenic purpura: A ten-year study, *J. Am. Med. Assoc.*, 226:644, 1973.

249. Rossi, E. C., D. Renaldo, and W. H. Barges: Thrombotic thrombocytopenic purpura: Survival following treatment with aspirin, dipyridamole and prednisone, *J. Am. Med. Assoc.*, 228:1141, 1974.

250. Cuttner, J.: Splenectomy, steroids, and dextran 70 in thrombotic thrombocytopenic purpura, *J. Am. Med. Assoc.*, 227:397, 1974.

251. Thompson, H. W., and L. J. McCarthy: Thrombotic thrombocytopenic purpura. Potential benefit of splenectomy after plasma exchange, *Arch. Intern. Med.*, 143:2117, 1983.

252. Zacharski, L. R., C. Walworth, and O. R. McIntyre: Antiplatelet therapy for thrombotic thrombocytopenic purpura, *N. Engl. J. Med.*, 285:408, 1971.

253. Eckel, R. H., E. B. Crowell, Jr., B. E. Waterhouse, and M. J. Bozdeh: Platelet inhibiting drugs in thrombotic thrombocytopenic purpura, *Arch. Intern. Med.*, 137:735, 1977.

254. Myers, T. J., C. J. Wakem, E. D. Ball, and S. J. Tremont: Thrombotic thrombocytopenic purpura: Combined treatment with plasmapheresis and antiplatelet agents, *Ann. Intern. Med.*, 92:149, 1980.

255. Rosove, N.H., W. G. Ho, and D. Goldfinger: Ineffectiveness of aspirin and dipyridamole in the treatment of thrombotic thrombocytopenic purpura, *Ann. Intern. Med.*, 96:27, 1982.

256. Aster, R. H.: Plasma therapy for thrombotic thrombocytopenic purpura, *N. Engl. J. Med.*, 312:985, 1985.

257. Ansell, J., R. S. Beaser, and L. Pechet: Thrombotic thrombocytopenic purpura fails to respond to fresh frozen plasma infusion, *Ann. Intern. Med.*, 89:647, 1978.

258. Bukowski, R. M., J. W. King, and J. S. Hewlett: Plasmapheresis in the treatment of thrombotic thrombocytopenic purpura, *Blood*, 50:413, 1977.

259. Harkness, D. R., J. J. Burnes, E. Lian, W. D. Williams, and G. T. Hensley: Hazard of platelet transfusion in thrombotic thrombocytopenic purpura, *J. Am. Med. Assoc.*, 246:1931, 1981.

260. Bonsib, S. M., L. Ercolani, D. Ngheim, and H. E. Hamilton: Recurrent thrombotic microangiopathy in a renal allograft, *Am. J. Med.*, 79:520, 1985.

261. Lieberman, E.: Haemolytic-uraemic syndrome, *J. Pediatr.*, 80:1, 1972.

262. Gianantonio, C. A., M. Vitacco, F. Mendilahharzu, and G. Gallo: The hemolytic-uremic syndrome: Renal status of 76 patients at long-term follow-up, *J. Pediatr.*, 72:757, 1968.

263. Kaplan, B. S., R. W. Chesney, and K. R. Drumond: Hemolytic-uremic syndrome in families, *N. Engl. J. Med.*, 292:1090, 1975.

264. Ray, C. G., V. L. Tucker, D. J. Harris, F. E. Cuppage, and T. D. Y. Chin: Enteroviruses associated with the hemolytic-uremic syndrome, *Pediatrics*, 46:378, 1970.

265. Mettler, N. E.: Isolation of a microtatobiote from patients with hemolytic-uremic syndrome and thrombotic thrombocytopenic purpura and from mites in the United States, *N. Engl. J. Med.*, 281:1023, 1969.

266. Moorthy, B., and S. P. Makker: Hemolytic-uremic syndrome associated with pneumococal sepsis, *J. Pediatr.*, 95:558, 1979.

267. Dolislager, D., and B. Tune: The hemolytic-uremic syndrome: Spectrum of severity and significance of prodrome, *Am. J. Dis. Child.*, 132:55, 1978.

268. Crisp, D. E., R. L. Siegler, J. F. Bale, and J. A. Thompson: Hemorrhagic cerebral infarction in the hemolytic-uremic syndrome, *J. Pediatr.*, 99:273, 1981.

269. Bale, J. F., C. Brasler, and R. L. Siegler: CNS manifestations of the hemolytic-uremic syndrome, *Am. J. Dis. Child.*, 134:869, 1980.

270. Powell, H. F., R. Rotenberg, A. L. Williams, and D. A. McCredie: Plasma renin activity in acute poststreptococcal glomerulonephritis and the haemolytic-uraemic syndrome, *Arch. Dis. Child.*, 49:802, 1974.

271. Siegler, R., P. L. Berry, and R. J. Hogg: Comparison of the epidemiologic and clinical features of endemic and sporadic forms of hemolytic uremic syndrome (HUS) in 220 USA children. Report of the Southwest Pediatric Nephrology Study Group, (abstract), *Kidney Int.*, 29:204, 1986.

272. Kaplan, B. S., D. Paed, J. Katz, S. Krawitz, and A. Lurie: An analysis of the results of therapy in 67 cases of hemolytic uremic syndrome, *J. Pediatr.*, 78:420, 1971.

273. Tune, B. M., T. J. Leavitt, and T. J. Gribble: The hemolytic-uremic syndrome in California: A review of 28 nonheparinized cases with long-term follow-up, *J. Pediatr.*, 82:304, 1973.

274. Kaplan, B. S., and K. N. Drummond: The hemolytic-uremic syndrome is a syndrome, *N. Engl. J. Med.*, 298:964, 1978.

275. Berry, P. L., R. L. Stiegler, and R. J. Hogg: A multicenter study of the outcome of children with the hemolytic-uremic syndrome (US). Report of the Southwest Pediatric Nephrology Study Group (abstract), *Kidney Int.*, 29:179, 1986.

276. Morris, A. J.: Management of hemolytic-uremic syndrome, *J. Pediatr.*, 81:424, 1972.

277. Taft, E. G., and S. T. Baldwin: Plasma exchange transfusion, *Semin. Thromb. Hemostas.*, 7:15, 1981.

278. Misiani, R., A. C. Appiani, A. Edefonti, E. Gatti, A. Bettinelli, M. Giani, M. Rossi, E. Rossi, F. Remuzzi, and G. Mecca: Haemolytic uraemic syndrome: Therapeutic effect of plasma infusion, *Br. Med. J.*, 285:1304, 1982.

279. Upadhyaya, K., K. Barwick, M. Fishaut, M. Kashgarian, and N. J. Siegel: The importance of nonrenal involvement in hemolytic-uremic syndrome, *Pediatrics*, 65:115, 1980.

280. Arenson, E. B., Jr., and C. S. August: Preliminary report: Treatment of the hemolytic-uremic syndrome with aspirin and dipyridamole, *J. Pediatr.*, 86:957, 1975.

281. O'Regan, S., R. W. Chesney, J.-G. Mongeau, and P. Robitaille: Aspirin and dipyridamole therapy in the hemolytic-uremic syndrome, *J. Pediatr.*, 97:473, 1980.

282. Beattie, T. J., A. V. Murphy, and M. L. N. Willoughby: Prolonged prostacyclin infusion in haemolytic uraemic syndrome in children, *Br. Med. J.*, 283:470, 1981.

283. Hebert, D., R. K. Sibley, and S. M. Mauer: Recurrence of hemolytic-uremic syndrome in renal transplant recipients, *Kidney Int.*, 30(suppl.):S-51, 1986.

284. Leithner, C., H. Sinzinger, E. Pohanka, M. Schwartz, G. Kretschemer, and G. Syre: Recurrence of haemolytic uraemic syndrome triggered by cyclosporine A after renal transplantation (letter), *Lancet*, 2:1470, 1982.

285. Karlsberg, R. P., J. W. Lacher, and C. E. Bartecchi: Adult hemolytic-uremic syndrome: Familial variant, *Arch. Intern. Med.*, 137:1155, 1977.

286. Laffay, D. L., R. R. Tubbs, M. D. Valenzuela, P. M. Hall, and L. J. McCormack: Chronic glomerular microangiopathy and metastatic carcinoma, *Hum. Pathol.*, 10:433, 1979.

287. Doll, D., A. F. List, A. Greco, J. D. Hainsworth, K. R. Hande, and D. H. Johnson: Acute vascular ischemic events after cisplatin-based combination chemotherapy for germ-cell tumors of the testis. *Ann. Intern. Med.*, 105:48, 1986.

288. Wolfe, J. A., R. L. McCann, and F. Sanfilippo: Cyclosporine-associated microangiopathy in renal transplantation: A severe but potentially reversible form of early graft injury, *Transplantation*, 41:541, 1986.

289. Shulman, H., G. Striker, H. J. Deeg, M. Kennedy, R. Storb, and E. D. Thomas: Nephrotoxicity of cyclosporin A after allogeneic marrow transplantation: Glomerular thrombosis and tubular injury, *N. Engl. J. Med.*, 305:1392, 1981.

290. Hows, J. M., P. M. Chipping, S. Fairhead, J. Smith, A. Baughan, and E. C. Gordon-Smith: Nephrotoxicity in bone marrow transplant recipients with cyclosporin A, *Br. J. Haematol.*, 54:69, 1983.

291. Atkinson, K., J. C. Biggs, J. Hayes, M. Ralston, A. J. Dodds, A. J. Concannon, and D. Naidos: Cyclosporin A associated nephrotoxicity in the first 100 days after allogeneic bone marrow transplantation: Three distinct syndromes, *Br. J. Haematol.*, 54:59, 1983.

292. Kohler, T. R., and N. L. Tilney: Microangiopathic hemolytic anemia associated with hyperacute rejection of a kidney allograft, *Transplant Proc.*, 14:444, 1982.

293. Date, A., R. Pulimood, C. K. Jacob, M. D. Kirubakaran, and J. C. M. Shastry: Haemolytic-uraemic syndrome complicating a snake bite, *Nephron*, 42:89, 1986.

294. Ponticelli, C., E. Rivolta, E. Imbasciati, E. Rossi, and P. M. Mannucci: Hemolytic uremic syndrome in adults, *Arch. Intern. Med.*, 140:353, 1980.

295. Cattran, D. C.: Adult hemolytic-uremic syndrome: Successful treatment with plasmapheresis, *Am. J. Kid. Dis.*, 3:275, 1984.

296. Chow, S., J. Roscoe, and D. C. Cattran: Plasmapheresis and antiplatelet agents in the treatment of the hemolytic uremic syndrome secondary to mitomycin, *Am. J. Kid. Dis.*, 7:407, 1986.

297. Winn, R., S. Mulgoakar, and M. G. Jacobs: Mitomycin-induced hemolytic-uremic syndrome: Successful treatment with corticosteroids and plasma exchange, *Arch. Intern. Med.*, 143:1617, 1983.

298. Gutterman, L. A., D. M. Levin, and B. S. George: The hemolytic-uremic syndrome: Recovery after treatment with vincristine, *Ann. Intern. Med.*, 98:612, 1983.

299. Grem, J. L., J. A. Merritt, and P. P. Carbone: Treatment of mitomycin-associated microangiopathic hemolytic anemia with vincristine, *Arch. Intern. Med.*, 146:566, 1986.

300. Verwey, J., E. Boven, J. van der Menlen, and H. M. Pinedo: Recovery from mitomycin C-induced hemolytic uremic syndrome, *Cancer*, 54:2878, 1984.

301. Giromini, M., C. A. Bouvier, R. Dami, M. Denizot, and M. Jeaknet: Effect of dipyridamole and aspirin in thrombotic microangiopathy, *Br. Med. J.*, 1:545, 1973.

302. Luke, R. G., W. Talbert, R. R. Siegel, and N. Holland: Heparin treatment for postpartum renal failure with microangiopathic hemolytic anaemia, *Lancet*, 2:750, 1970.

303. Ponticelli, C., E. Imbasciati, A. Farantino, and G. Graziano: Postpartum renal failure with microangiopathic haemolytic anemia, *Lancet*, 2:1034, 1970.

304. Arias-Rodrigues, M., J.-D. Sraer, O. Kowilsky, M. D. Smith, P. J. Veroust, A. Meyrier, H. Kuntziger, A. Kanfer, V. Neissim, G. Neuilly, L. Morel-Maroger, and G. Richet: Renal transplantation and immunologic abnormalities in thrombotic microangiopathy of adults, *Transplantation,* 23:360, 1977.

305. Hamilton, D. V., R. Y. Calne, and D. B. Evans: Haemolytic-uraemic syndrome and cyclosporin A (letter), *Lancet,* 2:151, 1982.

306. Walters, W. A. W., W. G. McGregor, and M. Hills: Cardiac output at rest during pregnancy and the puerperium, *Clin. Sci.,* 30:1, 1966.

307. Atherton, J. C., and R. Green: Renal function in pregnancy, *Clin. Sci.,* 65:449, 1983.

308. Lindheimer, M. D., and A. I. Katz: Sodium and diuretics in pregnancy, *N. Engl. J. Med.,* 288:891, 1973.

309. Lindheimer, M. D., and A. I. Katz: The kidney in pregnancy, in B. M. Brenner and F. C. Rector (eds.), *The Kidney,* 3d ed., Saunders, Philadelphia, 1986.

310. Davison, J. M., E. A. Gilmore, J. Durr, G. L. Robertson, and M. D. Lindheimer: Altered osmotic threshold for vasopressin secretion and thirst in human pregnancy, *Am. J. Physiol.,* 246:F105, 1984.

311. Kristensen, C. G., Y. Nakagawa, F. L. Coe, and M. D. Lindheimer: Effect of atrial natriuretic factor in rat pregnancy, *Am. J. Physiol.,* 250:R589, 1986.

312. Gant, N. F., G. L. Daley, S. Chand, P. J. Whalley, and P. C. MacDonald: A study of angiotensin II pressor response through primigravid pregnancy, *J. Clin. Invest.,* 52:2682, 1973.

313. Gant, N. F., R. J. Worley, R. Everett, and P. C. MacDonald: Control of vascular responsiveness during human pregnancy, *Kidney Int.,* 18:255, 1980.

314. Natrajan, P. G., H. H. G. McGarrigle, D. M. Lawrence, and G. C. L. Lachelin: Plasma noradrenaline and adrenaline levels in normal pregnancy and in pregnancy-induced hypertension, *Br. J. Obstet. Gynaecol.,* 89:1041, 1982.

315. Paller, M. S.: Mechanism of decreased pressor responsiveness to angiotensin II, norepinephrine, and vasopressin in the conscious pregnant cat, *Am. J. Physiol.,* 247:H100, 1984.

316. Walsh, S. W.: Preeclampsia: An imbalance in placental thromboxane production, *Am. J. Obstet. Gynecol.,* 152:335, 1985.

317. Magness, R. R., O. Kwabena, M. D. Mitchell, and C. R. Rosenfeld: In vitro prostacyclin production by uterine and systemic arteries, *J. Clin. Invest.,* 76:2206, 1985.

318. Everett, R. B., R. J. Worley, P. C. MacDonald, and N. F. Gant: Effect of prostaglandin synthetase inhibitors on pressor responsiveness to angiotensin

319. Cain, M. D., W. A. Walters, and K. J. Catt: Effects of oral contraceptive therapy on the renin-angiotensin system, *J. Clin. Endocrinol. Metab.,* 33:671, 1971.

320. Ferris, T. F.: The kidney and pregnancy, in L. E. Earley and C. W. Gottschalk (eds.), *Strauss and Welt's Diseases of the Kidney,* 3d ed., Little, Brown, Boston, 1979.

321. Ferris, T. F., J. H. Stein, and J. Kaufman: Uterine blood flow and uterine renin secretion, *J. Clin. Invest.,* 51:2827, 1972.

322. Weir, R. J., R. Fraser, A. F. Lever, J. J. Morton, J. J. Brown, A. Kraszewski, G. G. McIlwaine, J. I. S. Robertson, and M. Tree: Plasma renin, renin substrate, angiotensin II, and aldosterone in hypertensive disease of pregnancy, *Lancet,* 1:291, 1973.

323. Ferris, T. F., and E. K. Weir: Effects of captopril on uterine blood flow and prostaglandin E synthesis in the pregnant rabbit, *J. Clin. Invest.,* 71:809, 1983.

324. Davison, J. M., and M. C. B. Hoble: Serial changes in 24-hour creatinine clearance during normal menstrual cycles and the first trimester of pregnancy, *Br. J. Obstet. Gynaecol.,* 87:108, 1980.

325. Davison, J. M., W. Dunlop, and M. Ezimokhai: 24-hour creatinine clearances during the third trimester of normal pregnancy, *Br. J. Obstet. Gynaecol.,* 87:108, 1980.

326. Davison, J. M., and W. Dunlop: Renal haemodynamics and tubular function in normal human pregnancy, *Kidney Int.,* 18:152, 1980.

327. Dunlop, W.: Serial changes in renal haemodynamics during normal human pregnancy, *Br. J. Obstet. Gynaecol.,* 88:1, 1981.

328. Lim, V. S., A. I. Katz, and M. D. Lindheimer: Acid-base regulation in pregnancy, *Am. J. Physiol.,* 231:1764, 1976.

329. Lindheimer, M. D., and A. I. Katz: Hypertension in pregnancy, *N. Engl. J. Med.,* 313:675, 1985.

330. Pollak, V. E., and J. B. Nettles: The kidney in toxemia of pregnancy: A clinical and pathologic study based on renal biopsies, *Medicine,* 39:469, 1960.

331. Mautner, W., J. Churg, E. Grishman, and S. Dachs: Preeclamptic nephropathy: An electron microscopic study, *Lab. Invest.,* 11:518, 1962.

332. Vassali, R., R. H. Morris, and R. T. McCluskey: The pathogenic role of fibrin deposition in the glomerular lesions of toxemia of pregnancy, *J. Exp. Med.,* 118:467, 1963.

333. Heptinstall, R. H.: *Pathology of the Kidney,* 3d ed. Little, Brown, Boston, 1983, chap. 19.

334. Petrucco, O. M., N. M. Thompson, R. F. Lawrence,

and M. W. Weldon: Immunofluorescent studies in renal biopsies in preeclampsia, *Br. Med. J.,* 1:473, 1974.

335. Lindheimer, M. D., and A. I. Katz: *Renal Function and Disease in Pregnancy,* Lea & Febiger, Philadelphia, 1977.

336. McKay, D. G.: Clinical significance of the pathology of toxemia of pregnancy, *Circulation,* 30(suppl2):66, 1964.

337. Kitzmiller, J. L., and K. Benirschke: Immunofluorescent study of placental bed vessels in preeclampsia of pregnancy, *Am. J. Obstet. Gynecol.,* 115: 248, 1973.

338. Arias, F., and R. Mancilla-Jimenez: Hepatic fibrinogen deposits in pre-eclampsia: Immunofluorescent evidence, *N. Engl. J. Med.,* 295:578, 1976.

339. Cavanaugh, D., P. S. Rao, C. C. Tsai, and T. C. O'Connor: Experimental toxemia in the pregnant primate, *Am. J. Obstet. Gynecol.,* 128:75, 1977.

340. Abitbol, M. M., W. B. Ober, G. R. Gallo, S. G. Driscoll, and C. L. Pirani: Experimental toxemia of pregnancy in the monkey, with preliminary report on renin and aldosterone, *Am. J. Pathol.,* 86:573, 1977.

341. Gant, N. F., H. T. Hutchinson, P. K. Siiteri, and P. C. MacDonald: Study of the metabolic clearance rate of dehydroisoandrosterone sulfate in pregnancy, *Am. J. Obstet. Gynecol.,* 111:555, 1971.

342. Gant, N. F., Madden, J. D., P. K. Siiteri, and P. C. MacDonald: The metabolic clearance rate of dehydroisoandrosterone sulfate. IV. Acute effects of induced hypertension, and natriuresis in normal and hypertensive pregnancies, *Am. J. Obstet. Gynecol.,* 124:143, 1976.

343. Lunell, N. O., L. E. Nylund, R. Lewander, and B. Sarby: Uteroplacental blood flow in preeclampsia: Measurements with indium-113 and a computer-linked gamma camera, *Clin. Exp. Hypertens.,* 1: 105, 1982.

344. Becher, J. C.: Aetiology of eclampsia, *J. Obstet. Gynaecol. Br. Common.,* 55:746, 1948.

345. Frolich, J. C., and T. W. Wilson: Urinary prostaglandins: Identification and origin, *J. Clin. Invest.,* 55:763, 1975.

346. Bay, W. H., and T. F. Ferris: Factors controlling plasma renin and aldosterone during pregnancy, *Hypertension,* 1:410, 1979.

347. Paller, M. S., and T. F. Ferris: Prolactin, prostaglandins and pressor responsiveness to angiotensin II in pregnancy (abstract), *Hypertension,* 8:821, 1986.

348. Editorial: Prostaglandin synthesis inhibitors in obstetrics and after, *Lancet,* 2:185, 1980.

349. Downing, I., G. L. Shepherd, and P. J. Lewis: Reduced prostacyclin production in preeclampsia, *Lancet,* 1:442, 1981.

350. Pedersen, E. B., P. Christensen, N. J. Christensen, P. Johannsen, H. J. Korherup, S. Kristensen, J. G. Lauritsen, P. P. Leyssac, A. B. Rasmussen, and M. Wohlert: Prostaglandins, renin, aldosterone and catecholamines in preeclampsia, *Acta. Med. Scand.,* (suppl) 677:40, 1983.

351. Goodman, R. P., A. P. Killam, A. R. Brash, and R. A. Branch: Prostacyclin production during pregnancy: Comparison of production during normal pregnancy and pregnancy complicated by hypertension, *Am. J. Obstet. Gynecol.,* 142:817, 1982.

352. Gerber, J. G., N. A. Payne, and R. C. Murphy: Prostacyclin in pregnant human uterus, *Prostaglandins,* 17:113, 1979.

353. Makila, U.-M., L. Vinikka, and O. Ylikorkala: Increased thromboxane A$_2$ production but normal prostacyclin by the placenta in hypertensive pregnancies, *Prostaglandins,* 27:87, 1984.

354. Beaufils, M., S. Uzan, R. Donsimoni, and J. C. Colau: Prevention of pre-eclampsia by early antiplatelet therapy, *Lancet,* 1:840, 1985.

355. Wallenburg, H. C. S., J. W. Makovitz, G. A. Dekker, and P. Rotmans: Low-dose aspirin prevents pregnancy-induced hypertension and pre-eclampsia in angiotensin-sensitive primigravidae, *Lancet,* 1:1, 1986.

356. Vassali, P., G. Simon, and C. Rouiller: Production of ultrastructural glomerular lesions resembling those of toxaemia of pregnancy by thromboplastin infusion in rabbits, *Nature,* 199:1105, 1963.

357. Redman, C. W. G., K. W. E. Denson, L. J. Beilin, F. G. Bolton, and G. M. Stirrat: Factor VIII consumption in preeclampsia, *Lancet,* 2:1249, 1977.

358. Socol, M. L., C. P. Weiner, G. Louis, K. Rehnberg, and E. C. Rossi: Platelet activation in preeclampsia, *Am. J. Obstet. Gynecol.,* 151:494, 1985.

359. Redman, C. W. G., J. Bonnar, and L. Beilin: Early platelet consumption in preeclampsia, *Br. Med. J.,* 1:467, 1978.

360. Sraer, J. D., F. Delarue, S. Dard, R. de Seigneux, L. Morel-Maroger, and A. Kanfer: Glomerular fibrinolytic activity after thrombin perfusion in the rat. *Lab. Invest.,* 32:515, 1985.

361. Epstein, M. D., F. K. Beller, and G. W. Douglas: Kidney tissue activator of fibrinolysis in relation to pregnancy, *Obstet. Gynecol.,* 32:494, 1968.

362. Need, J. A.: Preeclampsia in pregnancies by different fathers: Immunological studies, *Br. Med. J.,* 1: 548, 1975.

363. Sinha, D., M. Wells, and W. P. Faulk: Immuno-

logic studies of human placentae: Complement components in preeclamptic chorionic villi, *Clin. Exp. Immunol.,* 56:175, 1984.

364. Moutquin, J. M., C. Rainville, L. Giroux, P. Raynauld, G. Amyot, R. Bilodeau, and N. Pelland: A prospective study of blood pressure in pregnancy: Prediction of preeclampsia, *Am. J. Obstet. Gynecol.,* 151:191, 1985.

365. Weinstein, L.: Syndrome of hemolysis, elevated liver enzymes, and low platelet count: A severe consequence of hypertension in pregnancy, *Am. J. Obstet. Gynecol.,* 142:159, 1982.

366. Wagnild, J. P., and F. D. Gutmann: Functional adaptation of nephrons in dogs with acute progressing to chronic glomerulonephritis, *J. Clin. Invest.,* 57:1575, 1976.

367. Kokko, J. P.: Effect of prostaglandins on renal epithelial electrolyte transport, *Kidney Int.,* 19:791, 1981.

368. Fadel, H. E., G. Northrop, and H. R. Misenhimer: Hyperuricemia in pre-eclampsia: A reappraisal, *Am. J. Obstet. Gynecol.,* 125:640, 1976.

369. Weinman, E. G., G. Eknoyan, and W. N. Suko: The influence of the extracellular fluid volume on the tubular reabsorption of uric acid, *J. Clin. Invest.,* 55:283, 1975.

370. Pritchard, J. A., F. G. Cunningham, and R. A. Mason: Coagulation changes in eclampsia: Their frequency and pathogenesis, *Am. J. Obstet. Gynecol.,* 124:855, 1976.

371. Dunlop, W., L. M. Hill, M. J. Landon, A. Oxley, and P. Jones: Clinical relevance of coagulation and renal changes in preeclampsia, *Lancet,* 2:346, 1978.

372. Beecham, J. B., W. J. Watson, and J. F. Clapp, III: Eclampsia, preeclampsia, and disseminated intravascular coagulation, *Obstet. Gynecol.,* 43:576, 1974.

373. McKay, D.: Hematologic evidence of disseminated intravascular coagulation in eclampsia, *Obstet. Gynecol. Survey,* 27:399, 1972.

374. Fisher, K. A., A. Luger, B. H. Spargo, and M. D. Lindheimer: Hypertension in pregnancy: Clinical-pathological correlations and late prognosis, *Medicine,* 60:267, 1981.

375. Oney, T., and H. Kaulhausen: The value of the angiotensin sensitivity test in the early diagnosis of hypertensive disorders in pregnancy, *Am. J. Obstet. Gynecol.,* 142:17, 1982.

376. Page, E. W. and R. Christianson: The impact of mean arterial pressure in the middle trimester upon the outcome of pregnancy, *Am. J. Obstet. Gynecol.,* 125:740, 1976.

377. Gant, N. F., S. Chand, R. J. Worley, P. J. Shalley, U. D. Crosby, and P. C. MacDonald: A clinical test useful for predicting the development of acute hypertension in pregnancy, *Am. J. Obstet. Gynecol.,* 120:1, 1974.

378. Gant, N. F., R. J. Worley, F. G. Cunningham, and P. J. Whalley: Clinical management of pregnancy-induced hypertension, *Clin. Obstet. Gynecol.,* 21:397, 1978.

379. Lazarchick, J., T. M. Stubbs, L. Romein, J. P. van Dorsten, and C. B. Loadholt: Predictive value of fibronectin levels in normotensive gravid women destined to become preeclamptic, *Am. J. Obstet. Gynecol.,* 154:1050, 1986.

380. Stubbs, T. M., J. Lazarchick, and E. O. Horger: Plasma fibronectin levels in preeclampsia: A possible biochemical marker for vascular endothelial damage, *Am. J. Obstet. Gynecol.,* 150:885, 1984.

381. Wickens, D., M. H. Wilkens, J. Lunec, G. Ball, and T. L. Dormandy: Free-radical oxidation (peroxidation) products in plasma in normal and abnormal pregnancy, *Ann. Clin. Biochem.,* 18:158, 1981.

382. Erskine, K. J., S. A. Iversen, and R. Davies: An altered ratio of 18:2 (9,11) to 18:2 (9,12) linoleic acid in plasma phospholipids as a possible predictor of preeclampsia, *Lancet,* 1:554, 1985.

383. Adams, E. M., and I. MacGillivray: Long-term effect of pre-eclampsia on blood pressure, *Lancet,* 2:1373, 1961.

384. Fay, R. A., D. R. Bromham, J. A. Brooks, and V. J. Debski: Platelets and uric acid in the prediction of preeclampsia, *Am. J. Obstet. Gynecol.,* 152:1038, 1985.

385. Chesley, L. C.: *Hypertensive Disorders in Pregnancy,* Appleton-Century-Crofts, New York, 1978.

386. Ober, W. E., D. E. Reid, S. L. Romney, and J. P. Merrill: Renal lesions and acute renal failure in pregnancy, *Am. J. Med.,* 21:781, 1956.

387. Smith, K., J. C. M. Browne, R. Shackman, and O. M. Wong: Acute renal failure of obstetric origin: An analysis of 70 patients, *Lancet,* 2:351, 1965.

388. Fried, A. M.: Hydronephrosis of pregnancy: Ultrasonographic study and classification of asymptomatic women, *Am. J. Obstet. Gynecol.,* 135:1066, 1979.

389. Homans, D. C., G. D. Blake, J. T. Harrington, and C. L. Cetrulo: Acute renal failure caused by ureteral obstruction by a gravid uterus, *J. Am. Med. Assoc.,* 246:1230, 1981.

390. Chesley, L. C.: Diagnosis of preeclampsia, *Obstet. Gynecol.,* 65:423, 1985.

391. Perkins, R. P.: The conservative management of toxemia: A brief report of effective perinatal concepts, *Obstet. Gynecol.,* 49:498, 1977.

392. Harvey, D., C. E. Parkinson, and S. Campbell: Risk of respiratory-distress syndrome, *Lancet*, 1:42, 1975.

393. Lamont, R. F., P. D. M. Dunlop, M. I. Levene, and M. G. Elder: Use of glucocorticoids in pregnancies complicated by severe hypertension and proteinuria, *Br. J. Obstet. Gynaecol.*, 90:199, 1983.

394. Sullivan, J. M.: *Hypertension and Pregnancy*, Year Book, Chicago, 1986, chap. 8.

395. Friedman, E. A., and R. K. Neff: Hypertension and hypotension in pregnancy, correlation with fetal outcome, *J. Am. Med. Assoc.*, 239:2249, 1978.

396. Page, E. W., and R. Christianson: The impact of mean arterial pressure in the middle trimester upon the outcome of pregnancy, *Am. J. Obstet. Gynecol.*, 125:740, 1976.

397. Feitelson, P. J., and M. D. Lindheimer: Management of hypertensive gravidas, *J. Reprod. Med.*, 8:111, 1972.

398. Sabai, B. M., T. N. Abdella, and G. D. Anderson: Pregnancy outcome in 211 patients with mild chronic hypertension, *Obstet. Gynecol.*, 61:571, 1983.

399. Cunningham, F. G., and J. S. Pritchard: How should hypertension during pregnancy be managed? Experience at Parkland Memorial Hospital, *Med. Clin. N. Am.*, 68:505, 1984.

400. Redman, C. W. G.: The management of hypertension in pregnancy, *Sem. Nephrol.*, 4:270, 1984.

401. Chesley, L. C.: Plasma and red cell volumes during pregnancy, *Am. J. Obstet. Gynecol.*, 112:440, 1972.

402. Gallery, E. D. M., S. M. Hunyor, and A. Z. Gyorty: Plasma volume concentration: A significant factor in both pregnancy-associated hypertension (preeclampsia) and chronic hypertension in pregnancy, *Q. J. Med.*, 48:593, 1979.

403. Perkins, R. P.: The conservative management of toxemia: A brief report of effective perinatal concepts, *Obstet. Gynecol.*, 49:498, 1977.

404. Hays, P. M., D. P. Cruikshank, and L. J. Dunn: Plasma volume determinants in normal and preeclamptic pregnancies, *Am. J. Obstet. Gynecol.*, 151:958, 1985.

405. Walters, B. N. J., and C. W. G. Redman: Treatment of severe pregnancy associated hypertension with the calcium antagonist nifedipine, *Br. J. Obstet. Gynaecol.*, 91:330, 1984.

406. Dudley, D. K. L.: Minibolus diazoxide in the management of severe hypertension in pregnancy, *Am. J. Obstet. Gynecol.*, 151:196, 1985.

407. Pipkin, F. B., S. R. Turner, and E. M. Symonds: Possible risk with captopril in pregnancy: Some animal data (letter), *Lancet*, 1:1256, 1980.

408. Turner, G., and E. Collins: Fetal effects of regular salicylate ingestion in pregnancy, *Lancet*, 2:338, 1975.

409. Chesley, L. C., J. E. Annitto, and R. A. Cosgrave: The remote prognosis of eclamptic women, *Am. J. Obstet. Gynecol.*, 124:446, 1976.

410. Bryans, C. I., Jr., W. L. Southerland, and F. P. Zuspan: Eclampsia: A long-term follow-up study, *Obstet. Gynecol.*, 21:701, 1963.

411. MacGillivray, I.: Some observations on the incidence of pre-eclampsia, *J. Obstet. Gynaecol. Br. Common.*, 65:536, 1958.

412. Schenker, J. G., and M. Granat: Pheochromocytoma and pregnancy: An updated appraisal, *Aust. N.Z. J. Obstet. Gynecol.*, 22:1, 1982.

413. Katz, A. I., J. M. Davison, J. P. Hayslett, E. Singoon, and M. D. Lindheimer: Pregnancy in women with kidney disease, *Kidney Int.*, 18:192, 1980.

414. Strauch, B. S., and J. P. Hayslett: Kidney disease and pregnancy, *Br. Med. J.*, 4:578, 1974.

415. Surian, M., E. Imbasciati, and P. Cosci: Glomerular disease and pregnancy: A study of 123 pregnancies in patients with primary and secondary glomerular diseases, *Nephron*, 36:101, 1984.

416. Hayslett, J. P.: Pregnancy does not exacerbate primary glomerular disease, *Am. J. Kid. Dis.*, 6:273, 1985.

417. Imbasciati, E., G. Pardi, P. Capetta, G. Ambroso, P. Bozzetti, B. Pagiari, and C. Ponticelli: Pregnancy in women with chronic renal failure, *Am. J. Nephrol.*, 6:193, 1986.

418. Hou, S. H.: Pregnancy in women with chronic renal disease, *N. Engl. J. Med.*, 312:836, 1985.

419. Baylis, C., and H. G. Rennke: Repetitive pregnancy: A physiologic model of hyperfiltration? (abstract), *Clin. Res.* 32:441a, 1984.

420. Becker, G. J., K. F. Fairley, and J. A. Whitworth: Pregnancy exacerbates glomerular disease, *Am. J. Kid. Dis.*, 6:266, 1985.

421. Rovati, C., M. C. Perrino, and G. Barbianodi-Belgiogoso: Pregnancy and the course of primary glomerular disease, *Contrib. Nephrol.*, 37:182, 1984.

422. Katz, A. I., and M. D. Lindheimer: Does pregnancy aggravate primary glomerular disease?, *Am. J. Kid. Dis.*, 6:261, 1985.

423. Hadi, H.: Pregnancy in renal transplant recipients: A review, *Obstet. Gynecol. Survey*, 41:264, 1986.

424. Rifle, G., and J. Traeger: Pregnancy after renal transplantation. An international review, *Transplant Proc.*, 7:723, 1975.

425. Wells, J. D., E. G. Margolin, and E. A. Gall: Renal cortical necrosis: Clinical and pathologic features in twenty-one cases, *Am. J. Med.*, 29:257, 1960.

426. Kleinknecht, D., J. P. Grunfeld, P. C. Gomez, J. F. Moreau, and R. Garcia-Torres: Diagnostic procedures and long-term prognosis in bilateral renal cortical necrosis, *Kidney Int.*, 4:390, 1973.

427. Matlin, R. A., and N. E. Gary: Acute cortical necrosis: Case report and review of literature, *Am. J. Med.*, 56:110, 1974.
428. Renal pathology forum: *Am. J. Nephrol.*, 5:305, 1985.
429. Heptinstall, R. H.: *Pathology of the Kidney*, 3d ed., Little, Brown, Boston, 1983, chap. 21.
430. McKay, D. G., S. J. Merrill, A. E. Weiner, A. T. Hertig, and D. E. Reid: The pathologic anatomy of eclampsia, bilateral renal cortical necrosis and other acute fatal complications of pregnancy and its possible relationship to the generalized Shwartzman phenomenon, *Am. J. Obstet. Gynecol.*, 66:507, 1953.
431. Conger, J. D., S. Falk, and S. J. Guggenheim: Glomerular dynamics and morphologic changes in the generalized Shwartzman reaction in postpartum rats, *J. Clin. Invest.*, 67:1334, 1981.
432. Sheehan, H. L., and J. C. Davis: Renal ischaemia with failed reflow, *J. Path. Bacteriol.*, 78:105, 1959.
433. Lauler, D. P., and G. E. Schreiner: Bilateral renal cortical necrosis, *Am. J. Med.*, 24:519, 1958.
434. Sefczek, R. J., I. Beckman, A. R. Lupetin, and N. Dash: Sonography of acute renal cortical necrosis, *Am. J. Roentgenol.*, 142:553, 1984.
435. Georgen, T. G., R. R. Lindstrom, H. Tan, and J. J. Lilley: CT appearance of acute renal cortical necrosis, *Am. J. Roentgenol.*, 137:176, 1981.
436. Smith, L. E., and R. D. Adelman: Early detection of renal calcification in acute renal cortical necrosis in a child, *Nephron*, 29:155, 1981.
437. Gelfand, M. C., and E. A. Friedman: Prognosis of renal allotransplants in patients with bilateral renal cortical necrosis, *Transplantation*, 10:442, 1970.
438. Hoxie, H. J., and C. B. Coggin: Renal infarction: Statistical study of two hundred and five cases and detailed report of an unusual case, *Arch. Intern. Med.*, 65:587, 1940.
439. Peterson, N. E., and D. F. McDonald: Renal embolization, *J. Urol.*, 100:140, 1968.
440. Lessman, R. K., S. F. Johnson, J. W. Coburn, and J. J. Kaufman: Renal artery embolism: Clinical features and long-term follow-up of 17 cases, *Ann. Intern. Med.*, 89:477, 1978.
441. Brachen, R. B., D. E. Johnson, H. M. Goldstein, S. Wallace, and A. G. Ayala: Percutaneous transfemoral renal artery occlusion in patients with renal carcinoma: Preliminary report, *Urology*, 6:6, 1975.
442. Cosby, R. L., P. D. Miller, and R. W. Schrier: Traumatic renal artery thrombosis, *Am. J. Med.*, 81:890, 1986.
443. Heptinstall, R. H., *Pathology of the Kidney*, 3d ed., Little, Brown, Boston, 1983, chap. 21.
444. Kassirer, J. P.: Thrombosis and embolization of the renal vessels, in L. E. Earley and C. W. Gottschalk

(eds.), *Strauss and Welt's Diseases of the Kidney*, 3d ed., Little, Brown, Boston, 1979.
445. Hoffman, R. M., K. W. Stieper, R. W. Johnson, and F. O. Belzer: Renal ischemic tolerance, *Arch. Surg.*, 109:550, 1974.
446. Myers, B. D., C. Miller, J. T. Mehigan, C. Olcott, IV, H. Golbetz, C. R. Robertson, R. Spencer, and S. Friedman: Nature of the renal injury following total renal ischemia in man, *J. Clin. Invest.*, 73:329, 1984.
447. Morris, G. C., Jr., C. F. Heider, and J. H. Moyer: The protective effect of subfiltration arterial pressure on the kidney, *Surg. Forum*, 6:623, 1955.
448. Brezis, M., S. Rosen, P. Silva, and F. H. Epstein: Renal ischemia: A new perspective, *Kidney Int.*, 26:375, 1984.
449. Schrimer, H. K. A.: The effect of intermittent and prolonged renal artery occlusion upon respiration and anaerobic glycolysis of dog kidney, *J. Urol.*, 94:511, 1965.
450. London, I. L., P. Hoffster, G. T. Perkoff, and T. G. Pennington: Renal infarction: Elevation of serum and urinary lactate dehydrogenase (LDH), *Arch. Intern. Med.*, 121:87, 1968.
451. Winzelberg, G. G., J. D. Hull, J. W. M. Agar, B. D. Rose, and P. G. Pletka: Elevation of serum lactate dehydrogenase levels in renal infarction, *J. Am. Med. Assoc.*, 242:268, 1979.
452. Anderson, C. B., M. A. Groce, R. N. Mohapatra, J. E. Codd, R. J. Graff, J. G. Gregory, and W. T. Newton: Serum lactic dehydrogenase and irreversible renal allograft rejection, *Surgery*, 79:161, 1976.
453. Janower, M. L., and A. L. Weber: Radiologic evaluation of acute renal infarction, *Am. J. Roentgenol. Radium Ther. Nucl. Med.*, 95:309, 1965.
454. Brest, A. N., R. Bower, and C. Heider: Renal functional recovery following anuria secondary to renal artery embolism *J. Am. Med. Assoc.*, 187:540, 1964.
455. Moyer, J. D., C. N. Rao, W. C. Wildrich, and C. A. Olson: Conservative management of renal artery embolus, *J. Urol.*, 109:138, 1973.
456. San Felippo, C. J., and A. Golden: Intra-arterial streptokinase and renal artery embolism, *Urology*, 11:62, 1978.
457. Fisher, C. P., J. W. Konnak, K. J. Cho, F. E. Eckhauser, and J. C. Stanley: Renal artery embolism: Therapy with intra-arterial streptokinase infusion, *J. Urol.*, 125:402, 1981.
458. Dhar, S. K., M. Konowitz, G. Fitzgerald, and J. W. Cristee: Acute oliguric renal failure due to bilateral renal artery emboli: Thrombolysis with intra-arterial streptokinase infusion, *J. Indiana State Med. Assoc.*, 75:802, 1982.
459. Steckel, A., J. Johnston, D. S. Fraley, F. J. Bruns,

D. P. Segel, and S. Adler: The use of streptokinase to treat renal artery thromboembolism, *Am. J. Kid. Dis.,* 4:166, 1984.

460. Cronan, J. J., and G. S. Dorfman: Low-dose thrombolysis: A nonoperative approach to renal artery occlusion, *J. Urol.,* 130:757, 1983.

461. Perkins, R. P., D. S. Jacobsen, F. P. Feder, E. O. Lipchik, and P. H. Fine: Return of renal function after late embolectomy, *N. Engl. J. Med.,* 276:1194, 1967.

462. Sheil, A. G., G. S. Stokes, D. J. Tiller, J. May, J. R. Johnson, and J. H. Stewart: Reversal of renal failure by revascularization of kidneys with thrombosed renal arteries, *Lancet,* 2:865, 1973.

463. Spark, R. F.: Renal trauma and hypertension, *Arch. Intern. Med.,* 136:1097, 1976.

464. Margolin, E. G., J. P. Merill, and J. H. Harrison: Diagnosis of hypertension due to occlusion of the renal artery, *N. Engl. J. Med.,* 292:1387, 1975.

465. Retan, J. W., and R. W. Miller: Microembolic complications of atherosclerosis: Literature review and report of a patient, *Arch. Intern. Med.,* 118:534, 1966.

466. Thurlbeck, W. M., and B. Castleman: Atheromatous emboli to the kidneys after aortic surgery, *N. Engl. J. Med.,* 138:1430, 1978.

467. Ramirez, G., W. M. O'Neill, Jr., R. Lambert, and A. Bloomer: Cholesterol embolization: A complication of angiography, *Arch. Intern. Med.,* 138:1430, 1978.

468. Harrington, J. T., S. C. Sommers, and J. P. Kassirer: Atheromatous emboli with progressive renal failure: Renal arteriography as the probable inciting factor, *Ann. Intern. Med.,* 68:152, 1968.

469. Sieniewicz, D. J., S. Moore, F. D. Moir, and D. F. McDade: Atheromatous emboli in the kidneys, *Radiology,* 92:1231, 1969.

470. Handler, F. D.: Clinical and pathologic significance of atheromatous embolization with emphasis on an etiology of renal hypertension, *Am. J. Med.,* 20: 366, 1956.

471. Kassirer, J. P.: Atheroembolic renal disease, *N. Engl. J. Med.,* 280:812, 1969.

472. Hollenhorst, R. W.: Significance of bright plaques in the retinal arterioles, *J. Am. Med. Assoc.,* 178:23, 1961.

473. McGowan, J. A., and A. Greenberg: Cholesterol atheroembolic renal disease. Report of 3 cases with emphasis on diagnosis by skin biopsy and extended survival, *Am. J. Nephrol.,* 6:135, 1986.

474. Kalter, D. C., A. Rudolph, and M. McGavran: Livedo reticularis due to multiple cholesterol emboli, *J. Am. Acad. Dermatol.,* 13:235, 1985.

475. Dalakos, T. G., D. H. P. Streeten, D. Jones, and A. Obeid: "Malignant" hypertension resulting from atheromatous embolization predominantly of one kidney, *Am. J. Med.,* 57:135, 1974.

476. Cosio, F. G., R. A. Zager, and H. M. Sharma: Atheroembolic renal disease causes hypocomplementaemia, *Lancet,* 2:118, 1985.

477. Firth, J. D., and J. P. North: Does atheroembolic renal disease cause hypocomplementaemia?, *Lancet,* 2:1133, 1985.

478. Bidani, A., B. S. Kasinath, H. L. Corwin, M. M. Schwartz, and E. J. Lewis: Eosinophilia in the diagnosis of atheroembolic renal disease, abstract, *Kidney Int.,* 27:134, 1985.

479. Case Records of the Massachusetts General Hospital: Case 30-1986. *N. Engl. J. Med.,* 315:308, 1986.

480. Clinicopathological Conference: Progressive renal failure with hematuria in a 62-year-old man, *Am. J. Med.,* 71:468, 1981.

481. Richards, A. M., R. S. Eliot, V. I. Kanjuh, R. D. Bloemendaal, and J. E. Edwards: Cholesterol embolism: A multiple-system disease masquerading as polyarteritis nodosa, *Am. J. Cardiol.,* 15:696, 1965.

482. Smith, M. C., M. K. Ghose, and A. R. Henry: The clinical spectrum of renal cholesterol embolization, *Am. J. Med.,* 71:174, 1981.

483. Motulsky, A. G.: Frequency of sickling disorders in U. S. Blacks, *N. Engl. J. Med.,* 288:31, 1973.

484. Statius van Eps, L. W., and L. E. Earley: The kidney in sickle cell disease, in L. E. Earley and C. W. Gottschalk (eds.), *Strauss and Welt's Diseases of the Kidney,* 3d ed., Little, Brown, Boston, 1979.

485. Buckalew, V. M., and A. Someren: Renal manifestations of sickle cell disease, *Arch. Intern. Med.,* 133: 660, 1974.

486. Statius, van Eps, L. W., C. Pinedo-Veels, G. H. de Vries, and J. de Koning: Nature of concentrating defect in sickle cell nephropathy, *Lancet,* 1:450, 1970.

487. de Jong, P. E., and L. W. Statius van Eps: Sickle cell nephropathy: New insights into its pathophysiology, *Kidney Int.,* 27:711, 1985.

488. Elfenbein, I., A. Patchefsky, A. W. Schwartz, and A. G. Weinstein: Pathology of the glomerulus in sickle cell anemia with and without the nephrotic syndrome, *Am. J. Pathol.,* 70:357, 1974.

489. Bernstein, J., and C. F. Whitten: A histological appraisal of the kidney in sickle cell anemia, *Arch. Pathol.,* 70:407, 1960.

490. Tejani, A., A. Nicastri, C. K. Chen, D. Sen, K. Phadke, and O. Adamson: Renal lesions in sickle cell nephropathy in children, *Nephron,* 39:352, 1985.

491. Pardo, V., J. Strauss, H. Kramer, T. Ozawa, and R. M. McIntosh: Nephropathy associated with sickle cell anemia: An autologous immune complex nephritis, III: Clinicopathologic study of seven patients, *Am. J. Med.,* 59:650, 1975.

492. McCoy, R. C.: Ultrastructural alterations in the kidney of patients with sickle cell disease and the nephrotic syndrome, *Lab. Invest.,* 21:85, 1969.

493. Humphreys, M. H., and A. C. Alfrey: Vascular diseases of the kidney, in B. M. Brenner, and F. C. Rector (eds.), *The Kidney,* 3d ed., Saunders, Philadelphia, 1986.

494. Keitel, H. G., D. Thompson, and H. A. Itano: Hyposthenuria in sickle cell anemia: A reversible renal defect, *J. Clin. Invest.,* 35:998, 1956.

495. Hatch, F. E., J. W. Culbertson, and L. W. Diggs: Nature of the renal concentrating defect in sickle cell disease, *J. Clin. Invest.,* 46:336, 1967.

496. Kong, H. H. P., and G. A. O. Alleyne: Defect in urinary acidification in adults with sickle-cell anemia, *Lancet,* 2:954, 1968.

497. De Fronzo, R. A., P. A. Taufield, H. Black, P. McPhedran, and C. R. Cooke: Impaired tubular potassium secretion in sickle cell disease, *Ann. Intern. Med.,* 90:310, 1979.

498. Harrow, B. R., J. A. Sloane, and N. C. Liebman: Roentgenologic demonstration of renal papillary necrosis in sickle-cell trait, *N. Engl. J. Med.,* 268:969, 1963.

499. Ettledorf, J. N., J. D. Smith, A. H. Tuttle, and L. W. Diggs: Renal hemodynamic studies in adults with sickle cell anemia, *Am. J. Med.,* 18:243, 1955.

500. Etteldorf, J. N., A. H. Tuttle, and G. W. Clayton: Renal Function studies in pediatrics. I. Renal haemodynamics in children with sickle cell anaemia, *Am. J. Dis. Child.,* 83:185, 1952.

501. Hatch, F. E., S. H. Azar, T. E. Ainsworth, J. M. Nardo, and J. W. Culbertson: Renal hemodynamic studies in sickle cell anemia, *J. Clin. Invest.,* 46:1067, 1967.

502. Morgan, A. G., and G. R. Serjeant: Renal function in patients over 40 with homozygous sickle cell disease, *Br. Med. J.,* 282: 1181, 1981.

503. Brenner, B. M.: Nephron adaptation to renal injury or ablation, *Am. J. Physiol.,* 249:F324, 1985.

504. Thomas, A. N., C. Pattison, and G. R. Serjeant: Causes of death in sickle cell disease in Jamaica, *Br. Med. J.,* 285:633, 1982.

505. Strauss, J., G. Zilleruelo, and C. Abitbol: The kidney and hemoglobin S, *Nephron,* 43:241, 1986.

506. Ozawa, T., M. F. Mass, S. Guggenheim, J. Strauss, and R. M. McIntosh: Autologous immune complex nephritis associated with sickle cell trait: Diagnosis of the hemoglobinopathy after renal structural and immunological studies, *Br. Med. J.,* 1:369, 1976.

507. Strauss, J., V. Pardo, M. N. Koss, W. Griswold, and R. M. McIntosh: Nephropathy associated with sickle cell anemia: An autologous immune complex nephritis. I. Studies on the nature of glomerular-bound antibody and antigen identification in a patient with sickle cell disease and immune deposit glomerulonephritis, *Am. J. Med.,* 58:382, 1975.

508. Alleyne, G. A. O., L. W. Statius van Eps, S. K. Addae, G. D. Nicholson, and H. Shouten: The kidney in sickle cell anemia, *Kidney Int.,* 7:371, 1975.

509. Chapman, Z. A., P. S. Reeder, I. A. Friedman, and L. A. Baker: Gross hematuria in sickle cell trait and sickle cell hemoglobin C disease, *Am. J. Med.,* 19: 773, 1955.

510. Lucas, W. M., and W. H. Bullock: Hematuria in sickle cell disease, *J. Urol.,* 83:733, 1960.

511. Mostofi, F. K., C. F. V. Bruegge, and L. W. Diggs: Lesions in kidneys removed for unilateral hematuria in sickle-cell disease, *Arch. Pathol.,* 63:336, 1957.

512. Allen, T. D.: Sickle cell disease and hematuria: A report of 29 cases, *J. Urol.,* 91:177, 1964.

513. River, G. L., A. B. Robbins, and S. O. Schwartz: S-C hemoglobin: A clinical study, *Blood,* 18:385, 1961.

514. Knochel, J. P.: Hematuria in sickle cell trait: The effect of intravenous administration of distilled water, urinary alkalinization, and diuresis, *Arch. Intern. Med.,* 123:160, 1969.

515. Bergin, J. J.: Complications of therapy with epsilon-aminocaproic acid, *Med. Clin. North Am.,* 50: 1669, 1966.

516. Kimmelstiel, P.: Vascular occlusion and ischemic infarction in sickle cell disease, *Am. J. Med. Sci.,* 216:11, 1948.

517. Femi-Pearse, D., and E. O. Odunjo: Renal cortical infarcts in sickle cell trait, *Br. Med. J.,* 3:34, 1968.

518. Miller, W. A., D. Peck, and R. M. Lowman: Perirenal hematoma in association with renal infarction in sickle cell trait, *Radiology,* 92:351, 1969.

519. Sickles, E. A., and M. Korobkin: Perirenal hematoma as a complication of renal infarction in sickle-cell trait, *Am. J. Roentgenol.,* 122:800, 1974.

520. Eckert, D. E., A. J. Jonutis, and A. J. Davidson: The incidence and manifestations of urographic papillary abnormalities in patients with S hemoglobinopathies, *Radiology,* 113:59, 1974.

521. Miller, R. E., E. C. Hartley, E. C. Clark, and C. H. Lupton: Sickle cell nephropathy, *Ala. J. Med. Sci.,* 1:233, 1964.

522. Statius van Eps, L. W., H. Schouten, L. W. la Porte-Wijsman, and A. M. Struyker-Boudier: The influ-

ence of red blood cell transfusion on the hyposthenuria and renal hemodynamics of sickle cell anemia, *Clin. Chim. Acta,* 17:449, 1967.

523. Levitt, M. F., A. D. Hauser, M. S. Levy, and D. Polimeros: The renal concentrating defect in sickle cell disease, *Am. J. Med.,* 29:611, 1960.

524. Hatch, F. E., J. W. Culbertson, and L. W. Diggs: Nature of renal concentrating defect in sickle cell disease, *J. Clin. Invest.,* 46:336, 1967.

525. Statius van Eps, L. W., H. Schouten, C. C. H. ter Haar Romeny-Wachter, and L. W. la Porte-Wijsman: The relation between age and renal concentrating capacity in sickle cell disease and hemoglobin SC disease, *Clin. Chim. Acta,* 27:501, 1970.

526. Ho Ping Kong, H., and G. A. O. Alleyne: Studies on acid excretion in adults with sickle cell anemia, *Clin. Sci.,* 41:505, 1971.

527. Goossens, J. F., L. W. Statius van Eps, H. Schouten, A. L. Giterson: Incomplete renal tubular acidosis in sickle cell disease, *Clin. Chim. Acta,* 41:149, 1972.

528. Oster, J. R., L. E. Lespier, S. M. Lee, E. L. Pellegrini, and C. A. Vaamonde: Renal acidification in sickle cell disease, *J. Lab. Clin. Med.,* 88:389, 1976.

529. Battle, I. D., K. Itsarayounggyuen, J. A. L. Arruda, and N. A. Kurtzman: Hyperkalemic hyperchloremic metabolic acidosis in sickle cell hemoglobinopathies, *Am. J. Med.,* 72:188, 1982.

530. Oster, J. R., D. C. Lanier, and C. A. Vaamonde: Renal response to potassium loading in sickle cell trait, *Arch. Intern. Med.,* 140:534, 1980.

531. Diamond, H. S., A. D. Meisel, E. Sharon, D. Holden, and A. Cacatian: Hyperuricosuria and increased tubular secretion of urate in sickle cell anemia, *Am. J. Med.,* 59:796, 1975.

532. Diamond, H. S., A. D. Meisel, and D. Holden: The natural history of urate overproduction in sickle cell anemia, *Ann. Intern. Med.,* 90:752, 1979.

533. de Jong, P. E., L. T. W. de Jong-van de Berg, and L. W. Statius van Eps: The tubular reabsorption of phosphate in sickle-cell nephropathy, *Clin. Sci. Mol. Med.,* 55:429, 1978.

534. Smith, E. C., K. S. Valika, J. E. Woo, J. G. O'Donnell, D. L. Gordon, and M. P. Westerman: Serum phosphate abnormalities in sickle cell anemia, *Proc. Soc. Exp. Biol. Med.,* 168:254, 1981.

535. Walker, B. R., F. Alexander, T. R. Birdsall, and R. L. Warren: Glomerular lesions in sickle cell nephropathy, *J. Am. Med. Assoc.,* 214:437, 1971.

536. Johnson, C. S., and A. J. Giorgio: Arterial blood pressure in adults with sickle cell disease, *Arch. Intern. Med.,* 141:891, 1981.

537. Grell, G. A. C., G. A. O. Alleyne, and G. R. Serjeant: Blood pressure with homozygous sickle cell disease, *Lancet,* 2:1166, 1981.

538. de Jong, P. E., H. Landman, L. W. Statius van Eps: Blood pressure in sickle cell disease, *Arch. Intern. Med.,* 142:1239, 1982.

539. Friedman, E. A., T. K. S. Rao, C. L. Sprung, A. Smith, T. Manis, R. Bessevue, K. M. H. Butt, R. D. Levere, and D. M. Holden: Uremia in sickle-cell anemia treated by maintenance hemodialysis, *N. Engl. J. Med.,* 291:1431, 1974.

540. Kunkler, P. B., R. F. Farr, and R. W. Luxton: The limit of renal tolerance to x-rays: An investigation into renal damage occurring following the treatment of tumors of the testis by abdominal baths, *Br. J. Radiol.,* 25:190, 1952.

541. Luxton, R. W.: Radiation nephritis: A long term study of 54 patients, *Lancet,* 2:1221, 1961.

542. Thompson, P. L., I. R. Mackay, G. S. M. Robson, and A. J. Wall: Late radiation nephritis after gastric x-irradiation for peptic ulcer, *Q. J. Med.,* 40:145, 1971.

543. Rubenstone, A. I., and L. B. Fitch: Radiation nephritis: A clinicopathologic study, *Am. J. Med.,* 33:545, 1962.

544. Keane, W. F., J. T. Crosson, N. A. Staley, W. R. Anderson, and F. L. Shapiro: Radiation-induced renal disease: A clinicopathologic study, *Am. J. Med.,* 60:127, 1976.

545. Avioli, L. V., M. Z. Lazor, E. Cotlove, K. C. Brace, and J. R. Roberts: Early effects of radiation on renal function in man, *Am. J. Med.,* 34:329, 1963.

546. Wilson, C., J. M. Ledingham, and M. Cohen: Hypertension following x-irradiation of the kidneys, *Lancet,* 1:9, 1958.

547. Shapiro, A. P., T. Cavallo, W. Cooper, D. Lapenas, K. Bron, and G. Berg: Hypertension in radiation nephritis: Report of a patient with unilateral disease, elevated renin activity levels, and reversal after unilateral nephrectomy, *Arch. Intern. Med.,* 137:848, 1977.

548. Asscher, A. W., C. Wilson, and S. G. Anson: Sensitisation of blood vessels to hypertensive damage by x-irradiation, *Lancet,* 1:580, 1961.

549. Steele, B. T., and D. J. Lirenman: Acute radiation nephritis and hemolytic uremic syndrome, *Clin. Nephrol.,* 11:272, 1979.

8

TUBULOINTERSTITIAL DISEASES

Burton D. Rose

Clinical Characteristics
Acute Interstitial Nephritis
Chronic Drug-Induced Interstitial Nephritis
Lithium
Cyclosporine
Nitrosoureas
Analgesic Abuse Nephropathy and Papillary Necrosis
Chronic Pyelonephritis and Reflux Nephropathy
Cystic Diseases of the Kidney
Polycystic Kidney Disease

Medullary Sponge Kidney
Medullary Cystic Kidney Disease
Acquired Cystic Disease
Simple Cysts
Myeloma Kidney
Uric Acid Renal Disease
Acute Uric Acid Nephropathy
Chronic Urate Nephropathy
Uric Acid Nephrolithiasis
Hypercalcemic Nephropathy
Sarcoidosis
Calcium Balance
Granulomatous Interstitial Nephritis
Glomerulonephritis
Miscellaneous
Intratubular Obstruction
Infiltrative Diseases
Heavy Metal Toxicity
Hypokalemic Nephropathy
Primary Immunologic Disorders
Balkan Nephropathy
Secondary Tubulointerstitial Disease

Involvement of the tubules and interstitium is a frequent finding in renal disease. In many cases, the major problem is glomerulonephritis, vascular disease, or urinary tract obstruction with tubulointerstitial damage occurring as a secondary event. There are, however, a variety of disorders that primarily affect the tubules or interstitium (Table 8–1). These conditions are important causes of both acute and chronic renal insufficiency. Acute tubular necrosis (see Chap. 3) and acute drug-induced interstitial nephritis are among the more common conditions that produce acute renal failure. Tubulointerstitial diseases may also account for as many as 25 percent of cases of chronic renal failure.[1] This is most commonly due to chronic pyelonephritis (in

which bacterial infection of the kidney is associated with an anatomic abnormality such as vesicoureteral reflux), polycystic kidney disease, or analgesic abuse nephropathy.

The aim of this chapter is to review the disorders responsible for primary tubulointerstitial disease. Only the more common conditions are discussed in detail; rarer diseases will be reviewed briefly at the end of the chapter.

CLINICAL CHARACTERISTICS

As can be appreciated from Table 8–1, a variety of mechanisms may be responsible for tubular or interstitial damage. Although the

TABLE 8-1. Causes of Primary Tubulointerstitial Kidney Disease

Mechanism	Relatively Common	Rare
Toxins	Acute tubular necrosis Analgesic abuse nephropathy Cyclosporine	Lithium Lead Nitrosoureas Balkan nephropathy
Tubular obstruction	Hypercalcemia Multiple myeloma Uric acid nephropathy	Hyperoxaluria Certain drugs
Developmental abnormalities	Polycystic kidney disease Simple renal cysts Medullary sponge kidney	Medullary cystic kidney disease
Infection	Acute and chronic pyelonephritis	Acute interstitial nephritis
Immunologic factors	Acute interstitial nephritis Transplant rejection	Systemic lupus erythematosus Sjögren's syndrome Goodpasture's syndrome
Infiltrative diseases		Sarcoidosis Lymphoma Leukemia
Ischemia	Acute tubular necrosis	
Miscellaneous	Acquired cystic disease	Urate nephropathy Hypokalemia Idiopathic interstitial nephritis

glomeruli are not primarily involved, tubulointerstitial disease can lead to a fall in GFR and progressive renal failure due, for example, to tubular obstruction (as in multiple myeloma) or to interference with nephron blood supply (as with the increased interstitial pressure induced by polycystic kidney disease).

Regardless of the underlying mechanism, tubulointerstitial diseases tend to share several clinical characteristics. First, the urinalysis is frequently normal or only mildly abnormal in chronic conditions, usually revealing sterile pyuria or mild proteinuria with few cells or casts. Protein excretion is generally under 1.5 g/day and can result from two mechanisms: (1) the excretion of *normally filtered* low-molecular-weight proteins due either to increased production (as with immunoglobulin light chains in multiple myeloma) or to decreased proximal tubular reabsorp-

tion due to tubular damage (as with β_2-microglobulin)[2,3]; or (2) the excretion of albumin and other *usually nonfiltered* macromolecules because of secondary glomerular injury, most often due to hemodynamic mechanisms (see Chap. 4).[4]

In comparison, the urine may be quite abnormal in the more acute tubulointerstitial diseases such as acute tubular necrosis (tubular cells, granular and tubular cell casts), acute interstitial nephritis (hematuria, pyuria with eosinophiluria, white cell casts), and bacterial pyelonephritis (pyuria with white cell casts). In addition, episodes of infection or gross hematuria can complicate polycystic kidney disease, medullary sponge kidney, or analgesic abuse nephropathy.

Second, the primary tubular damage can lead to impaired proximal and distal tubular function relatively early in the course of the disease.[5] Distal defects can be manifested by decreased concentrating ability, sodium wasting of varying degree, metabolic acidosis, and hyperkalemia.[6-9] For example, chronic tubulointerstitial diseases are, along with diabetic nephropathy, the major cause of hyperkalemia due to hyporeninemic hypoaldosteronism.[9]

On the other hand, impaired proximal function can lead to different abnormalities including renal glucosuria, aminoaciduria, and proximal (type 2) renal tubular acidosis.[5] For example, multiple myeloma, in which the filtered light chains appear to be toxic to the tubular cells, is one of the most common causes of proximal renal tubular acidosis in adults.[10]

ACUTE INTERSTITIAL NEPHRITIS

Acute interstitial nephritis generally represents a hypersensitivity reaction to a drug.[11,12] This has been described most often with methicillin,[13-15] occurring in up to 17 percent of patients who are treated for more than 10 days.[16,17] Many other drugs have also been associated with this problem,[11,12] with the most common being other β-lactam antibiotics (natural and synthetic penicillins and cephalosporins), nonsteroidal anti-inflamma-

tory drugs, cimetidine, sulfa drugs (including the combination of sulfamethoxazole-trimethoprim and sulfonamide diuretics such as furosemide and the thiazides), and rifampin (Table 8–2).[18-30]

In addition to drugs, infection is a less frequent cause of acute interstitial nephritis. This complication has been described with streptococcal infections, *Legionella,* leptospirosis, and rarely with viruses.[31-36] In some patients, however, no cause of the interstitial nephritis can be identified.[31,37]

PATHOLOGY

The major histologic changes in this disorder are interstitial edema and an interstitial infiltrate consisting primarily of lymphocytes and monocytes (Fig. 8–1).[12] Eosinophils, plasma cells, neutrophils, and basophils may also be found, but are generally less prominent. The severity of the interstitial infiltrate is variable, being most prominent in patients with more severe disease. In addition, tubular damage is also commonly present, with actual tubular necrosis and regeneration occurring in some patients.

The glomeruli and blood vessels are usually spared in this disorder. In some cases, however, the interstitial nephritis is accompanied

TABLE 8-2. Drugs Association with Acute Interstitial Nephritis*

Strong Association	Probable Association	Weak Association
Methicillin	Carbenicillin	Phenytoin
Penicillins	Cephalosporins	Tetracycline
Cephalothin	Oxacillin	Probenecid
Nonsteroidal anti-inflammatory drugs	Ampicillin	Captopril
Cimetidine	Sulfonamides	Allopurinol
	Rifampin	Erythromycin
	Thiazides	Chloramphenicol
	Furosemide	Clofibrate
	Leukocyte interferon	
	Phenindione	

*Adapted from S. G. Adler, A. H. Cohen, and W. A. Border, *Am. J. Kid. Dis.,* 5:75, 1985.

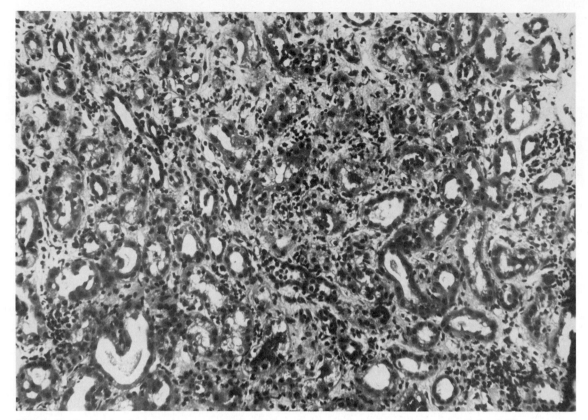

FIG. 8–1. Histologic changes in acute interstitial nephritis. There is a prominent cellular infiltration (composed predominantly of mononuclear cells) and interstitial edema, as evidenced by the space separating the tubules from one another. The glomeruli, which are not shown in this field, are typically spared. (*Courtesy of Dr. Jerome B. Jacobs.*)

by heavy proteinuria and glomerular changes typical of minimal change disease (primarily consisting of diffuse fusion of the epithelial cell foot processes; see Chap. 6). This has been most commonly described with nonsteroidal anti-inflammatory drugs[23,24] but also may rarely occur with ampicillin, rifampin, or recombinant leukocyte interferon.[19,38,39]

PATHOGENESIS

The mechanism by which the hypersensitivity reaction involves the kidney is incompletely understood. The observation that the interstitial infiltrate is composed predominantly of thymic-derived lymphocytes (T cells) is compatible with a primary role for cell-mediated immunity.[40–42] Further evidence in support of this hypothesis comes from the demonstration in isolated cases that circulating lymphocytes display increased in vitro blast transformation or release more macrophage inhibition factor when incubated with the offending drug.[25,43,44] In addition to producing tubulointerstitial damage, the activated T cells could also release soluble mediators that could account for the eosinophilic infiltration (by chemotaxis)[42] and for the occasional occurrence of minimal change disease, which is also thought to be a T-cell disorder (see Chap. 6). With the non-steroidal anti-inflammatory drugs, for example, inhibition of the cyclooxygenase pathway may facilitate the conversion of arachidonic acid to leukotrienes,[23] a change that could promote the activation of helper T cells.[45]

Accumulation of the inciting antigen (drug or drug-hapten complex) within the kidney, where it can interact with activated T cells, may also be an important determinant of tubulointerstitial damage. In patients with methicillin nephritis, for example, a methicillin-derived antigen dimethoxyphenylpenicilloyl (DPO) can be found along the tubular basement membranes (TBM).[13,46] However, DPO deposition also occurs in patients without renal disease, indicating the concurrent need for an immune response directed against the drug.[46]

Although cell-mediated immunity may play a primary role in most patients, humoral mechanisms can also produce tubulointerstitial disease. In occasional patients with methicillin nephritis, linear deposition of IgG, DPO, and C3 (by immunofluorescence) along the TBM and circulating anti-TBM antibodies have been found.[47] It has been postulated that antibodies were formed to the DPO-TBM conjugate, resulting in antibody and complement deposition along the TBM and tubular injury. It is also possible, however, that the formation of anti-TBM antibodies is merely a secondary event, resulting from tubular damage induced in some other way, e.g., by cellular mechanisms.[48] Anti-TBM antibody-mediated disease has also been described in isolated cases of idiopathic acute interstitial nephritis and in patients with concurrent anti-GBM antibody-induced glomerulonephritis.[49-51]

The deposition of circulating antigen-antibody complexes along the TBM does not appear to be important in drug-induced interstitial nephritis. It may, however, be present and contribute to tubulointerstitial damage in many patients with systemic lupus erythematosus.[52]

CLINICAL PRESENTATION

The clinical features of drug-induced acute interstitial nephritis have been best characterized with methicillin nephritis.[11-15] The patient initially responds to methicillin therapy with defervescence and improvement in symptoms. After a latent period that usually is greater than 10 days (but may be as short as 3 days), however, fever recurs and is infrequently accompanied by a rash. At this time, peripheral eosinophilia is usually present, and the urinalysis reveals hematuria which is often grossly visible, pyuria with occasional eosinophiluria (which can be appreciated by the bilobed appearance of the eosinophils on Wright's stain of the urine sediment), white cell casts, and mild proteinuria. These changes in the urine sediment can precede any decline in the GFR by as much as 1 week.[16] A somewhat surprising finding is that the fractional excretion of sodium may remain under 1 percent, despite the presence of tubular damage.[53,54]

Other causes of drug-induced interstitial nephritis can produce a somewhat different picture. With nonsteroidal anti-inflammatory drugs, for example, the latent period can be as long as 18 months, there is frequently no eosinophilia or eosinophiluria, and nephrotic range proteinuria and edema may also be present.[23,24,54] Although almost any of the nonsteroidal anti-inflammatory drugs can produce this disorder, it most commonly occurs with the propionic acid derivatives, particularly fenoprofen.[23,24,40,54] The allergic findings (eosinophilia, eosinophiluria, and rash) also tend to be absent with postinfectious or idiopathic interstitial nephritis.[31,37]

DIAGNOSIS

The history and physical examination are clearly important in identifying a possible offending drug (Table 8–2), the presence of an allergic skin rash, or the signs or symptoms of a systemic infection such as streptococcal pharyngitis, pneumonia due to *Legionella*, or myalgias and jaundice induced by leptospirosis.[31-35] In the appropriate clinical setting, the characteristic urinary findings frequently provide confirmatory evidence of the diagnosis of acute interstitial nephritis.

However, glomerulonephritis or vasculitis also must be excluded in any patient with acute renal failure, hematuria, and proteinuria. This distinction can be illustrated by the major types of renal disease that can occur in bacterial endocarditis. In this setting, drug-induced interstitial nephritis must be differentiated from an immune-complex glomerulonephritis induced by the bacterial infection (see p. 230). The timing of the onset of renal disease may be helpful in arriving at the correct diagnosis. In the glomerulonephritis, the degree of renal failure is typically maximal at or soon after the initiation of appropriate antimicrobial therapy. Red cell casts and hypocomplementemia are also frequently present. In comparison, the interstitial nephritis is characterized by late onset after therapy has been started, normal complement levels, eosinophilia, eosinophiluria, and the absence of red cell casts.[14,16]

Two other factors may lead to difficulty in differential diagnosis. First, the acutely ill patient is frequently receiving many potentially nephrotoxic drugs and may be hemodynamically unstable, both of which can promote the development of renal failure due to acute tubular necrosis. The urinalysis may be helpful in this setting, since the sediment in acute tubular necrosis typically consists of free tubular epithelial cells and muddy brown granular and epithelial cell casts (see Chap. 3). These findings are substantially different from those usually seen with acute interstitial nephritis. It has also been suggested that gallium scanning may be helpful in distinguishing between these disorders, being negative in acute tubular necrosis but markedly positive in most cases of acute interstitial nephritis (by an unknown mechanism).[55]

Second, drugs that produce acute interstitial nephritis may also produce other renal lesions. As examples, nonsteroidal anti-inflammatory drugs can exacerbate prerenal disease (see p. 82),[23,24] rifampin can lead to acute tubular necrosis,[30] and the penicillins and sulfa derivatives can produce a hypersensitivity vasculitis in which skin purpura is typically present (see Chap. 7).[56] The urinalysis is usually helpful in distinguishing these disorders from acute interstitial nephritis.

COURSE AND THERAPY

The mainstay of therapy is to discontinue the responsible drug or to treat the inciting infection. Renal function will improve in most patients, but it is not uncommon for there to be some residual renal insufficiency (as evidenced by a plasma creatinine concentration that is higher than the previous baseline value).[15] The degree of functional recovery and the rate at which it occurs appear to vary with the severity of renal involvement. Clearing of the urine sediment may occur within several days in patients without azotemia. On the other hand, recovery may take as long as 2 to 4 months in patients who have already developed renal insufficiency.[15,31]

The role of corticosteroids in this disorder is uncertain. In an uncontrolled study of patients with methicillin-induced disease, prednisone (beginning in a dose of 60 mg/day and then rapidly tapering as a response occurred) appeared to result in a more complete and more rapid (9 days versus 54 days in untreated patients) resolution of the disease.[15] However, a relapse may occur as the prednisone is being discontinued. Since at least partial spontaneous recovery is the rule, it seems reasonable to use corticosteroids only in those patients with methicillin nephritis who develop substantial renal insufficiency (plasma creatinine concentration above 2.5 to 3.0 mg/dL).

It is not known how applicable these uncontrolled findings are to other causes of acute interstitial nephritis. There is little evidence, for example, that prednisone is effective when a nonsteroidal anti-inflammatory drug is the offending agent,[23] and prednisone probably should not be used with postinfectious causes where treatment of the underlying infection is of primary importance.[31] A trial of prednisone therapy may be indicated, however, in patients with relatively severe disease who have clinical evidence of an allergic reaction (eosinophilia, rash) or who have idiopathic interstitial nephritis.[37]

There is even less information concerning the use of cytotoxic agents such as cyclophosphamide, chlorambucil, or azathioprine. These agents appear to be effective in experimental interstitial nephritis[57] and have been tried in patients with persistent renal insufficiency despite a course of prednisone therapy.[31,44] The apparent improvement that occurred in this setting is difficult to interpret, considering the small number of patients involved and the tendency for spontaneous recovery to occur.

CHRONIC DRUG-INDUCED INTERSTITIAL NEPHRITIS

A variety of drugs which are given for prolonged periods of time can produce chronic tubulointerstitial damage, presumably due to cumulative injury to the tubules or the renal microcirculation. The most common include lithium, cyclosporine, the nitrosoureas, and analgesic abuse nephropathy, which will be considered separately below.

LITHIUM

The renal toxicity of lithium is presumably related to toxic damage to the proximal and cortical collecting tubules, sites at which filtered lithium is reabsorbed.[58-60] The most common manifestation of lithium nephropathy is polyuria and polydipsia due to nephrogenic diabetes insipidus. This problem seems to result from the entry of filtered lithium into the collecting tubular cells via the sodium channel in the luminal membrane.[60] Within the cells, lithium impairs both the antidiuretic hormone-induced generation of cyclic AMP (perhaps by reducing the activity of adenyl cyclase)[60,61] and possibly the subsequent ability of cyclic AMP to increase water permeability.[58] The net effect is that maximum concentrating ability is impaired in up to 50 percent of patients,[62] being severe enough to produce symptomatic polyuria in as many as 15 to 30 percent.[58,63] These symptoms may appear as early as 8 to 12 weeks after drug use, and the concentrating defect may be irreversible if therapy is prolonged.[64] It has recently been suggested that the potassium-sparing diuretic amiloride can partially reverse this abnormality and possibly protect against its development,[65] probably by closing the sodium channel through which filtered lithium enters the collecting tubule cell.[60,65]

Somewhat more controversial is the development of interstitial fibrosis, tubular atrophy, and the formation of tubular microcysts following chronic lithium therapy.[66 68] These findings are difficult to interpret since patients taking lithium are frequently taking other psychoactive drugs which could also be responsible for renal injury. Although this issue is not completely resolved, it is likely that lithium is capable of producing some chronic tubulointerstitial damage. Long-term follow-up, however, reveals that this is rarely of clinical importance since the GFR is generally well-maintained.[62,69]

CYCLOSPORINE

Cyclosporine is a unique immunosuppressive agent that has dramatically improved the results of organ transplantation and holds promise for the treatment of autoimmune diseases such as rheumatoid arthritis, uveitis, and insulin-dependent (type 1) diabetes mellitus.[70-75] Its use, however, has been complicated by the development of nephrotoxicity in up to two-thirds of patients.[71-75] For example, the plasma creatinine concentration in stable renal transplant recipients is approximately 0.6 mg/dL higher in patients treated with cyclosporine when compared to those treated with only prednisone and azathioprine.[74] This rise in the plasma creatinine concentration tends to occur within the first few months of therapy, is associated with a relatively benign urinalysis, and typically remains stable with continuing usage.[74] The decline in renal function is usually reversible, as evidenced by a fall in the plasma creatinine concentration if azathioprine is substituted for cyclosporine.[74,75] However, end-stage renal failure requiring maintenance dialysis may occur if high doses are used for a prolonged period of time.[76]

The pathologic changes in cyclosporine nephropathy include focal or diffuse interstitial fibrosis, tubular injury with giant mitochondria in the proximal tubules, and, less commonly, arterial and arteriolar lesions similar to those in the hemolytic-uremic syndrome (see Chap. 7).[72,77,78] These findings were initially described in renal transplant recipients, making it difficult to exclude a contribution from transplant rejection.* They have, however, also been seen in cyclosporine-treated patients with uveitis, rheumatoid arthritis, or a heart transplant (who have no primary renal disease), suggesting a specific toxic effect of cyclosporine.[72,73,76]

The pathogenesis of these lesions is uncertain as is the primary site of involvement.

*The diagnosis of cyclosporine nephrotoxicity in the renal transplant is one of exclusion, being made on the basis of impaired renal function and the absence both of the characteristic pathologic changes of transplant rejection and of any other apparent cause of renal disease.

Active renal vasoconstriction and direct damage to the arterioles and the proximal tubules have been demonstrated.[79,80] The relative importance of these changes is at present unclear.

Cyclosporine nephrotoxicity currently limits the use of this potentially valuable drug. Studies are being performed to ascertain if lower doses are less nephrotoxic but maintain adequate immunosuppressive activity. Pending the results of these studies, some renal transplant centers are evaluating the use of cyclosporine for the first 3 to 6 months (the time when acute rejection is most likely to occur), followed by conversion to long-term maintenance therapy with azathioprine.[75]

NITROSOUREAS

The nitrosoureas (methyl-CCNU, BCNU, and streptozotocin) are alkylating agents used in cancer chemotherapy. Patients (particularly children) receiving a total of more than 1200 to 1500 mg/m^2 of methyl-CCNU or BCNU run a relatively high risk of developing a chronic interstitial nephritis (characterized histologically by tubular atrophy and interstitial fibrosis) that may progress to renal failure.[81-83] The onset of clinically apparent disease is frequently delayed for as long as several months to up to several years after therapy has been discontinued. As a result, careful long-term follow-up is essential. Mild proteinuria or an asymptomatic elevation in the plasma creatinine concentration is usually the first sign of disease, since the urine sediment generally is normal or near-normal with few cells or casts.

The mechanism of nephrotoxicity of these drugs is unknown. Alkylation of tubular cell proteins may be involved since nitrosourea metabolites are excreted by the kidneys.[12] There is no known therapy for this disorder.

ANALGESIC ABUSE NEPHROPATHY AND PAPILLARY NECROSIS

Renal disease associated with analgesic abuse was first described in Switzerland in 1953. However, increasing awareness of this problem has led to the recognition that analgesic abuse nephropathy (AAN) is a relatively common cause of chronic renal failure. The incidence with which this occurs is variable, depending in part upon regional differences in analgesic consumption. Thus, AAN accounts for approximately 1 to 2 percent of cases of end-stage renal failure in the United States as a whole, up to 10 percent in northwestern North Carolina, and 20 percent or more in Australia.[84-86] Early diagnosis is particularly important since progressive renal failure can usually be prevented by discontinuing analgesic intake.[86,87]

PATHOLOGY

Analgesic abuse nephropathy primarily affects the renal medulla. The earliest changes are in the inner medulla (papilla) and consist of patchy areas of necrosis of cells in the loop of Henle and the interstitium, with prominent hyaline thickening of the vasa recta capillaries.[88,89] These vascular changes are also found in the renal pelvis and ureter and have been considered to represent an "analgesic microangiopathy."[90]

Progression of the disease, due at least in part to occlusive changes in the vasa recta, leads to enlarging areas of necrosis, extending through the papilla into the outer medulla. Total papillary necrosis is the eventual result. The necrotic papillary tissue may remain in place, or fragments may slough into the calyx and then pass into the renal pelvis and ureter. At this stage, an intravenous pyelogram (IVP) may show the characteristic radiographic findings of papillary necrosis (see below).

Histologic changes also may be found in the renal cortex, including tubular atrophy, interstitial fibrosis, and mononuclear cell infiltration.[88,89] These changes are thought to be secondary to the papillary disease and usually overlie areas of papillary necrosis. Focal or diffuse glomerulosclerosis may be seen in the later stages of the disease and in part represent hemodynamically mediated injury (see Chap. 4).

PATHOGENESIS

In humans, AAN is usually associated with the ingestion of analgesics containing *both* phenacetin and aspirin.[91,92] For example, a prospective 10-year study of women with heavy consumption of combination analgesics revealed that 12 percent developed an elevation in the plasma creatinine concentration (versus 1.4 percent in the control group).[93] In comparison, papillary necrosis leading to renal insufficiency is extremely rare in patients taking aspirin, phenacetin, or acetaminophen (the primary metabolite of phenacetin) alone.[86,92] This can be illustrated by studies of patients with rheumatoid arthritis. Despite taking daily aspirin in high doses for many years, these patients typically have little change in renal function.[94-96] There are, however, occasional patients who develop papillary necrosis after the ingestion of nonsteroidal anti-inflammatory drugs.[23,24,97] The degree of renal damage is relatively mild in this setting, and renal insufficiency is unusual.

The quantity of analgesics required to induce AAN is variable. In general, patients with clinical evidence of renal disease have ingested more than 2 to 3 kg each of phenacetin and aspirin,[91,92] although mild abnormalities in renal function (such as decreased concentrating ability or a small reduction in GFR) can be detected after the cumulative intake of as little as 1 kg.[92] Considering these dosage requirements, the time required to produce renal disease can be appreciated from the following simple calculations. Most compound analgesics (which are now much less available) contain 130 to 160 mg of phenacetin. Therefore, clinical evidence of AAN may develop after 5 to 8 years if a patient takes 6 to 8 tablets (or about 1 g) a day.

The mechanism by which phenactin and aspirin induce renal injury is not completely understood.[98,99] In the liver, phenacetin is converted primarily to acetaminophen, which then accumulates in the kidney along the medullary osmotic gradient.[100] As a result, the highest concentrations are achieved at the papillary tip, the site of the initial pathologic lesion. Experimental models suggest that this distribution is important since lessening the medullary gradient with a water diuresis protects against the development of papillary necrosis.[101]

In the medulla, acetaminophen can be metabolized by local hydroperoxidases to a reactive intermediate that can induce tissue damage by causing lipid peroxidation.[98,99] In this setting, aspirin can contribute to the development of AAN in two ways: it can interfere with the hexose monophosphate shunt, thereby lowering the concentration of glutathione, which normally inactivates the reactive acetaminophen metabolites; and it can cause medullary ischemia by inhibiting the local production of vasodilator prostaglandins.

It is unclear whether the tubular cells or vascular endothelium is the primary site of injury. The hyaline thickening of the vasa recta capillaries described above[90] and the early finding of medullary ischemia[102] are compatible with a vascular origin for the disease, but this hypothesis remains unproven.

CLINICAL PRESENTATION

Many patients with AAN present with a fairly typical history (Table 8–3). The disease primarily affects middle-aged women who have a history of chronic headaches or back pain requiring the use of analgesics.[91,92] A psychoneurotic disorder frequently is present as is

TABLE 8–3. Typical Clinical Features of Analgesic Abuse Nephropathy

Age range (30 to 70)
Females (70 to 85 percent)
Headaches
Ulcerlike symptoms
Psychiatric disturbances
Urinary tract infection
Hypertension
Urinalysis
  Sterile pyuria, mild proteinuria, or normal
Intravenous pyelogram
  Papillary necrosis (25 to 40 percent)
  Normal (5 to 15 percent)
  Small kidneys (50 to 65 percent)

peptic ulcer disease, due in part to chronic aspirin ingestion. The patient may also complain of symptoms directly referable to the kidney disease. These include: (1) flank pain or hematuria due to passage of a sloughed papilla into the renal pelvis or ureter; (2) weakness, lethargy, and anorexia resulting from the insidious onset of uremia; and (3) dysuria, back pain, and fever due to a urinary tract infection, which occurs with increased frequency in AAN.[103]

The findings on the physical examination and routine laboratory tests are nonspecific.[91,92] Hypertension, anemia, and an elevated plasma creatinine concentration are commonly present. The urinalysis may be normal or reveal sterile pyuria with mild proteinuria, usually not exceeding 1.5 g/day. However, microscopic or gross hematuria may be present during episodes of acute papillary necrosis.

The primary medullary involvement can also lead to the early development of subtle, asymptomatic renal functional abnormalties. These include impairments in concentrating ability, urinary acidification, and the ability to lower urinary sodium excretion to a normal minimum of less than 15 meq/day in the presence of volume depletion.[92,104,105]

DIAGNOSIS

The diagnosis of AAN can be made only if the physician considers this disorder in the differential diagnosis. AAN should be suspected in any patient, particularly a woman who presents with *chronic renal insufficiency and a urinalysis that is normal or shows only sterile pyuria.* Other features of the charactersitic symptom complex depicted in Table 8–3 also may be present. Confirmation of the diagnosis requires a history of analgesic ingestion. However, some patients will deny such a history even after careful evaluation. In this setting, questioning family and friends may be helpful.

An IVP may be of diagnostic importance in AAN.[106,107] Although papillary necrosis is present in almost all cases on histologic examination, this change can be detected radiographically only if part or all of the papilla has been sloughed (Fig. 8–2). Thus, only 25 to 40 percent of patients will show partial or complete papillary necrosis, and 50 to 65 percent will show small kidneys and/or blunted calyces as seen in chronic pyelonephritis (see Fig. 8–3).[91,103,108]

The demonstration of papillary necrosis is not pathognomonic of AAN since similar changes can also occur in a variety of other diseases, particularly diabetes mellitus, acute pyelonephritis, urinary tract obstruction, sickle cell disease, and renal tuberculosis.[106,109–111] These disorders can usually be distinguished from AAN by the history and appropriate laboratory tests.

COURSE

The decline in renal function can be expected to progress, eventually to end-stage renal failure, if analgesic abuse continues. In contrast, most patients who discontinue analgesics have stabilization of or a mild improvement in renal function.[86,87,91,112,113] Those patients whose renal function continues to deteriorate usually have uncontrolled hypertension or

hemodynamically mediated glomerular injury (see Chap. 4), or they are surreptitiously continuing analgesics. It is important to be aware that even aspirin alone may be deleterious in a patient who already has AAN.[91,112,113] The only commonly used analgesics that have not been associated with papillary necrosis are propoxyphene and codeine.[92,114]

In addition to renal failure, AAN may also be complicated by transitional cell carcinomas (which may be multiple and bilateral) of the renal pelves, ureters, and bladder[115–119] and less often by renal cell carcinoma.[118] Analgesic abuse is, for example, the most common cause of bladder cancer in young women (under the age of 50).[117] These tumors appear to develop in as many as 8 to 10 percent of patients, although uroepithelial atypia has been found in *almost 50 percent* of nephrectomy specimens obtained prior to renal transplantation.[119]

It is presumed that the development of malignancy is related to the accumulation of toxic metabolites of phenacetin.[117] In general, these tumors appear after 15 to 25 years of phenacetin use; they may occur several years after analgesics have been discontinued as well as after renal transplantation has been performed.[115,119] The most common presenting sign is microscopic or gross hematuria, which occurs in 90 percent of patients.[115] Thus, the new onset of hematuria is an important finding and should be investigated with urinary cytology, intravenous pyelography, and, if necessary, cystoscopy with retrograde pyelography. It is also prudent to obtain urinary cytology yearly, since this test reveals tumor cells in approximately 75 percent of patients with a malignancy,[120] and to remove the native kidneys in patients who receive a renal transplant.[119]

Prophylactic screening for malignancy is clearly more difficult in patients on maintenance dialysis who frequently have little or no urine output. It may be desirable in this setting to perform retrograde pyelography at

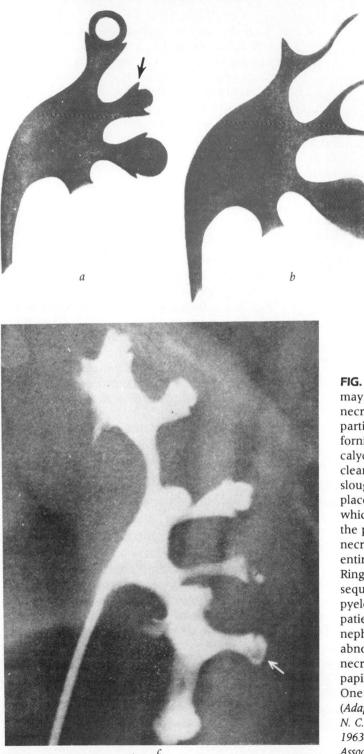

FIG. 8-2. Radiographic findings which may be present in renal papillary necrosis. (*a*) Depiction of the findings in partial papillary necrosis as the calyceal fornices are intact (arrow). The three calyces reveal a medullary ring (the clear area representing a portion of the sloughed papilla which has remained in place) and a small and large cavity which are due to partial sloughing of the papilla. (*b*) In complete papillary necrosis, the fornices are also lost as the entire papillary surface is destroyed. Ring shadows are again due to sequestered papillae. (*c*) Retrograde pyelogram of the left kidney from a patient with analgesic abuse nephropathy. All the calyces are abnormal with complete papillary necrosis in the lower calyx and partial papillary necrosis in the other calyces. One medullary ring is present (arrow). (*Adapted from B. R. Harrow, J. A. Sloane, and N. C. Liebman, J. Am. Med. Assoc., 184:445, 1963. By permission of the American Medical Association, copyright 1963.*)

periodic intervals,[119] although the value of this regimen has not been proven.

PROGNOSIS

In the absence of neoplasms, the prognosis is relatively good in those patients in whom renal function can be stabilized by the discontinuation of analgesics. There is, however, an increased incidence of arteriosclerotic disease (including myocardial and cerebral infarction) and premature aging and graying.[87,92] The mechanism by which this occurs is not known since there does not appear to be an increased incidence of other risk factors such as hypertension in patients with AAN (when compared to those with other forms of renal disease). It is possible that the analgesic microangiopathy described above plays an important role.[90]

PREVENTION

It is likely that AAN can be prevented by limiting the intake of medications containing both phenacetin and aspirin. The incidence of new cases of this disorder, for example, has generally dropped markedly when phenacetin has been removed from over-the-counter analgesic compounds.[85,86,113,121] These compounds have largely been replaced by aspirin alone (or with caffeine), ibuprofen, or acetaminophen. As described above, papillary necrosis is extremely unusual with the use of these single agents.

CHRONIC PYELONEPHRITIS AND REFLUX NEPHROPATHY

Chronic pyelonephritis refers to progressive renal damage (associated with parenchymal scarring on IVP) that is induced by recurrent or persistent infection of the kidneys. It is important to note, however, that this disorder is *generally unrelated to acute pyelonephri-*

tis. Women with acute renal infection typically have no anatomic abnormality in the urinary tract[122] and have little long-term morbidity and no decline in renal function.[123] In comparison, *chronic* pyelonephritis occurs in patients with urinary tract infection who also have a major anatomic abnormality such as vesicoureteral reflux (VUR), obstruction, or renal calculi (which act as foreign bodies and prevent elimination of bacteria).[1,124,125]

PATHOGENESIS

Chronic pyelonephritis, which is associated with prominent renal scarring, is primarily a *disease of children with VUR.* The importance of reflux can be appreciated from the following statistics: VUR is present in 30 to 45 percent of young children with a urinary tract infection[126-128] and in almost all children with renal scars (Fig. 8-3).[127-130] Children with gross reflux (reflux back to the renal pelvis plus ureteral dilatation) are at greatest risk, since the incidence of renal scarring in this setting can exceed 60 percent.[125] The net effect is that chronic pyelonephritis due to reflux (also called *reflux nephropathy*) accounts for about 20 to 30 percent of cases of end-stage renal failure in children.[124]

VUR is usually a congenital defect that results from incompetence of the functional ureterovesical valve, most often due to a short intramural segment.* The degree of reflux is important in terms of prognosis since only gross reflux extending up to the renal pelvis and then *into the renal parenchyma* (intrarenal reflux) is associated with renal scarring (Fig. 8-4).[124,132,133] Lesser degrees of reflux, e.g., one-third of the way up the ureter, do

---

*VUR and renal scarring can also be seen with chronic infection and a flaccid bladder in patients with a spinal cord injury.[131] The frequent association with struvite (or infection) stones may be important in this setting. These stones can lead to urinary obstruction; the ensuing rise in pressure proximal to the obstruction can produce the intrarenal reflux that appears to be required for scarring to occur (Fig. 8-4).

not appear to produce renal damage and usually disappear spontaneously.[132]

The evidence supporting the importance of intrarenal reflux (IRR) can be summarized by the following observations:

1. There is a high correlation between scars and IRR in children under the age of 5. In comparison, VUR without IRR is much less likely to be associated with scarring.[133]
2. Most renal scars occur at the upper and lower poles (in the absence of an obstructing lesion such as urethral values).[132] IRR also occurs at the poles where the papillary collecting duct orifices in young children are wide open, not slitlike as in the middle calyces.[134]
3. Almost all renal scars in children with VUR occur before the age of 5 to 6.[124,126,130,135] Since IRR can be demonstrated only in this age group,[133] spontaneous cessation of IRR, probably due to renal growth, could account for the general lack of new scar formation in older children, even though VUR persists and contraction of old scars may continue.

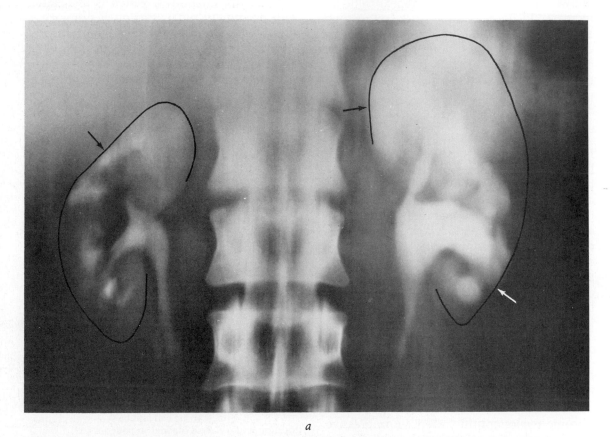

a

FIG. 8-3. Radiographic changes in chronic pyelonephritis. (*a*) IVP in a 32-year-old man demonstrates blunting of the calyces (more prominent in the left kidney) and scarring with loss of parenchyma in both upper poles and the left lower pole (arrows). (*b*) A voiding cystourethrogram on the same patient demonstrates gross reflux up to the left renal collecting system. Although reflux was not demonstrable on the right, cystoscopy revealed changes at the ureteral orifice compatible with previous reflux.

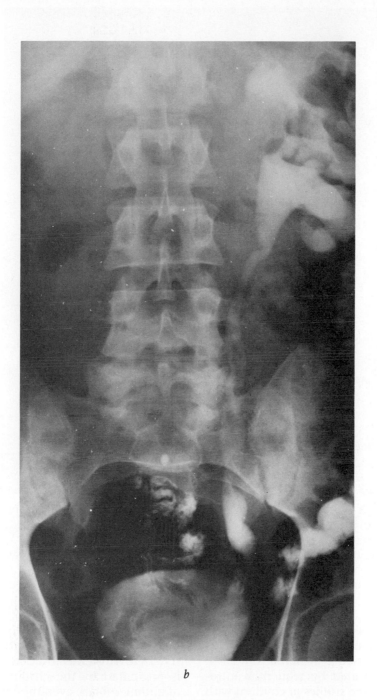

b

FIG. 8-3 (Continued).

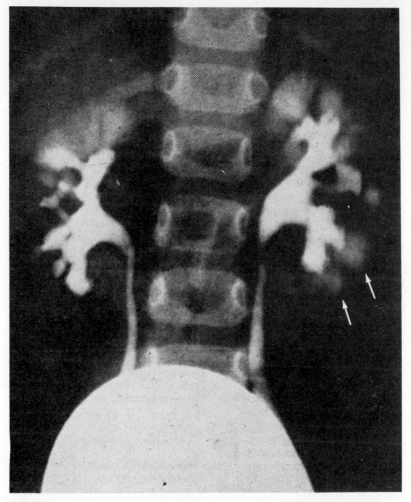

FIG. 8-4. Voiding cystourethrogram in a 4-year-old girl with recurrent urinary tract infections. Gross reflux is demonstrable into the renal collecting systems *and* the renal parenchyma bilaterally. Arrows demonstrate the intrarenal reflux in lower pole of the left kidney. (*From A. D. Amar, J. Am. Med. Assoc., 213:293, 1970. Copyright, American Medical Association, 1970.*)

It is generally believed that it is the *reflux of infected urine* into the renal parenchyma that is responsible for scarring in humans.[127-130,133] This can be illustrated by sequential intravenous pyelographic studies in children with VUR. New scars form only in those children who develop a urinary tract infection.[129,130,136] In comparison, new scars do not occur and renal growth tends to be normal if infection is prevented by the chronic administration of antimicrobials, even though VUR may persist.[137]

The pathologic changes associated with chronic pyelonephritis are typical of other interstitial nephritides: interstitial fibrosis with mononuclear cell infiltration and tubular atrophy. In addition, progressive glomerular sclerosis occurs in advanced chronic pyelonephritis.[125,138,139] It seems likely that this late change is due primarily to hemodynamically mediated glomerular injury (see Chap. 4).[140] According to this theory, the initial infection-induced nephron loss leads to compensatory increases in glomerular capillary pressure and filtration rate in the relatively unaffected nephrons. The intraglomerular hypertension then appears to produce glomerular injury and eventual sclerosis.

CLINICAL PRESENTATION

The clinical history in chronic pyelonephritis varies with the underlying disorder. Many infants or children with VUR present with a urinary tract infection. The diagnosis can easily be missed in infants, however, who may display such nonspecific findings as fever, failure to thrive, abdominal distress, or loss of bladder control.[141] If the diagnosis is not made or the infections are asymptomatic, the patient may not seek medical care until there are signs and symptoms directly due to advanced renal failure such as pallor, weakness, anorexia, nocturia, hypertension, or anemia.

In comparison, patients with chronic pyelonephritis due to nephrolithiasis may have findings related to stone disease. These include a history of passing stones, episodes of renal colic or hematuria, or, with persistently infected struvite stones, a history of symptomatic urinary tract infections with urease-producing organisms and chronic vague back or flank pain.

The urinalysis in chronic pyelonephritis typically reveals pyuria and less often white cell casts. Bacteriuria will be seen only if the patient is infected at the time of presentation.

Protein excretion is usually less than 1 g/day in patients with relatively mild disease. However, proteinuria can reach the nephrotic range in patients with renal insufficiency, a finding that presumably reflects the development of hemodynamically mediated focal glomerulosclerosis.[138-140]

DIAGNOSIS

The diagnosis of chronic pyelonephritis is established by an IVP which reveals the characteristic changes of decreased renal size, blunting and dilatation of the calyces, and segmental cortical scarring over the affected calyces (Fig. 8-3). Ureteral dilatation may also be seen in patients who have had marked reflux.

These findings are relatively specific for chronic pyelonephritis, although not necessarily for infection with common bacteria. Urinary tuberculosis can produce similar renal changes, but ureteral strictures and a contracted bladder (due to scarring at sites of tuberculous infection) are also frequently found. This combination of *upper and lower tract abnormalities* is highly suggestive of tuberculosis.[142] In addition, men with genital involvement may have calcifications in the vas deferens, seminal vesicles, and prostate. Renal scarring also may occur with vascular diseases such as nephrosclerosis. In this setting, however, the scars are randomly distributed and the calyces are normal.

Once the diagnosis of chronic pyelonephritis is established by IVP, a young child should have a voiding cystourethrogram to see if VUR is present (Fig. 8-3). In many patients, however, VUR can no longer be demonstrated. This is most likely to occur after puberty, as the increased length of the submucosal portion of the terminal ureter leads to the spontaneous disappearance of reflux.[137,143] In this setting, cystoscopy, if performed, still reveals changes at the ureteral orifices that are compatible with previous reflux.[144]

A somewhat separate issue is how to evaluate children who have a urinary tract infection, 30 to 45 percent of whom will have VUR.[126-128] Children over the age of 5 should have at least a plain film of the abdomen (looking for stones) and a renal ultrasound which, if the study is adequate, should detect significant renal scarring.[145,146] No further evaluation is necessary if scarring is absent, since the loss of intrarenal reflux in this age group makes the likelihood of forming new scars very small.[124,126,130,135] An IVP should be performed if scarring appears to be present or there is suboptimal visualization of the kidneys on the ultrasound examination.

The evaluation is somewhat different in younger children who may still be at risk of developing new scars. In this setting, a plain film, renal ultrasound, and voiding cystourethrogram should be part of the initial evaluation and an IVP performed if indicated.[145,146]

It is also important to recognize the familial nature of VUR. A prospective evaluation of 104 siblings of 78 children with reflux revealed that 32 percent had VUR, usually without a history of a symptomatic urinary tract infection.[147] Fifteen percent of the siblings with reflux (or 5 percent of all siblings) also had renal scars. Thus, it may be reasonable to perform a screening renal ultrasound in siblings of children with chronic pyelonephritis.

COURSE AND THERAPY

Chronic pyelonephritis not infrequently progresses to end-stage renal failure. Two factors appear to be important in those patients who progress: recurrent infection[129,130,136] and glomerulosclerosis that is presumably mediated by hemodynamic factors.[125,138-140] The benefit of preventing infection has been illustrated by the continuous prophylactic use of low-dose therapy with trimethoprim-sulfamethoxazole or nitrofurantoin.[137] If continued for 5 to 10 years, this regimen is associated with normal renal growth and no new scars

in over 90 percent of refluxing kidneys, and cessation of reflux in 80 percent of refluxing ureters, including many with gross reflux.

Focal glomerulosclerosis is a relatively late finding in chronic pyelonephritis, with the plasma creatinine concentration usually being above 2 mg/dL[125,138,139] The major clinical clue to its presence is protein excretion that exceeds 1 g/day.[125] This is an important diagnosis to make since neither control of infection nor surgical correction of reflux appears to prevent progressive renal failure once glomerulosclerosis is present.[125,148,149] The major therapeutic objective at this time is control of the compensatory *intraglomerular* hypertension with a converting enzyme inhibitor and/or dietary protein restriction (see Chap. 4). The safety of the latter, however, is uncertain in children since a low-protein diet could impair growth.

Medical versus Surgical Therapy. The role for surgical correction of VUR is a source of controversy in the management of patients with chronic pyelonephritis.[150-152] Although surgery is of relatively little risk and is highly effective in reversing reflux, it is not clear that surgery alters the course of the disease as long as infection can be prevented. In adults with VUR and scarring, for example, surgery can decrease the incidence of episodes of acute pyelonephritis but has no effect on kidney size, scarring, proteinuria, or the GFR when compared to patients managed conservatively.[153,154] Similar results have been found in older children (6 to 15 years of age) in whom progressive renal failure did not usually occur in the absence of infection.[155]

This lack of efficacy of surgery in older children and adults is not surprising since intrarenal reflux ceases after the age of 5.[133] As a result, new scar formation is unusual (in the absence of severe infection)[124,126,130,135] and a continued decline in renal function is generally due to glomerulosclerosis. As described above, chronic antimicrobial therapy can prevent infection and allow normal renal growth to occur, with VUR frequently disappearing spontaneously by puberty.[137,143] Surgery is also not necessary, if infection can be controlled, in patients with unilateral VUR and scarring since the normal kidney plus continued growth in the affected kidney permit the maintenance of good overall renal function.[156]

The major indication for surgery is the presence of gross reflux and ureteral dilatation in a young child (particularly if under the age of 1 to 2), since scarring may develop in as many as 60 percent of patients in this group.[125] Surgery is also indicated in children with progressive scarring, who usually become infected[129,130,136] due to poor compliance with antimicrobial therapy, and in patients with large staghorn calculi due to infected struvite stones.[157] Antimicrobials are generally ineffective in the latter setting (because the bacteria are embedded in the stone), and persistence of the stone can lead to progressive renal damage. Although stone removal is the procedure of choice, the affected kidney may be virtually nonfunctional in some patients and nephrectomy may be indicated for control of infection.

A typical example of the course of severe reflux nephropathy is illustrated by the following case history.

Case History 8–1. A 21-year-old woman with a chief complaint of weakness is found to be anemic on routine laboratory evaluation. Her past history is unremarkable except for a urinary tract infection at age 3 that was treated with antimicrobials but was not evaluated further. She has had no subsequent symptoms suggest of recurrent infection. Her physical examination is normal except for pallor and a blood pressure of 140/100.

Blood tests reveal that the hematocrit is 29 percent, blood urea nitrogen (BUN) 79 mg/dL, and plasma creatinine concentration 5.8 mg/dL. The urinalysis shows 3+ protein and 15 to 20 white cells per high power field. The urine culture is negative; 24-h urine protein excretion is 4.4 g. An IVP demonstrates small kidneys and the typical changes of chronic pyelonephritis with marked cortical scarring. A voiding cystourethrogram shows bilateral reflux.

Comment. This young woman undoubtedly had gross reflux and infection as a child, leading to marked renal damage. Although she had only one detected urinary tract infection, it is likely that she had other infections that were either asymptomatic or missed because of atypical symptoms. She now presents with advanced renal insufficiency and probably glomerulosclerosis, considering the presence of proteinuria. At this time, corrective surgery will neither restore nor preserve renal function. The only therapy that might be effective is attempting to minimize further hemodynamic damage by lowering the systemic blood pressure (preferentially with a converting enzyme inhibitor) and/or dietary protein restriction.

CYSTIC DISEASES OF THE KIDNEY

Cystic diseases in the renal tubule occur in a variety of disorders. These include polycystic kidney disease, medullary sponge kidney, medullary cystic kidney disease, acquired cystic disease in patients with chronic renal failure, and single or multiple simple cysts. The last disorder is usually asymptomatic and is detected only as an incidental finding on a radiologic examination. In contrast, the first three conditions have characteristic pathologic and clinical abnormalities (Table 8–4).

POLYCYSTIC KIDNEY DISEASE

The most common form of polycystic kidney disease (PKD) is the adult type. This disorder is inherited as an autosomal dominant with

TABLE 8–4. Clinical Characteristics of Cystic Diseases of the Kidney

	Polycystic Kidney Disease, Adult Type	Medullary Sponge Kidney	Medullary Cystic Kidney Disease
Heredity	Autosomal dominant or sporadic	Usually not familial	Variable—autosomal recessive or dominant or not familial
Location of cysts	Throughout nephron	Terminal collecting ducts	Primarily at corticomedullary junction
Flank pain	Common	Only with complications	Absent
Hypertension	Common	Unusual	Unusual
Hematuria	Frequent	Only with complications	Absent
Intravenous pyelography	Large kidneys with cysts	Papillary cavities, stones	Small kidneys
Azotemia after onset	Frequent	Only with complications	Invariable
Age at uremia	Usually greater than 50	Not present	20 to 40

SOURCE: From S. H. Goldman, S. R. Walker, T. C. Merigan, Jr., K. D. Gardner, Jr., and J. M. C. Bull, *N. Engl. J. Med.*, 274:984, 1966. Reprinted by permission from the *New England Journal of Medicine*.

virtually complete penetrance if the patient lives to 80 years of age.[158-161] A sporadic form also occurs that tends to have a more benign clinical course.[162] It is possible, however, that some of these cases represent familial PKD in which delayed expression masked the diagnosis in affected relatives.[160]

Adult PKD is a common disorder, occurring in approximately 1 in every 1250 live births.[161] It also accounts for 10 to 12 percent of cases of end-stage renal disease, a finding that is related to the almost uniformly progressive nature of the disease.[161]

Infantile and childhood forms of PKD also occur.[163,164] These rare disorders, which will not be discussed further, are transmitted as an autosomal recessive trait. Renal failure and hepatic cirrhosis (due to cysts and fibrosis) frequently develop and are the major causes of death. In some patients, only one kidney is affected.[164] This abnormality may remain undetected or be discovered incidentally as the kidney appears hypoplastic or dysplastic.

PATHOLOGY AND PATHOGENESIS

The kidneys in adult PKD eventually become enlarged by the presence of multiple cysts of varying size throughout the renal parenchyma. Cysts can occur at any site in the nephron,[158,165] each of which is a localized distension of an intact functioning tubule. As a result, the composition of the cyst fluid reflects that segment of the nephron in which the cyst is formed: similar to plasma in the proximal tubule and low-sodium–high-potassium concentration in the distal nephron.[166,167]

The anatomic abnormalities in PKD are not limited to the kidney.[158-160] Cysts may also be found in the liver and less commonly in the pancreas, spleen, and other organs. In addition, structural weakness of the walls of the cerebral arteries can lead to aneurysm formation and intracerebral or subarachnoid hemorrhage in about 10 percent of patients.[168] Other findings that may occur with increased frequency in PKD include colonic diverticula, inguinal hernias, and aortic regurgitation due to dilatation of the aortic root and annulus.[169-171]

The genetic defect in PKD has been localized to an abnormality on the short arm of chromosome 16.[172] However, the factors responsible for cyst formation are unclear. In experimental animals, the administration of toxins such as diphenylamine and diphenylthiazole can lead to a cystic disease similar to PKD.[173,174] It has been postulated that these toxins produce a structural defect in the tubular basement membrane (TBM). The ensuing weakening of the TBM could, in the presence of normal intratubular pressures, lead to segmental distension of the tubule and cyst formation. This hypothesis may also be applicable to humans, except that the abnormal basement membrane would result from a genetic rather than a toxic source.[159,174] A primary basement membrane defect has the additional advantage of also being able to explain the extrarenal manifestations of PKD, such as aneurysm formation, cysts in other organs, and colonic diverticula.

Alternatively, PKD could result from primary hyperplasia of the tubular cells with subsequent tubular obstruction.[159,174] The associated rise in tubular pressure proximal to the obstruction would then promote cyst formation.

CLINICAL PRESENTATION

Excluding patients who are evaluated at any early age because of a positive family history, the diagnosis of PKD is not usually made until the age of 30 to 50, the time at which symptoms typically first appear. Flank pain, vague abdominal complaints, symptoms of a urinary tract infection, episodes of gross hematuria, and the incidental discovery of

hypertension are common presenting problems.[158,160] In contrast, a sense of abdominal fullness due to enlarged kidneys (which are frequently palpable on physical examination) occurs relatively late in the course of the disease.

Hypertension eventually occurs in up to 70 percent of patients, usually before the onset of renal failure.[175-177] Focal compression of the intrarenal arteries by the cysts may be of primary importance in this setting by promoting renin secretion and subsequent sodium retention.[175]

The laboratory data at the time of presentation are variable. The BUN and plasma creatinine concentration are usually somewhat elevated, although rare patients may have advanced renal failure. The urinalysis may be relatively normal or reveal hematuria, pyuria (if infection is present), or mild proteinuria. The hematocrit is occasionally higher than would be expected from the degree of renal insufficiency.[177] This may be seen even in nonazotemic patients, as about 5 percent of men have a hemoglobin concentration above 18 g/dL.[170] Increased production of erythropoietin, perhaps resulting from local ischemia induced by the cysts, is thought to be responsible for these findings.

DIAGNOSIS

The diagnosis of PKD may be suspected from a positive family history or the presence of palpable kidneys on physical examination. Confirmation of the diagnosis is made by radiologic studies. Although intravenous pyelography may be useful, this test has largely been replaced by ultrasonography and CT scanning, which are better able to detect smaller cysts (Fig. 8–5). In general, cysts as small as 1 to 1.5 cm in diameter can be seen by ultrasonography and 0.5 cm by CT scanning.[178]

When ultrasonography or CT scanning is used to screen for early PKD, the criteria for

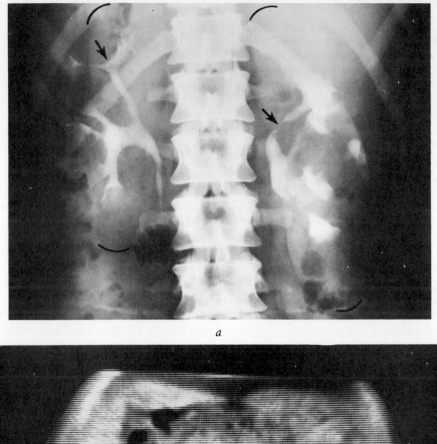

a

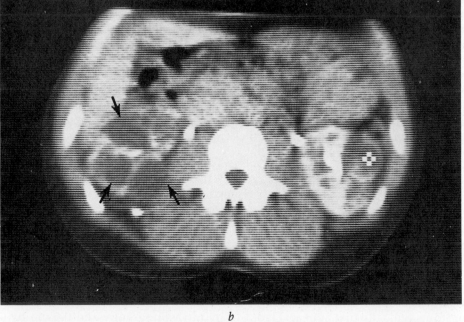

b

FIG. 8–5. Radiographic changes in polycystic kidney disease. (*a*) IVP reveals enlarged kidneys (20.5 cm on left, 18 cm on right) with splaying of the calyces (arrows) due to deforming effects of the cysts. (*b*) CT scan reveals multiple cysts in each kidney (arrows demonstrate cysts in right kidney).

a positive test are at least one cyst in each kidney, with at least one of the kidneys having two or more cysts.[172,179] In the absence of a positive family history of PKD, however, these findings are not diagnostic since they may also be seen with multiple simple cysts (see below). The latter usually occur in older patients (above the age of 50), a time at which patients with PKD generally have had symptoms and have radiologic changes that are much more prominent than the minimal criteria described above. These include renal enlargement due to bilateral and diffuse cyst formation, with areas of normal parenchyma between the cysts frequently not visualized.

If asymptomatic first-degree relatives of patients with PKD are evaluated by ultrasonography, the likelihood of detecting the disease increases with age. It has been estimated, for example, that the probability of a positive test in subjects who will ultimately develop PKD is approximately 8 percent below the age of 10, 70 to 80 percent between the ages of 20 and 30, and almost 100 percent above the age of 35 to 40.[179] Thus, although ultrasonography is an excellent screening procedure, a negative test cannot reliably exclude this disease under the age of 40.[178] CT scanning can detect some of the patients missed by ultrasonography, but a negative test can still occur in patients with the disease who are under 30 years of age.

COURSE

In most patients with PKD, there is a slow decline in renal function over many years.[158,177,180] It is likely that only a minority of nephrons form cysts, with the decline in renal function being due to obstruction or atrophy of the nonaffected nephrons by the expanding cysts.[159] End-stage renal failure is uncommon below the age of 40 but occurs in about 25 percent of patients by age 50, and 70 percent by age 65.[177,180] The prognosis may be better in patients with the sporadic form of

PKD in whom renal failure appears to be uncommon.[162]

In addition to progressive renal failure, the course of PKD can be complicated by a variety of other problems including gross hematuria due to bleeding into a cyst, urinary tract infections, severe pain resulting from an enlarged cyst, nephrolithiasis, renal cell carcinoma, and subarachnoid or intracerebral hemorrhage.[158-161,168,181] Infected cysts occur more often in women, are typically due to ascending infection, and may follow urinary tract instrumentation, which should be avoided if possible.[161,177,182] Effective treatment requires the use of antimicrobials that are able to penetrate the infected cyst. This is an important issue since drugs such as the aminoglycosides, cephalosporins, and ampicillin achieve low concentrations in the cyst and are generally unable to cure the infection.[183,184] Potentially effective antimicrobials in this setting include trimethoprim-sulfamethoxazole, chloramphenicol, clindamycin, and erythromycin.[183-185] The urine culture results should determine which agent is used.

Severe flank pain is usually a transient problem related to bleeding into or gradual enlargement of a cyst. In patients with marked or persistent pain, however, decompression of the cyst may be required. This can be achieved most easily by percutaneous puncture, although fluid accumulation and pain frequently recur within 3 to 12 weeks.[186] In this setting, surgery may be required for permanent relief of the pain.

Renal cell carcinoma is an infrequent complication of PKD.[161,181] It may be bilateral in some patients, suggesting the presence of multiple foci of cellular proliferation. Why this occurs is not known. The diagnosis of renal cell carcinoma can easily be missed because typical presenting findings such as hematuria and a flank mass are also commonly seen in uncomplicated PKD. Thus, only systemic symptoms or signs (anorexia, fatigue, weight loss, anemia) that are out of proportion to the degree of renal insufficiency are likely to suggest the presence of a malignancy. CT scanning and arteriography may be required to establish the diagnosis.

The 10 to 13 percent incidence of ruptured intracerebral aneurysm is an important cause of morbidity and mortality in PKD.[158,168] Nevertheless, routine cerebral arteriography does not appear to be indicated, considering the invasive nature of this procedure and the fact that a negative test does not preclude development of an aneurysm at a later time.[168] It is possible, however, that CT scanning of the brain can be used as a screening procedure in patients with a family history of intracerebral hemorrhage.

TREATMENT

Therapy in PKD is largely supportive since the as yet unidentified underlying defect cannot be corrected. There is, however, preliminary evidence suggesting that attempting to prevent hemodynamically mediated glomerular injury by a low-protein diet and control of hypertension (particularly with a converting enzyme inhibitor) can slow the rate of decline in renal function (see Chap. 4).[187-189] Control of the systemic blood pressure might also be expected to reduce the incidence of cerebral aneurysm rupture. Dialysis and transplantation can be performed in those patients who progress to end-stage renal failure.[190,191]

MEDULLARY SPONGE KIDNEY

Medullary sponge kidney (MSK) is characterized by malformation of the collecting ducts with cyst formation.[192,193] Although these changes appear to be congenital, evidence for genetic transmission is lacking in most patients.

The relationship between MSK and other cystic diseases of the kidney is uncertain. Examination of relatives of patients with medullary cystic disease has in some instances revealed a high incidence of MSK.[194,195] Similarly, MSK and PKD have been described both within a single family and together in the same patient.[196-198] The significance of these findings is uncertain; it is possible, for example, that at least in some patients MSK may be a *forme fruste* of the more serious cystic diseases.

PATHOLOGY

Medullary sponge kidney is primarily a disease of the terminal collecting ducts in the pericalyceal region of the renal pyramids. Both macroscopic and microscopic cysts may be present. In contrast to PKD, the renal cortex is spared and the degree of cyst formation may be limited. Although the cysts are usually diffuse and bilateral, unilateral changes may be seen involving all or only isolated pyramids in the affected kidney.[199]

Calculi are frequently present within the cysts. These stones are primarily composed of calcium salts which precipitate in part because of stasis within the abnormal tubules.[200,201] Hypercalciuria or hyperuricosuria make stone formation more likely, but the incidence of these metabolic abnormalities is similar to that in stone formers without MSK.[200]

CLINICAL PRESENTATION AND COURSE

Many patients with MSK have no symptoms, and the diagnosis is never made unless an IVP is performed for some other reason. Symptoms occur only if infection develops or if the passage of a stone results in flank pain or hematuria. The urinary findings usually vary with the clinical state, ranging from normal to hematuria or pyuria during symptomatic episodes.

In contrast to PKD or medullary cystic disease, renal function does not usually deteriorate in MSK. Thus, the GFR is normal unless a stone has led to urinary tract obstruction.

DIAGNOSIS

The diagnosis of MSK is made by intravenous pyelography. As a result of the dilated terminal collecting ducts, opacifications are seen in the pericalyceal areas of some or all calyces which have the appearance of a brush radiating outward from the calyx (Fig. 8–6). Calculi also may be visualized; they are small and characteristically bunched around the affected calyces.

These changes, although relatively diagnostic, may appear similar to those seen with papillary necrosis. Differentiating between these disorders is generally not difficult since a cause of papillary necrosis (diabetes mellitus, analgesic abuse, obstruction) can usually be identified. In patients in whom the diagnosis is in doubt, retrograde pyelography may be helpful, since the calyces are usually normal in MSK but grossly distorted in papillary necrosis.[199]

TREATMENT

MSK is a benign disease that typically requires no specific treatment except during episodes of urinary tract infection or stone passage. Patients who are recurrent stone formers may require therapy with thiazide diuretics, allopurinol, potassium citrate, or oral phosphate depending upon the biochemical abnormality that is present.[202,203]

MEDULLARY CYSTIC KIDNEY DISEASE

Medullary cystic kidney disease (MCD) is a rare disorder of children that invariably progresses to end-stage renal failure.[192,204–206] Another condition which develops at a somewhat older age, familial juvenile nephronophthisis, appears to be histologically and clinically indistinguishable from MCD. These disorders can occur sporadically or, more commonly, as an inherited disorder.[205,206]

The mode of inheritance is variable as autosomal recessive, autosomal dominant, and, less often, X-linked forms have been described.

PATHOLOGY

Medullary cystic disease is characterized by cysts ranging in size from less than 1 mm to 1 cm. These cysts arise from structurally intact distal and collecting tubules and are primarily located at the corticomedullary junction and in the medulla. Microscopic examination also reveals interstitial inflammation and fibrosis, tubular atrophy, and eventually glomerular sclerosis.

CLINICAL PRESENTATION

There are no early symptoms associated with MCD since stone formation, infection, and hypertension usually do not occur. As a result, patients typically present with nocturia (due to loss of concentrating ability) or symptoms of uremia such as anorexia, nausea, and fatigue. The age at which renal failure develops is variable, usually occurring before the age of 20 in autosomal recessive MCD and as old as 40 to 50 in autosomal dominant familial juvenile nephronophthisis.[205,206]

The urinalysis is characteristically normal in this disorder, a reflection of the noninflammatory nature of the disease. However, abnormal tubular function can lead to a relatively early impairment in concentrating ability and to sodium wasting. The latter is usually not important clinically as long as sodium intake is maintained. Nevertheless, signs and symptoms of volume depletion (fatigue, muscle cramps, postural dizziness) can occur if intake is reduced.

DIAGNOSIS

The diagnosis of MCD is most often made by inference from the clinical presentation and, if present, a positive family history. In a child

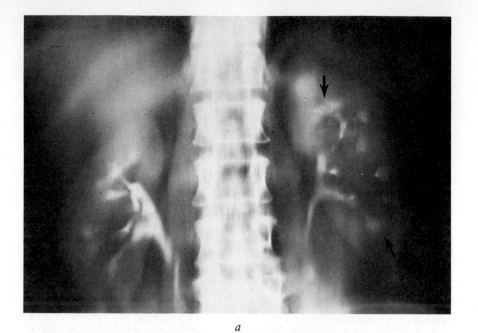

a

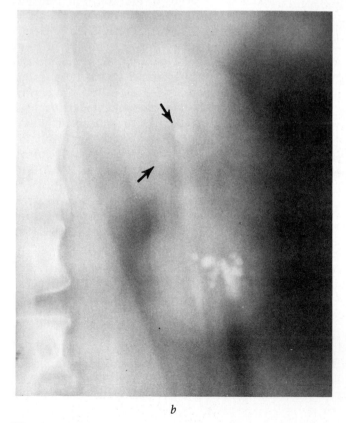

b

FIG. 8-6. Radiologic findings in medullary sponge kidney. (*a*) All the calyces are abnormal as evidenced by brushlike appearance radiating outward from the calyces (arrows). (*b*) Calcium stones are bunched around upper (arrows) and lower calyces in a patient in whom these were the only involved pyramids.

or young adult with advanced renal failure and a normal urinalysis, the primary causes other than MCD are obstructive uropathy and chronic pyelonephritis. These conditions have characteristic radiologic changes (hydronephrosis and segmental scarring with blunted calyces, respectively) that allow them to be differentiated from MCD, where multiple small cysts may be seen at the corticomedullary junction by ultrasonography or CT scanning. Renal biopsy is usually not indicated, since the kidneys are small. If a biopsy is performed, however, the typical cystic changes in the medulla can generally be identified.

COURSE AND TREATMENT

Medullary cystic disease invariably progresses to end-stage renal failure, requiring dialysis or transplantation. There is no known therapy that alters the course of the disease.

ACQUIRED CYSTIC DISEASE

It has recently been recognized that patients with chronic renal failure frequently develop a unique form of acquired cystic disease.[161,207–209] This disorder is particularly common in patients who have been hemodialyzed for more than 3 years, reaching an incidence that can exceed 35 to 45 percent.

The cysts are small, multiple, and bilateral and can arise from tubular cells in both the proximal and distal nephron.[209] They may be associated with cellular proliferation and adenoma formation in up to one-quarter of patients.[161,208] The mechanism by which these changes occur is not understood. Three theories have been proposed, each of which may play a contributory role: (1) the loss of renal function can lead to the retention of renotropic or toxic factors that promote epithelial cell hyperplasia or weakening of the tubular basement membranes; (2) the compensatory increase in nephron glomerular filtration rate (GFR) in the relatively unaffected nephrons results in enhanced flow within the nephron that, in the presence of basement membrane abnormalities, can favor cyst formation; and (3) plasticizers or other substances associated with dialysis or dialysis tubing may have a toxic effect on the cells or the basement membranes.[161,208] The observation that cyst size falls after successful renal transplantation is compatible with all these hypotheses, since they are all reversed by the restoration of relatively normal renal function.[161,208]

The cysts are most often an incidental finding and produce no symptoms. In some patients, however, rupture of unsupported blood vessels within the cyst can lead to pain and gross hematuria. Even more serious is the development of *carcinoma*. This potentially fatal complication occurs in 1 to 4 percent of patients with acquired cysts, an incidence much higher than that in the general population.[161,208]

As a result of the risk of malignancy and the increasing incidence of acquired cystic disease with time on dialysis, it has been recommended that patients who have been dialyzed for more than 3 years should have screening renal ultrasonography at yearly intervals.[161,208] Once cystic disease is found, a CT scan should be performed at periodic intervals to screen for the development of an intracystic tumor.

SIMPLE CYSTS

Simple renal cysts are the most common renal masses, accounting for about 65 to 70 percent of cases.[210,211] They are particularly frequent in patients over the age of 50, up to one-half of whom may have cystic disease (as determined from postmortem examination).[211] Simple cysts can lead to abdominal or flank pain in some patients,[211] but they are most often asymptomatic and discovered as an incidental finding on a plain film of the abdomen, IVP, or renal ultrasound. They may be solitary, or multiple and bilateral.

The major concern is distinguishing simple

cysts from more serious disorders such as PKD (see above) and solid masses such as a renal carcinoma or abscess. Ultrasonography and CT scanning are usually able to make this distinction.[212] The criteria for a cyst on ultrasonography include:

1. The mass is sharply marginated with smooth walls.
2. There are no echoes (anechoic) within the mass.
3. There is a strong posterior wall echo indicating good transmission through the cyst.

If all three of these findings is present, no further evaluation is indicated since the likelihood of a malignancy is extremely small. A CT scan should be performed, however, if the ultrasonogram is equivocal, if calcifications or septa are seen, or if multiple cysts are clustered in a pattern that could mask an underlying carcinoma. A simple cyst is considered to be present if, on CT scan:

1. The cyst is sharply demarcated from the surrounding parenchyma and has a smooth, thin wall.
2. Fluid within the cyst is homogeneous with a density of 0 to 20 Hounsfield units.
3. There is no enhancement of the cyst fluid following the administration of radiocontrast media.

The accuracy of these radiologic procedures has led to a marked reduction in the necessity for cyst puncture (which can lead to complications such as a perirenal hematoma or gross hematuria in up to 4 percent of patients)[211] or for renal arteriography in the evaluation of a renal mass.[212] These tests may be required in patients who fulfill some but not all the criteria for a benign cyst. This topic is reviewed in detail elsewhere.[212]

MYELOMA KIDNEY

Renal disease progressing to renal failure is a common occurrence in multiple myeloma and, after infection, is the leading cause of death.[213–215] A variety of factors can contribute to the decline in renal function, including the excretion of immunoglobulin light chains in the urine (so-called *myeloma kidney*), hypercalcemia, primary amyloidosis or light chain deposition disease, and, rarely, hyperuricemia or plasma cell invasion of the renal parenchyma.[214–217]

PATHOLOGY

The pathologic changes in myeloma kidney are most prominent in the tubules, particularly the distal and collecting tubules. The primary abnormalities are glassy, eosinophilic casts, and tubular atrophy and degeneration (Fig. 8–7).[214–216] Although it had been thought that the tubular casts represented only precipitated light chains, immunofluorescent studies have indicated that other filtered proteins (albumin, fibrinogen, and intact gamma globulins) and Tamm-Horsfall mucoprotein are also present.[218,219] The glomeruli are usually spared unless amyloidosis or light chain deposition disease is also present.

PATHOGENESIS

The malignant plasma cells in multiple myeloma may produce both monoclonal intact globulins (which are not nephrotoxic) and free light chains. Monomeric free light chains, which are normally produced in slight excess of heavy chains, have a molecular weight of approximately 22,000. They are freely filtered across the glomerulus and then largely reabsorbed by and catabolized in the proximal tubular cells.[220] As a result, light chain excretion is normally less than 30 mg/day. However, proximal reabsorptive capacity can be exceeded when the production and subsequent filtration of light chains is enhanced, as occurs in approximately one-half of patients with multiple myeloma.[213,221] In this setting, the excretion of light chains (or Bence Jones proteins) is increased, ranging from 100 mg/day to more than 20 g/day.

Myeloma kidney is directly related to the

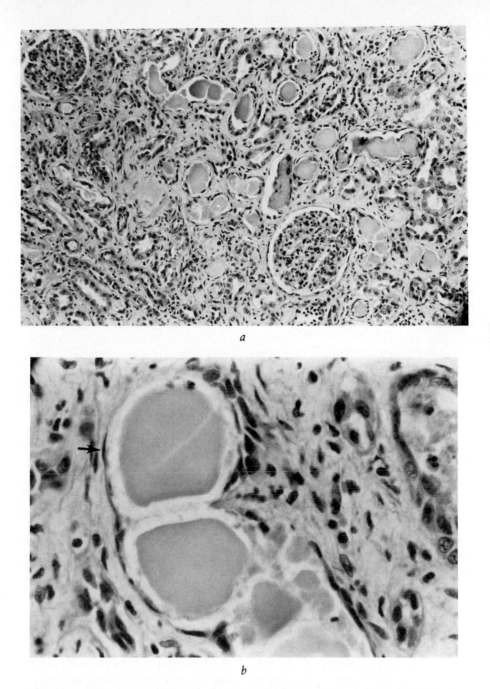

FIG. 8–7. Pathologic findings in myeloma kidney. (*a*) Many of the tubules are filled with hyaline material which primarily contains precipitated light chains. Interstitial edema, fibrosis, and mononuclear cell infiltration are also present. The glomeruli are normal. (*b*) A high power view also demonstrates tubular atrophy with marked flattening of the tubular epithelium (arrow).

urinary excretion of light chains, which usually exceeds 1 g per day in patients who develop renal insufficiency.[214,222] However, some patients excrete much larger quantities without developing a fall in GFR, suggesting that light chains in different patients have variable degrees of nephrotoxicity.[214,223,224]

The mechanism by which light chains produce renal disease is incompletely understood. *Tubular obstruction* by the precipitated casts appears to be one important factor. It has been suggested that light chains with a high isoelectric point (pI > 5.8–6.0) are most likely to lead to renal failure.[225-227] At the acid urine pH in the distal nephron, these light chains would have a positive charge, allowing them to interact with anionic Tamm-Horsfall mucoprotein (pI $= 3.2$), thereby forming obstructing casts.[225,226,228] The observation that alkalinization of the urine with sodium bicarbonate protects against myeloma kidney in animals is consistent with this hypothesis, since at a high urine pH both the light chain and Tamm-Horsfall mucoprotein will be negatively charged and therefore less likely to coprecipitate.[228]

Tubular obstruction, however, cannot explain the entire picture of myeloma kidney. Renal function has been noted to correlate best with the degree of tubular atrophy and not with cast formation, which is relative mild in some patients.[214,229] Furthermore, not all investigators have been able to document the preferential toxic effects of light chains with a high pI.[230,231]

Taken together, these findings suggest that *direct tubular toxicity* may be of primary importance in myeloma kidney.[214,229,231] Such a change could interact positively with the tubular obstruction model. Suppose, for example, that the excess filtered light chains are reabsorbed by and accumulate in the proximal tubular cells.[220] These toxic proteins could impair tubular function, leading to a subsequent reduction in reabsorptive capacity. As a result, more filtered light chains are delivered distally, favoring the formation of obstructing tubular casts. A similar increase in distal delivery could result from the initial loss of functioning nephrons, creating a vicious cycle that promotes progressive renal failure. As described in Chap. 4, nephron loss leads to compensatory hyperfiltration in the remaining less affected nephrons. This elevation in nephron GFR also enhances the filtration of light chains producing more tubular toxicity and obstruction.

In addition to promoting the development of renal failure, tubular toxicity can lead to a variety of abnormalities in both the proximal and distal nephron segments.[232,233] These include the Fanconi syndrome (characterized in part by proximal renal tubular acidosis and aminoaciduria) and distal defects such as sodium-wasting and impaired concentrating and acidifying ability.

It is important to note that excess production of light chains also can produce *glomerular lesions* due to primary amyloidosis or light chain deposition disease (see p. 208) as well as myeloma kidney. Furthermore, patients with one of the first two disorders do not typically develop extensive tubular cast formation.[222]

These observations suggest an important role for the *biochemical characteristics* (in addition to the isoelectric point) of the excess light chains that are produced. For example lambda (λ) light chains, particularly those containing the λ_{VI} variable region, are much more likely to form the characteristic β-pleated amyloid fibrils than are kappa (κ) light chains.[234,235] In comparison, light chain deposition disease primarily involves κ light chains.[236] In both of these disorders, the excess light chains must be able to be taken up by and degraded in macrophages, which then secrete the fragments that are deposited in the tissues.[237] It is possible that these fragments are less nephrotoxic and less likely to promote intratubular obstruction than the intact light chains in myeloma kidney.

The ability of the light chain to be filtered is another potential determinant of the type of renal disease that can occur. Polymerized or highly anionic (low pI) light chains may be relatively poorly filtered because of the size and charge restriction to the filtration of macromolecules across the glomerulus (see p. 13).[222] In this setting, myeloma kidney would not occur, but the nonfiltered light chains would accumulate in the plasma and could then undergo tissue deposition as in amyloidosis.

CLINICAL MANIFESTATIONS AND DIAGNOSIS

The common clinical and laboratory manifestations of multiple myeloma include weakness, bone pain, anemia, lytic lesions on x-ray, hypercalcemia, and renal insufficiency in approximately one-half of patients at the time of diagnosis.[213] Impaired renal function is particularly common in patients with light chain myeloma (who do not produce excess intact globulins), probably due to the uniform presence of Bence Jones proteinuria in this setting.[238] The urine sediment in mycloma kidney is typically normal, and albuminuria (as detectable by the dipstick which senses only albumin) is mild or absent. In comparison, marked albuminuria (with a positive dipstick reading) is suggestive of amyloidosis or light chain deposition disease.

The diagnosis of multiple myeloma is more strongly suggested by the demonstration of a paraprotein in the plasma or urine. A monoclonal globulin is present in the plasma in 75 to 90 percent of patients and can be detected by protein electrophoresis. Most of the remaining patients produce only light chains (light chain myeloma).[213,238] These light chains can be detected by *immunoelectrophoresis* of the plasma or urine but not by routine protein electrophoresis.

However, a plasma or urine paraprotein is not specific for multiple myeloma, also being found in some patients with primary amyloidosis, Waldenström's macroglobulinemia, malignant lymphoma, and chronic lymphocytic leukemia*,[213,215,221] and as an idiopathic condition which frequently evolves into overt multiple myeloma over a period of many years.[224] As a result, examination of a bone marrow specimen is required to establish the diagnosis.

It is important to note that the finding of *polyclonal* light chains (both λ and κ) in the urine is nonspecific and does not suggest an underlying hematologic malignancy.[221] This abnormality can be seen in renal failure (as tubular damage impairs the proximal reabsorption of normally filtered light chains) and in disorders associated with a generalized increase in globulin synthesis, such as collagen vascular diseases and neoplasms.

Several screening tests that are simpler to perform than immunoelectrophoresis are available to detect Bence Jones proteinuria. If the urine is gradually heated, Bence Jones proteins characteristically precipitate at 45 to 55°C, redissolve at 100°C, and then precipitate again as the urine cools.[221] Another method of detecting nonalbumin protcins (but not specifically light chains) is to test the urine with both the dipstick and sulfosalicyclic acid (see p. 14). A more positive test with sulfosalicylic acid is typically found in patients with myeloma kidney (versus an equivalent degree of positivity when albuminuria is present). Both the heat and sulfosalicylic acid tests, however, are much less sensitive than immunoelectrophoresis, not being positive unless the concentration of light chains is greater than 1 to 1.5 g/L.[215,240]

The importance of routinely using sulfosalicyclic acid in the evaluation of patients with renal disease can be illustrated by the following case history:

Case History 8–2. A 63-year-old man with a 10-year history of inadequately controlled

---

*Rarely, patients with one of these disorders can develop renal failure due to myeloma kidney.[239]

hypertension complains of increasing weakness and anorexia. The remainder of the history is unremarkable, and the physical examination reveals only a blood pressure of 180/110, arteriolar narrowing and arteriovenous crossing changes in the fundi, and a fourth heart sound.

The following laboratory data are obtained: BUN 140 mg/dL; plasma creatinine concentration 8.9 mg/dL; and hematocrit 28 percent. No previous measurements are available. The electrocardiogram is compatible with left ventricular hypertrophy. The urinalysis is within normal limits except for 4^+ proteinuria by sulfosalicylic acid and only 1^+ with the dipstick.

Comment. The history of hypertension, presence of cardiac and retinal changes, and normal urinalysis are suggestive of hypertensive nephrosclerosis, with the anemia being due to the renal disease. Only the more positive test with sulfosalicylic acid points to the correct diagnosis of multiple myeloma.

COURSE AND TREATMENT

Renal insufficiency is commonly present at the time of presentation in patients with multiple myeloma.[213] The decline in renal function is frequently precipitated by a superimposed problem such as infection, dehydration, the administration of radiocontrast media (usually performed with prior fluid restriction), or hypercalcemia.[213,215,217,228,241,242] The first three of these problems appear to promote tubular cast formation by slowing the rate of urine flow within the nephron and, with radiocontrast media, by possible direct interaction with the urinary light chains.[228] Initial therapy usually consists of saline rehydration and loop diuretics in an attempt to wash out obstructing tubular casts. In some patients, renal function continues to deteriorate, presumably due to persistent light chain filtration. In this setting, the light chain load can be substantially reduced by lowering the plasma concentration with plasmapheresis.[243-245] This regimen has led to improved renal function in selected patients with acute renal failure.[244,245]

Once renal function is stabilized, the subsequent course of the renal disease is dependent upon several factors. Most important is the response of the malignant plasma cells to chemotherapy, e.g., with prednisone and melphalan. The prognosis is clearly improved if the tumor mass and therefore the rate of light chain production are reduced. However, slowly progressive renal failure may ensue if there is not a satisfactory response to treatment. Prevention of volume depletion and maintenance of a high fluid intake (2 to 3 L/day) may help preserve renal function in these patients by minimizing the likelihood of cast formation within the tubules.[246]

Either hemodialysis or peritoneal dialysis can be used in those patients who develop end-stage renal failure. These modalities are most useful in untreated patients with acute, potentially reversible renal dysfunction who may also have a positive response to chemotherapy.[247,248] On the other hand, using dialysis to prolong life makes little sense in a debilitated patient with refractory disease. There is limited experience with renal transplantation, which has been performed in selected patients who had previously undergone a prolonged remission of their myeloma.[248,249]

URIC ACID RENAL DISEASE

Three types of renal disease may be associated with abnormalities in uric acid metabolism: (1) acute uric acid nephropathy; (2) chronic urate nephropathy; and (3) uric acid nephrolithiasis.[250] The conditions in which these disorders are likely to occur are related to the chemical characteristics of *undissociated* uric acid and its urate salt:

$$\text{Urate}^- + \text{H}^+ \rightleftharpoons \text{uric acid}$$

The relative amounts of uric acid and urate present in the urine (where the pK_a is about 5.35) can be determined from the Henderson-Hasselbach equation[251]:

$$pH = 5.35 + \log \frac{[urate]}{[uric\ acid]}$$

Thus, the normal acidification of the urine, from the pH of 7.40 in the filtrate to as low as 4.5 to 5.0 in the collecting tubules, results in the progressive conversion of urate (the predominant circulating form) to uric acid. This is important clinically because *undissociated uric acid* has a solubility in human urine of only about 100 mg/L (Fig. 8–8), whereas *urate* is much more soluble.[251,252]

These relationships indicate that *concentration and pH* are the main determinants of the likelihood of uric acid precipitation in the urine. Within the kidney, uric acid handling involves four sequential steps: filtration; almost total reabsorption in the early proximal tubule; secretion by the proximal organic acid secretory pathway, the source of most of the excreted uric acid; and partial postsecretory reabsorption.[253,254] The highest solute concentrations in both the tubules and interstitium are achieved within the medulla (because of the countercurrent mechanism). The combination of high concentration and acid urine pH in the collecting tubules favors intratubular precipitation of uric acid at this site in susceptible subjects. The result can be acute renal failure or the formation of uric acid stones. In contrast, *urate* deposition occurs only in the medullary interstitium where the pH and therefore the urate concentration are relatively high. This can potentially lead to microtophus formation and chronic interstitial nephritis.[250]

ACUTE URIC ACID NEPHROPATHY

Acute uric acid nephropathy (UAN) is a disorder characterized by acute renal failure due to uric acid precipitation within the tubules. It is typically associated with a marked increase in the production of uric acid (from the metabolism of purines; see Fig. 8–9) and its subsequent excretion in the urine. En-

FIG. 8–8. Nomogram showing undissociated uric acid concentration at different values of urine pH and total uric acid concentration (uric acid plus urate). The cross-hatched bars depict the solubility limit for uric acid in urine (about 100 mg/L). At an acid urine pH of 4.5 to 5.0, there is more uric acid than urate (since the pK_a is 5.35). As a result, the solubility of uric acid can be exceeded at total urinary uric acid concentrations under 200 mg/L. In contrast, more than 1200 mg/L remains soluble when the urine pH is 6.5 because almost all the urinary uric acid exists as the more soluble urate. (*From F. L. Coe, Kidney Int., 24:392, 1983. Reprinted by permission from Kidney International.*)

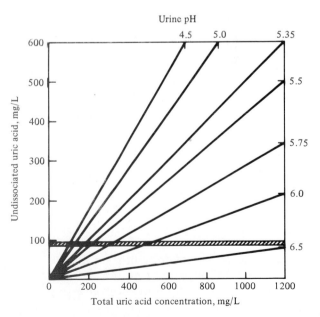

hanced tissue breakdown is usually the inciting event, most commonly occurring in lymphoproliferative and myeloproliferative diseases (lymphomas, leukemias, polycythemia vera), particularly after chemotherapy or radiation has induced rapid cell lysis.[255-257] Seizures, tissue ischemia, and the treatment of solid tumors also can result in tissue catabolism and UAN.[258,259] In addition, there is a primary increase in uric acid production in 20 to 25 percent of patients with primary gout and in the rare syndrome of hypoxanthine-guanine phosphoribosyl transferase (HGPRTase) deficiency.[260-262] In these patients, episodes of poor fluid intake can lead to the formation of a concentrated urine and intratubular uric acid deposition.[262]

PATHOLOGY AND PATHOGENESIS

In both human and experimental UAN, the major pathologic findings are widespread obstruction of the collecting tubules by uric acid crystals, resulting in dilatation of the more proximal segments.[250,263] Uric acid sludge may also be present in the renal pelves and occasionally the ureters.

A high urinary uric acid concentration (promoted by dehydration as well as overproduction) and an acid urine pH are required for the development of UAN. As depicted in Fig. 8–8, a urine pH of 6.5 will usually keep the undissociated uric acid concentration below the solubility limit, even in the presence of marked hyperuricosuria.

It must be emphasized that only the urinary uric acid concentration is important in this disorder. Thus, UAN will not develop in patients with hyperuricemia due to reduced urinary excretion as occurs in renal failure or after the use of diuretics.

CLINICAL PRESENTATION

UAN is usually associated with the relatively abrupt onset of oliguria or anuria. There are typically no other symptoms referable to the urinary tract, although flank pain due to ureteral obstruction can occasionally occur.

The laboratory data reveal progressive elevations in the BUN and plasma creatinine concentration. The initial plasma total uric acid concentration (comprised mostly of urate at the systemic pH of 7.40) generally exceeds 15 mg/dL (range 10 to greater than 50 mg/dL). In comparison, the plasma urate concentration in uncomplicated renal failure is less than 12 mg/dL.[264] The urinalysis may be normal or reveal uric acid crystals and amorphous urates, findings that are suggestive but not diagnostic of UAN.

Tissue breakdown also is associated with the release of intracellular constituents other than purines. As a result, patients with UAN may have marked elevations in the plasma concentrations of potassium, urea, phosphorus (leading to the precipitation of calcium phosphate and hypocalcemia), and lactate dehydrogenase.[256,257,265,266]

DIAGNOSIS

The combination of marked hyperuricemia and acute renal failure should always raise the possibility of UAN. The diagnosis is not difficult to make when this follows the treatment of lymphoma or leukemia or occurs in a patient with a rapid increase in tumor mass. No other cause of renal failure is usually apparent in this setting since neither tumor invasion of the kidney nor urinary tract obstruction due to metastatic disease is typically associated with a dramatic rise in the plasma urate concentration. Measurement of the urine uric acid/creatinine ratio on a random urine specimen can help to confirm the diagnosis.[257,267] This value is characteristically above 1.0 in overexcretors with UAN but is generally below 0.60 to 0.75 in normals and patients with other forms of renal failure.

Radiologic studies are generally not very helpful in UAN. Ultrasonography shows no obstruction, and intravenous pyelography reveals only poor or no calyceal visualization. Retrograde pyelography will be positive only when there is uric acid sludge in the renal pelves or ureters and is therefore not routinely performed. It may be useful, however, in selected patients with flank pain or prolonged oliguria in whom washing out of the sludge (in part by perfusion with an alkaline solution) can lead to improved renal function.[256]

There are two other disorders that can produce acute renal failure and hyperuricemia that are *much more common* than UAN. First, prerenal disease (as with diuretic therapy) is associated with enhanced proximal sodium reabsorption in an attempt to conserve sodium and restore euvolemia. Net uric acid reabsorption is also increased in this condition since it is indirectly linked to the reabsorption of sodium.[268] As a result, excretion falls, leading to a rise in the plasma urate concentration.[269] This disorder can usually be distinguished from UAN by the absence of a relevant clinical history, the low urine uric acid/creatinine ratio, and the characteristic laboratory findings of prerenal disease (low urine sodium concentration, low fractional excretion of sodium, and high urine osmolality; see p. 65).

Second, trauma or hypotension can lead to renal failure due to ATN, as well as tissue breakdown and hyperuricemia. The correct diagnosis may be suggested by the urinary findings of renal tubular epithelial cells and granular and epithelial cell casts and the less marked degree of hyperuricemia (usually below 12 to 15 mg/dL).

A final consideration is that the renal failure seen in the tumor lysis syndrome may be due in part or, in patients pretreated with allopurinol, mostly to calcium phosphate not uric acid deposition within the kidney.[266,270] This is an important diagnosis to establish since alkalinization of the plasma and urine may be beneficial in UAN but can exacerbate calcium phosphate deposition. The latter should be suspected when marked hyperphosphatemia and hypocalcemia are also present.[265,266,270]

COURSE AND THERAPY

Despite the severity of the renal failure, the prognosis in UAN is excellent if treatment is initiated rapidly.[256,257] Therapy consists of attempting to maintain a high urine volume (to wash out the obstructing uric acid crystals) with a loop diuretic and fluids, and decreasing further uric acid production with allopurinol, an inhibitor of xanthine oxidase (Fig. 8–9). Alkalinization of the urine by the administration of acetazolamide (250 mg intravenously) and sodium bicarbonate should be tried only if there is an adequate urine output and it is felt that calcium phosphate precipitation is not playing a major role. In those patients in whom a diuresis cannot be achieved, lowering the plasma urate concentration with hemodialysis (which is 10 to 20 times more rapid than peritoneal dialysis) hastens the recovery of renal function.[256]

Every effort should also be made to prevent UAN. The administration of allopurinol (in higher than normal doses of 600 to 900 mg/day) plus maintenance of an alkaline diuresis (of over 2.5 to 3 L/day if possible) with sodium bicarbonate should minimize uric acid precipitation in patients who are about to receive chemotherapy for lymphoma, leukemia, or other rapidly growing malignancy. Even with optimal therapy, however, the degree of tumor lysis may be so large that UAN still occurs.[256,271]

Prophylactic therapy may also be effective in patients who chronically overproduce uric acid and who may develop acute renal failure during periods of dehydration.[250,262] This can occur in patients with an untreated hematologic malignancy or less commonly with primary gout or HGPRTase deficiency. It is important to be aware that the initial response to increased uric acid production is to min-

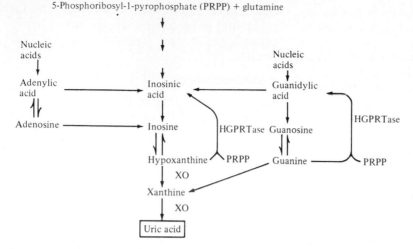

5-Phosphoribosyl-1-pyrophosphate (PRPP) + glutamine

FIG. 8-9. Formation of uric acid from purine metabolism. XO = xanthine oxidase; HGPRTase = hypoxanthine-guanine phosphoribosyltransferase.

imize the degree of hyperuricemia by enhanced proximal tubular secretion and subsequent urinary excretion. As a result, urinary uric acid excretion will be increased earlier and to a greater extent than the plasma urate concentration.[263] Thus, *marked hyperuricosuria can occur when there is only mild to moderate hyperuricemia.* As a result, 24-h urinary uric acid excretion should be measured in a patient with one of the above disorders when there is even a minor elevation in the plasma urate concentration. The risk of uric acid precipitation is enhanced if daily excretion exceeds 900 to 1000 mg/day.[252,261,262] Although the value of prophylactically treating patients with asymptomatic hyperuricemia and marked hyperuricosuria has not been proven, it seems prudent in this setting to maintain a high fluid intake, to limit dietary purine ingestion, and either to alkalinize the urine to a pH of 6.5 (preferably with potassium bicarbonate or citrate; see below) or to lower uric acid production with allopurinol.[252,272]

CHRONIC URATE NEPHROPATHY

Chronic urate nephropathy, which is currently an unusual problem, occurs over a period of many years in patients with persistent hyperuricemia, most often as a consequence of primary gout.[273] It is not known if the secondary hyperuricemia associated with diuretics or renal failure[269,274] can also lead to urate nephropathy and a decline in renal function (see below).

PATHOLOGY AND PATHOGENESIS

The primary histologic finding in urate nephropathy is the deposition of monosodium urate crystals in the medullary interstitium with a surrounding giant cell reaction (Fig. 8–10).[250,273] These changes eventually lead to interstitial fibrosis and tubular atrophy and dilatation. Vascular thickening and glomerular sclerosis may also be present, due at least in part to the frequent association with hypertension.[273,275,276]

The major factors determining monosodium urate deposition are the concentrations of sodium and urate. As with other solutes, a high concentration of sodium and urate is achieved in the renal medulla, the latter primarily by diffusion out of the vasa recta capillaries.[277] This distribution could promote local tophus formation.

CLINICAL PRESENTATION

There are no symptoms associated with interstitial urate deposition, and the urinalysis is relatively benign. Thus, the presence of renal disease is usually discovered by routine measurement of the BUN and plasma creatinine concentration. A history of gouty arthritis is frequently obtained and, rarely, palpable tophi are present.

The only laboratory finding suggestive of urate nephropathy is an elevation in the plasma urate concentration out of proportion to the degree of renal insufficiency. This has been defined, in patients with mild to moderate renal disease, as a plasma urate concentration exceeding 9 mg/dL if the plasma creatinine concentration (P_{cr}) is 1.5 mg/dL or less, 10 mg/dL if the P_{cr} is between 1.5 and 2.0 mg/dL, and 12 mg/dL if the P_{cr} is between 2.1 and 3.0 mg/dL.[1]

DIAGNOSIS

The diagnosis of urate nephropathy is always *one of exclusion* supported by the findings described above. The differential diagnosis of chronic renal failure with a benign urinalysis includes benign nephrosclerosis secondary to hypertension, obstructive uropathy, and the other tubulointerstitial diseases discussed in this chapter. Only hyperuricemia points to the presence of urate nephropathy.

Recent observations, however, have cast doubt on the prevalence of this disorder. Long-term studies in patients with primary gout have revealed that progressive renal failure (out of proportion to the decline in GFR that normally occurs with aging) is unusual[276,278] and when present is likely to be due to nephrosclerosis.[276] These findings suggest that urate nephropathy is uncommon unless *marked* hyperuricemia (plasma urate concentration greater than 13 mg/dL in men and 10 mg/dL in women) persists for several decades.[278]

If these observations are correct, then another explanation is required for the oc-

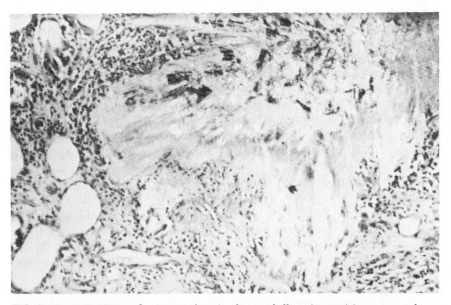

FIG. 8-10. Formation of microtophus in the medullary interstitium around birefringent crystals of sodium urate in a patient with HGPRTase deficiency. (*From B. T. Emmerson and P. G. Row, Kidney Int., 8:65, 1975. Reprinted by permission from Kidney International.*)

casional association of hyperuricemia and renal insufficiency without other apparent cause. One likely possibility is *chronic lead intoxication* which both damages the tubules and reduces uric acid excretion, possibly by diminishing proximal tubular secretion by an unknown mechanism.[279] Two different studies evaluated patients with chronic renal insufficiency, with and without a history of gouty arthritis.[280,281] Measurement of urinary lead excretion after the administration of EDTA (ethylenediaminetetraacetic acid) was performed in each patient, with increased excretion being an indicator of elevated body lead stores. Almost all patients with gout but only an occasional patient without gout had a positive EDTA test. These findings suggest that, at the present time when tophaceous gout is rare, the clinical findings of urate nephropathy may be most often due to lead intoxication.[280,281] Sources of lead in adults include the ingestion of moonshine whiskey and occupational exposure.

In addition to the EDTA test, two other factors may help distinguish lead intoxication from primary gout. Approximately 20 to 25 percent of patients with primary gout are overproducers with elevated urinary uric acid excretion[261]; a similar percentage (although not necessarily representing the same patients) develop uric acid stones.[251,261] Neither of these findings occur in lead nephropathy since urinary uric acid excretion is in the low-normal range.[279]

TREATMENT

Optimal therapy is uncertain given the likely low incidence of true urate nephropathy. Patients who in the past appeared to have urate nephropathy with interstitial tophi (Fig. 8–10) also tended to have severe tophaceous gout,[273] a clear indication for therapy aimed at lowering the plasma urate concentration. Other possible indications for hypouricemic therapy with allopurinol are similar to those described

above: uric acid stones or overproduction as evidenced by 24-h urine uric acid excretion above 900 to 1000 mg/day.[252,272] Asymptomatic patients with secondary hyperuricemia due to diuretic therapy or renal insufficiency are at very little renal risk and do not require active therapy.

Appropriate treatment is different in patients shown to have lead intoxication. In this setting, further exposure should be avoided, and the primary therapy consists of increasing lead excretion with a chelating agent such as EDTA.[282]

URIC ACID NEPHROLITHIASIS

A general discussion of renal stone disease is beyond the scope of this text. Nevertheless, it is useful to review the pathogenesis of uric acid stones (which are nonopaque on radiologic examination). These stones occur in approximately 20 percent of patients with primary gout and occasionally in patients with other disorders (such as polycythemia vera and chronic diarrhea).[251,261,283]

An acid urine pH and an elevated urinary uric acid concentration (due to overproduction or the use of uricosuric agents such as probenicid or aspirin) are the major factors promoting stone formation.[261,283] In primary gout, for example, the incidence of stone disease rises with the rate of uric acid excretion, reaching 40 to 50 percent in patients excreting 1000 mg or more per day.[261,283] However, less than one-half of all stone formers with primary gout have increased uric acid excretion. In these patients, a persistent acid urine pH (usually below 5.5) is the predominant abnormality,[261,283] allowing uric acid precipitation to occur at normal urinary concentrations (see Fig. 8–8). The importance of pH and concentration can also be illustrated in patients with chronic diarrhea in whom volume depletion and metabolic acidosis also may be present. As a result, the urine tends to be acid and concentrated, a combination that promotes uric acid precipitation even though uric acid excretion is in the low-normal range.[284,285]

Optimal therapy depends upon the factors that are leading to uric acid stone formation. Patients who are overproducers should probably be treated with a high-fluid–low-purine intake and either alkalinization of the urine (to a pH above 6.5 for at least part of the day) or allopurinol.*[,251,283,287] Fluids and urinary alkalinization (both of which reduce the concentration of undissociated uric acid which is relatively insoluble; see Fig. 8–8) are probably preferable in patients in whom uric acid excretion is normal. Potassium bicarbonate or citrate (which is metabolized to bicarbonate) appears to have a more desirable overall effect than the comparable sodium salt, since sodium loading tends to raise urinary calcium excretion.[251,287] This is of practical importance because urinary uric acid can also promote the formation of calcium oxalate stones.[251,288]

HYPERCALCEMIC NEPHROPATHY

Renal insufficiency, abnormalities in tubular function, and nephrolithiasis are frequent complications of hypercalcemia. These changes are independent of etiology, other than nephrolithiasis which is seen only with chronic hypercalcemia, as in primary hyperparathyroidism or sarcoidosis.

Hypercalcemia is most often due to increased bone resorption but can also result from enhanced intestinal absorption or reduced renal excretion. The major causes of

---

*Allopurinol has some unusual, although rare, complications in this setting. The administration of this drug leads to increased production and excretion of xanthine (since xanthine oxidase is inhibited; see Fig. 8–9) and oxypurinol, the major metabolite of allopurinol. In selected patients, xanthine or oxypurinol stones can occur.[285,286]

hypercalcemia are malignancies (solid tumors, multiple myeloma, lymphoma) and primary hyperparathyroidism.[289,290] The increase in bone resorption with malignancy can be due to direct erosion by tumor cells or to the release of humoral substances such as osteoclast activating factor, a parathyroid hormone (PTH)-like peptide, or rarely prostaglandins or 1,25-dihydroxyvitamin D (the most active metabolite of vitamin D).[290,291] Less common causes of chronic hypercalcemia include sarcoidosis (see below), hypervitaminosis D, and the milk-alkali syndrome.[289]

PATHOLOGY AND PATHOGENESIS

The earliest histologic changes of hypercalcemic nephropathy are found in the distal and collecting tubules.[292,293] Calcification, degeneration, and necrosis of the tubular epithelial cells leads to sloughing and subsequently to tubular obstruction with dilatation of the more proximal segments. Later changes include tubular atrophy and interstitial fibrosis and calcification (nephrocalcinosis). Calcium deposits may also be found in the proximal tubules, glomeruli, and blood vessels.

The obstructing cellular and calcium casts undoubtedly contribute to the development of renal insufficiency. However, other factors also appear to play a role, particularly the renal hemodynamic changes induced by hypercalcemia.[293] Renal vasoconstriction, most likely due to a direct effect of calcium on vascular tone, can lead to reductions in renal blood flow and GFR.[294] Furthermore, both hypercalcemia and, if present, increased levels of parathyroid hormone can lower the permeability coefficient of the glomerular capillary wall, further impairing glomerular filtration.[295]

CLINICAL PRESENTATION

Hypercalcemia is now most often discovered as an incidental finding on routine laboratory examination. Many patients, however, can present with symptoms referable to nephrolithiasis (flank pain, hematuria) or to hypercalcemia.* The latter include anorexia, nausea, vomiting, weight loss, lethargy, constipation, and polyuria and polydipsia.[289] The last two symptoms are due primarily to the development of nephrogenic diabetes insipidus in which the kidney is relatively unresponsive to the action of antidiuretic hormone (ADH).[292,296] Cyclic AMP generation is impaired in this setting, an effect that may involve the ADH receptor in the cell membrane or the ability of the hormone-receptor complex to activate adenyl cyclase.[297,298] Two other factors in addition to ADH antagonism can contribute to the hypercalcemia-induced increase in urine output: decreased sodium chloride reabsorption in the loop of Henle and a primary increase in water intake due to stimulation of thirst.[299,300]

The physical examination may reveal hypertension, signs of an underlying malignancy, and calcium deposition along the lateral and medial margins of the cornea (band keratopathy), which is best detected by slit-lamp examination. The laboratory findings, other than hypercalcemia, are nonspecific. The BUN and plasma creatinine concentration may be elevated, due to hypercalcemia and frequent concomitant volume depletion. Both of these problems are in part minimized by the secretion of vasodilator prostaglandins and, therefore, can be exacerbated by the use of nonsteroidal anti-inflammatory drugs.[294]

In addition to the decrease in concentrating ability, a variety of other tubular functions may also be abnormal. These defects can lead to inappropriate losses of sodium, potassium, and phosphate, potentially producing hypovolemia, hypokalemia, and hypophosphatemia.[292,301,302] These changes may disappear spontaneously with the develop-

*This discussion will include only the general findings associated with hypercalcemia. The historical, physical, and laboratory changes characteristic of the specific causes of hypercalcemia are reviewed elsewhere.[289]

ment of renal insufficiency, as the fall in filtration rate minimizes solute wasting.

The urinalysis is usually normal or near-normal in patients with hypercalcemic nephropathy. However, hematuria may occur in patients with kidney stones or in those with hypercalciuria alone in whom microcalculi or tubular damage from crystalluria are thought to be of etiologic importance.[303]

DIAGNOSIS

The presumptive diagnosis of hypercalcemic nephropathy requires only the demonstration of renal insufficiency and hypercalcemia. If the plasma calcium concentration has not already been measured, this disorder should be suspected in any patient with renal insufficiency and either a normal urinalysis or an underlying malignancy. Once hypercalcemia has been confirmed, a plain film of the abdomen should be obtained, looking for nephrolithiasis or nephrocalcinosis.

TREATMENT

In most patients, renal function can be markedly improved by lowering the plasma calcium concentration. This improvement is due to reversal of the hemodynamic effects of hypercalcemia and to washing out the obstructing tubular casts. Patients with chronic hypercalcemia, however, may have persistent renal insufficiency due to irreversible interstitial fibrosis and tubular atrophy.

The mainstay of therapy is to augment urinary calcium excretion with a loop diuretic and intravenous saline (or a high salt diet).[290,304] The rationale behind this regimen is that the reabsorption of calcium in the proximal tubule and loop of Henle is primarily passive, following gradients established by the reabsorption of sodium and water.[305] Thus, decreasing sodium transport in the proximal tubule (by saline-induced volume expansion) and the loop of Henle (with the loop diuretic) also diminishes calcium reabsorption, leading to a marked calciuresis. The aim is to maintain the urine output above 2.5 L/day. However, increasing the urine output with a high water intake is inadequate in this setting, since neither sodium nor calcium reabsorption will be affected.

Corticosteroids also may lower the plasma calcium concentration in certain patients. This is most likely to occur in two settings: in neoplastic disorders, particularly hematologic malignancies, in which steroids appear to act by antagonizing the bone resorptive effect of osteoclast activating factors[290,306]; and in hypervitaminosis D and sarcoidosis, disorders in which high vitamin D levels enhance intestinal calcium absorption (see "Sarcoidosis," below).[307-309] In these conditions, corticosteroids may both directly diminish intestinal calcium absorption[310,311,] and decrease the circulating levels of 1,25-dihydroxyvitamin D.[312] In contrast, steroids are ineffective in primary hyperparathyroidism, the other major cause of hypercalcemia.

If saline, a loop diuretic, and corticosteroids are unable to control the plasma calcium concentration, other modalities that may be effective include intravenous mithramycin or calcitonin (both of which directly reduce bone resorption), oral phosphate (which complexes with intestinal and circulating calcium), and possibly diphosphonates.[290,304,313] The use of intravenous phosphate (which can lead to widespread calcium phosphate deposition) or hemodialysis to treat severe hypercalcemic crisis is rarely necessary.[313-315]

Patients in whom the underlying disorder cannot be corrected (primarily due to malignancy) require chronic hypocalcemic therapy. A high-salt diet, a loop diuretic, oral phosphate, and, in the appropriate setting, oral corticosteroids all may be effective. In addition, selected patients in whom a tumor is releasing a bone-resorbing prostaglandin may respond to a nonsteroidal anti-inflammatory drug.[290,316]

SARCOIDOSIS

Clinically important renal involvement occasionally occurs in sarcoidosis.[317-319] The primary problem is usually related to hypercalciuria and hypercalcemia, but granulomatous involvement of the interstitium or a glomerulopathy also may be seen.

CALCIUM BALANCE

Hyperabsorption of dietary calcium leading to hypercalciuria occurs in up to one-half of patients with sarcoidosis.[317,320] Initial studies in this disorder demonstrated that this abnormality was due to increased sensitivity to the calcium-retaining effects of oral vitamin D.[320] It was subsequently shown that the primary problem is enhanced formation of 1,25-dihydroxyvitamin D,[308,309] which occurs not in the kidney,[321] but in the lung and lymph nodes of patients with diffuse sarcoidosis by activated mononuclear cells (particularly macrophages).[322,323] Why this occurs is uncertain, but vitamin D has been shown to have immunomodulatory functions[324] and may therefore be involved in the inflammatory process. Monocytes, for example, have receptors for 1,25-dihydroxyvitamin D; this hormone may promote conversion of these cells to activated macrophages.[324] The ability of activated mononuclear cells to produce 1,25-dihydroxyvitamin D may also explain the occasional association of hypercalcemia both with other granulomatous diseases such as tuberculosis, berylliosis, and post-silicon implantation[325] and rarely with malignant lymphoma.[291]

The excess calcium is initially excreted in the urine, resulting in hypercalciuria but not hypercalcemia. This may be manifested clinically by nephrolithiasis, nephrocalcinosis, or polyuria due to reduced concentrating ability.[317] Hypercalcemia eventually develops in 15 to 20 percent of patients (who tend to have higher 1,25-dihydroxyvitamin D levels than those with a normal plasma calcium concentration),[322] and can lead to renal insufficiency typical of hypercalcemic nephropathy (see "Hypercalcemic Nephropathy," above).[317,326]

Treatment of these disturbances consists of a low calcium diet* and corticosteroids, which rapidly reduce intestinal calcium absorption and therefore hypercalciuria and hypercalcemia.[312,320] This is associated with a fall in circulating 1,25-dihydroxyvitamin D levels toward normal,[312] presumably due to decreased synthesis by the activated monocytes and macrophages.[322] If corticosteroids are ineffective, another cause of hypercalcemia should be suspected, particularly primary hyperparathyroidsim which may occur with increased frequency in sarcoidosis.[326,328] Plasma parathyroid hormone levels are usually able to differentiate between these disorders, being elevated in primary hyperparathyroidism but appropriately reduced by the hypercalcemia in uncomplicated sarcoidosis.[328]

GRANULOMATOUS INTERSTITIAL NEPHRITIS

Interstitial granuloma formation in the kidneys is common in sarcoidosis, although involvement severe enough to produce renal insufficiency is unusual. When this does occur, there is typically evidence of generalized sarcoidosis.[319,329] Some patients, however, present with renal insufficiency with only minimal extrarenal manifestations.[330]

---

*A low calcium diet alone (or combined with oral phosphate in patients with persistent hypercalcemia) is not entirely protective in patients who form calcium oxalate stones. The decrease in free calcium in the intestine (due both to reduced intake and to complexing with phosphate), results in less calcium to combine with dietary oxalate. Consequently, more intestinal oxalate remains soluble, leading to increased absorption, hyperoxaluria, and an unchanged or even elevated tendency to calcium oxalate stone formation.[327] Addition of dietary oxalate restriction protects against this problem.

Laboratory evaluation in this disorder is nonspecific.[319,329] The urinalysis is typical of other tubulointerstitial diseases: sterile pyuria, minimal or absent hematuria, and no or mild proteinuria. Signs of tubular dysfunction may also be present, including nephrogenic diabetes insipidus, renal glucosuria, and renal tubular acidosis.[329] In the absence of nephrocalcinosis or stone formation, the IVP or renal ultrasonogram are unremarkable. Renal biopsy will usually show normal glomeruli, noncaseating granulomas in the interstitium, tubular damage, and interstitial infiltration and fibrosis. Corticosteroid therapy tends to return renal function to normal, although a relapse may occur as the steroids are discontinued.[326,329]

GLOMERULONEPHRITIS

Glomerulonephritis is another form of renal disease that can occur in sarcoidosis. A wide variety of histologic patterns have been described, including proliferative or crescentic glomerulonephritis, membranous nephropathy, and focal glomerulosclerosis.[318,319,331,332] The urinary findings are typical of other glomerulonephrides and include proteinuria which can reach the nephrotic range, hematuria, and cellular casts. As with other forms of sarcoid renal disease, corticosteroid therapy appears to improve renal function.

The pathogenesis of these changes is not well understood. It has been postulated that primary tubular damage could lead to the release of previously "unseen" tubular antigens into the systemic circulation, with subsequent antibody and immune complex formation (see p. 181).

MISCELLANEOUS

A variety of other disorders are uncommon causes of tubulointerstitial disease and are discussed only briefly at this time (Table 8–1).

INTRATUBULAR OBSTRUCTION

Intratubular obstruction appears to be of major importance in the development of renal failure in acute tubular necrosis and multiple myeloma (see Chap. 3 and above). Renal disease can also result from intratubular precipitation in several other settings including the administration of intravenous acyclovir,[333] methotrexate,[334] sulfonamide antibiotics,[335,336] and low-molecular-weight dextran.[337]

Hyperoxaluria can also produce a similar problem. This can be seen in several clinical settings:

1. Oxalate production can be increased by the intake of substances that are metabolized in part to oxalate. Thus, acute renal failure has been seen with very high doses of vitamin C,[338,339] the ingestion of ethylene glycol (in which toxic effects of other metabolites such as glycolate can also contribute to the renal disease),[340,341] the anesthetic methoxyflurane (in which fluoride toxicity also may play a role),[342] and glycerol used to treat cerebral edema.[343]

   Overproduction of oxalate can also result from an enzymatic defect, as occurs in primary hyperoxaluria.[344,345] Patients with this disorder usually present with kidney stones, with renal failure generally occurring before the age of 20. Tubular and interstitial oxalate deposits with marked scarring are prominent histologic findings. There is some suggestion that these problems can be minimized by a high fluid intake, neutral phosphate (leading to the excretion of pyrophosphate which inhibits calcium oxalate precipitation), and high doses of pyridoxine (which favor the conversion of glyoxalate into glycine rather than oxalate).[345,346]

2. Hyperoxaluria can also be induced by increased intestinal absorption of dietary oxalate, which is normally limited (to 5 to 7 percent of intake) in part by the intraluminal formation of insoluble calcium oxalate.[347,348] However, absorption can reach 35 to 40 percent of intake in chronic diarrheal states with malabsorption,[347] leading to increased oxalate excretion, calcium oxalate stones (in up to 10 percent of patients),[347] and, rarely, acute renal failure.[349] Both binding of intestinal calcium to fat (thereby leaving oxalate in a soluble form, rather than complexed to calcium) and a toxic effect of nonabsorbed bile salts to increase colonic permeability may contribute to the hyperoxaluria in this setting.[347,350] A low oxalate diet effectively reverses the hyperoxaluria in these patients.

INFILTRATIVE DISEASES

Infiltration of the kidney by granulomatous and neoplastic diseases is relatively common. However, involvement severe enough to impair renal function is unusual and is most likely to occur with sarcoidosis (see "Sarcoidosis," above) or a rapidly growing malignancy such as lymphoma or acute leukemia (but only rarely solid tumors).[351,352] These patients generally present with renal failure of recent onset, a relatively benign urinalysis, and enlarged kidneys that may be palpable.

The differential diagnosis includes other causes of renal insufficiency associated with hematologic neoplasms such as hypercalcemia, urinary tract obstruction, hyperuricemia, and the toxic effects of chemotherapeutic drugs. The presence of tumor infiltration is suggested by the finding of large kidneys without hydronephrosis on renal ultrasonography. Similar radiologic findings can be produced by acute renal vein thrombosis. This disorder, however, usually causes flank pain and hematuria and is not typically associated with leukemia or lymphoma.

The prognosis is dependent upon the responsiveness of the underlying malignancy to chemotherapy or radiation. With responsive diseases, there may be a rapid reduction in renal size (within days) and a return of renal function toward normal.[351,352] These patients are, however, at risk from the tumor lysis syndrome, as the marked degree of cell breakdown can lead to marked hyperuricemia, hyperphosphatemia, and hypocalcemia. These problems can be minimized by the maintenance of a high fluid intake and the prior administration of high doses of allopurinol (see "Acute Uric Acid Nephropathy," above).

HEAVY METAL TOXICITY

Heavy metals can lead to several different types of renal disease including: (1) the nephrotic syndrome (gold, mercury) (see Chap. 6); (2) acute tubular necrosis (cisplatin, arsenic, mercury, uranium) (see Chap. 3); and (3) chronic tubulointerstitial nephritis, which is most often due to lead or cadmium.[353-357]

These problems have been thought to be relatively uncommon (in the absence of a direct occupational exposure), but recent studies suggest that chronic lead intoxication may be more prevalent than generally appreciated. Patients with this disorder may present with abdominal pain, peripheral neuropathy, or anemia. The initial renal findings typically include subtle proximal tubular abnormalities such as aminoaciduria and renal glucosuria.[355,356] This defect is probably due to proximal reabsorption of filtered lead with subsequent accumulation in the proximal tubular cells. Histologic examination is consistent with this hypothesis, revealing proximal tubular degeneration with intranuclear inclusion bodies composed of a lead-protein complex. In comparison to other proximal defects (including that due to cadmium),[357] however, lead nephropathy is associated with reduced rather than increased uric acid excretion, perhaps due to diminished tubular secretion.[279]

Continued lead exposure produces a chronic interstitial nephritis. The renal disease at this time is usually characterized by the triad of renal insufficiency, hypertension, and gout[354-356] and therefore can be confused with either hypertensive nephrosclerosis or chronic urate nephropathy (see p. 423). At least some patients who were thought to have one of these disorders have been shown to have lead nephropathy instead.[280,281,355] This diagnosis is best established by demonstrating an abnormally large increase in urinary lead excretion after a standard infusion of EDTA.[282,355] However, the diagnosis of this potentially treatable disorder *will not be made unless it is suspected* on the basis of gout, otherwise unexplained renal insufficiency, and a history of exposure due to occupation, the ingestion of moonshine whiskey, or children living near a major highway (when leaded gasoline was in widespread use).[355] Therapy consists of removing the source of lead and increasing urinary lead excretion by the chronic administration of a chelating agent such as EDTA.[282,355]

HYPOKALEMIC NEPHROPATHY

Chronic potassium depletion can affect a variety of tubular functions, producing one or more of the following: polyuria and polydipsia due to ADH resistance and perhaps a primary stimulus to thirst; impaired urinary acidification, and increased sodium and bicarbonate reabsorption.[358,359] These changes may be associated with vacuolar lesions in the tubular cells of the proximal and less commonly the distal nephron.[359] Both the functional and histologic abnormalities are corrected within a few weeks after potassium repletion has been achieved.

The GFR is usually normal or mildly reduced in patients with hypokalemia. Permanent renal insufficiency with interstitial fibrosis and tubular atrophy is rare but apparently can occur.[360]

PRIMARY IMMUNOLOGIC DISORDERS

Primary immunologic disorders, in addition to those induced by drugs, are uncommon causes of tubulointerstitial disease. These conditions can produce renal injury by one of three mechanisms: immune complex deposition, antibodies directed against the TBM, and cell-mediated cytotoxicity.[12,361]

IMMUNE COMPLEX DEPOSITION

Systemic lupus erythematosus (SLE) is the most common disorder associated with tubular immune complex deposition. These complexes, some of which contain DNA, can be found along the TBM (by immunofluorescent and electron microscopy) in approximately 50 percent of patients with SLE.[52,362] In most patients, the number of tubular deposits is relatively small and the associated tubulointerstitial damage is probably secondary to the glomerular disease. Selected patients, however, present with renal insufficiency, minimal proteinuria, a benign sediment, and, on biopsy, severe tubulointerstitial nephritis, minor glomerular changes, and immunoglobulin and complement deposition along the TBM and in the interstitium.[363-365] It appears likely that at least these patients have primary tubulointerstitial disease. Corticosteroids seem to be beneficial in this setting, usually leading to an improvement in renal function.[363]

Similar mechanisms may be operative in Sjögren's syndrome, a condition that may be associated with an interstitial nephritis or rarely an immune complex glomerulonephritis.[366-368] The interstitial nephritis is characterized by a variable (but generally mild) reduction in GFR, a relatively benign urinalysis, and prominent abnormalities in tubular function including the Fanconi syndrome, distal renal tubular acidosis, and nephrogenic diabetes insipidus.[366,369] Histologic examination typically reveals minimal glomerular changes, tubular atrophy, interstitial fibrosis, and an interstitial infiltrate composed of lymphocytes and plasma cells that is similar to that found in the salivary, parotid, and lacrimal glands. Immune complexes have been demonstrated along the TBM and could reflect the combination of antibody, perhaps produced locally by the interstitial mononuclear cells, with in situ tubular antigens.[367] Alternatively, cell-mediated damage, not antibody formation, may be the primary event responsible for tubular injury. This could result in the exposure of previously "unseen" tubular antigens and secondary antibody formation. Regardless of the mechanism, corticosteroids are frequently beneficial.[367,368]

ANTI-TBM ANTIBODY DISEASE

Tubulointerstitial disease due to the deposition of circulating anti-TBM antibodies is characterized by the presence of linear immunofluorescence along the TBM. This problem is most often seen in patients who also have anti-GBM antibody-induced glomerulonephritis (as occurs in Goodpasture's syndrome).[51,361,362] The observation that tubulointerstitial changes (interstitial infiltrate and fibrosis, tubular atrophy) are more prominent in those patients with anti-GBM antibody disease who also have anti-TBM antibodies suggests that these antibodies are pathogenetically important.[51]

Anti-TBM antibodies have also been demonstrated in selected patients with methicillin nephritis,[47,362,370] concurrent membranous nephropathy,[371] and idiopathic interstitial nephritis.[49,50,370] In at least some patients with idiopathic disease, the antibody is directed against a glycoprotein tubular antigen that is similar to the inciting antigen in experimental anti-TBM antibody disease,[49] produced by the injection of heterologous tubular basement membranes in Freund's adjuvant.[57] This finding suggests that exposure of a specific antigen may be of primary importance in this disorder.

Circulating anti-TBM antibodies with linear deposits of immunoglobulin and complement along the TBM have also been found in less than 5 percent of renal transplant recipients.[48] These patients, however, frequently have no evidence of tubulointerstitial disease, raising doubt about the contribution of these antibodies to renal injury in this setting.

CELL-MEDIATED DAMAGE

Acute transplant rejection is the major disorder thought to be initiated by a cell-mediated reaction.[372] In this condition, sensitized lymphocytes react against the foreign tissue antigens present in the transplanted kidney.

It is also possible that cellular mechanisms play a role in Sjögren's syndrome and in at least some patients with acute drug-induced interstitial nephritis in whom sensitized mononuclear cells may react against drug antigens deposited in the kidney.[25,43,44]

BALKAN NEPHROPATHY

Balkan nephropathy is a form of chronic interstitial nephritis that occurs in a limited geographic area within the Danube River basin.[12,373] This disorder typically becomes clinically evident between the ages of 30 and 60, and can affect up to 10 to 30 percent of the adult population in endemic areas. People who move into these areas appear to have a latent period of at least 15 years before developing clinical signs of the disease.

Balkan nephropathy is characterized histologically by progressive interstitial fibrosis (with little mononuclear cell infiltration) and tubular atrophy.[373] The primary site of involvement in this disorder is not known. Mitochondrial swelling and degeneration in the proximal tubule is a relatively early finding.

In addition, the first detectable clinical abnormality appears to be increased excretion of low-molecular-weight proteins (such as β_2-microglobulin),[374] a finding that is also compatible with primary proximal tubular damage, since this is the segment in which these proteins are normally reabsorbed.

The etiology of Balkan nephropathy is incompletely understood. The epidemiologic data raise the possibility of a toxin that is limited to the endemic area; some studies suggest that ochratoxin A, produced by fungi of the *Penicillium* species in stored barley, may be the inciting factor.[373,375]

The clinical picture in Balkan nephropathy is one of progressive renal insufficiency, with most patients developing end-stage renal disease within 10 years of diagnosis.[373] An important complicating feature is an apparently increased incidence in the development of transitional cell tumors of the renal pelvis, ureter, and bladder.[373,376] These malignancies may be multiple and bilateral. The mechanism by which they occur is not known, but a carcinogenic effect of the mycotoxin is possible.

SECONDARY TUBULOINTERSTITIAL DISEASE

This chapter has dealt with primary tubulointerstitial diseases. However, tubular and interstitial damage is also a prominent feature of glomerular and vascular diseases, such as chronic glomerulonephritis and benign nephrosclerosis.[1] The mechanism by which these changes occur is uncertain, as secondary ischemic damage has been considered to be important in at least some patients. A recent hypothesis suggests an alternative explanation.[377] Nephron loss initially leads to compensatory hypertrophy in the remaining normal or less damaged nephrons (see Chap. 4). This adaptation is characterized by an increase both in nephron GFR and in a variety of tubular functions, including the production of ammonia in an attempt to excrete the daily acid load. This can lead to increased tissue levels of ammonia, which is capable of reacting with C3 to form a convertase of the alternate complement pathway. The ensuing activation of complement can directly damage the tubular cells and, via the release of chemotactic factors, promote the infiltration of mononuclear cells.

Evidence in favor of this hypothesis has come from experiments in which renal insufficiency was produced by surgical removal of 85 to 90 percent of the renal mass.[377] This is typically followed by progressive glomerulosclerosis and marked tubulointerstitial disease.[4] If, however, sodium bicarbonate is given to diminish the net acid load and therefore ammonia production, the degree of tubulinterstitial damage and local complement deposition is substantially reduced. If these intriguing results are confirmed, the administration of alkali may become a standard part of therapy in patients with any form of chronic progressive renal disease.

REFERENCES

1. Murray, T., and M. Goldberg: Chronic interstitial nephritis: Etiologic factors, *Ann. Intern. Med.*, 82:453, 1975.
2. Peterson, A., E. Evrin, and I. Berggard: Differentiation of glomerular, tubular, and normal proteinuria: Determinations of urinary excretion of β_2-microglobulin, albumin, and total protein, *J. Clin. Invest.*, 48:1189, 1969.
3. Portman, R. J., J. M. Kissane, and A. M. Robson: Use of β_2-microglobulin to diagnose tubulointerstitial renal lesions in children, *Kidney Int.*, 30:91, 1986.
4. Brenner, B. M.: Nephron adaptation to renal injury or ablation, *Am. J. Physiol.*, 249:F324, 1985.
5. Cogan, M. G.: Tubulo-interstitial nephropathies—A pathophysiologic approach, *West. J. Med.*, 132:134, 1980.
6. Gilbert, R. M., H. Weber, L. Turchin, L. G. Fine, J. J. Bourgoignie, and N. S. Bricker: A study of the intrarenal recycling of urea in the rat with chronic experimental pyelonephritis, *J. Clin. Invest.*, 58:1348, 1976.
7. Danovitch, G. M., J. J. Bourgoignie, and N. S. Bricker: Reversibility of the "salt-losing" tendency of chronic renal failure, *N. Engl. J. Med.*, 296:14, 1977.
8. Morris, R. C., Jr., and A. Sebastian: Renal tubular acidosis and the Fanconi syndrome, in J. B. Stanbury, J. B. Wyngaarden, D. S. Fredrickson, J. L. Goldstein, and M. S. Brown (eds.), *The Metabolic Basis of Inherited Disease*, 5th ed., McGraw-Hill, New York, 1983.
9. DeFronzo, R. A.: Hyperkalemia in hyporeninemic hypoaldosteronism, *Kidney Int.*, 17:118, 1980.
10. Maldonado, J. E., J. A. Velosa, R. A. Kyle, R. D. Wagoner, D. E. Holley, and R. M. Salassa: Fanconi syndrome in adults: A manifestation of a latent form of myeloma, *Am. J. Med.*, 58:354, 1975.
11. Adler, S. G., A. H. Cohen, and W. A. Border: Hypersensitivity phenomena and the kidney: Role of drugs and environmental agents, *Am. J. Kid. Dis.*, 5:75, 1985.
12. Cotran, R. S., R. H. Rubin, and N. E. Tolkoff-Rubin: Tubulointerstitial diseases, in B. M. Brenner and F. C. Rector, Jr. (eds.), *The Kidney*, 3d ed., Saunders, Philadelphia, 1986.
13. Baldwin, D. S., B. B. Levine, R. T. McCluskey, and G. R. Gallo: Renal failure and interstitial nephritis due to penicillin and methicillin, *N. Engl. J. Med.*, 279:1245, 1968.
14. Ditlove, J., P. Weidmann, M. Bernstein, and S. G. Massry: Methicillin nephritis, *Medicine*, 56:483, 1977.
15. Galpin, J. E., J. H. Shinaberger, T. M. Stanley, M. J. Bluemenkrantz, A. S. Bayer, G. S. Friedman, J. Z. Montgomerie, L. B. Guze, J. W. Coburn, and R. J. Glassock: Acute interstitial nephritis due to methicillin, *Am. J. Med.*, 65:756, 1978.
16. Nolan, C. M., and R. S. Abernathy: Nephropathy associated with methicillin therapy: Prevalence and determinants in patients with staphylococcal bacteremia, *Arch. Intern. Med.*, 137:997, 1977.
17. Sanjad, S. A., G. G. Haddad, and V. H. Nassar: Nephropathy, an underestimated complication of methicillin therapy, *J. Pediatr.*, 84:873, 1974.
18. Ruley, E. J., and L. N. Lisi: Interstitial nephritis and renal failure due to ampicillin, *J. Pediatr.*, 84:878, 1974.

19. Rennke, H. G., P. C. Roos, and S. G. Wall: Drug-induced interstitial nephritis with heavy glomerular proteinuria (letter), *N. Engl. J. Med.*, 302:691, 1980.

20. Parry, M. F., W. D. Ball, J. E. Conte, Jr., and S. N. Cohen: Nafcillin nephritis, *J. Am. Med. Assoc.*, 225:178, 1973.

21. Burton, J. R., N. S. Lichtenstein, R. B. Colvin, and N. E. Hyslop, Jr.: Acute interstitial nephritis from oxacillin, *Bull. Johns Hopkins Hosp.*, 134:58, 1974.

22. Burton, J. R., N. S. Lichtenstein, R. B. Colvin, and N. E. Hyslop, Jr.: Acute renal failure during cephalothin therapy, *J. Am. Med. Assoc.*, 229:679, 1974.

23. Clive, D. M., and J. S. Stoff: Renal syndromes associated with nonsteroidal antiinflammatory drugs, *N. Engl. J. Med.*, 310:563, 1984.

24. Garella, S., and R. A. Matarese: Renal effects of prostaglandins and clinical adverse effects of nonsteroidal anti-inflammatory drugs. *Medicine*, 63:165, 1984.

25. Watson, A. J., M. H. Dalbow, I. Stachura, J. A. Fragola, M. F. Rubin, R. M. Watson, and E. Bourke: Immunologic studies in cimetidine-induced nephropathy and polymyositis, *N. Engl. J. Med.*, 308:142, 1983.

26. Payne, C. R., P. Ackrill, and A. J. Ralston: Acute renal failure and rise in alkaline phosphatase activity caused by cimetidine, *Br. Med. J.*, 285:100, 1982.

27. Richmond, J. M., J. A. Whitworth, K. F. Fairley, and P. Kincaid-Smith: Co-trimoxazole nephrotoxicity, *Lancet*, 1:493, 1979.

28. Lyons, H., V. W. Pinn, S. Cortell, J. J. Cohen, and J. T. Harrington: Allergic interstitial nephritis causing reversible renal failure in four patients with idiopathic nephrotic syndrome, *N. Engl. J. Med.*, 288:124, 1973.

29. Magil, A. B., H. S. Ballon, E. C. Cameron, and A. Rae: Acute interstitial nephritis associated with thiazide diuretics. Clinical and pathologic observations in three cases, *Am. J. Med.*, 69:939, 1980.

30. Nessi, R., G. L. Bonoldi, B. Redaelli, and G. D. Filippo: Acute renal failure after rifampicin: A case report and survey of the literature, *Nephron*, 16:148, 1976.

31. Ellis, D., W. A. Fried, E. J. Yunis, and E. B. Blau: Acute interstitial nephritis in children: A report of 13 cases and review of the literature, *Pediatrics*, 67:867, 1981.

32. Case Records of the Massachusetts General Hospital (Case 17-1978), *N. Engl. J. Med.*, 298:1014, 1978.

33. Poulter, N., R. Gabriel, K. A. Porter, C. Bartlett, M. Kershaw, G. D. W. McKendrick, and R. Venkataraman: Acute interstitial nephritis complicating Legionnaires' disease, *Clin. Nephrol.*, 15:216, 1981.

34. Winearls, C. G., L. Chan, J. D. Coghlan, and D. O. Oliver: Acute renal failure due to leptospirosis: Clinical features and outcome in six cases, *Q. J. Med.*, 53:487, 1984.

35. Pecchini, F., M. Borghi, U. Bodini, B. Copercini, C. G. d'Auria, G. L. Romanini, and C. Romano: Acute renal failure from leptospirosis. New trends of treatment (letter), *Clin. Nephrol.*, 18:164, 1982.

36. Rosen, S., W. Harmon, A. M. Krensky, P. J. Edelson, B. L. Padgett, B. W. Grinnell, M. J. Rubino, and D. L. Walker: Tubulo-interstitial nephritis associated with polyomavirus (BK type) infection, *N. Engl. J. Med.*, 308:1192, 1983.

37. Chazan, J. A., S. Garella, and A. Esparaza: Acute interstitial nephritis: A distinct clinico-pathological entity, *Nephron*, 9:10, 1972.

38. Neugarten, J., G. R. Gallo, and D. S. Baldwin: Rifampin-induced nephrotic syndrome and acute interstitial nephritis, *Am. J. Nephrol.*, 3:38, 1983.

39. Averbuch, S. D., H. A. Austin III, S. A. Sherwin, T. Antonovych, P. A. Bunn, Jr., and D. L. Longo: Acute interstitial nephritis with the nephrotic syndrome following recombinant leukocyte A interferon therapy for mycosis fungoides, *N. Engl. J. Med.*, 310:32, 1984.

40. Finkelstein, A., D. S. Fraley, I. Stachura, H. A. Feldman, D. R. Gandy, and E. Bourke: Fenoprofen nephropathy: Lipoid nephrosis and interstitial nephritis. A possible T-lymphocyte disorder, *Am. J. Med.*, 72:81, 1982.

41. Bender, W. L., A. Whelton, W. E. Beschorner, M. O. Darwish, M. Hall-Craggs, and K. Solez: Interstitial nephritis, proteinuria, and renal failure caused by nonsteroidal anti-inflammatory drugs. Immunologic characterization of the inflammatory infiltrate, *Am. J. Med.*, 76:1004, 1984.

42. Wilson, D. B., and R. C. Blantz: Nephroimmunopathology and pathophysiology, *Am. J. Physiol.*, 248:F319, 1985.

43. Sheth, K. J., J. T. Casper, and T. A. Good: Interstitial nephritis due to phenytoin hypersensitivity, *J. Pediatr.*, 91:438, 1977.

44. Rosenfeld, J., V. Gura, G. Boner, M. Ben-Bassat, and E. Livni: Interstitial nephritis with acute renal failure after erythromycin, *Br. Med. J.*, 286:938, 1983.

45. Goodwin, J. S., D. Atluru, S. Sierakowsky, and E. A. Lianos: Mechanism of action of glucocorticosteroids. Interference of T cell proliferation and interleukin 2 production by hydrocortisone is re-

versed by leukotriene B₄, *J. Clin. Invest.*, 77:1244, 1986.

46. Colvin, R. B., J. R. Burton, N. E. Hyslop, Jr., L. Spitz, and N. S. Lichtenstein: Penicillin-associated interstitial nephritis, *Ann. Intern. Med.*, 81:404, 1974.

47. Border, W. A., D. H. Lehman, J. D. Egan, H. J. Sass, J. E. Globe, and C. B. Wilson: Antitubular basement-membrane antibodies in methicillin-associated interstitial nephritis, *N. Engl. J. Med.*, 291:381, 1974.

48. Rotellar, C., L. H. Noel, D. Droz, H. Kreis, and J. Berger: Role of antibodies directed against tubular basement membranes in human renal transplantation, *Am. J. Kid. Dis.*, 7:157, 1986.

49. Clayman, M. D., L. Michaud, J. Brentjens, G. A. Andres, N. A. Kefalides, and E. G. Neilson: Isolation of the target antigen of human anti-tubular basement membrane antibody-associated interstitial nephritis, *J. Clin. Invest.*, 77:1143, 1986.

50. Bergstein, J., and N. Litman: Interstitial nephritis with anti-tubular-basement-membrane antibody, *N. Engl. J. Med.*, 292:875, 1975.

51. Andres, G., J. Brentjens, R. Kohli, R. Anthone, S. Anthone, T. Baliah, M. Montes, B. K. Mookerjee, A. Prezyna, M. Sepulveda, R. Venuto, and C. Elwood: Histology of human tubulo-interstitial nephritis associated with antibodies to renal basement membranes, *Kidney Int.*, 13:480, 1978.

52. Brentjens, J. R., M. Sepulveda, T. Baliah, C. Bentzel, B. F. Erlanger, C. Elwood, M. Montes, K. C. Hsu, and G. A. Andres: Interstitial immune complex nephritis in patients with systemic lupus erythematosus, *Kidney Int.*, 7:342, 1975.

53. Case Records of the Massachusetts General Hospital (Case 42-1982), *N. Engl. J. Med.*, 309:970, 1983.

54. Abraham, P. A., and W. F. Keane: Glomerular and interstitial disease induced by nonsteroidal anti-inflammatory drugs, *Am. J. Nephrol.*, 4:1, 1984.

55. Linton, A. L., J. M. Richmond, W. F. Clark, R. M. Lindsay, A. A. Dreidger, and L. M. Lamki: Gallium scintigraphy in the diagnosis of acute renal disease, *Clin. Nephrol.*, 24:84, 1985.

56. Mullick, F. G., H. A. McAllister, Jr., B. M. Wagner, and J. J. Fenoglio, Jr.: Drug related vasculitis: Clinicopathologic correlations in 30 patients, *Hum. Pathol.*, 10:313, 1979.

57. Agus, D., R. Mann, M. Clayman, C. Kelly, L. Michaud, D. Cohn, and E. G. Neilson: The effects of daily cyclophosphamide administration on the development and extent of primary experimental interstitial nephritis in rats, *Kidney Int.*, 29:635, 1986.

58. Cox, M., and I. Singer: Lithium and water metabolism, *Am. J. Med.*, 59:153, 1975.

59. Walker, R. G., M. Escott, I. Birchall, J. P. Dowling, and P. Kincaid-Smith: Chronic progressive renal lesions induced by lithium, *Kidney Int.*, 29:875, 1986.

60. Cogan, E., and M. Abramow: Inhibition by lithium of the hydroosmotic action of vasopressin in the isolated perfused cortical collecting tubule of the rabbit, *J. Clin. Invest.*, 77: 1507, 1986.

61. Christensen, S., E. Kusano, A. N. Yusufi, N. Murayama, and T. P. Dousa: Pathogenesis of nephrogenic diabetes insipidus due to chronic administration of lithium in rats, *J. Clin. Invest.*, 75:1869, 1985.

62. Wallin, L., C. Alling, and M. Aurell: Impairment of renal function in patients on long-term lithium treatment, *Clin. Nephrol.*, 18:23, 1982.

63. Baylis, P. H., and D. A. Heath: Water disturbances in patients treated with oral lithium carbonate, *Ann. Intern. Med.*, 88:607, 1978.

64. Simon, N. M., E. Garber, and A. J. Arieff: Persistent nephrogenic diabetes insipidus after lithium carbonate, *Ann. Intern. Med.*, 86:446, 1977.

65. Batlle, D. C., A. B. von Riotte, M. Gaviria, and M. Grupp: Amelioration of polyuria by amiloride in patients receiving long-term lithium therapy, *N. Engl. J. Med.*, 312:408, 1985.

66. Hestbech, J., H. H. Hansen, A. Amdisen, and S. Olsen: Chronic renal lesions following long-term treatment with lithium, *Kidney Int.*, 12:205, 1977.

67. Hansen, H. E., J. Hestbech, J. I. Sorensen, K. Norgaard, J. Heilskov, and A. Amdisen: Chronic interstitial nephropathy in patients on long-term lithium treatment, *Q. J. Med.*, 48:577, 1979.

68. Aurell, M., C. Svalander, L. Wallin, and C. Alling: Renal function and biopsy findings in patients on long-term lithium treatment, *Kidney Int.*, 20:663, 1981.

69. Coppen A., M. E. Bishop, J. E. Bailey, W. R. Cattell, and R. G. Price: Renal function in lithium and non-lithium treated patients with affective disorders, *Acta Psychiatr. Scand.*, 62:343, 1980.

70. Kahan, B. D.: Cyclosporine: A powerful addition to the immunosuppressive armamentarium, *Am. J. Kid. Dis.*, 3:444, 1984.

71. Cohen, D. J., R. Loertscher, M. F. Rubin, N. L. Tilney, C. B. Carpenter, and T. B. Strom: Cyclosporine: A new immunosuppressive agent for organ transplantation, *Ann. Intern. Med.*, 101:667, 1984.

72. Palestine, A. G., H. A. Austin, III, J. E. Balow, T. T. Antonovych, S. G. Sabnis, H. G. Preuss, and R. B.

Nussenblatt: Renal histopathologic alterations in patients treated with cyclosporine for uveitis, *N. Engl. J. Med.,* 314:1293, 1986.

73. Berg, K. J., O. Forre, F. Bjerkhoel, E. Amundsen, O. Djoseland, H. E. Rugstad, and B. Westre: Side effects of cyclosporin A treatment in patients with rheumatoid arthritis, *Kidney Int.,* 29:1180, 1986.

74. The Canadian Multicentre Transplant Study Group: A randomized clinical trial of cyclosporin in cadaveric renal transplantation: Analysis at 3 years, *N. Engl. J. Med.,* 314:1219, 1986.

75. Rocher, L. L., E. L. Milford, R. L. Kirkman, C. B. Carpenter, T. B. Strom, and N. L. Tilney: Conversion from cyclosporine to azathioprine in renal allograft recipients, *Transplantation,* 38:669, 1984.

76. Myers, B. D., J. Ross., L. Newton, J. Luetscher, and M. Perlroth: Cyclosporine-associated chronic nephropathy, *N. Engl. J. Med.,* 311:699, 1984.

77. Mihatsch, M. J., G. Thiel, V. Basler, B. Ryffel, J. Landmann, J. von Overbeck, and H. U. Zollinger: Morphologic patterns in cyclosporin-treated renal transplant recipients, *Transpl. Proc.,* 17(suppl. 1):101, 1985.

78. Bergstrand, A., S. O. Bohman, A. Farnsworth, et al.: Renal histopathology in kidney transplant recipients immunosuppressed with cyclosporin A: Results of an international workshop, *Clin. Nephrol.,* 24:107, 1985.

79. Thiel, G.: Experimental cyclosporine A nephrotoxicity: A summary of the International Workshop, *Clin. Nephrol.,* 25(suppl. 1):205, 1986.

80. Humes, H. D., N. M. Jackson, R. P. O'Connor, D. A. Hunt, and M. D. White: Pathogenetic mechanisms of nephrotoxicity: Insights into cyclosporine nephrotoxicity, *Transpl. Proc.,* 17(suppl. 1):51, 1985.

81. Harmon, W. E., H. J. Cohen, E. E. Schneeberger, and W. E. Grupe: Chronic renal failure in children treated with methyl CCNU, *N. Engl. J. Med.,* 300:1200, 1979.

82. Micetich, K. C., M. Jensen-Akula, J. C. Mandard, and R. I. Fisher: Nephrotoxicity of semustine (methyl-CCNU) in patients with malignant melanoma receiving adjuvant chemotherapy, *Am. J. Med.,* 71:967, 1981.

83. Perry, D. J., and R. B. Weiss: Nephrotoxicity of streptozotocin (letter), *Ann. Intern. Med.,* 96:122, 1982.

84. Consensus Conference: Analgesic-associated kidney disease, *J. Am. Med. Assoc.,* 251:3123, 1984.

85. Goldberg, M.: Analgesic-associated nephropathy: An important cause of chronic renal failure in the United States, *Am. J. Kid. Dis.,* 7:162, 1986.

86. Buckalew, V. M., Jr., and H. M. Schey: Renal disease from habitual antipyretic analgesic consump-tion: An assessment of the epidemiologic evidence, *Medicine,* 65:291, 1986.

87. Kincaid-Smith, P.: Analgesic abuse and the kidney, *Kidney Int.,* 17:250, 1980.

88. Gloor, F. J.: Changing concepts in pathogenesis and morphology of analgesic nephropathy as seen in Europe, *Kidney Int.,* 13:27, 1978.

89. Burry, A.: Pathology of analgesic nephropathy, *Kidney Int.,* 13:34, 1978.

90. Mihatsch, M. J., H. O. Hofer, F. Gudat, C. Knusli, J. Torhorst, and H. U. Zollinger: Capillary sclerosis of the urinary tract and analgesic nephropathy, *Clin. Nephrol.,* 20:285, 1983.

91. Murray, T. G., and M. Goldberg: Analgesic-associated nephropathy in the U.S.A.: Epidemiologic, clinical and pathogenetic features, *Kidney Int.,* 13:64, 1978.

92. Nanra, R. S., J. Stuart-Taylor, A. H. deLeon, and K. H. White: Analgesic nephropathy: Etiology, clinical syndrome, and clinicopathologic correlations in Australia, *Kidney Int.,* 13:79, 1978.

93. Dubach, V. C., B. Rosner, and E. P. Pfister: Epidemiologic study of abuse of analgesics containing phenacetin. Renal morbidity and mortality (1968–1979), *N. Engl. J. Med.,* 308:357, 1983.

94. New Zealand Rheumatism Association Study: Aspirin and the kidney, *Br. Med. J.,* 1:593, 1974.

95. Emkey, R. D., and J. A. Mills: Aspirin and analgesic nephropathy, *J. Am. Med. Assoc.,* 247:55, 1982.

96. Aykol, S. M., M. Thompson, and D. N. Kerr: Renal function after prolonged consumption of aspirin, *Br. Med. J.,* 284:631, 1982.

97. Allen, R. C., R. E. Petty, D. S. Lirenman, P. N. Malleson, and R. M. Laxer: Renal papillary necrosis in children with chronic arthritis, *Am. J. Dis. Child.,* 140:20, 1986.

98. Bach, P. H., and T. L. Hardy: Relevance of animal models to analgesic-associated renal papillary necrosis in humans, *Kidney Int.,* 28:605, 1985.

99. Duggin, G. G.: Mechanisms in the development of analgesic nephropathy, *Kidney Int.,* 18:553, 1980.

100. Bleumle, L. W., Jr., and M. Goldberg: Renal accumulation of salicylate and phenacetin: Possible mechanisms in the nephropathy of analgesic abuse, *J. Clin. Invest.,* 47:2507, 1968.

101. Sabatini, S., S. Koppera, J. Manaligod, J. A. Arruda, and N. A. Kurtzman: Role of urinary concentrating ability in the generation of toxic papillary necrosis, *Kidney Int.,* 23:705, 1983.

102. Nanra, R. S., P. Chirawong, and P. Kincaid-Smith: Medullary ischaemia in experimental analgesic nephropathy—The pathogenesis of renal papillary necrosis, *Aust. N. Z. J. Med.,* 3:580, 1973.

103. Brod, J., K. W. Kuhn, H. S. Stender, and E. Stolle:

Phenacetin abuse and chronic pyelonephritis, *Nephron,* 19:311, 1977.

104. Steele, T. W., A. Z. Gyory, and K. D. G. Edwards: Renal function in analgesic nephropathy, *Br. Med. J.,* 2:213, 1969.

105. Cove-Smith, J. R., and M. S. Knapp: Sodium handling in analgesic nephropathy, *Lancet,* 2:70, 1973.

106. Harrow, B. R., J. A. Sloane, and N. C. Liebman: Renal papillary necrosis and analgesics: Roentgen differentiation from sponge kidney and other disease, *J. Am. Med. Assoc.,* 184:445, 1963.

107. Hartman, G. W., V. E. Torres, G. F. Leago, B. Williamson, Jr., and R. R. Hattery: Analgesic-associated nephropathy. Pathophysiologic and radiological correlation, *J. Am. Med. Assoc.,* 251:1734, 1984.

108. Cove-Smith, J. R., and M. S. Knapp: Analgesic nephropathy: An important cause of chronic renal failure, *Q. J. Med.,* 47:49, 1978.

109. Eknoyan, G., W. Y. Qunibi, R. T. Grissom, S. N. Tuma, and J. C. Ayus: Renal papillary necrosis: An update, *Medicine,* 61:55, 1982.

110. Harrow, B. R., J. A. Sloane, and N. C. Liebman: Roentgenologic demonstration of renal papillary necrosis in sickle-cell trait, *N. Engl. J. Med.,* 268:969, 1963.

111. Simon, H. B., A. J. Weinstein, M. S. Pasternak, M. N. Swartz, and L. J. Kunz: Genito-urinary tuberculosis: Clinical features in a general hospital population, *Am. J. Med.,* 63:410, 1977.

112. Murray, R. M., D. H. Lawson, and A. L. Linton: Analgesic nephropathy: Clinical syndrome and prognosis, *Br. Med. J.,* 1:479, 1971.

113. Gault, M. H., and D. R. Wilson: Analgesic nephropathy in Canada: Clinical syndrome, management, and outcome, *Kidney Int.,* 13:58, 1978.

114. Shelley, J. H. L.: Pharmacologic mechanisms of analgesic nephropathy, *Kidney Int.,* 13:15, 1978.

115. Bengtsson, U., S. Johansson, and L. Angervall: Malignancies of the urinary tract and their relation to analgesic abuse, *Kidney Int.,* 13:107, 1978.

116. Gonwa, T. A., V. M. Buckalew, and W. T. Corbett: Analgesic nephropathy and urinary-tract carcinoma, *Ann. Intern. Med.,* 90:432, 1979.

117. Piper, J. M., J. Tonascia, and G. M. Matanoski: Heavy phenacetin use and bladder cancer in women aged 20 to 49 years, *N. Engl. J. Med.,* 313:292, 1985.

118. McCredie, M., J. H. Stewart, J. J. Carter, J. Turner, and J. F. Mahony: Phenacetin and papillary necrosis: Independent risk factors of renal pelvic cancer, *Kidney Int.,* 30:81, 1986.

119. Blohme, I., and S. Johansson: Renal pelvic neoplasms and atypical urothelium in patients with end-stage analgesic nephropathy, *Kidney Int.,* 20:671, 1981.

120. Eriksson, O., and S. Johansson: Urothelial neoplasms of the upper urinary tract: A correlation between cytologic and histologic findings in 43 patients with urothelial neoplasms of the renal pelvis or ureter, *Acta Cytol.,* 20:20, 1976.

121. Murray, R. M.: Analgesic nephropathy: Removal of phenacetin from proprietary analgesics, *Br. Med. J.,* 4:131, 1972.

122. Evans, J. A., M. A. Meyers, and M. A. Bosniak: Acute renal and perirenal infections, *Semin. Roentgenol.,* 6:274, 1971.

123. Parker, J., and C. Kunin: Pyelonephritis in young women: A 10- to 20-year follow-up, *J. Am. Med. Assoc.,* 224:585, 1973.

124. Hodson, J.: Reflux nephropathy, *Med. Clin. N. Am.,* 62:1201, 1978.

125. Cotran, R. S.: Glomerulosclerosis in reflux nephropathy, *Kidney Int.,* 21:528, 1982.

126. MacGregor, M. E., and P. Freeman: Childhood urinary infection associated with vesicoureteric reflux, *Q. J. Med.,* 44:481, 1975.

127. Shah, K. J., D. G. Robins, and R. H. R. White: Renal scarring and vesicoureteric reflux, *Arch. Dis. Child,* 53:210, 1978.

128. Smellie, J. M., I. C. Normand, and G. Katz: Children with urinary infection: Comparison of those with and those without vesicoureteric reflux, *Kidney Int.,* 20:717, 1981.

129. Smellie, J. M., and I. C. S. Normand: Bacteriuria, reflux, and renal scarring, *Arch. Dis. Child.,* 50:581, 1975.

130. Smellie, J. M., P. G. Ransley, I. C. Normand, N. Prescod, and D. Edwards: Development of new renal scars: A collaborative study, *Br. Med. J.,* 290:1957, 1985.

131. Warren J. W., H. L. Muncie, Jr., G. J. Bergquist, and J. M. Hoopes: Sequelae and management of urinary infection in the patient requiring chronic catheterization, *J. Urol.,* 125:1, 1981.

132. Rolleston, G. L., R. T. Shannon, and W. L. F. Utley: Relationship of infantile vesicoureteric reflux to renal damage, *Br. Med. J.,* 1:460, 1970.

133. Rolleston, G. L., T. M. J. Maling, and C. J. Hodson: Intrarenal reflux and the scarred kidney, *Arch. Dis. Child.,* 49:531, 1974.

134. Ransley, P. G., and R. A. Risdon: Renal papillae and intrarenal reflux in the pig, *Lancet,* 2:1114, 1974.

135. Cardiff-Oxford Bacteriuria Study Group: Sequelae of covert bacteriuria in schoolgirls, *Lancet,* 1:889, 1978.

136. Huland, H., and R. Busch: Pyelonephritic scarring in 213 patients with upper and lower urinary tract infections: Long-term follow-up, *J. Urol.,* 132:936, 1984.

137. Edwards, D., I. C. S. Normand, N. Prescod, and J. M. Smellie: Disappearance of vesicoureteric reflux during long-term prophylaxis of urinary tract infection in children, *Br. Med. J.,* 2:285, 1977.

138. Bhathena, D. B., J. H. Weiss, N. H. Holland, R. G. McMorrow, J. J. Curtis, B. A. Lucas, and R. G. Luke: Focal and segmental glomerular sclerosis in reflux nephropathy, *Am. J. Med.,* 68:886, 1980.

139. Torres, V. E., J. A. Velosa, K. E. Holley, P. P. Kelalis, G. B. Stickler, and S. B. Kurtz: The progression of vesicoureteral reflux nephropathy, *Ann. Intern. Med.,* 92:776, 1980.

140. Steinhardt, G. F.: Reflux nephropathy, *J. Urol.,* 134:855, 1985.

141. Smellie, J. M., C. J. Hodson, D. Edwards, and I. C. S. Normand: Clinical and radiological features of urinary infection in childhood, *Br. Med. J.,* 2:1222, 1964.

142. Kollins, S. A., G. W. Hartman, D. T. Carr, J. W. Segura, and R. R. Hattery: Roentgenographic findings in urinary tract tuberculosis, *Am. J. Roentgenol. Rad. Ther. Nucl. Med.,* 121:487, 1974.

143. Lenaghan, D., J. G. Whitaker, F. Jensen, and F. D. Stephens: The natural history of reflux and long-term effects of reflux on the kidney, *J. Urol.,* 115:728, 1976.

144. Vermillion, C. D., and W. F. Heale: Position and configuration of the ureteral orifice and its relationship to renal scarring in adults, *J. Urol.,* 109:579, 1973.

145. Sherwood, T., and R. H. Whitaker: Initial screening of children with urinary tract infections: Is plain film radiography and ultrasonography enough?, *Br. Med. J.,* 288:827, 1984.

146. Whitaker, R. H., and T. Sherwood: Another look at diagnostic pathways in children with urinary tract infection, *Br. Med. J.,* 288:839, 1984.

147. Jerkins, G. R., and H. N. Noe: Familial vesicoureteral reflux: A prospective study, *J. Urol.,* 128:774, 1982.

148. Senkkjian, H. O., B. J. Stinebaugh, C. A. Mattioli, and W. N. Suki: Irreversible renal failure following vesicoureteral reflux, *J. Am. Med. Assoc.,* 241:160, 1979.

149. Salvatierra, O., S. L. Kountz, and F. O. Belzer: Primary vesicoureteral reflux and end-stage renal disease, *J. Am. Med. Assoc.,* 226:1454, 1973.

150. Report of the International Reflux Study Committee: Medical versus surgical treatment of primary vesicoureteral reflux: A prospective international reflux study in children, *J. Urol.,* 125:277, 1981.

151. Woodward, J. R.: Vesicoureteral reflux: A surgical perspective, *Am. J. Kid. Dis.,* 3:136, 1983.

152. Duckett, J. W.: Vesicoureteral reflux: A "conservative" analysis, *Am. J. Kid. Dis.,* 3:139:1983.

153. Malek, R. S., J. Svensson, R. J. Neves, and V. E. Torres: Vesicoureteral reflux in the adult, III. Surgical correction: Risks and benefits, *J. Urol.,* 130:882, 1983.

154. Neves, R. J., V. E. Torres, R. S. Malek, and J. Svensson: Vesicoureteral reflux in the adult. IV. Medical versus surgical management, *J. Urol.,* 132:882, 1984.

155. Kincaid-Smith, P.: Reflux nephropathy, *Br. Med. J.,* 286:2002, 1983.

156. Claesson, I., B. Jacobsson, U. Jodal, and J. Winberg: Compensatory kidney growth in children with urinary tract infection and unilateral renal scarring: An epidemiologic study, *Kidney Int.,* 20:759, 1981.

157. Griffith, D. P.: Infection-induced renal calculi, *Kidney Int.,* 21:422, 1982.

158. Dalgaard, O. Z.: Bilateral polycystic disease of the kidney: A follow-up of two hundred and eighty-four patients and their families, *Acta Med. Scand.,* 158(suppl. 328):1, 1957.

159. Grantham, J. J.: Polycystic kidney disease: A predominance of giant nephrons, *Am. J. Physiol.,* 244:F3, 1983.

160. Suki, W. N.: Polycystic kidney disease, *Kidney Int.,* 22:571, 1982.

161. Gardner, K. D., Jr., and A. P. Evan: Cystic kidneys: An enigma evolves, *Am. J. Kid. Dis.,* 3:403, 1984.

162. Hatfield, P. M., and R. C. Pfister: Adult polycystic disease of the kidneys (Potter type 3), *J. Am. Med. Assoc.,* 222:1527, 1972.

163. Osathanondh, V., and E. L. Potter: Pathogenesis of polycystic kidneys: Type 1 due to hyperplasia of interstitial portions of collecting tubules, *Arch. Pathol.,* 77:466, 1964.

164. Osathanondh, V., and E. L. Potter: Pathogenesis of polycystic kidneys: Type 2 due to inhibition of ampullary activity, *Arch. Pathol.,* 77:474, 1964.

165. Osathanondh, V., and E. L. Potter: Pathogenesis of polycystic kidneys: Type 3 due to multiple abnormalities of development, *Arch. Pathol.,* 77:485, 1964.

166. Huseman, R., A. Grady, D. Welling, and J. J. Grantham: Macropuncture study of polycystic disease in adult human kidneys, *Kidney Int.,* 18:375, 1980.

167. Gardner, K. D., Jr.: Composition of fluid in twelve cysts of a polycystic kidney, *N. Engl. J. Med.,* 281:985, 1969.

168. Levey, A. S., S. G. Pauker, and J. P. Kassirer: Occult intracranial aneurysms in polycystic kidney disease. When is cerebral arteriography indicated?, *N. Engl. J. Med.,* 308:986, 1983.

169. Scheff, R. T., G. Zuckerman, H. Harter, J. Delmez, and R. Koehler: Diverticular disease in patients with chronic renal failure due to polycystic kidney disease, *Ann. Intern. Med.,* 92:202, 1980.
170. Gabow, P. A., D. W. Ikle, and J. H. Holmes: Polycystic kidney disease: Prospective analysis of non-azotemic patients and family members, *Ann. Intern. Med.,* 101:238, 1984.
171. Leier, C. V., P. B. Baker, J. W. Kilman, and C. F. Wooley: Cardiovascular abnormalities associated with adult polycystic kidney disease, *Ann. Intern. Med.,* 100:683, 1984.
172. Reeders, S. T., M. H. Breuning, G. Corney, S. J. Jeremiah, P. Meera Khan, K. E. Davies, D. A. Hopkinson, P. L. Pearson, and D. J. Weatherall: Two genetic markers closely linked to adult polycystic kidney disease on chromosome 16, *Br. Med. J.,* 292:851, 1986.
173. Evan, A. P., and K. D. Gardner, Jr.: Comparison of human polycystic and medullary cystic kidney disease with diphenylamine-induced cystic disease, *Lab. Invest.,* 35:93, 1976.
174. Gardner, K. D., Jr., and A. P. Evan: Renal cystic disease induced by diphenylthiazole, *Kidney Int.,* 24:43, 1983.
175. Nash, D. A., Jr.: Hypertension in polycystic kidney disease without renal failure, *Arch. Intern. Med.,* 137:1571, 1977.
176. Calabrese, G., G. Vagelli, C. Cristofano, and G. Barsotti: Behaviour of arterial pressure in different stages of polycystic kidney disease, *Nephron,* 32:207, 1982.
177. Milutinovic, J., P. J. Fialkow, L. Y. Agodoa, L. A. Phillips, T. G. Rudd, and J. I. Bryant: Autosomal dominant polycystic kidney disease: Symptoms and clinical findings, *Q. J. Med.,* 53:511, 1984.
178. Editorial: Adult polycystic disease of the kidneys, *Br. Med. J.,* 282:1097, 1981.
179. Bear, J. C., P. McManamon, J. Morgan, R. H. Payne, H. Lewis, M. H. Gault, and D. N. Churchill: Age at clinical onset and at ultrasonographic detection of adult polycystic kidney disease: Data for genetic counselling. *Am. J. Med. Genet.,* 18:45, 1984.
180. Churchill, D. N., J. C. Bear, J. Morgan, R. H. Payne, P. J. McManamon, and M. H. Gault: Prognosis of adult onset polycystic kidney disease re-evaluated. *Kidney Int.,* 26:190, 1981.
181. Kumar, S., A. I. Cedarbaum, and P. G. Pletka: Renal cell carcinoma in polycystic kidneys: Case report and review of literature, *J. Urol.,* 124:708, 1980.
182. Waters, W. B., H. Hershman, and L. A. Klein: Management of infected polycystic kidneys, *J. Urol.,* 122:383, 1979.
183. Muther, R. S., and W. M. Bennett: Cyst fluid antibiotic concentrations in polycystic kidney disease: Differences between proximal and distal cysts, *Kidney Int.,* 20:519, 1981.
184. Bennett, W. M., L. Elzinga, J. P. Pulliam, A. L. Rashad, and J. M. Barry: Cyst fluid antibiotic concentrations in autosomal-dominant polycystic kidney disease, *Am. J. Kid. Dis.,* 6:400, 1985.
185. Schwab, S.: Efficacy of chloramphenicol in refractory cyst infections in autosomal dominant polycystic kidney disease, *Am. J. Kid. Dis.,* 5:258, 1985.
186. Bennett, W. M., and J. M. Barry: Reduction of cyst volume for symptomatic management of autosomal dominant polycystic disease (abstract), *Kidney Int.,* 29:179, 1986.
187. Oldrizzi, L., C. Rugiu, E. Valvo, A. Lupo, C. Loschiavo, L. Gammaro, N. Tessitore, A. Fabris, G. Panzetta, and G. Maschio: Progression of renal failure in patients with renal disease of diverse etiology on protein-restricted diet, *Kidney Int.,* 27:553, 1985.
188. Gretz, N., E. Korb, and M. Strauch: Low-protein diet supplemented by ketoacids in chronic renal failure: A prospective controlled study, *Kidney Int.,* 24(suppl. 16):S-263, 1983.
189. Rosman, J. B., P. M. ter Wee, S. Meiser, T. Ph.M. Piers-Becht, W. J. Sluiter, and Ab. J. M. Donker: Prospective randomized trial of early dietary protein restriction in chronic renal failure, *Lancet,* 2:1291, 1984.
190. Chester, A. C., W. P. Argy, Jr., T. A. Rakowski, and G. E. Schreiner: Polycystic kidney disease and chronic hemodialysis, *Clin. Nephrol.,* 10:129, 1978.
191. Mendez, R., R. G. Mendez, J. E. Payne, and T. V. Berne: Renal transplantation in adult patients with end-stage polycystic kidney disease, *Urology,* 5:26, 1975.
192. Welling L. W., and J. J. Grantham: Cystic and developmental diseases of the kidney, in B. M. Brenner and F. C. Rector, Jr. (eds.), *The Kidney,* 3d ed., Saunders, Philadelphia, 1986.
193. Morris, R. C., Jr., H. Yamauchi, A. J. Palubinskas, and H. J. Howenstine: Medullary sponge kidney, *Am. J. Med.,* 38:883, 1965.
194. Kliger, A. S., and R. L. Schler: Familial disease of the renal medulla: A study of progeny in a family with medullary cystic disease, *Ann. Intern. Med.,* 85:190, 1976.
195. Bennett, W. B.: Kindred coexistence of medullary sponge kidney and medullary cystic disease, *Ann. Intern. Med.,* 85:829, 1976.
196. Fairley, K. F., P. W. Leighton, and P. Kincaid-

Smith: Familial visual defects associated with polycystic kidney and medullary sponge kidney, *Br. Med. J.,* 1:1060, 1963.

197. Nemoy, N. J., and L. Forsberg: Polycystic renal disease presenting as medullary sponge kidney, *J. Urol.,* 100:408, 1968.

198. Abreo, K., and T. H. Steele: Simultaneous medullary sponge and adult polycystic kidney disease: The need for accurate diagnosis, *Arch. Intern. Med.,* 142:163, 1982.

199. Emmett, J. L., and D. M. Witten: *Clinical Urography: An Atlas and Textbook of Roentgenologic Diagnosis,* 3d ed., Saunders, Philadelphia, 1971, chap. 9.

200. O'Neill, M., N. A. Breslau, and C. Y. C. Pak: Metabolic evaluation of nephrolithiasis in patients with medullary sponge kidney, *J. Am. Med. Assoc.,* 245:1233, 1981.

201. Parks, J. H., F. L. Coe, and A. L. Strauss: Calcium nephrolithiasis and medullary sponge kidney in women, *N. Engl. J. Med.,* 306:1088, 1982.

202. Pak, C. Y. C., P. Peters, G. Hurt, M. Kadesky, M. Fine, D. Reisman, F. Splann, C. Caramela, A. Freeman, F. Britton, K. Sakhaee, and N. A. Breslau: Is selective therapy of recurrent nephrolithiasis possible, *Am. J. Med.,* 71:615, 1981.

203. Pak, C. Y. C., and C. Fuller: Idiopathic hypocitraturic calcium-oxalate nephrolithiasis successfully treated with potassium citrate, *Ann. Intern. Med.,* 104:33, 1986.

204. Strauss, M. B., Clinical and pathological aspects of cystic disease of the renal medulla: An analysis of eighteen cases, *Ann. Intern. Med.,* 57:373, 1962.

205. Burke, J. R., J. A. Inglis, P. W. Craswell, K. R. Mitchell, and B. T. Emmerson: Juvenile nephronophthisis and medullary cystic disease—the same disease (report of a large family with medullary cystic disease associated with gout and epilepsy), *Clin. Nephrol.,* 18:1, 1982.

206. Case Records of the Massachusetts General Hospital (Case 48-1981), *N. Engl. J. Med.,* 305:1334, 1981.

207. Bommer, J., R. Waldherr, G. von Kaick, L. Strauss, and E. Ritz: Acquired renal cysts in uremic patients—In vivo demonstration by computed tomography, *Clin. Nephrol.,* 14:299, 1980.

208. Grantham, J. J., and E. Levine: Acquired cystic disease: Replacing one kidney disease with another, *Kidney Int.,* 28:99, 1985.

209. Mickisch, O., J. Bommer, S. Bachmann, R. Waldherr, J. F. Mann, and E. Ritz: Multicystic transformation of kidneys in chronic renal failure, *Nephron,* 38:93, 1984.

210. Pollack, H. M., B. B. Goldberg, J. O. Morales, and M. Bogash: A systematized approach to the differential diagnosis of renal masses, *Radiology,* 113:653, 1974.

211. Clayman, R. V., V. Surya, R. P. Miller, D. B. Reinke, and E. E. Fraley: Pursuit of the renal mass. Is ultrasound enough?, *Am. J. Med.,* 77:218, 1984.

212. Bosniak, M. A.: The current radiologic approach to renal cysts, *Radiology,* 158:1, 1986.

213. Kyle, R. A.: Multiple myeloma: Review of 869 cases, *Mayo Clin. Proc.,* 50:29, 1975.

214. DeFronzo, R. A., C. R. Cooke, J. R. Wright, and R. L. Humphrey: Renal function in patients with multiple myeloma, *Medicine,* 57:151, 1978.

215. Fang, L.-S.: Light-chain nephropathy, *Kidney Int.,* 27:582, 1985.

216. DeFronzo, R. A., R. L. Humphrey, J. R. Wright, and C. R. Cooke: Acute renal failure in multiple myeloma, *Medicine,* 54:209, 1975.

217. Cohen, D. J., W. H. Sherman, E. F. Osserman, and G. B. Appel: Acute renal failure in patients with multiple myeloma, *Am. J. Med.,* 76:247, 1984.

218. Border, W. A., and A. H. Cohen: Renal biopsy diagnosis of clinically silent multiple myeloma, *Ann. Intern. Med.,* 93:43, 1980.

219. Levi, D., R. C. Williams, Jr., and F. D. Lindstrom: Immunofluorescent studies of the myeloma kidney with special reference to light chain disease, *Am. J. Med.,* 44:922, 1968.

220. Kaysen, G. A., B. D. Myers, W. G. Couser, R. Rabkin, and J. M. Felts: Mechanisms and consequences of proteinuria, *Lab. Invest.,* 54:479, 1986.

221. Perry, M. C., and R. A. Kyle: The clinical significance of Bence Jones proteinuria, *Mayo Clin. Proc.,* 50:234, 1975.

222. Hill, G. S., L. Morel-Maroger, J-P. Méry, J. C. Brouet, and F. Mignon: Renal lesions in multiple myeloma: Their relationship to associated protein abnormalities, *Am. J. Kid. Dis.,* 2:423, 1983.

223. Hayes, J. S., N. Jankey, A. L. Cuthbert, and P. M. Das: Massive proteinuria in light chain disease, *Arch. Intern. Med.,* 138:785, 1978.

224. Kyle, R. A., and P. R. Greipp: "Idiopathic" Bence Jones proteinuria: Long-term follow-up in seven patients, *N. Engl. J. Med.,* 306:564, 1982.

225. Clyne, D. H., A. J. Pesce, and R. E. Thompson: Nephrotoxicity of Bence Jones proteins in the rat: Importance of protein isoelectric point, *Kidney Int.,* 16:345, 1979.

226. Melcion, C., B. Mougenot, R. Baudouin, P. Ronco, L. Moulanguet-Doleris, P. H. Vanhille, M. Beaufils, L. Morel-Maroger, P. Verroust, and G. Richet: Renal failure in myeloma: Relationship with isoelectric point of immunoglobulin light chains, *Clin. Nephrol.,* 22:138, 1984.

227. Coward, R. A., I. W. Delamore, N. P. Mallick, and E. L. Robinson: The importance of urinary immunoglobulin light chain isoelectric point (PI) in nephrotoxicity in multiple myeloma, *Clin. Sci.,* 66: 229, 1984.

228. Holland, M. D., J. H. Galla, P. W. Sanders, and R. G. Luke: Effect of urinary pH and diatrizoate on Bence Jones protein nephrotoxicity in the rat, *Kidney Int.,* 27:46, 1985.

229. Hamblin, T. J.: The kidney in myeloma, *Br. Med. J.,* 292:2, 1986.

230. Smolens, P., M. Venkatachalam, and J. H. Stein: Myeloma kidney cast nephropathy in a rat model of multiple myeloma, *Kidney Int.,* 24:192, 1983.

231. Weiss, J. H., R. H. Williams, J. H. Galla, J. L. Gottschall, E. D. Rees, D. Bhathena, and R. G. Luke: Pathophysiology of acute Bence Jones protein nephrotoxicity in the rat, *Kidney Int.,* 20:198, 1981.

232. Smithline, N., J. P. Kassirer, and J. J. Cohen: Lightchain nephropathy: Renal tubular dysfunction associated with light-chain proteinuria, *N. Engl. J. Med.,* 294:71, 1976.

233. Maldonado, J. E., J. A. Velosa, R. A. Kyle, R. D. Wagoner, K. E. Holley, and R. M. Salassa: Fanconi syndrome in adults: A manifestation of a latent form of myeloma, *Am. J. Med.,* 58:354, 1975.

234. Glenner, G. G.: Amyloid deposits and amyloidosis. The β-fibrilloses. *N. Engl. J. Med.,* 302:1283, 1333, 1980.

235. Solomon, A., B. Frangione, and E. C. Franklin: Bence Jones proteins and light chains of immunoglobulins. Preferential association of the $V_{\lambda VI}$ subgroup of human light chains with amyloidosis AL (λ), *J. Clin. Invest.,* 70:453, 1982.

236. Caneval, D., L-H. Noel, J-L. Preud'Homme, D. Droz, and J-P. Grunfeld: Light-chain deposition disease: Its relation with AL-type amyloidosis, *Kidney Int.,* 26:1, 1984.

237. Durie, B. G. M., B. Persky, B. J. Soehnlen, T. M. Grogan, and S. E. Salmon: Amyloid production in human myeloma stem-cell culture, with morphologic evidence of amyloid secretion by associated macrophages, *N. Engl. J. Med.,* 307:1689, 1982.

238. Stone, M. J., and E. P. Frenkel: The clinical spectrum of light chain myeloma: A study of 35 patients with special reference to the occurrence of amyloidosis, *Am. J. Med.,* 58:601, 1975.

239. Burke, J. F., Jr., R. Flis, N. Lasker, and M. Simenhoff: Malignant lymphoma with "myeloma kidney" acute renal failure, *Am. J. Med.,* 60:1055, 1976.

240. Lindstrom, F. D., R. C. Williams Jr., W. R. Swaim, and E. F. Freier: Urinary light-chain excretion in myeloma and other disorders—An evaluation of

the Bence Jones test, *J. Lab. Clin. Med.,* 71:812, 1968.

241. Coward, R. A., N. P. Mallick, and I. W. Delamore: Should patients with renal failure associated with myeloma be dialysed?, *Br. Med. J.,* 287:1575, 1983.

242. Morgan, C., Jr., and W. J. Hammack: Intravenous urography in multiple myeloma, *N. Engl. J. Med.,* 275:77, 1966.

243. Russell, J. A., B. M. Fitzharris, R. Corringham, D. A. Darcy, and R. L. Powles: Plasma exchange v peritoneal dialysis for removing Bence Jones protein, *Br. Med. J.* 2:1397, 1978.

244. Misiani, R., G. Remuzzi, T. Bertami, R. Licini, P. Levoni, A. Crippi, and G. Mecca: Plasmapheresis in the treatment of acute renal failure in multiple myeloma, *Am. J. Med.,* 66:684, 1979.

245. Zucchelli, P., S. Pasquali, L. Cagnoli, and C. Rovinetti: Plasma exchange therapy in acute renal failure due to light chain myeloma. *Trans. Am. Soc. Artif. Int. Org.,* 30:36, 1984.

246. MRC Working Party on Leukemia in Adults: Analysis and management of renal failure in fourth MRC myelomatosis trial., *Br. Med. J.,* 288:1411, 1984.

247. Johnson, W. J., R. A. Kyle, and P. J. Dahlberg: Dialysis in the treatment of multiple myeloma, *Mayo Clin. Proc.,* 55:65, 1980.

248. Cosio, F. G., T. V. Pence, F. L. Shapiro, and C. M. Kjellstrand: Severe renal failure in multiple myeloma, *Clin. Nephrol.,* 15:206, 1981.

249. Humphrey, R. L., J. R. Wright, J. B. Zachary, S. Sterioff, and R. A. DeFronzo: Renal transplantation in multiple myeloma: A case report, *Ann. Intern. Med.,* 83:651, 1975.

250. Emmerson, B. T., and P. G. Row: An evaluation of the pathogenesis of the gouty kidney, *Kidney Int.,* 8:65, 1975.

251. Coe, F. L.: Uric acid and calcium oxalate nephrolithiasis, *Kidney Int.,* 24:392, 1983.

252. Rodman, J. S., J. J. Williams, and C. M. Peterson: Dissolution of uric acid calculi, *J. Urol.,* 131:1039, 1984.

253. Boss, G. R., and J. E. Seegmiller: Hyperuricemia and gout: Classification, complications and management, *N. Engl. J. Med.,* 300:1459, 1979.

254. Guggino, S. E., and P. S. Aronson: Paradoxical effects of pyrazinoate and nicotinate on urate transport in dog renal microvillus membranes, *J. Clin. Invest.,* 76:543, 1985.

255. Rieselbach, R. E., C. J. Bentzel, E. Cotlov, E. Frei, and E. J. Freireich: Uric acid excretion and renal function in the acute hyperuricemia of leukemia:

Pathogenesis and therapy of uric acid nephropathy, *Am. J. Med.,* 37:872, 1964.

256. Kjellstrand, C. M., D. C. Campbell, B. von Hartitzch, and T. J. Buselmeier: Hyperuricemic acute renal failure, *Arch. Intern. Med.,* 133:349, 1974.

257. Kelton, J., W. N. Kelley, and E. N. Holmes: A rapid method for the diagnosis of acute uric acid nephropathy, *Arch. Intern. Med.,* 138:612, 1978.

258. Warren, D. J., A. G. Leitch, and R. J. E. Leggett: Hyperuricaemic renal failure after epileptic seizures, *Lancet,* 2:385, 1975.

259. Crittenden, D. R., and G. L. Ackerman: Hyperuricemic acute renal failure in disseminated carcinoma, *Arch. Intern. Med.,* 137:97, 1977.

260. Wyngaarden, J. B., and W. N. Kelley: Gout, and Clinical syndromes associated with hypoxanthine-guanine phosphoribosyltransferase deficiency, in J. B. Stanbury, J. B. Wyngaarden, D. S. Fredrickson, J. L. Goldstein, and M. S. Brown (eds.), *The Metabolic Basis of Inherited Disease,* 5th ed., McGraw-Hill, New York, 1983.

261. Yu, Ts.-F., and A. B. Gutman: Uric acid nephrolithiasis in gout: Predisposing factors, *Ann. Intern. Med.,* 67:1133, 1967.

262. Emmerson, B. T., and L. Thompson: The spectrum of hypoxanthine-guanine phosphoribosyltransferase deficiency, *Q. J. Med.,* 42:423, 1973.

263. Conger, J. D., S. A. Falk, S. J. Guggenheim, and T. J. Burke: A micropuncture study of the early phase of acute urate nephropathy, *J. Clin. Invest.,* 58:681, 1976.

264. Steele T. H., and R. E. Rieselbach: The contribution of residual nephrons within the chronically diseased kidney to urate homeostasis in man, *Am. J. Med.,* 43:876, 1967.

265. Zusman, J., D. M. Brown, and M. E. Nesbit: Hyperphosphatemia, hyperphosphaturia, and hypocalcemia in acute lymphoblastic leukemia, *N. Engl. J. Med.,* 289:1335, 1973.

266. Manballyu, J., P. Zachee, R. Verberckmoes, and M. A. Boogaerts: Transient acute renal failure due to tumor-lysis-induced severe phosphate load in a patient with Burkitt's lymphoma, *Clin. Nephrol.,* 22:47, 1984.

267. Wortmann, R. L., and I. H. Fox: Limited value of uric acid to creatinine ratios in estimating uric acid excretion, *Ann. Intern. Med.,* 93:822, 1980.

268. Weinman, E. G., G. Eknoyan, and W. N. Suki: The influence of the extracellular fluid volume on the tubular reabsorption of uric acid, *J. Clin. Invest.,* 55:283, 1975.

269. Steele, T. H., and S. Oppenheimer: Factors affecting urate excretion following diuretic administration in man, *Am. J. Med.,* 47:564, 1969.

270. Kanfer, A., G. Richet, J. Roland, and F. Chatelet: Extreme hyperphosphatemia causing acute anuric nephrocalcinosis in lymphosarcoma, *Br. Med. J.,* 1:1320, 1979.

271. Masera, G., M. Jankovic, M. G. Zurlo, A. Locasciulli, M. R. Rossi, C. Uderzo, and M. Recchia: Urate-oxidase prophylaxis of uric acid-induced renal damage in childhood leukemia, *J. Pediatr.,* 100:152, 1982.

272. Liang, M. H., and J. F. Fries: Asymptomatic hyperuricemia: The case for conservative management, *Ann. Intern. Med.,* 88:666, 1978.

273. Talbott, J. H., and K. L. Terplan: The kidney in gout, *Medicine,* 39:405, 1960.

274. Steele, T. H., and R. E. Rieselbach: The contribution of residual nephrons within the chronically diseased kidney to urate homeostasis in man, *Am. J. Med.,* 43:876, 1967.

275. Barlow, K. A., and L. J. Beilin: Renal disease in primary gout, *Q. J. Med.,* 37:79, 1968.

276. Yu, Ts.-F., and L. Berger: Impaired renal function in gout. Its association with hypertensive vascular disease and intrinsic renal disease, *Am. J. Med.,* 72:95, 1982.

277. Epstein, F. H., and G. Pigeon: Experimental urate nephropathy: Studies of the distribution of urate in renal tissue, *Nephron,* 1:144, 1964.

278. Fessel, W. J.: Renal outcomes of gout and hyperuricemia, *Am. J. Med.,* 67:74, 1979.

279. Yu, Ts-F.: Lead nephropathy and gout, *Am. J. Kid. Dis.,* 2:555, 1983.

280. Batuman, V., J. K. Maesaka, B. Haddad, E. Tepper, E. Landy, and R. P. Wedeen: The role of lead in gout nephropathy, *N. Engl. J. Med.,* 304:520, 1981.

281. Craswell, P. W., J. Price, P. D. Boyle, V. J. Heazlewood, H. Baddeley, H. M. Lloyd, B. J. Thomas, and B. W. Thomas: Chronic renal failure with gout, *Kidney Int.,* 26:319, 1984.

282. Weeden, R. P., D. K. Mallik, and V. Batuman: Detection and treatment of occupational lead nephropathy, *Arch. Intern. Med.,* 139:53, 1979.

283. Yu, Ts.-F.: Urolithiasis in hyperuricemia and gout, *J. Urol.,* 126:424, 1981.

284. Deren, J. J., J. C. Porush, M. F. Levitt, and M. T. Khilvani: Nephrolithiasis as a complication of ulcerative colitis and regional enteritis, *Ann. Intern. Med.,* 56:843, 1962.

285. Stote, R. N., L. H. Smith, J. W. Dubb, T. P. Moyer,

F. Alexander, and J. L. Roth: Oxypurinol nephrolithiasis in regional enteritis secondary to allopurinol therapy, *Ann. Intern. Med.,* 92:384, 1980.

286. Band, P. R., D. S. Silverberg, J. F. Ulan, R. H. Wensel, T. K. Banerjee, and A. S. Little: Xanthine nephropathy in a patient with lymphosarcoma treated with allopurinol, *N. Engl. J. Med.,* 283:354, 1970.

287. Pak, C. Y. C., K. Sakhaee, and C. Fuller: Successful management of uric acid nephrolithiasis with potassium citrate, *Kidney Int.,* 30:422, 1986.

288. Coe, F. L.: Treated and untreated recurrent calcium nephrolithiasis in patients with idiopathic hypercalciuria, hyperuricosuria, or no metabolic disorder, *Ann. Intern. Med.,* 87:404, 1977.

289. Parfitt, A. M., and M. Kleerekoper: Clinical disorders of calcium, phosphorus, and magnesium metabolism, in M. H. Maxwell and C. R. Kleeman (eds.), *Clinical Disorders of Fluid and Electrolyte Metabolism,* 3d ed., McGraw-Hill, New York, 1980.

290. Mundy, G. R., K. J. Ibbotson, S. M. D'Souza, E. L. Simpson, J. W. Jacobs, and T. J. Martin: The hypercalcemias of cancer. Clinical implications and pathogenic mechanisms, *N. Engl. J. Med.,* 310:1718, 1984.

291. Breslau, N. A., J. L. McGuire, J. E. Zerwekh, E. P. Frenkel, and C. Y. C. Pak: Hypercalcemia associated with increased serum calcitriol levels in three patients with lymphoma, *Ann. Intern. Med.,* 100:1, 1984.

292. Schwartz, W. B., and A. S. Relman: Effects of electrolyte disorders on renal structure and function, *N. Engl. J. Med.,* 276:452, 1967.

293. Benabe, J. E., and M. Martinez-Maldonado: Hypercalcemic nephropathy, *Arch. Intern. Med.,* 138:777, 1978.

294. Levi, M., M. A. Ellis, and T. Berl: Control of renal hemodynamics and glomerular filtration rate in chronic hypercalcemia. Role of prostaglandins, renin-angiotensin system and calcium, *J. Clin. Invest.,* 71:1624, 1983.

295. Humes, H. D., I. Ichikawa, J. L. Troy, and B. M. Brenner: Evidence for parathyroid hormone-dependent influence of calcium on the glomerular ultrafiltration coefficient, *J. Clin. Invest.,* 61:32, 1978.

296. Goldfarb, S., and Z. S. Agus: Mechanism of the polyuria of hypercalcemia, *Am. J. Nephrol.,* 4:69, 1984.

297. Beck, N., H. Singh, S. W. Reed, H. V. Murdaugh, and B. B. Davis: Pathogenic role of cyclic AMP in

the impairment of urinary concentrating ability in acute hypercalcemia, *J. Clin. Invest.,* 54:1049, 1974.

298. Wiesmann, W., S. Sinha, and S. Klahr: Effects of ionophore A23187 on base-line and vasopressin-stimulated sodium transport in the toad bladder, *J. Clin. Invest.,* 59:418, 1977.

299. Levi, M., L. Peterson, and T. Berl: Mechanism of concentrating defect in hypercalcemia. Role of polyuria and prostaglandins, *Kidney Int.,* 23:489, 1983.

300. Galla, J. H., B. B. Booker, and R. G. Luke: Role of the loop segment in the concentrating defect of hypercalcemia, *Kidney Int.,* 29:977, 1986.

301. Aldinger, K. A., and N. A. Samaan: Hypokalemia with hypercalcemia: Prevalence and significance in treatment, *Ann. Intern. Med.,* 87:571, 1977.

302. Powell, D., F. R. Singer, T. M. Murray, C. Minkin, and J. T. Potts, Jr.: Nonparathyroid humoral hypercalcemia in patients with neoplastic diseases, *N. Engl. J. Med.,* 289:176, 1973.

303. Stapleton, F. B., S. Roy, III, H. N. Noe, and G. Jenkins: Hypercalciuria in children with hematuria, *N. Engl. J. Med.,* 310:1345, 1984.

304. Stewart, A. F.: Therapy of malignancy-associated hypercalcemia: 1983, *Am. J. Med.,* 74:475, 1983.

305. Ng, R. C. K., R. A. Peraino, and W. N. Suki: Divalent cation transport in isolated tubules, *Kidney Int.,* 22:492, 1982.

306. Mundy, G. R., M. E. Rick, R. Turcotte, and M. A. Kowalski: Pathogenesis of hypercalcemia in lymphosarcoma cell leukemia: Role of an osteoclast activating factor-like substance and a mechanism of action for glucocorticoid therapy, *Am. J. Med.,* 65:600, 1978.

307. Hughes, M. R., D. J. Baylink, P. G. Jones, and M. R. Haussler: Radioligand receptor assay for 25-dihydroxyvitamin D_2/D_3 and $1\alpha,25$-dihydroxyvitamine D_2/D_3: Application to hypervitaminosis D, *J. Clin. Invest.,* 58:61, 1976.

308. Stern, P. H., J. de Olazabal, and N. H. Bell: Evidence for abnormal regulation of $1\alpha,25$-dihydroxyvitamin D in patients with sarcoidosis and normal calcium metabolism, *J. Clin. Invest.,* 66:852, 1980.

309. Sandler, L. M., C. G. Winearls, L. J. Fraher, T. L. Clemens, R. Smith, and J. L. H. O'Riordan: Studies of the hypercalcaemia of sarcoidosis: Effect of steroids and exogenous vitamin D_3 on the circulating concentrations of 1,25-dihydroxy vitamin D_3, *Q. J. Med.,* 53:165, 1984.

310. Hahn, T. J., L. R. Halstead, and D. T. Baran: Effects of short term glucocorticoid administration on in-

testinal calcium absorption and circulating vitamin D metabolite concentrations in man, *J. Clin. Endocrinol. Metab.,* 52:111, 1981.

311. Seeman, E., R. Kumar, G. G. Hunder, M. Scott, H. Heath, III, and B. L. Riggs: Production, degradation, and circulating levels of 1,25-dihydroxyvitamin D in health and in chronic glucocorticoid excess, *J. Clin. Invest.,* 66:664, 1980.

312. Sandler, L. M., C. G. Winearls, L. J. Fraher, T. L. Clemens, R. Smith, and J. L. H. O'Riordan: Studies of the hypercalcemia of sarcoidosis: Effects of steroids and exogenous vitamin D_3 on the circulating concentration of 1,25-dihydroxy vitamin D_3, *Q. J. Med.,* 53:165, 1984.

313. Mazzaferri, E. L., T. M. O'Dorisio, and A. F. Lobuglio: Treatment of hypercalcemia associated with malignancy, *Semin. Oncol.,* 5:141, 1978.

314. Goldsmith, R. S., H. Bartos, S. B. Hulley, S. H. Ingbar, and W. C. Maloney: Phosphate supplementation as an adjunct in the therapy of multiple myeloma, *Arch. Intern. Med.,* 122:128, 1968.

315. Carey, R. W., G. W. Schmitt, H. H. Kopald, and P. A. Kantrowitz: Massive extraskeletal calcification during phosphate treatment of hypercalcemia, *Arch. Intern. Med.,* 122:150, 1968.

316. Seyberth, H. W., G. V. Serge, J. L. Morgan, B. J. Sweetman, J. T. Potts, Jr., and J. A. Oates: Prostaglandins as mediators of hypercalcemia associated with certain types of cancer, *N. Engl. J. Med.,* 293:1278, 1975.

317. Muther, R. S., D. A. McCarron, and W. M. Bennett: Renal manifestations of sarcoidosis, *Arch. Intern. Med.,* 141:643, 1981.

318. Goldszer, R. C., E. G. Galvanek, and J. M. Lazarus: Glomerulonephritis in a patient with sarcoidosis. Report of a case and review of the literature, *Arch. Pathol. Lab. Med.,* 105:478, 1981.

319. Korzets, A., M. Schneider, R. Taragon, J. Bernheim, and J. Bernheim: Acute renal failure due to sarcoid granulomatous infiltration of the renal parenchyma, *Am. J. Kid. Dis.,* 6:250, 1978.

320. Bell, N. H., J. R. Gill, Jr., and F. C. Bartter: On the abnormal calcium absorption in sarcoidosis: Evidence for increased sensitivity to vitamin D, *Am. J. Med.,* 36:500, 1964.

321. Barbour, G. L., J. W. Coburn, E. Slatopolsky, A. W. Norman, and R. L. Horst: Hypercalcemia in an anephric patient with sarcoidosis: Evidence for extrarenal generation of 1,25-dihydroxyvitamin D, *N. Engl. J. Med.,* 305:441, 1981.

322. Adams, J. S., O. P. Sharma, M. A. Gacod, and F. R. Singer: Metabolism of 25-hydroxyvitamin D_3 by cultured pulmonary alveolar macrophages in sarcoidosis, *J. Clin. Invest.,* 72:1856, 1983.

323. Mason, R. S., T. Frankel, Y.-L. Chan, D. Lissner, and S. Posen: Vitamin D conversion by sarcoid lymph node homogenate, *Ann. Intern. Med.,* 100:59, 1984.

324. Manolagas, S. C., and L. J. Deftos: The vitamin D endocrine system and the hematolymphopoietic tissue, *Ann. Intern. Med.,* 100:144, 1984.

325. Kozeny, G. A., A. L. Barbato, V. K. Bansal, L. L. Vertuno, and J. E. Hano: Hypercalcemia associated with silicone-induced granulomas, *N. Engl. J. Med.,* 311:1103, 1984.

326. Romer, F. K.: Renal manifestations and abnormal calcium metabolism in sarcoidosis, *Q. J. Med.,* 49:233, 1980.

327. Kogan, B. A., J. W. Konnak, and K. Lau: Marked hyperoxaluria in sarcoidosis during orthophosphate therapy, *J. Urol.,* 127:339, 1982.

328. Cushard, W. G., Jr., A. B. Simon, J. M. Canterbury, and E. Reiss: Parathyroid function in sarcoidosis, *N. Engl. J. Med.,* 286:395, 1972.

329. Muther, R. S., D. A. McCarron, and W. M. Bennett: Granulomatous sarcoid nephritis: A cause of multiple renal tubular abnormalities, *Clin. Nephrol.,* 14:190, 1980.

330. King, B. P., A. R. Esparza, S. I. Kahn, and S. Garella: Sarcoid granulomatous nephritis occurring as isolated renal failure, *Arch. Intern. Med.,* 136:241, 1976.

331. McCoy, R. C., and C. C. Tisher: Glomerulonephritis associated with sarcoidosis, *Am. J. Pathol.,* 68:339, 1972.

332. Taylor, R. G., C. Fisher, and B. I. Hoffbrand: Sarcoidosis and membranous glomerulonephritis: A significant association, *Br. Med. J.,* 284:1297, 1982.

333. Brigden, D., A. E. Rosling, and N. C. Woods: Renal function after acyclovir intravenous injection, *Am. J. Med.,* 73(1A):182, 1982.

334. Pitman, S. W., and E. Frei, III: Weekly methotrexate-calcium leukovorin rescue. Effect of alkalinization on nephrotoxicity; pharmacokinetics in the CNS; and use in CNS non-Hodgkin's lymphoma, *Cancer Treat. Rep.,* 61:695, 1977.

335. Dorfman, L. E., and J. P. Smith: Sulfonamide crystalluria: A forgotten disease, *J. Urol.,* 104:482, 1970.

336. Buchanan, N.: Sulphamethoxazole, hypoalbuminemia, crystalluria, and renal failure, *Br. Med. J.,* 2:172, 1978.

337. Mailloux, L., C. D. Swartz, R. Capizzi, K. E. Kim, G. Onesti, O. Ramirez, and A. N. Brest: Acute renal failure after administration of low-molecular-weight dextran, *N. Engl. J. Med.,* 277:1113, 1967.

338. Swartz, R. D., J. R. Wesley, M. G. Somermeyer,

and K. Lau: Hyperoxaluria and renal insufficiency due to ascorbic acid administration during total parenteral nutrition, *Ann. Intern. Med.,* 100:530, 1984.

339. McAllister, C. J., E. R. Scowden, F. L. Dewberry, and A. Richman: Renal failure secondary to massive infusion of vitamin C (letter), *J. Am. Med. Assoc.,* 252:1684, 1981.

340. Case Records of Massachusetts General Hospital (Case 38-1979), *N. Engl. J. Med.,* 301:650, 1979.

341. Bove, K. E.: Ethylene glycol toxicity, *Am. J. Clin. Pathol.,* 45:46, 1966.

342. Mazze, R. I., J. R. Trudell, and M. J. Cousins: Methoxyflurane metabolism and renal dysfunction: Clinical correlation in man, *Anesthesiology,* 35:247, 1971.

343. Krausz, T., M. Scllyei, and I. Abranyi: Renocerebral oxalosis after intravenous glycerol infusion, *Lancet,* 2:89, 1977.

344. Williams, H. E.: Oxalic acid and the hyperoxaluric syndromes, *Kidney Int.,* 13:410, 1978.

345. Yendt, E. R., and M. Cohanim: Response to a physiologic dose of pyridoxine in type I primary hyperoxaluria, *N. Engl. J. Med.,* 312:953, 1985.

346. Scheinman, J. I., J. S. Najarian, and S. M. Mauer: Successful strategies for renal transplantation in primary oxalosis, *Kidney Int.,* 25:804, 1984.

347. Earnest, D. L., G. Johnson, H. E. Williams, and W. H. Admirand: Hyperoxaluria in patients with ileal resections: An abnormality in dietary oxalate absorption, *Gastroenterology,* 66:1114, 1974.

348. Barilla, D. E., C. Notz, D. Kennedy, and C. Y. C. Pak: Renal oxalate excretion following oral oxalate loads in patients with ileal disease and with renal and absorptive hypercalciuria: Effects of calcium and magnesium, *Am. J. Med.,* 64:579, 1978.

349. Mandell, I., E. Krauss, and J. C. Millan: Oxalate-induced acute renal failure in Crohn's disease, *Am. J. Med.,* 69:628, 1980.

350. Kathpalia, S. C., M. J. Favus, and F. L. Coe: Evidence for size and charge permselectivity of rat ascending colon. Effects of ricinoleate and bile salts on oxalic acid and neutral sugar transport, *J. Clin. Invest.,* 74:805, 1984.

351. Coggins, C. H.: Renal failure in lymphoma, *Kidney Int.,* 17:847, 1980.

352. Lundberg, W. B., E. D. Cadman, S. C. Finch, and R. L. Capizzi: Renal failure secondary to leukemic infiltration of the kidneys, *Am. J. Med.,* 62:636, 1977.

353. Wedeen, R. P.: Occupational renal disease, *Am. J. Kid. Dis.,* 3:241, 1981.

354. Humes, H. D., and J. M. Weinberg: Toxic ne-

phropathies, in B. M. Brenner and F. C. Rector, Jr. (eds.), *The Kidney,* 3d ed., Saunders, Philadelphia, 1986.

355. Bennett, W. M.: Lead nephropathy, *Kidney Int.,* 28:212, 1985.

356. Emmerson, B. T.: Chronic lead nephropathy, *Kidney Int.,* 4:1, 1973.

357. Adams, R. G., J. F. Harrison, and P. Scott: The development of cadmium-induced proteinuria, impaired renal function and osteomalacia in alkaline battery workers, *Q. J. Med.,* 38:425, 1969.

358. Rose, B. D.: *Clinical Physiology of Acid Base and Electrolyte Disorders,* 2d ed., McGraw Hill, New York, 1985, chap. 27.

359. Schwartz, W. B., and A. S. Relman: Effects of electrolyte disorders on renal structure and function, *N. Engl. J. Med.,* 276:383, 1967.

360. Riemenschneider, Th., and A. Bohle: Morphologic aspects of low-potassium and low-sodium nephropathy, *Clin. Nephrol.,* 19:271, 1983.

361. Andres, G. A., and R. T. McCluskey: Tubular and interstitial renal disease due to immunologic mechanisms, *Kidney Int.,* 7:271, 1975.

362. Lehman, D. H., C. B. Wilson, and F. J. Dixon: Extraglomerular immunoglobulin deposits in human nephritis, *Am. J. Med.,* 58:765, 1975.

363. Case Records of the Massachusetts General Hospital (Case 2-1976), *N. Engl. J. Med.,* 294:100, 1976.

364. Cunningham, E., T. Provost, J. Brentjens, M. Reichlin, and R. C. Venuto: Acute renal failure secondary to interstitial lupus nephritis, *Arch. Intern. Med.,* 138:1560, 1978.

365. Tron, F., D. Ganeval, and D. Droz: Immunologically-mediated acute renal failure of non-glomerular origin in the course of SLE, *Am. J. Med.,* 67:259, 1979.

366. Tu, W. J., M. A. Shearn, J. C. Lee, and J. Hopper, Jr.: Interstitial nephritis in Sjögren's syndrome, *Ann. Intern. Med.,* 69:1163, 1968.

367. Winer, R. L., A. H. Cohen, A. S. Sawhney, and J. T. Gorman: Sjögren's syndrome with immune-complex tubulointerstitial renal disease, *Clin. Immunol. Immunopathol.,* 8:494, 1974.

368. Mountsopoulos, H. M., J. E. Balow, T. J. Lawley, N. I. Stahl, T. T. Antonovych, and T. M. Chused: Immune complex glomerulonephritis in sicca syndrome, *Am. J. Med.,* 64:955, 1978.

369. Walker, B. R., F. Alexander, and P. J. Tannenbaum: Fanconi syndrome with renal tubular acidosis and light chain proteinuria, *Nephron,* 8:103, 1971.

370. Cattran, D. C.: Circulating anti-tubular basement membrane antibody in a variety of human renal

diseases. Detection and significance, *Nephron,* 26:13, 1980.

371. Levy, M., M. F. Gagnadoux, A. Beziau, and R. Habib: Membranous glomerulonephritis associated with antitubular and alveolar basement membrane antibodies, *Clin. Nephrol.,* 10:158, 1978.

372. Carpenter, C. B., and E. L. Milford: Renal transplantation: Immunobiology, in B. M. Brenner and F. C. Rector, Jr. (eds.). *The Kidney,* 3d ed., Saunders, Philadelphia, 1986, pp. 1908–1914.

373. Berndt, W. O., A. W. Hayes, and R. D. Phillips: Effects of mycotoxins on renal function: Mycotoxic nephropathy, *Kidney Int.,* 18:656, 1980.

374. Hall, P. W., and M. Vasiljevic: Beta$_2$-microglobulin excretion as an index of renal tubular disorders with special reference to endemic Balkan nephropathy, *J. Lab. Clin. Med.,* 81:897, 1973.

375. Barnes, J. M., P. K. C. Austwick, R. L. Carter, F. V. Flynn, G. C. Peristianis, and W. N. Aldridge: Balkan (endemic) nephropathy and a toxin-producing strain of *Pencillium verrucosum* var *cyclopium*: An experimental model in rats, *Lancet,* 1:671, 1977.

376. Sattler, T. A., T. S. Dimitrov, and P. W. Hall: Relation between endemic (Balkan) nephropathy and urinary-tract tumours, *Lancet,* 1:278, 1977.

377. Nath, K. A., M. K. Hostetter, and T. H. Hostetter: Pathophysiology of chronic tubulointerstitial disease in rats. Interactions of dietary acid load, ammonia, and complement component C3, *J. Clin. Invest.,* 76:667, 1985.

9

URINARY TRACT OBSTRUCTION

Laurence A. Turka

Urinary tract obstruction (UTO) is a relatively common cause of renal disease, with variable clinical manifestations including pain, hematuria, infection, and renal insufficiency. Both the symptoms and renal function can usually be improved by relief of the obstruction. It is therefore essential to recognize the situations in which UTO should be suspected and to develop a sequential approach to diagnosis and therapy.

ETIOLOGY

Obstruction to the flow of urine can arise at any site in the urinary tract. The most common causes are listed in Table 9-1. The frequency with which these disorders occur is dependent on the age and sex of the patient. UTO in children is most often due to anatomic abnormalities. Included in this group are urethral valves or stricture, meatal stenosis, and stenosis at the ureterovesical or ureteropelvic junction.[1,2] In comparison, acquired disorders predominate in adults. Obstructing calculi are most common in young patients. Although calculi can also occur in older patients, prostatic hypertrophy or carcinoma and retroperitoneal or pelvic neoplasms (lymphoma; carcinoma of the bladder, cervix, uterus, ovary, or colon; metastatic carcinoma, particularly breast) become increasingly prevalent.

TABLE 9-1. Major Causes of Urinary Tract Obstruction

Level of Obstruction	Disease Process
Renal pelvis	Calculus
	Sloughed papillary tissue
	Stricture or aberrant vessel at ureteropelvic junction
Ureter	Prostate, bladder, or pelvic carcinoma
	Calculus
	Retroperitoneal lymphoma, metastatic carcinoma, or fibrosis
	Sloughed papillary tissue
	Ureterocele
	Primary ureteral neoplasms
	Accidental surgical ligation
	Edema at ureterovesical junction after retrograde catheterization
	Regional enteritis
	Pregnancy
	Blood clot
	Stricture
Urethra or bladder neck	Benign prostatic hypertrophy
	Carcinoma of the prostate or bladder
	Urethral valves, stricture or meatal stenosis
	Neurogenic bladder
	Calculus

PATHOGENESIS

CHANGES IN INTRARENAL PRESSURES AND GLOMERULAR HEMODYNAMICS

The changes in the urinary collecting system and in renal function that occur with UTO are dependent upon the degree (partial versus complete, unilateral versus bilateral) and duration of obstruction. The *initial event* with marked or complete obstruction is a rise in pressure proximal to the obstruction, due to the combination of continued glomerular filtration and the impedance to urinary flow. The elevation in hydrostatic pressure in the collecting system induces corresponding anatomic changes. For example, ureteral obstruction leads to dilatation of the proximal ureter (hydroureter) and renal pelvis (hydronephrosis). These changes are important clinically because their detection by ultrasonography is the major noninvasive method of diagnosing UTO (see below).

The increase in intrarenal pressure also produces important hemodynamic changes.

The transmission of the elevation in pressure back to the proximal tubule reduces the trans-glomerular pressure gradient (glomerular capillary pressure minus tubular hydrostatic pressure), leading to an immediate fall in glomerular filtration rate (GFR). If the obstruction is complete, the proximal tubular pressure will rise until glomerular filtration essentially ceases. With partial obstruction, however, the elevation in tubular pressure is usually not sufficient to stop the GFR.

Important alterations in arteriolar resistance and renal perfusion also occur. Initially, there is a transient increase in renal blood flow that lasts for 1 to 2 h.[3-5] This early renal hyperemia appears to be mediated by vasodilator prostaglandins, which may be released in response to medullary ischemia induced by the rise in intrarenal pressure.[5,6] If, however, complete obstruction is maintained beyond 4 to 5 h, the increase in intratubular pressure induces *arteriolar vasoconstriction*, leading to a fall in renal blood flow below baseline, a decrease in glomerular capillary pressure, and a further decline in GFR (Fig. 9-1*a*).[7] These events appear to be humorally mediated with thromboxane A_2 and angiotensin II contributing to the vasoconstriction, an effect that is partially offset by the release of vasodilator prostaglandins.[3,8-11] The factors responsible for these humoral changes are not well understood; it is possible that an alteration in macula densa flow plays an important role.[7]

Micropuncture studies indicate that these microvascular changes are *regulated locally* by the individual obstructed nephrons.[7,12] If, for example, single nephrons are obstructed, glomerular hemodynamics remain normal in adjacent nonobstructed nephrons.[7] Thus, the changes in arteriolar resistance that are induced by obstruction can be viewed as an adaptive mechanism that serves to shift perfusion away from obstructed, nonfiltering nephrons.

The reduction in GFR in obstructed nephrons eventually lowers the intratubular pressure. After 12 to 24 h in the rat, for example, the intrapelvic and intratubular pressures have returned to near normal levels with complete unilateral obstruction, and have fallen by about 50 percent from their peak values with complete bilateral obstruction (Fig. 9–1b).[3-5] The persistent elevation in pressure in the latter setting may be related to the retention of unidentified vasodilating substances that are normally excreted in the urine.[13]

Similar changes appear to occur in humans as the intrapelvic pressure falls to normal by 28 days of complete obstruction (Fig. 9–2a).[14] In comparison, the intrapelvic pressure with *partial* obstruction is initially lower than with complete obstruction but remains elevated with time (Fig. 9–2b). This continued increase in pressure with partial obstruction is probably related to the persistence of glomerular filtration, an effect that may be mediated in part by vasodilator prostaglandins.[15] It should also be noted that, despite the reduction in

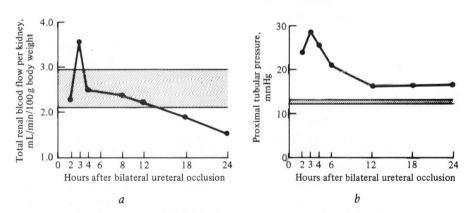

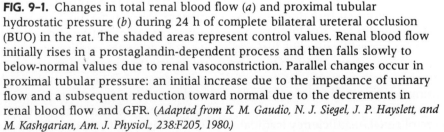

FIG. 9–1. Changes in total renal blood flow (*a*) and proximal tubular hydrostatic pressure (*b*) during 24 h of complete bilateral ureteral occlusion (BUO) in the rat. The shaded areas represent control values. Renal blood flow initially rises in a prostaglandin-dependent process and then falls slowly to below-normal values due to renal vasoconstriction. Parallel changes occur in proximal tubular pressure: an initial increase due to the impedance of urinary flow and a subsequent reduction toward normal due to the decrements in renal blood flow and GFR. (*Adapted from K. M. Gaudio, N. J. Siegel, J. P. Hayslett, and M. Kashgarian, Am. J. Physiol., 238:F205, 1980.*)

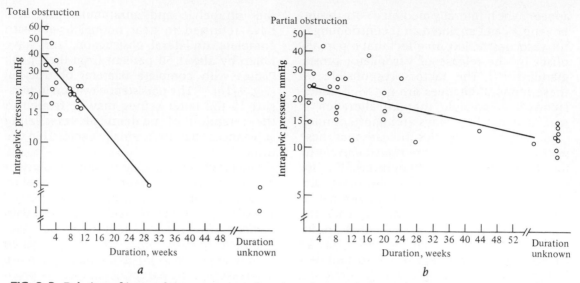

FIG. 9–2. Relation of intrapelvic pressure to duration of ureteral obstruction in patients with complete (*a*) or partial (*b*) obstruction. "Duration unknown" indicates obstruction present for at least 1 year. [*From G. Michaelson, Acta. Med. Scand. (suppl.), 559:1, 1974.*]

intrapelvic pressure, hydonephrosis persists, presumably due to increased compliance produced by chronic distention.

CLINICAL CHANGES IN RENAL FUNCTION

Urinary tract obstruction can produce a variety of changes in renal function, particularly a reduction in GFR. The impairment in total GFR is dependent upon the degree and duration of obstruction. With unilateral obstruction, there is at most a 50 percent fall in GFR and a doubling of the plasma creatinine concentration (assuming both kidneys previously had roughly equal function). In fact, the change is generally less marked because of compensatory hyperfiltration in the contralateral kidney (see Chap. 4). With bilateral obstruction, there is a variable decrease in GFR, including anuric renal failure if the obstruction is complete.

The degree of renal insufficiency is initially less severe with partial obstruction. However, irreversible renal failure may eventually occur as a result of tubular atrophy and necrosis and/or secondary bacterial infection (see "Complications," below).[16]

In addition to lowering the GFR, the elevation in intratubular pressure also can affect tubular function.[3] With acute bilateral obstruction, the reduction in tubular flow rate is associated with increased sodium and water reabsorption, leading to a low urine sodium concentration and a high urine osmolality, findings similar to those in prerenal disease.[17] However, tubular function (particularly in the distal nephron) eventually becomes impaired, presumably due to the increase in hydrostatic pressure. As might be expected, this can lead to defects in the ability to conserve sodium, concentrate or acidify the urine, and secrete potassium.[3,18–20] For example, both decreased sodium chloride reabsorption in the loop of Henle and reduced responsiveness of the collecting tubules to antidiuretic hormone can contribute to the impairment in concentrating ability.[18]

The clinical consequences of these abnormalities in tubular function can include hyperkalemia, a hyperchloremic metabolic acidosis with an inappropriately high urine pH (distal or type 1 renal tubular acidosis), and either hypo- or hypernatremia depending upon the patient's intake of sodium and water. The decreases in sodium and water reabsorption account in part for the observation that the urine output is most often normal (i.e., equal to intake) in patients with chronic UTO, despite a reduction in GFR. Oliguria or anuria does not occur unless the obstruction becomes complete or prolonged partial obstruction leads to end-stage renal failure.

CLINICAL PRESENTATION

HISTORY

The symptoms and signs directly produced by UTO are dependent upon the site and cause of obstruction and the rapidity with which the obstruction has occurred (Table 9–2). For example, pain frequently causes the patient with UTO to seek medical care. This symptom is usually the result of distention of the bladder, collecting system, or renal capsule, and it is more closely related to the rate of distention than the degree of dilatation. Thus, pain is commonly associated with acute obstruction. The pain can be excruciating, and patients frequently describe it as "the worst pain in my life." In contrast, chronic obstruction results in gradual distention and may produce no symptoms or lead to only vague abdominal, back, or flank discomfort.

When pain occurs, its location is determined by the site of obstruction. Obstruction of the renal pelvis or upper ureter most often causes flank pain and tenderness. With lower ureteral obstruction, the pain may radiate to the testicles or labia, and occasionally this may be the sole sight of discomfort. Ureteral obstruction may also induce a paralytic ileus, resulting in abdominal distention and gastrointestinal symptoms.

The presence of symptoms is related both to the degree of obstruction and to the urinary flow rate. In some patients with partial obstruction of the ureteropelvic junction, for example, pain may occur primarily during periods of high fluid intake. In this setting

TABLE 9–2. Symptoms and Signs That May Occur with Urinary Tract Obstruction*

Level of Obstruction	Typical Symptoms and Signs
Renal pelvis or ureter	Acute: flank pain and tenderness, renal colic with ureteral obstruction, occasional gross hematuria, paralytic ileus Chronic: may have vague back, flank, or abdominal discomfort; frequently asymptomatic unless infection or renal failure supervenes; polyuria or nocturia if partial and bilateral; enlarged kidney may be palpable; occasional gross hematuria
Bladder neck or urethra	Acute: suprapubic pain, anuria or decreased caliber of urinary stream, palpable bladder, enlarged prostate Chronic: hesitancy, frequency, postvoid dribbling, decreased caliber of urinary stream, nocturia, incontinence; pelvic mass or enlarged bladder or prostate may be palpable; may present with renal insufficiency

*In addition to the findings listed in this table, the symptoms and signs associated with infection may complicate any form of UTO.

the increase in urine output in the presence of a fixed obstruction causes acute hydronephrosis and back pain.[21]

The range of symptoms that can occur with obstruction can be illustrated by the findings in prostatic hypertrophy. In patients presenting acutely, the primary symptoms are a marked decrease or cessation in urine output and severe suprapubic pain due to the rapid increase in bladder size. These patients usually have a prior history compatible with partial chronic urethral obstruction, such as hesitancy, frequency, nocturia, postvoid dribbling, and diminished force and caliber of the urinary stream. In comparison, men with chronic obstruction from prostatic disease may never develop acute symptoms and may present only with frequency, nocturia, and/or renal insufficiency. In such instances, the markedly enlarged bladder causes no symptoms due to the prolonged period of time over which it developed.

Although they are an unusual cause of UTO, bladder stones may give rise to a characteristic set of symptoms that are due to direct irritation of the bladder wall and to obstruction of the urethral orifice. These changes may be manifested clinically by sudden interruption of the urinary stream, terminal hematuria (since the stone is closest to the bladder wall at the end of micturition), or suprapubic pain exacerbated by exercise (which increases the movement of the stone against the bladder wall). Bladder stones should be strongly suspected, when part or all of this triad is present.

In addition to the symptoms directly referable to obstruction, it is important to look for findings related to the underlying disease. Thus, the physician should inquire about a history or symptoms suggestive of malignancy; previous abdominal, pelvic or genitourinary surgery; renal calculi; one of the disorders associated with papillary necrosis such as diabetes mellitus, sickle cell disease, or anal-

gesic abuse nephropathy (although obstruction itself can cause papillary necrosis); migraine headaches treated with methysergide, a drug that can cause retroperitoneal fibrosis; or symptoms of inflammatory bowel disease, since the right ureter is occasionally obstructed by fistula or abscess formation in regional enteritis.[22]

PHYSICAL EXAMINATION

As with the history, the findings on physical examination are also related to the duration and the location of the obstruction. Acute upper UTO, for example, is usually associated with flank tenderness on the affected side. In comparison, chronic upper tract obstruction generally produces no abnormalities on physical examination.

The findings are different with lower UTO in which a distended, palpable bladder is the most common abnormality. Pelvic and rectal examinations should always be performed in this setting since they may reveal a local malignancy or prostatic enlargement as the cause of obstruction.

LABORATORY DATA

The routine laboratory findings with UTO are nonspecific. The elevations in the BUN and plasma creatinine concentration are dependent upon the degree of obstruction and whether one or both kidneys is involved. The urinalysis may be relatively normal or reveal hematuria, particularly with stone disease,[23] or pyuria and bacteriuria if infection is present. Although cystine crystals are diagnostic of cystinuria, other crystals may be found normally and are not indicative of stone formation. In patients with prolonged obstruction and chronic renal insufficiency, the urine will tend to be isosthenuric, and the urine sodium concentration will exceed 20 meq/L,[17,19,24] findings that are typical of any chronic renal disease.

COMPLICATIONS

In addition to the direct effects of obstruction outlined above, a variety of complications may occur including infection, hypertension, renal failure, stone formation, papillary necrosis, and dehydration.

INFECTION

There is an increased incidence of infection when urinary stasis develops behind an area of obstruction. This is particularly true with lower tract obstruction, since bladder washout is the primary natural defense against infection.[25] The symptoms that may occur again depend upon the site involved. Infection in the bladder is usually manifested by dysuria, frequency, small voidings, and cloudy urine. These complaints are also present with acute pyelonephritis, but the additional findings of flank pain, nausea, vomiting, and fever suggest upper tract infection, although accurate differentiation on clinical grounds alone is often not possible.[26,27] The urinalysis usually reveals pyuria, bacteriuria, and, in some patients with pyelonephritis, white blood cell casts. The organism responsible for the infection can be identified by urine culture and appropriate antimicrobial therapy instituted. In acutely ill patients, antimicrobials will often have been started empirically before culture results are available. In such cases, drug susceptibility testing will allow the physician to narrow the antimicrobial coverage to the least toxic medication(s).

Although urinary tract infections are relatively common, particularly cystitis in females, there are certain clues that point toward the possible presence of some anatomic abnormality in the urinary tract. These include infection in males, recurrent or persistent infection, and infection with an unusual organism, such as *Candida* or *Pseudomonas*. In these settings, correction of the anatomic abnormality may be required before sterilization of the urine can be achieved, since persistent urinary stasis may prevent eradication of the infection even with appropriate antimicrobial therapy.[28]

HYPERTENSION

Hypertension is an occasional finding in patients with UTO. The mechanism responsible for the elevation in blood pressure (BP) appears to vary with the duration and type of obstruction.[29] In patients with *acute unilateral obstruction,* renin secretion is usually enhanced, and lateralizing renal vein renin studies similar to those in unilateral renal artery stenosis (see Chap. 12) are often found.[29-31] In this setting, a reduction in BP can be achieved with relief of the obstruction.

In contrast, renin secretion is usually normal in patients with *bilateral obstruction* (including obstruction of a solitary kidney).[31,32] In this condition, renal failure leading to volume expansion is commonly present.[31-33] As a result, the elevation in BP may be volume-mediated, since relief of the obstruction usually leads to loss of the excess fluid and a fall in BP.

The mechanism by which *chronic unilateral obstruction* raises the BP frequently cannot be determined. The plasma renin activity and renal vein renins are usually normal,[31] and both renal failure and volume expansion are prevented by the contralateral, nonobstructed kidney. In this setting, relief of the obstruction may not correct the hypertension,[31] except in the infrequent patient in whom renal vein renins are lateralizing.[29] These findings suggest that there may have been some subtle permanent damage to the kidney or that the hypertension is unrelated to the obstruction.

RENAL FAILURE

Progressive renal failure occurs only with bilateral obstruction. Although recovery of renal function can be achieved if the obstruction is relieved relatively soon after onset, prolonged severe obstruction can lead to irreversible tubulointerstitial changes characterized by tubular dilatation and atrophy, and interstitial fibrosis with mononuclear cell infiltration (see "Prognosis," below).[34]

STONES AND PAPILLARY NECROSIS

Stone formation and papillary necrosis may occasionally result from obstruction. The former is most likely to occur in patients who become infected with a urease-producing organism, such as *Proteus mirabilis*. The ensuing alkaline urine favors the formation of magnesium-ammonium-phosphate (struvite) stones, typically in the renal pelvis. This can then lead to further obstruction. Bladder stone formation also may occur in obstructed patients, due either to lower UTO or to the passage of stones from the kidney down through the ureter.[35]

Obstruction can also cause (as well as be produced by) papillary necrosis (see Chap. 8).[36] This is seen primarily with severe obstruction, and is thought to reflect ischemic damage.[37,38] It has been suggested that medullary ischemia, due to partial occlusion of the vasa recta capillaries, may result from the obstruction-induced rise in hydrostatic pressure in the renal pelvis and medullary interstitium.

DEHYDRATION

The reductions in maximum sodium conservation and concentrating ability are not usually severe enough to lead to negative sodium and water balance as long as adequate intake is maintained. However, hypernatremia or volume depletion may ensue when intake is diminished (which may occur because of pain and nausea or an intercurrent illness).[39]

DIAGNOSIS

Early diagnosis of UTO is important since most cases are treatable, and a delay in therapy can lead to irreversible renal damage. When a patient presents with recurrent or persistent urinary tract infections, or with the symptoms and signs outlined above, the possibility of UTO is readily apparent. It is important to remember, however, that some patients with relatively long-standing obstruction present only with renal insufficiency (either discovered on routine blood tests or because of signs and symptoms referrable to uremia).

The degree to which the physician pursues the diagnosis will depend in part upon the initial index of suspicion. However, the accuracy of ultrasonography, a noninvasive screening test, has shifted the burden onto the clinician to exclude UTO in all cases where the cause of renal failure is unknown. Nonetheless, superfluous tests can be avoided if the physician is aware of clinical situations that point toward (or away from) the possibility of obstruction.

First, the urinalysis in UTO is generally normal or reveals only minor abnormalities such as a few red or white cells per high power field or mild proteinuria. Findings such as red cell casts, or nephrotic range proteinuria point to a glomerular disease, not obstruction.

Second, the urine volume may be helpful. *Anuria* strongly suggests the possibility of complete bilateral obstruction. Of all the causes of renal failure, only a few others are associated with no urine output. Included in this group are shock and, much less commonly, bilateral major vascular occlusion, renal cortical necrosis, and infrequent cases of acute glomerulonephritis, hemolytic-uremic syndrome, or acute tubular necrosis. In these disorders, the history, physical examination, and urinalysis usually point to the correct diagnosis. In contrast, the urine output is usually well maintained with chronic, partial UTO because of the decrease in tubular sodium and water reabsorption. Thus, a normal or high urine output should not exclude the possibility of UTO.

Third, the timing of onset of disease may be important in the patient with acute renal failure. Most forms of UTO that are associated with decreased renal function are chronic, and both kidneys usually must be involved to produce more than a twofold increase in the plasma creatinine concentration. As a result, renal failure *developing in the hospital* is not likely to be caused by obstruction (except for acute prostatic obstruction). In contrast, UTO should be considered as a possible etiology in any patient presenting with renal disease of unknown cause.

Finally, obstruction should be strongly suspected when renal insufficiency develops in any patient with an underlying malignancy. Hypercalcemia, hyperuricemia, prerenal disease (due to reduced intake or gastrointestinal losses), toxic nephropathy secondary to chemotheraputic agents (especially cisplatin), and tumor infiltration of the kidney also may be important in this setting, and they can all present with nonspecific urinary findings.

SEQUENTIAL EVALUATION

The evaluation for obstruction should begin with catheterization of the bladder if there is any reason to suspect that bladder neck obstruction may be present. Clues suggesting this problem include suprapubic pain, a history of neurogenic bladder, a palpable bladder, or an older man with otherwise unexplained renal insufficiency. If urethral obstruction or a neurogenic bladder is indeed the primary problem, catheterization will lead

to a brisk diuresis. A diuresis, however, should not be taken as conclusive evidence that obstruction was the cause of the renal insufficiency. There are occasional patients in whom catheterization produces a large volume of urine, yet whose renal failure is not secondary to UTO. The physician must verify that a fall in the plasma creatinine concentration accompanies the increased urine output.

The rate at which an enlarged bladder should be decompressed has been a source of misunderstanding. Two complications can be induced by the sudden reduction in pressure within the bladder: gross hematuria (due to stretching of the distended bladder veins) and rarely reflex hypotension. As a result, it has been suggested that it is safer to avoid rapid emptying of the bladder by partially clamping the catheter after the initial 500 to 1000 mL has been removed, thereby allowing the bladder to drain slowly over many hours. However, the pressure within a tense bladder is *extremely sensitive to very small reductions in volume*, beginning to fall after the removal of only 5 to 15 mL of urine, and falling by about 50 percent after the removal of 100 mL.[40] Consequently, partial clamping of the catheter is not likely to be beneficial unless the physician is prepared to remove only 25 to 50 mL at a time, an unrealistic approach in an attempt to prevent a self-limited complication.

If catheterization of the bladder is performed and does not result in a large output, then UTO, if present, must be at the level of the ureters or above. In order to diagnose or exclude obstruction, most procedures rely almost exclusively on their ability to detect dilatation of the collecting system (Fig. 9–3). Therefore, it is important to remember that *UTO can occur without hydronephrosis*. This finding is seen primarily in three situations:

1. Early in the course of obstruction (1 to 3 days), before the collecting system has had time to dilate

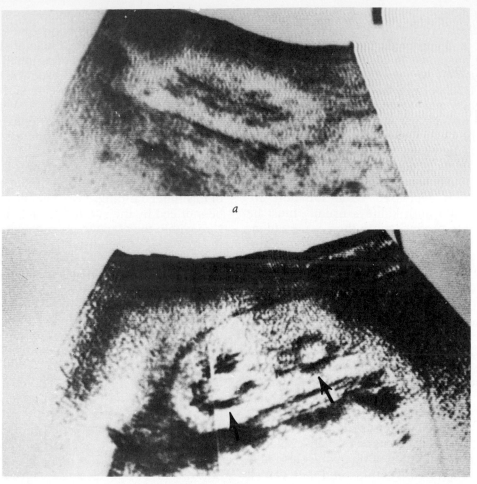

a

b

FIG. 9–3. Ultrasonographic detection of hydronephrosis. (*a*) In the normal kidney, the collecting structures (black areas in the middle of the kidney) are closely bunched together. (*b*) In contrast, the collecting structures can be seen to be distended (arrows) by fluid (which is sonolucent and appears white) in the presence of hydronephrosis.

2. When there is encasement of the collecting system in the retroperitoneum by local tumor or fibrosis[41,42]
3. When there is mild obstruction which produces minimal dilatation (and usually no renal insufficiency)

There are also patients in whom hydronephrosis can be found in the *absence of ob-*struction. Perhaps the most common example is severe vesicoureteral reflux (see p. 399), in which collecting system dilatation results from increased pressure transmitted from the bladder via the ureters. A parapelvic cyst can also give the appearance of calyceal dilatation although pelvic dilatation will not be seen.

The initial radiologic evaluation in most patients consists of a plain film of the abdomen (to detect calculi) and ultrasonography (Table 9–3).[43,44] This combination has the advantages of being noninvasive and of avoiding the need for radiocontrast media which are potentially nephrotoxic (see Chap. 3)[45,46] and can in rare patients cause an anaphylactoid reaction.

In the majority of patients, the ultrasound and plain film will be able to exclude UTO, diagnose obstruction and its cause, or demonstrate another potential etiology of renal failure (such as polycystic kidney disease).[44] Computed tomography should be performed if there is inadequate visualization (due, for example, to obesity) or equivocal results on ultrasonography, or if the cause of obstruction cannot be identified. CT scanning also may be helpful if ultrasonography suggests mild dilatation of the collecting system, a finding that may represent a false-positive test.

The combination of a plain film of the abdomen, ultrasonography, and computed tomography (if needed) will be adequate for diagnostic purposes in about 90 percent of all patients with UTO.[44] An intravenous pyelogram is needed only in patients with cysts or staghorn calculi (since obstruction may

not be detectable by other modalities in this setting) or when CT scanning cannot identify the level of obstruction.

Retrograde or antegrade pyelography should be performed as a diagnostic test when the above modalities are inconclusive, despite a history strongly suggestive of obstruction (as might occur when retroperitoneal tumor prevents dilation of the collecting system).[41,42] In this setting, a negative ultrasonogram cannot confidently exclude the disease.[47] Therefore, if the prior probability of obstruction is great (e.g., an elderly man with known prostatic carcinoma who presents with new and otherwise unexplained renal insufficiency and anuria), retrograde (or antegrade) pyelography may be required even when other studies "rule out" obstruction.[41-44]

More commonly, these procedures are used therapeutically to relieve the obstruction. Retrograde pyelography requires general or spinal anesthesia in men (and in some women) and is usually done in the operating suite. The aim is to pass a catheter into the ureter, thus bypassing the obstruction. In the antegrade pyelogram, a small needle is introduced percutaneously into the renal pelvis, and radiocontrast material is injected (after an appropriate amount of urine is withdrawn). This is most likely to succeed when the collecting system is dilated. If obstruction is found, a nephrostomy tube can be placed in the pelvis (and occasionally into the ureter past the obstruction), allowing decompression of the urinary tract.

TABLE 9–3. Sequential Evaluation for UTO

1. Bladder catheterization (if history is suggestive)
2. Ultrasonography and plain film of the abdomen
3. Computed tomography if
   a. Inadequate visualization by ultrasonography
   b. Ultrasonography shows obstruction but is unable to identify cause
4. Intranvenous pyelography if
   a. Cysts are demonstrated by ultrasonography or CT scanning
   b. Staghorn calculi are present
   c. Site of obstruction cannot be identified
5. Retrograde or antegrade pyelography if
   a. Hydronephrosis is not demonstrated with above studies, but a strong clinical suspicion exists, without any other cause for renal failure

TREATMENT

The necessity for treatment and the rapidity with which it should be instituted are dependent upon the clinical setting and whether the obstruction is complete or partial. *Immediate* relief of obstruction is required only in patients with generalized sepsis due to infection behind the obstruction. In this situation, antimicrobial therapy alone frequently will be ineffective. Pain, recurrent infections or bleeding, hypertension, or progressive impairment in renal function are other indications for correction of obstruction, although emergent therapy is not required. For example, dialysis may precede any diagnostic studies or therapy in a patient presenting with renal failure and severe biochemical abnormalities. The short delay in relieving the obstruction will not lead to any irreversible deterioration in renal function, and the rapid improvement in the patient's metabolic (and possibly hemodynamic) status may be crucial.

In contrast, treatment may be unnecessary with partial obstruction, particularly if unilateral. Many patients with congenital strictures (of moderate severity) at the ureteropelvic junction will be asymptomatic, with neither hypertension nor deterioration in renal function despite the presence of hydronephrosis.[21,48] In this setting major abdominal surgery, which may be associated with recurrent stricture formation, is not indicated.[21]

RENAL PELVIS AND URETER

The most common causes of obstruction of the upper urinary tract are calculi and neoplasms.

CALCULI

The approach to patients with nephro- or ureterolithiasis is dependent upon the size of the stone. As a general guideline, calculi larger than 10 mm in diameter will not pass spontaneously, those 5 to 10 mm in size may pass, and those smaller than 5 mm will usually be excreted. A renal pelvic calculus that is causing symptoms and is too large to pass spontaneously or a completely obstructing ureteral stone should be removed. In the past, this would be done surgically. Now, ultrasonic or shock-wave lithotripsy may

offer a less invasive alternative for renal or proximal ureteral calculi.[49-51]

Stones reaching the lower ureter are usually smaller and often pass spontaneously. Thus, the patient can be observed for as long as 4 to 8 weeks if infection is absent and pain can be controlled. If removal is necessary, a basket extraction may be attempted before surgery is considered. Similar guidelines apply to other causes of intraluminal obstruction such as a sloughed papilla or blood clot.

NEOPLASMS

Neoplasms can result in upper tract obstruction via direct encasement of the ureter by the primary tumor (in which case urinary tract dilation may not occur), enlarged retroperitoneal lymph nodes, or involvement of the bladder, particularly in the area adjacent to the ureterovesicular junction. Once the diagnosis of obstruction is made, there are several options available, and ultimately the approach will be tailored to the needs of the individual patient.

Ureteral Stents.   In most cases, the initial procedure will be placement of a ureteral stent via cystoscopy.[52-54] The catheter can be left in place for several weeks, during which time more definitive therapy can be undertaken. More prolonged use of the stent is frequently prevented by catheter occlusion, possibly due to precipitation of calcium salts.[54] Furthermore, the stent is a foreign body, and can serve as a nidus for infection. As a result, the use of chronic stent insertion is generally limited to patients with refractory tumor and a poor long-term prognosis.

Antegrade Nephrostomy.   In many patients, a stent cannot be placed via cystoscopy because the ureteral catheter cannot bypass the obstruction or the ureters cannot be entered because of tumor invasion of the bladder. In this setting, the obstruction can be relieved by placement of a nephrostomy tube in the renal pelvis, either percutaneously under ultrasonic guidance[55] or, less preferably, by a surgical approach.[56] In critically ill patients, percutaneous nephrostomy may be done before cystoscopy, since it can be performed at the bedside.

Prolonged use of a nephrostomy tube is associated with an increased risk of infection.[55,56] As a result, percutaneous nephrostomy is generally a temporizing measure until more definitive therapy can be undertaken. However, the nephrostomy tube can be left in on a long-term basis in patients with advanced and refractory disease.

Approach to Bilateral UTO. A frequent question in patients with bilateral UTO is whether one or both kidneys should be decompressed. This is an important issue, since many patients with bilateral obstruction have asymmetric involvement with one kidney being more severely affected. The aim of therapy in such a patient is to regain the maximum amount of renal function at the minimum risk to the patient. Thus, asymptomatic renal obstruction does not have to be relieved if there is strong reason to suspect that there will be little functional recovery, as suggested, for example, by a marked reduction in parenchymal width on ultrasonography (see "Prognosis," below). In this setting, treatment of the less involved kidney is frequently adequate since it will lead to a substantial recovery of renal function. In comparison, the obstruction to both sides should be relieved when both kidneys appear viable.

Functional Recovery. The most important factors determining functional recovery are the duration and the severity of the obstruction. A complete return to baseline renal function is the rule in patients with uncomplicated acute obstruction (less than 1 to 2 weeks). However,

irreversible renal damage will occur with prolonged complete or severe partial obstruction. In this setting, the degree of functional recovery diminishes as the duration of obstruction increases.[16,21,57-59] Little or no improvement should be expected after more than 12 weeks of complete obstruction.[59]

Functional recovery can also be predicted by radiologic studies. Good prognostic findings include relatively normal parenchymal width (the distance between the calyces and the renal capsule) on ultrasonography, and calyceal visualization on intravenous pyelogram (IVP) (if performed). Radionuclide scans to assess cortical blood flow have also been used to predict recovery.[60,61] At present, however, they appear to have limited utility, since return of renal function has occurred even after total nonvisualization (see "Prognosis," below).[62]

Renal function can continue to improve for at least 10 days after the relief of obstruction.[59] Therefore management decisions which are based on the "new baseline" plasma creatinine concentration should be appropriately deferred.

Urinary Diversion. If the cause of the ureteral obstruction is not amenable to primary treatment (with chemotherapy, surgery, or radiation therapy), then a urinary diversion procedure may be performed. Before proceeding with this modality, two factors should be considered. First, the previously obstructed kidney should have adequate function to justify chronic relief of the obstruction. This can be estimated by measuring the creatinine clearance from the urine draining from the ureteral catheter or nephrostomy tube. A creatinine clearance of 10 mL/min, although markedly reduced, is usually sufficient to maintain life without dialysis and therefore represents a level of function that should be retained. In contrast, chronic relief of the obstruction will be of little benefit if the creatinine clearance is much less than 10 mL/min. In this setting, nephrectomy may be considered if persistent pain or infection is present.

Second, the prognosis of the patient with a nonresponsive malignancy should be taken into account. In patients with widespread disease in whom palliative urinary diversions are performed, the mortality rate is approximately 50 percent at 3 months and 90 percent at 1 year, with as much as 64 percent of survival time being spent in the hospital.[56,63] Given this information, some severely debilitated patients may choose to die painlessly from uremia.

For a urinary diversion procedure to be successful, there must be enough healthy ureter proximal to the obstruction to allow for mobilization and reanastomosis. Therefore, patients who undergo this type of procedure generally have either bladder carcinoma or tumor occlusion of the ureter near the ureterovesicular junction. Once the decision has been made to proceed with urinary diversion, there are still a number of choices that must be made regarding the type of procedure.

The first operation for urinary diversion involved the insertion of the ureters into the intact sigmoid colon, thus creating a ureterosigmoidostomy. Although this had the advantage of maintaining continence and not requiring an ostomy bag, complications were common, particularly acute pyelonephritis (due to reflux of colonic bacteria into the kidney), loss of renal function (secondary to scarring from recurrent infections), and hyperchloremic metabolic acidosis (due to exchange of urinary chloride for bicarbonate by the colonic mucosa).[64]

Long-term follow-up has revealed another, more serious, complication, *colon carcinoma.* It has been estimated that colon carcinoma is roughly 500 times more prevalent in patients who have undergone ureterosigmoidostomy.[65] The mean lag time seems to be bimodal, being 8 to 9 years in patients over 40, and 21 years in those under 40.[65]

The precise reason for this increased risk of malignancy is not completely clear. In a rat model, ureterosigmoidostomy was associated with a significant incidence of colon carcinoma at or adjacent to the ureteral anastomosis.[66] Three factors were required for this complication to occur: urine, stool, and a suture line (an area of high cell turnover). If, for example, the mixture of urine and stool was prevented by performing a colonic diversion proximal to the ureterosigmoidostomy, malignancy did not occur. One possible explanation for the requirement for both urine and stool is that the urine may serve to activate fecal carcinogens.[67,68] Alternatively, fecal bacteria may convert harmless substances excreted in the urine (such as nitrates) to potentially dangerous compounds (such as nitrites, which can combine into nitrosamines).[69] This hypothesis is supported by the fact that fecal material can cause uroepithelial metaplasia.[64]

Another, perhaps less likely, theory proposes that the increased risk of malignancy results from chronic irritation of the bowel mucosa.[70,71] In this case, the anastomotic site may serve as a pseudopolyp, which undergoes malignant change after years of trauma.

Physicians caring for patients who have previously undergone ureterosigmoidostomy should maintain a high index of suspicion for carcinoma of the colon. Serial testing for fecal blood should be routine, and some have suggested that periodic colonoscopy be performed as well. The colonoscopist should be aware that the anastomotic site may resemble a polyp, since it is obviously important that it not be mistakenly removed.

Neoplasia (as well as the other complications mentioned above) has limited the utility of ureterosigmoidostomy, which has now largely been replaced by ileal and colon conduits (also called loops). These procedures involve the creation of a blind loop (which prevents the mixture of stool with urine) of ileum or colon to which the ureter is anastomosed. The distal end of the loop is brought out via a stoma onto the abdominal wall.

Creation of an ileal loop does not preserve continence, but it does reduce the incidence of pyelonephritis (since the ileum is usually sterile) and metabolic acidosis (since the rapid drainage of urine into the ostomy bag leads to a contact time that is too short for substantial chloride-bicarbonate exchange to occur). There is, however, free reflux up the ureter because the ileal wall has an insufficient muscular layer to allow the creation of a nonrefluxing submucosal tunnel. Thus, recurrent urinary tract infections can still be a problem, as well as a high incidence of anatomic complications such as stomal stenosis, and stone disease (particularly after infection with urease-producing organisms).[72-74] Although hyperchloremic acidosis is usually not a problem with a normally functioning loop, it can occur when contact time is prolonged because of excess conduit length.[73]

Colonic loops are less susceptible to stomal stenosis (since they are wider), and infection (and hence stone formation) is less common since the thick muscular wall of the colon allows for the creation of an antirefluxing anastomosis. However, colonic loops are more difficult to construct surgically and are not totally free of the problems to which ileal conduits are prone.[73,75] They are therefore preferred only in situations where the patient can tolerate a longer operation and is expected to survive long enough to benefit from the lower complication rate.

Since a conduit does not maintain continence, it is generally a palliative procedure. A patient with a good performance status (for whom a chronic ureteral stent or a nephrostomy would be impractical) but a relatively poor long-term prognosis is an ideal candidate. An example would be a man with irreversible obstruction from a slow-growing prostatic malignancy that is unresponsive to any form of therapy. In this instance, a simple procedure such as an ileal loop can significantly improve the quality of life. An alternative continence maintaining operation (see below) is probably not justified because the increased complexity of the procedure with its concomitantly greater morbidity and mortality would not provide enough benefit in the short term to outweigh the added risks.

In individuals with either cured or potentially curable disease, a continent form of urinary diversion (other than ureterosigmoidostomy) should be considered. There are a number of alternatives that generally fall into one of three categories: (1) bladder replacement using hollow abdominal viscera; (2) continent abdominal wall stoma; and (3) a prosthetic bladder.[76] For example, the Kock pouch, a type of continent abdominal wall stoma, is widely used in patients undergoing urinary diversion for bladder cancer, a malignancy causing obstruction at the ureterovesical junction, or a neurogenic bladder.[76] This procedure creates a nonrefluxing ileal loop, and anastomoses it to the abdominal wall with a nipple valve that maintains continence; the pouch is intermittently emptied via self-catheterization. It is an attractive alternative for the patient with cured or very limited disease.

NONMALIGNANT DISEASES

Treatment of other forms of upper UTO (see Table 9–1) varies with the underlying disorder. Anatomic abnormalities such as ureteropelvic junction stricture or a ureterocele can be corrected directly by surgery.[1] In patients with retroperitoneal fibrosis, the ureteral obstruction can be relieved by dissecting the ureters free of the fibrotic process (ureterolysis) and recurrent retroperitoneal obstruction then prevented by bringing the ureters into the peritoneum or by moving them laterally and interposing retroperitoneal fat between the ureters and the fibrotic process.[77]

BLADDER

Other than neoplasms, a neurogenic bladder (in either adults or children) or congenital exstrophy of the bladder are the most common bladder disorders that can interfere with urine flow. Although urinary diversion had been used as the primary treatment for these disorders,[78] this procedure is now performed infrequently, and only when other measures have failed. Primary closure, if possible, is preferred for patients with exstrophy of the bladder, whereas intermittent self-catheterization several times daily (to substitute for normal bladder emptying) is effective in most patients with a flaccid bladder.[79–82] If performed properly, self-catheterization can prevent infections and renal scarring and is not associated with the anatomic complications frequently seen with urinary diversion procedures.[80] The Crede maneuver (manual compression of the bladder over the suprapubic area) may also be helpful, either as a primary measure or as an adjunct to catheterization.

Pharmacological agents may also be effective in selected patients. If the bladder is spastic for example, anticholinergic drugs (such as atropine) can relax the bladder wall and allow for continence. In the more common case of a partially paralytic bladder, strict avoidance of all anticholinergic drugs and, if necessary, the addition of a cholinergic agonist (such as bethanechol chloride) may prove sufficient either to forego the need for catheterization or to reduce its frequency.[79,81]

BLADDER NECK AND URETHRA

The major cause of bladder neck obstruction in men is benign prostatic hypertrophy or carcinoma. Urethral catheterization will generally provide immediate relief of pain or renal insufficiency. Surgery is ultimately required to relieve the obstruction.

In contrast, bladder neck or urethral obstruction is unusual in women. Procedures such as urethral dilation (to help prevent recurrent episodes of cystitis) should be performed only when urethral stenosis has been well documented.

In children, urethral valves or stricture can lead to recurrent infections, bleeding, or upper tract dilatation. These problems can be corrected with electrocautery or urethral dilation, respectively.[1] Patients with congenital urethral abnormalities also may have other urinary tract changes that require correction, such as vesicoureteral reflux or ureteropelvic junction strictures.

Finally, bladder stones causing intermittent obstruction can be removed in one of two ways.[35] If the stones are relatively small and soft, they may be able to be crushed during cystoscopic examination, thereby allowing the fragments to be passed spontaneously through the urethra. Larger, harder stones must be removed via suprapubic cystotomy.

POSTOBSTRUCTIVE DIURESIS

The brisk diuresis that follows the relief of bilateral obstruction is initially due to urine that has been trapped in the dilated collecting system. Frequently, a high rate of urine output persists for a variable length of time. As a therapeutic guide, it is important to distinguish between a diuresis that is *appropriate*, or physiologic, and one that is *inappropriate*, or pathologic. Many patients will have a marked negative sodium and water balance for the first few days after relief of obstruction.[83,84] In the vast majority of these cases, the losses represent sodium and water that were retained during the period of obstruction.[83–87] In this sense, the diuresis (and natriuresis) is *appropriate* for the patient's volume status. It lasts only until the excess fluid has been excreted and does not induce signs of volume depletion such as postural hypotension, decreased skin turgor, or a further increase in the blood urea nitrogen and plasma creatinine concentration. As a result, fluid replacement above maintenance is generally not required during a postobstructive diuresis. If the urinary losses are replaced milliliter for milliliter, a persistent diuresis that can exceed 10 L/day may ensue because of continued volume expansion.

The nature of the driving forces for this usually *physiologic diuresis* is not completely defined but probably involves several mechanisms:

1. Volume expansion can produce hormonal changes that promote sodium excretion, such as reduced secretion of aldosterone or increased release of atrial natriuretic peptide.
2. The urea that accumulates during the period of obstruction can act as an endogenous osmotic diuretic once glomerular filtration is reestablished.[86]
3. Circulating, perhaps nonspecific, natriuretic substances that are normally excreted in the urine may be retained with bilateral obstruction.[3,88–90]

The inability to demonstrate an inappropriate diuresis does not necessarily mean that tubular function is normal. Decreased ability to conserve sodium or to concentrate the urine maximally has been demonstrated both in experimental animals and humans after the relief of urinary tract obstruction. However, these tubular defects (which may be reversible) are usually counterbalanced by a persistent reduction in GFR, an abnormality that prevents marked polyuria.[4,13,24]

In perhaps 5 percent of patients or less,[87] the fluid losses seen after relief of obstruction are inappropriate, and volume depletion with hemodynamic compromise will develop if the urine output is not replaced.[83,87,91–93] This is most likely to occur after the correction of *bilateral* obstruction but can rarely be seen in patients with *unilateral* disease.[24,94,95] The pathogenesis of this pathologic type of postobstructive diuresis is poorly understood. In some patients, the GFR rapidly returns to normal or near normal; in this setting, the tubular defects in sodium and water reabsorption can be unmasked and an inappropriate diuresis can ensue, even with the relief of unilateral obstruction.[94,95]

It is also possible that an exaggerated response to urea or other natriuretic factors could be important in some patients, since inappropriate fluid losses generally last for only a few days.[84,93] However, the diuresis may persist for several weeks or months in rare cases[83,91] long after any retained substances have been excreted. Severe tubular damage is presumably responsible for this problem.

In summary, a postobstructive diuresis is appropriate in most patients and results in the excretion of sodium and water retained during the period of obstruction. If these losses are automatically replaced, the diuresis will persist indefinitely. Thus, a rational plan for treatment of a postobstructive diuresis must allow the patient to have a period of negative sodium and water balance while he or she is observed closely for signs of volume depletion. One approach is to give only standard replacement fluids (such as 50 to 75 mL/h of half-isotonic saline) during the initial diuresis. Marked fluid restriction should be avoided, since the ability to conserve sodium and water maximally is likely to be abnormal, at least in the early recovery period.[24,94,95] Treated in this fashion, most patients will return to a euvolemic state uneventfully.

PROGNOSIS

The prognosis for recovery of renal function following obstructive uropathy is variable, depending primarily on the severity and duration of obstruction (see p. 459). Other important factors include the possible presence of preexisting renal disease, infection above the level of obstruction, nephrolithiasis, hypertension, and papillary necrosis.

The use of radiologic studies to predict

functional recovery has not proven to be very accurate. Normal parenchymal width (the distance between the calyces and the renal capsule) on ultrasonography and adequate cortical perfusion on radionuclide scanning are good prognostic findings. However, substantial return of renal function can occur even in patients with total nonvisualization (on radionuclide scan) or marked parenchymal thinning.[62,94]

Even the recovery of a normal GFR (as estimated clinically by the plasma creatinine concentration) does not mean that there has been no permanent renal damage.[3,96,97] In a rat model in which unilateral UTO was induced

for only 24 h, up to 15 percent of nephrons were nonfunctional as late as 60 days after release, a change that was presumed to be permanent.[96] Despite this loss of functioning renal mass, the total GFR was normal, indicative of hyperfiltration in the remaining nephrons. If this model is applicable to humans, transient UTO, which is relieved with a return of the plasma creatinine concentration to normal may actually leave the patient with significant permanent nephron loss. If so, these patients could be at risk for progressive renal failure over many years secondary to hemodynamically mediated glomerular sclerosis (see Chap. 4).

REFERENCES

1. Hendren, W. H.: Pediatric surgery, *N. Engl. J. Med.,* 289:562, 1973.
2. Warshaw, B. L.: Progression to end stage renal disease in children with obstructive nephropathy, *J. Pediatr.,* 100:83, 1982.
3. Klahr, S.: Pathophysiology of obstructive nephropathy, *Kidney Int.,* 23:414, 1983.
4. Wilson, D. R.: Pathophysiology of obstructive nephropathy, *Kidney Int.,* 18:281, 1980.
5. Gaudio, K. M., N. J. Siegel, J. P. Hayslett, and M. Kashgarian: Renal perfusion and intratubular pressure during ureteral occlusion in the rat, *Am. J. Physiol.,* 238:F205, 1980.
6. Allen, J. T., E. D. Vaughan, Jr., and J. Y. Gillenwater: The effect of indomethacin on renal blood flow and ureteral pressure in unilateral ureteral obstruction in awake dogs, *Invest. Urol.,* 15:324, 1978.
7. Tanner, G. A.: Effects of kidney tubule obstruction on glomerular function in rats, *Am. J. Physiol.,* 237:F379, 1979.
8. Cadnapaphornchai P., N. P. Bondar, and F. D. McDonald: Effect of imidazole on the recovery from bilateral ureteral obstruction in dogs, *Am. J. Physiol.,* 243:F532, 1982.
9. Balint, P., and K. Laszol: Effect of imidazole and indomethacin on hemodynamics of the obstructed canine kidney, *Kidney Int.,* 27:892, 1985.
10. Ichikawa, I., M. L. Purkerson, J. Yates, and S. Klahr: Dietary protein intake conditions the degree of renal vasoconstriction in acute renal failure caused by ureteral obstruction, *Am. J. Physiol.,* 249:F54, 1985.
11. Klotman, P. E., S. R. Smith, B. D. Volpp, T. M. Coffman, and W. E. Yarger: Thromboxane inhibition improves function of hydronephrotic rat kidneys, *Am. J. Physiol.,* 250:F282, 1986.
12. Arendshorst, W. J., W. F. Finn, and C. W. Gottschalk: Nephron stop-flow response to obstruction for 24 hours in the rat kidney, *J. Clin. Invest.,* 53:1497, 1975.
13. Yarger, W. E., H. S. Aynedjian, and N. Bank: A micropuncture study of postobstructive diuresis in the rat, *J. Clin. Invest.,* 51:625, 1972.
14. Michaelson, G.: Percutaneous puncture of the renal pelvis, intrapelvic pressure and the concentrating capacity of the kidney in hydronephrosis, *Acta Med. Scand.* (suppl.), 559:1, 1974.
15. Ichikawa, I., and B. M. Brenner: Local intrarenal vasoconstrictor-vasodilator interactions in mild partial ureteral obstruction, *Am. J. Physiol.,* 236:F131, 1979.
16. Olbrich, O., E. Woodford-Williams, R. E. Irvine, and D. Webster: Renal function in prostatism, *Lancet,* 1:1322, 1957.
17. Hoffman, L. M., and W. N. Suki: Obstructive uropathy mimicking volume depletion, *J. Am. Med. Assoc.,* 236:2096, 1976.

18. Hanley M. J., and K. Davidson: Isolated nephron segments from rabbit models of obstructive nephropathy, *J. Clin. Invest.,* 69:165, 1982.

19. Berlyne, G. M.: Distal tubular function in chronic hydronephrosis, *Q. J. Med.,* 30:339, 1961.

20. Batlle, D. C., J. T. Sehy, M. K. Roseman, J. A. L. Arruda, and N. A. Kurtzman: Hyperkalemic distal renal tubular acidosis associated with obstructive uropathy, *N. Engl. J. Med.,* 304:373, 1981.

21. Klahr, S., J. Buerkert, and A. Morrison: Urinary tract obstruction, in B. M. Brenner and F. C. Rector, Jr. (eds.), *The Kidney,* 3d ed., Saunders, Philadelphia, 1986.

22. Block, G. E., W. E. Enker, and J. B. Kirsner: Significance and treatment of occult obstructive uropathy complicating Crohn's disease, *Ann. Surg.,* 178:322, 1973.

23. Burkholder, G. V., L. N. Dotin, W. B. Thomason, and O. D. Beach: Unexplained hematuria: How extensive should the evaluation be?, *J. Am. Med. Assoc.,* 210:1729, 1969.

24. Gillenwater, J. Y., F. B. Westervelt, Jr., E. D. Vaughan, Jr., and S. S. Howards: Renal function after release of chronic unilateral hydronephrosis in man, *Kidney Int.,* 7:179, 1975.

25. Lapides, J.: Mechanisms of urinary tract infection, Urology, 14:217, 1979.

26. Andriole V. T.: Current concepts of urinary tract infections, in L. Weinstein and B. N. Fields (eds.), *Seminars in Infectious Disease,* vol. III, Thieme-Stratton, New York, 1980.

27. Komaroff, A. L.: Urinalysis and urine culture in women with dysuria, *Ann. Intern. Med.,* 104:212, 1986.

28. Kauffman, C. A., and J. S. Tan: *Torulopsis glabrata* renal infection, *Am. J. Med.,* 57:217, 1974.

29. Weidmann, P., C. Beretta-Picoli, D. Hirsh, F. C. Reubi, and S. G. Massry: Curable hypertension with unilateral hydronephrosis, *Ann. Intern. Med.,* 87:437, 1977.

30. Belman, A. B., K. A. Kropp, and N. M. Simon: Renal-pressor hypertension secondary to unilateral hydronephrosis, *N. Engl. J. Med.,* 278:1133, 1968.

31. Vaughan, E. D., Jr., F. R. Buhler, and J. H. Laragh: Normal renin secretion in hypertensive patients with primarily unilateral chronic hydronephrosis, *J. Urol.,* 112:153, 1974.

32. Palmer, J. M., F. G. Zweiman, and T. A. Assaykeen: Renal hypertension due to hydronephrosis with normal plasma renin activity, *N. Engl. J. Med.,* 283:1032, 1970.

33. Muldowney, F. P., G. J. Duffy, D. G. Kelly, F. A. Duff, C. Harrington, and R. Freaney: Sodium diuresis after relief of obstructive uropathy, *N. Engl. J. Med.,* 274:1294, 1966.

34. Heptinstall, R. H.: *Pathology of the Kidney,* 3d ed., Little, Brown, Boston, 1983, chap. 28.

35. Drach, G. W.: Urinary lithiasis, in P. C. Walsh, R. F. Gittes, A. D. Perlmutter, and T. A. Stamey (eds.), *Campbell's Urology,* 5th ed., Saunders, Philadephia, 1986.

36. Eknoyan, G., W. Y. Qunibi, R. T. Grissom, S. N. Tuma, and J. C. Ayus: Renal papillary necrosis: An update, *Medicine,* 61:55, 1982.

37. Muirhead, E. E., J. Vanatta, and A. Grollman: Papillary necrosis of the kidney: A clinical and experimental condition, *J. Am. Med. Assoc.,* 142:627, 1950.

38. Solez, K., S. Ponchak, R. A. Buono, N. Vernon, P. M. Finer, M. Miller, and R. H. Heptinstall: Inner medullary plasma flow in the kidney with ureteral obstruction, *Am. J. Physiol.,* 231:1315, 1976.

39. Landsberg, L.: Hypernatremia complicating partial urinary-tract obstruction, *N. Engl. J. Med.,* 283:746, 1970.

40. Osius, T. G., and F. Hynman, Jr.: Dynamics of acute urinary retention: A manometric, radiographic and clinical study, *J. Urol.,* 90:702, 1963.

41. Rascoff, J. H., R. A. Golden, B. S. Spinowitz, and C. Charytan: Nondilated obstructive nephropathy, *Arch. Intern. Med.,* 143:696, 1983.

42. Laville, M., P. J. Maillet, D. Pelle-Francey, J. Finaz de Villaire, J. Traeger, and A. Pinet: Non-dilated obstructive acute renal failure (abstract), *Kidney Int.,* 28:694, 1985.

43. Arafa, N. M., M. M. Fathi, M. Safwat, H. Moro, H. Torky, M. Kenawi, and M. Abdel-Wahab: Accuracy of ultrasound in the diagnosis of nonfunctioning kidneys, *J. Urol.,* 128:1165, 1982.

44. Webb, J. A. W., R. H. Reznek, S. E. White, W. R. Cattell, I. K. Fry, and L. R. I. Baker: Can ultrasound and computed tomography replace high-dose urography in patients with impaired renal function, *Q. J. Med.,* 53:411, 1984.

45. Berloseth, R. O., and C. M. Kjellstrand: Radiologic contrast-induced nephropathy, *Med. Clin. N. Am.,* 68:351, 1984.

46. Byrd, L., and R. L. Sherman: Radiocontrast-induced acute renal failure, *Medicine,* 58:270, 1979.

47. Griner, P. F., R. J. Mayewski, A. I. Mushlin, and P. Greenland: Selection and interpretation of diagnostic tests and procedures, *Ann. Intern. Med.,* 94:553, 1981.

48. Kelalis, P. P., O. S. Culp, G. B. Stickler, and E. C. Burke: Ureteropelvic obstruction in children: Experiences with 109 cases, *J. Urol.,* 106:418, 1971.

49. Finlayson, B., and W. C. Thomas, Jr.: Extracorporeal

shock-wave lithotripsy, *Ann. Intern. Med.,* 101:387, 1984.

50. Riehle, R. A. Jr., W. R. Fair, and E. D. Vaughan, Jr.: Extracorporeal shock-wave lithotripsy for upper urinary tract calculi, *J. Am. Med. Assoc.,* 255:2043, 1986.

51. Chaussy, C., and E. Schmiedt: Shock wave treatment for stones in the upper urinary tract, *Urol. Clin. N. Am.,* 10:743, 1983.

52. Gibbons, R. P., R. J. Correa, Jr., K. B. Cummings, and J. T. Mason: Experience with indwelling ureteral stent catheter, *J. Urol.,* 115:22, 1976.

53. Singh, B., H. Kim, and S. H. Wax: Stent versus nephrostomy: Is there a choice?, *J. Urol.,* 121:268, 1979.

54. Andriole, G. L., M. A. Bettman, M. B. Garnick, and J. P. Richie: Indwelling double-J ureteral stent for temporary and permanent urinary drainage: Experience with 87 patients, *J. Urol.,* 131:239, 1984.

55. Reznek, R. H., and L. B. Talner, Percutaneous nephrostomy, *Radiol. Clin. N. Am.,* 22:393, 1984.

56. Holden, S., M. McPhee, and H. Grabstald: Rationale of urinary diversion in cancer patients, *J. Urol.,* 121:19, 1979.

57. Pridgen, W. R., D. M. Woodhead, and R. K. Younger: Alterations in renal function produced by ureteral obstruction: Determination of critical obstruction time in relation to renal survival, *J. Am. Med. Assoc.,* 178:563, 1961.

58. Garret, J., S. L. Polse, and J. W. Morrow: Ureteral obstruction and hypertension, *Am. J. Med.,* 49:271, 1970.

59. Better, O. S., A. I. Arieff, S. G. Massry, C. R. Kleeman, and M. H. Maxwell: Studies on renal function after relief of complete unilateral obstruction of three month's duration in man, *Am. J. Med.,* 54:234, 1973.

60. Kalika, V., R. H. Bard, A. Iloreta, L. M. Freeman, S. Heller, and M. D. Blaufox: Prediction of renal functional recovery after relief of upper urinary tract obstruction, *J. Urol.,* 126:301, 1981.

61. Belis, J. A.: Radionuclide determination of individual kidney function in the treatment of chronic renal obstruction, *J. Urol.,* 127:636, 1982.

62. McAfee, J. G., A. Singh, and J. P. O'Callaghan: Nuclear imaging supplementary to urography in obstructive uropathy, *Radiology,* 137:487, 1980.

63. Brin, E. N., M. Schiff, Jr., and R. M. Weiss: Palliative urinary diversion for pelvic malignancy, *J. Urol.,* 113:619, 1975.

64. Duckett, J. W., and J. M. Gazak: Complications of ureterosigmoidostomy, *Urol. Clin. N. Am.,* 10:473, 1983.

65. Leadbetter, G. W., Jr, P. Zickerman, and E. Pierce: Ureterosigmoidostomy and carcinoma of the colon, *J. Urol.,* 121:732, 1979.

66. Crissey, M. M., G. D. Steele, and R. F. Gittes: Rat model for carcinogenesis in ureterosigmoidostomy, *Science,* 207:1079, 1980.

67. Crissey, M. M., G. D. Steele, Jr., and R. F. Gittes: Carcinoma in the colonic urinary diversion in rats, *Surg. Forum,* 30:554, 1979.

68. Harguindey, S. S., R. C. Colbeck, and E. D. Bransome, Jr.: Ureterosigmoidostomy and cancer: New observations (letter), *Ann. Intern. Med.,* 83:833, 1975.

69. Chiang, M. S., J. P. Minton, K. Clausen, H. W. Clatworthy, and H. A. Wise, III: Carcinoma in a colon conduit urinary diversion, *J. Urol.,* 127:1185, 1982.

70. Rivard, J.-Y., A. Bedard, and L. Dionne: Colonic neoplasms following ureterosigmoidostomy, *J. Urol.,* 113:781, 1975.

71. Gillman, J. C.: Adenomatous polyp of the bowel following ureterocolic anatomosis. *Br. J. Urol.,* 36:263, 1964.

72. Pitts, W. R., Jr., and E. C. Muecke: A 20-year experience with ileal conduits: The fate of the kidneys, *J. Urol.,* 122:154, 1979.

73. Hendren, W. H., and D. Radopoulis: Complications of ileal loop and colon conduit urinary diversion, *Urol. Clin. N. Am.,* 10:451, 1983.

74. Dretler, S. P.: The pathogenesis of urinary tract calculi occurring after ileal conduit diversion, *J. Urol.,* 109:204, 1973.

75. Althausen, A. F., K. Hagen-Cook, and W. H. Hendren III: Non-refluxing colon conduit: Experience with 70 cases, *J. Urol.,* 120:35, 1978.

76. Goldwasser, B., and G. D. Webster: Continent urinary diversion, *J. Urol.,* 134:227, 1985.

77. Lepor, H., and P. C. Walsh: Idiopathic retroperitoneal fibrosis, *J. Urol.,* 122:1, 1979.

78. Middleton, A. W., Jr., and W. H. Hendren: Ileal conduits in children at the Massachusetts General Hospital from 1955 to 1970, *J. Urol.,* 115:591, 1976.

79. Lapides, J., A. C. Diokno, F. R. Gould, and B. S. Lowe: Further observations on self-catheterization, *J. Urol.,* 116:169, 1976.

80. Crooks, K. K., and B. G. Enrile: Comparison of the ileal conduit and clean intermittent catheterization for myelomeningocele, *Pediatrics,* 72:203, 1983.

81. Rhame, F. S., and I. Perkash: Urinary tract infections occurring in recent spinal cord injury patients on intermittent catheterization, *J. Urol.,* 122:669, 1979.

82. Retik, A.: Urinary tract disorders in children: New approaches, *Hosp. Pract.,* 19(8):121, 1984.

83. Eismann, B., C. Vivian, and J. Vivian: Fluid and electrolyte changes following the relief of urinary obstruction, *J. Urol.,* 74:222, 1955.

84. Howards, S. S.: Post-obstructive diuresis: A misunderstood phenomenon, *J. Urol.,* 110:537, 1973.

85. Persky, L., J. W. Benson, S. Levery, and W. E. Abbott: Metabolic alterations in surgical patients, X: The benign course of the average patient with acute urinary retention, *Surgery,* 42:290, 1957.

86. Sophasan, S., and S. Sorrasuchart: Factors inducing post-obstructive diuresis in rats, *Nephron,* 38:125, 1984.

87. Bishop, M. C.: Diuresis and renal functional recovery in chronic retention, *Br. J. Urol.,* 57:1, 1985.

88. Wilson, D. R., and U. Honroth: Cross-circulation study of natriuretic factors in post-obstructive diuresis, *J. Clin. Invest.,* 57:380, 1976.

89. Harris, R. H., and W. E. Yarger: Urine-reinfusion natriuresis: Evidence for potent natriuretic factors in rat urine, *Kidney Int.,* 11:93, 1977.

90. Harris, R. H., and W. E. Yarger: The pathogenesis of post-obstructive diuresis, *J. Clin. Invest.,* 56:880, 1975.

91. Bricker, N. S., E. I. Shwayri, J. B. Reardon, D. Kellog, J. P. Merrill, and J. H. Holmes: An abnormality in renal function resulting from urinary tract obstruction, *Am. J. Med.,* 23:554, 1957.

92. Witte, M. H., F. A. Short, and W. Hollander, Jr.,: Massive polyuria and natriuresis following relief of urinary tract obstruction, *Am. J. Med.,* 37:320, 1964.

93. Maher, J. F., G. E. Schreiner, and T. J. Waters: Osmotic diuresis due to retained urea after release of obstruction, *N. Engl. J. Med.,* 268:1099, 1963.

94. Green, J., Y. Vardy, M. Munichor, and O. S. Better: Extreme unilateral hydronephrosis with normal glomerular filtration rate: Physiological studies in a case of obstructive uropathy, *J. Urol.,* 136:361, 1986.

95. Schlossberg, S. M., and E. D. Vaughan, Jr.: The mechanism of unilateral postobstructive diuresis, *J. Urol.,* 131:534, 1984.

96. Bander, S. J., J. E. Buerkert, D. Martin, and S. Klahr: Long-term effects of 24-hour unilateral obstruction on renal function in the rat, *Kidney Int.,* 28:614, 1985.

97. Wilson, D. R.: Nephron functional heterogeneity in the postobstructive kidney, *Kidney Int.,* 7:19, 1974.

10

PATHOGENESIS OF ESSENTIAL HYPERTENSION

Burton D. Rose

Definition
Determinants of Blood Pressure
Determinants of Hypertension
   Systemic Hemodynamics
   Plasma Volume
   Renin-Angiotensin System
   Sympathetic Nervous System
   Role of the Kidney
   Dietary Factors
   Heredity and Race
Summary

Hypertension is one of the major problems confronting the physician. The basic aspects of this disorder can be appreciated by the following observations. First, hypertension is extremely common, as 20 to 25 percent of white adults and about 30 percent of black adults have a blood pressure (BP) of 160/90 mmHg or greater.[1] The prevalence of hypertension is also age-dependent, being higher in older patients. If isolated systolic hypertension is included (in which the BP is >160/<90), the incidence of hypertension rises from approximately 16 percent in patients who are 35 to 44 years of age to about 55 percent in patients over the age of 64.[1] Second, a chronically elevated BP can lead to a variety of serious complications including cerebrovascular accidents, congestive heart failure, myocardial infarction, renal failure, and death. Third, the overall morbidity and mortality of hypertension can be reduced by restoring normal BP through the use of diet and antihypertensive medications (Fig. 10–1).[2-6]

In order to attain this therapeutic benefit, a proper approach to the diagnosis, compli-

cations, and therapy of hypertension is required. Before discussing these topics in the next chapter, this chapter reviews the factors that contribute to the elevation in BP.

DEFINITION

The distribution of BP within the general population forms a continuum with no discernible dividing line between normal and elevated BP (Fig. 10–2).[7] As a result, a strict definition of hypertension cannot be made. Since our major concern is the accelerated development of cardiovascular and renal diseases, hypertension could be defined as that BP at which the risk of complications first becomes apparent. However, actuarial studies indicate that survival is inversely related to BP at all levels above 111/70.[8] Thus, a 35-year-old man with a BP of 120/80 will live 4 years longer on the average than a similar subject with a BP of 130/90, even though both pressures are considered normal.[7] These

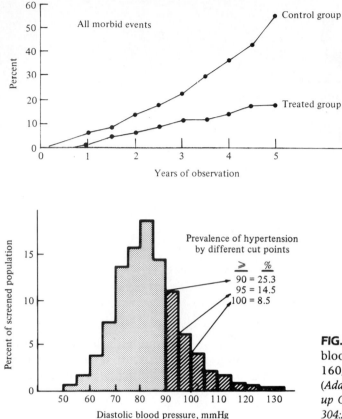

FIG. 10–1. Estimated cumulative incidence of all (nonfatal plus fatal) morbid events over a 5-year period in treated and untreated (control) patients with initial diastolic blood pressure between 105 and 114 mmHg. (*From Veterans Administration Cooperative Study on Antihypertensive Agents, J. Am. Med. Assoc., 213:1143, 1970, Copyright 1970, American Medical Association.*)

FIG. 10–2. Frequency distribution of diastolic blood pressure at screening of almost 160,000 persons, 30 to 69 years of age. (*Adapted from Hypertension Detection and Follow-up Cooperative Group, Ann. N.Y. Acad. Sci., 304:254, 1979.*)

statistics make it unrealistic to define hypertension in terms of increased risk in the untreated subject.

A more helpful approach involves examining the efficacy of therapy in reducing hypertensive complications. This topic will be reviewed in detail in the next chapter but can be briefly summarized at this time. Long-term studies have demonstrated that therapy is most effective when the diastolic pressure is above 104 mmHg,[2,3] is probably effective between 95 and 104 mmHg,[4,6] and is of uncertain benefit between 90 and 94 mmHg.[4,6,9,10] Although these studies grouped patients according to their diastolic pressure, systolic hypertension is a separate and perhaps greater

risk factor for morbidity and mortality (Fig. 10–3).[11-13] As a result of these findings, *a BP of 160/95 or more* (taken on at least three occasions) is generally considered to represent treatable hypertension[14,15] although many physicians will treat a diastolic pressure at or above 90 mmHg.[6] This distinction is important clinically since treating a diastolic BP of 90 rather than 95 mmHg means that an extra 11 percent of adults will require antihypertensive therapy (Fig. 10–2).

There are two groups of patients who have blood pressures lower than the average adult and who therefore require a different definition of hypertension: children and pregnant women. The approximate upper limit of

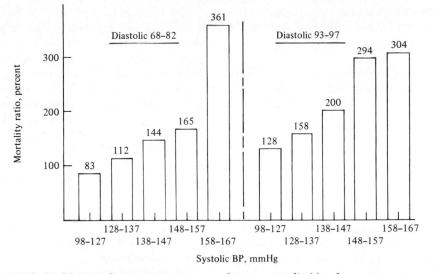

FIG. 10-3. Mortality experience according to systolic blood pressure at specified levels of diastolic BP in men, ages 40 to 49. (*From W. B. Kannel, Prog. Cardiovasc. Dis.,* 17:5, 1974. Reprinted by permission.)

normal for BP in children (with the ages in parentheses) are 110/75 (0 to 5), 120/80 (6 to 9), 125/85 (10 to 13), and 130/90 (14 to 17).[1,16] Low BP is also seen in the second trimester of pregnancy due to vasodilatation, which lowers the systemic vascular resistance. In this setting, a BP exceeding 120/80 is associated with a marked increase in the rate of stillbirth and in the development of preeclampsia in the third trimester.[17]

DETERMINANTS OF BLOOD PRESSURE

The BP, which is generated by cardiac contraction against a resistance, reaches its peak during systole (systolic BP) and its nadir at the end of cardiac relaxation (diastolic BP). The mean arterial pressure (MAP) lies between the systolic (SBP) and diastolic (DBP) pressures and can be estimated from the DBP plus one-third of the pulse pressure (the difference between the systolic and diastolic pressures)*:

$$MAP = DBP + \frac{SBP - DBP}{3}$$

For example, the MAP at a BP of 120/80 is approximately 93 mmHg.

The relationship between the MAP and its major determinants, the cardiac output (CO)

---

*The pulse pressure is divided by one-third rather than one-half since the duration of diastole is normally about twice as long as that of systole. Thus, the MAP is affected twice as much by the DBP:

$$MAP = \frac{2 \times DBP + SBP}{3}$$

If $(3 \times DBP - DBP)$ is substituted for $2 \times DBP$, then

$$MAP = \frac{3 \times DBP + (SBP - DBP)}{3}$$

$$= DBP + \frac{(SBP - DBP)}{3}$$

and the systemic vascular resistance (SVR), can be expressed by the following formula*:

$$MAP = CO \times SVR$$

Since the cardiac output is equal to the product of the stroke volume (SV) and the heart rate (HR),

$$MAP = SV \times HR \times SVR$$

The net BP that is seen in the hypertensive patient is dependent upon which of these variables is altered. When the MAP is elevated by increments in heart rate or SVR, there will usually be proportionate increases in both the systolic and diastolic pressures. There are, however, several settings in which the pulse pressure is elevated, producing a preferential rise in the systolic BP. This can occur *with an increase in either the stroke volume or the rapid ejection phase or with a reduction in arterial compliance.*[18,19] The first two changes increase the systolic pressure because blood is pumped more rapidly into the arterial tree. In contrast, compliance, which can be defined as the change in pressure seen with a given change in volume, affects the BP by a different mechanism. In a highly compliant arterial system, the increase in arterial volume during ejection produces a relatively small rise in pressure because the elasticity in the major blood vessels allows them to expand. The result is a pulse pressure that is normally 40 to 50 mmHg. In contrast, arterial compliance frequently falls with age, due both to decreased elasticity and to superimposed atherosclerosis. In this setting, elastic expansion is reduced, and the same stroke volume now produces a larger increment in pressure with a larger elevation in the systolic BP.

---

*The product of the CO and the SVR actually equals the pressure drop across the circulation, i.e., the MAP minus the venous pressure. However, the mean venous pressure (normal equals 1 to 6 mmHg) is generally so much lower than the MAP that only a slight error results from ignoring the venous pressure.

The clinical importance of the factors affecting the pulse pressure can be appreciated from studies in patients with isolated systolic hypertension.[19] In young patients (mean age 26, average BP 174/83), the primary abnormality is an increase in the rate of ejection during early systole. This problem is due at least in part to enhanced sympathetic tone and can be largely corrected by the administration of a β-adrenergic blocker. This therapy, however, is relatively ineffective in older patients (mean age 51, average BP 183/85) in whom decreased arterial compliance is primarily responsible for the elevation in systolic BP. In this setting, the BP can be effectively lowered by the administration of a direct vasodilator.[19]

It is important to note that *compliance is not synonymous with SVR.* Compliance is a function of the elasticity of the larger arteries, particularly the aorta, whereas the primary site of vascular resistance is at the level of the large and small arterioles.[18,20] Consequently, compliance can be diminished without a necessary increase in arteriolar resistance or therefore in total SVR. In this setting, the mean arterial pressure will be unchanged, but the rise in pulse pressure (due to the fall in compliance) will produce systolic hypertension and *diastolic hypotension.* For example, an elevated mean arterial pressure of 125 mmHg due to an increase in SVR might be associated with a BP of 155/110 in a 20-year-old with normal aortic elasticity. In contrast, the same mean arterial pressure in a 65-year-old might result in a BP of 185/95, due to the reduction in compliance. Thus, hypertension in older patients is frequently characterized by a preferential rise in systolic BP.[21]

DETERMINANTS OF HYPERTENSION

The underlying abnormality responsible for the development of hypertension can be detected in only a minority of patients. As examples, angiotensin II is largely responsible for the elevation in BP in unilateral renal artery stenosis and norepinephrine for that seen with a pheochromocytoma. In both of these disorders, the humoral agents act primarily by augmenting the SVR.

In contrast, the etiology is not apparent in over 90 percent of adults who are therefore said to have primary or essential hypertension. At the present time, the pathogenesis of this disorder is somewhat confusing since *no single abnormality has been identified that can solely account for the rise in BP.* To the contrary, essential hypertension is probably heterogeneous, with a variety of factors, both acquired and genetic, making a contribution (Table 10–1). Furthermore, the role of any specific factor is variable, being important in some patients but not in others.

The remainder of this chapter reviews the current evidence supporting the role of these factors in the development of essential hypertension. Some of this discussion is, of necessity, speculative in an attempt to describe areas in which future research might lead.

SYSTEMIC HEMODYNAMICS

The primary hemodynamic pattern in *established* essential hypertension is an elevation in SVR with the cardiac output usually being normal. This may not be the initial pattern, however. The major abnormality in many younger patients with intermittent or borderline hypertension is an increase in cardiac output which, as described above, may be related to enhanced sympathetic tone.[19,22-24] With time, the cardiac output spontaneously returns to normal in these patients and the rise in BP is sustained by an elevation in SVR.[22,23]

An example of this transition from output- to resistance-mediated hypertension is illustrated in Fig. 10–4. The development of vol-

TABLE 10–1. Factors Contributing to Development of Essential Hypertension

Systemic hemodynamics
Plasma volume
Renin-angiotensin system
Sympathetic nervous system
Role of the kidney
Dietary factors
    Sodium
    Calcium
    Potassium
    Obesity
    Alcohol
Heredity
Race

ume expansion in an anephric patient initially leads to an elevation in BP that is associated with a rise in cardiac output. Within 3 weeks, the cardiac output returns to baseline while an increase in SVR maintains the hypertension. The factors responsible for this change in resistance are incompletely understood. It has been postulated that a circulating natriuretic hormone that inhibits the sodium-potassium–activated adenosine triphosphatase (Na-K-ATPase) pump may play an important role in this phenomenon (see Fig. 10–14, below). Alternatively, the rise in SVR may be related to a local autoregulatory response in which constriction of the precapillary sphincter maintains capillary flow and pressure at a relatively constant level.[25] This would be different from the autoregulation that follows an acute change in BP, since the increase in resistance in the acute setting occurs within minutes. Arteriolar hyperplasia induced by hypertension, rather than local metabolic factors, may be responsible for the chronic form of autoregulation.[25]

PLASMA VOLUME

The plasma volume, which may be an important determinant of the cardiac output, is inversely related to the BP in most *untreated* patients with essential hypertension,* being lowest in those patients with the most marked elevations in BP (Fig. 10–5).[28,29] This apparently paradoxical effect is thought to reflect an increase in capillary hydrostatic pressure, which would favor the movement of fluid from the vascular space into the interstitium. The intracapillary hypertension could result from venous constriction (induced by enhanced sympathetic tone)[29] or from incomplete autoregulation by the precapillary sphincters, which would allow some of the elevation in BP to be transmitted to the capillary.

Despite the reduction in plasma volume in untreated subjects, it should not be assumed that the plasma volume is unimportant in BP regulation in hypertensive subjects. Although the initial plasma volume may be low, *changes in the plasma volume* in a given patient typically results in parallel changes in BP (Fig. 10–6). For example, lowering the plasma volume with a low-sodium diet or diuretic therapy frequently reduces the BP. On the other hand, a rise in plasma volume is typically associated with both an elevation in BP and diminished effectiveness of most nondiuretic antihypertensive agents.[30–32]

The degree to which volume expansion produces hypertension is dependent in part upon the activity of the sympathetic nervous system. Those patients who are able to normally diminish sympathetic tone may show little or no change in BP, in part because venous dilatation permits the extra fluid to be stored in the vascular space without alter-

*A reduced plasma volume is not found in all hypertensives. For example, the plasma volume may be somewhat increased in blacks and in obese patients.[26,27] The mechanism by which this occurs is not known. In obesity, a high plasma volume and cardiac output is required to perfuse the excessive amount of adipose tissue. Thus, the plasma volume is enhanced even in normotensive patients (in whom vascular resistance is reduced to maintain a normal BP). With the development of hypertension, however, the plasma volume in obesity tends to fall toward normal,[27] a directional change that is similar to that in nonobese patients.

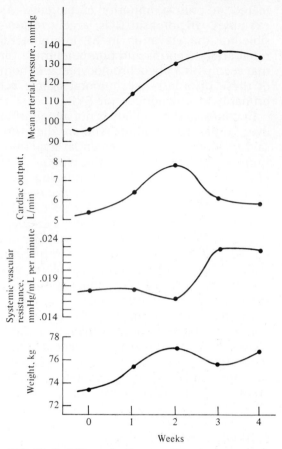

FIG. 10–4. Effect of volume expansion on mean arterial pressure, cardiac output, and systemic vascular resistance in an anephric 22-year-old woman. (*From T. G. Coleman, H. J. Granger, and A. C. Guyton, Circ. Res., 28 (suppl. 2):76, 1971. By permission of the American Heart Association, Inc.*)

ing systemic hemodynamics. If, however, sympathetic tone cannot be changed, the excess volume can lead to increases in both cardiac output and BP.[33,34]

RENIN-ANGIOTENSIN SYSTEM

The renin-angiotensin system plays an important role in many patients with essential hypertension. Renin is a proteolytic enzyme

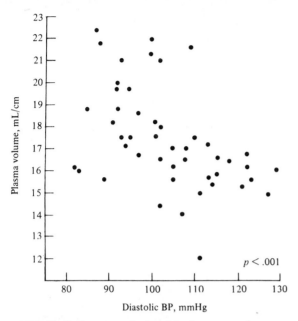

FIG. 10-5. Inverse relationship between plasma volume (in milliliters per centimeter of height) and diastolic blood pressure in *untreated* men with essential hypertension. [*From H. P. Dustan, R. C. Tarazi, E. L. Bravo, and R. A. Dart, Circ. Res., 32 (suppl. 1):73, 1973. By permission of the American Heart Association, Inc.*]

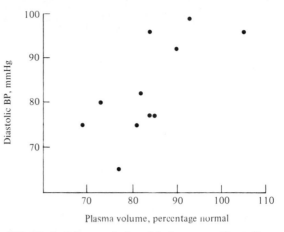

FIG. 10-6. Direct relationship between diastolic blood pressure and plasma volume in 11 essential hypertensive patients *during chronic diuretic treatment.* A similar relationship between diastolic blood pressure and plasma volume can be demonstrated with changes in sodium intake or the administration of sympathetic blocking agents. (*From H. P. Dustan, E. L. Bravo, and R. C. Tarazi, Am. J. Cardiol., 31:606, 1973.*)

secreted by the juxtaglomerular cells in the afferent arteriole of the glomerulus. A decrease in mean renal perfusion pressure, produced by effective volume depletion or stenosis in the renal arterial tree, and increased sympathetic activity are the major stimuli to renin release and initiate the sequence illustrated in Fig. 10-7.[35] Renin cleaves a decapeptide, angiotensin I, from renin substrate, an α_2 globulin produced in the liver. Angiotensin I is then converted into an octapeptide, angiotensin II. This reaction is catalyzed by *angiotensin converting enzyme,* which is located in many organs, including the lung, the luminal membrane of vascular endothelial cells, and the juxtaglomerular apparatus itself.[36]

Angiotensin II has two important effects which tend to elevate the BP; (1) it promotes renal sodium and water retention both by stimulating the secretion of aldosterone and by directly affecting the renal tubule; and (2) it is a potent vasoconstrictor, thereby increasing the SVR.[35,37] The latter effect may also be mediated in part by enhanced release of or sensitivity to norepinephrine.[38,39]

The role of angiotensin II in the maintenance of BP has been elucidated by the use of two classes of drugs: analogues of angiotensin II (such as saralasin) that are competitive antagonists of the native hormone; and, more importantly, converting enzyme inhibitors (CEI) that block the formation of angiotensin II from angiotensin I. The results obtained from the use of these drugs can be summarized by the following observations. Angiotensin II is of little importance in BP regulation in euvolemic subjects on a regular diet.[40,41] If, however, renin secretion is enhanced by the induction of volume depletion with a low-sodium diet or diuretics, the

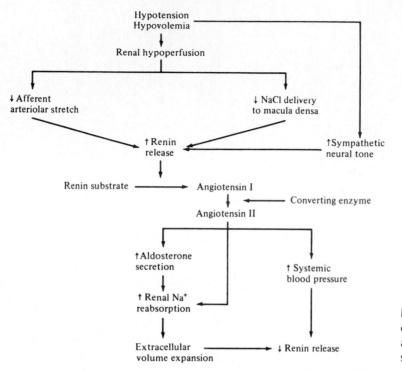

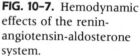

FIG. 10–7. Hemodynamic effects of the renin-angiotensin-aldosterone system.

resulting increase in angiotensin II production plays an important role in BP maintenance as evidenced by a hypotensive response to saralasin or CEI (Fig. 10–8).[40] A reduction in BP following angiotensin II inhibition is also seen in other normotensive conditions associated with effective circulating volume depletion and high renin secretion such as heart failure and hepatic cirrhosis.[42-44]

Similar results have been seen in essential hypertension. Most patients have a normal (70 percent) or mildly elevated plasma renin activity (PRA).[45] This finding can be considered to be inappropriate, since the elevation in BP should suppress renin secretion. Furthermore, angiotensin II appears to contribute to the hypertension as demonstrated by a fall in BP[46] and improvement in renal perfusion[47] in many patients following the administration of a CEI or an angiotensin antagonist.

The mechanisms responsible for renin secretion in hypertension are unclear; it is likely that renal ischemia or increased sympathetic tone are important in at least some patients. Untreated patients with high plasma renin levels tend to have enhanced sympathetic activity[48,49]; the administration of a β-adrenergic blocker such as propranolol is capable of both reducing renin release and lowering the BP in this setting.[48,50] The factors responsible for the hyperadrenergic state are uncertain (see below).

In addition to its effect in the untreated patient, angiotensin II may become more important in the maintenance of BP after the institution of antihypertensive therapy. The use of diuretics and vasodilators results in enhanced renin secretion; the ensuing increase in angiotensin II tends to blunt the antihypertensive effect of these drugs.[51,52]

The above discussion has considered the physiologic importance of the renin-angiotensin system in terms of the plasma renin activity. However, the chronic response to CEI treatment is not directly related to the baseline PRA; even patients with low renin levels may have a good hypotensive response,[53-55] *including bilaterally nephrectomized patients who have no renal renin.*[56] This effect may in part be due to increased production of vasodilator prostaglandins induced in an unknown manner by CEI.[53,57] It is also possible, however, that *extrarenal angiotensin II production* may be important in some patients. Complete renin-angiotensin systems have been identified in the central nervous system, the vascular endothelium, and the zona glomerulosa, the site of aldosterone production in the adrenal gland.[58-61] The activity of these systems may be regulated independent of renal renin release. For example, the local generation of angiotensin II may be an im-

portant determinant of vascular resistance.[59,60] This might explain at least in part the efficacy of CEI in hypertensive patients who have low plasma renin levels.[53-56]

There is also evidence that *intrarenal* angiotensin II may be physiologically important at a time when circulating levels are relatively low. Approximately 40 percent of patients with essential hypertension do not normally increase renal blood flow and urinary sodium excretion following a sodium load.[62] When these "nonmodulators" are compared to those with a normal response, the former have a greater increase in BP with volume expansion but suppress *plasma* renin, angiotensin II, and aldosterone levels to the same degree. Despite the reduced circulating concentration of angiotensin II, the abnormal renal and blood pressure responses in nonmodulators are reversed with the administration of a CEI, suggesting that the underlying problem may be enhanced intrarenal angiotensin II activity. Why this might occur is unknown.

A possible animal model of the nonmodulator is illustrated in Fig. 10–9. The chronic infusion of a subpressor dose of angiotensin II to a dog induces marked sodium sensitivity, as the BP rises with increments in sodium intake. This response, which is not seen in control dogs, may occur because the angiotensin II-induced *renal* vasoconstriction obligates a higher than normal systemic BP to excrete the extra dietary sodium (see "Role of the Kidney," below). It is possible, however, that increased release of aldosterone (which is not seen in the nonmodulator) could also contribute to the sodium sensitivity in this experiment.

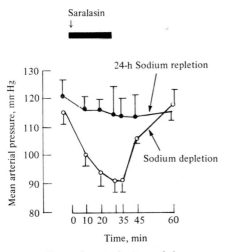

FIG. 10–8. Effect of an infusion of the angiotensin II inhibitor saralasin on the mean arterial pressure in sodium-repleted and sodium-depleted rats. A hypotensive response is seen only with sodium depletion. (*From H. Gavras, H. R. Brunner, E. D. Vaughan, Jr., and J. H. Laragh, Science, 180:1369, 1973. Copyright 1973 by the American Association for the Advancement of Science.*)

SYMPATHETIC NERVOUS SYSTEM

Sympathetic neural tone and the secretion of catecholamines from the adrenal medulla play an important role in the regulation of

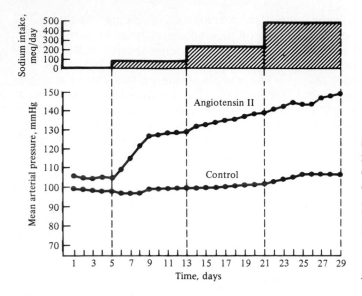

FIG. 10–9. Effect of changes in sodium intake on mean arterial pressure in control dogs and in those infused chronically with a low dose of angiotensin II. A significant rise in blood pressure with increasing sodium intake occurred only in the dogs given angiotensin II. (*From T. E. Hall, A. C. Guyton, M. J. Smith, Jr., and T. G. Coleman, Am. J. Physiol., 239:F271, 1980.*)

circulatory hemodynamics. In the presence of volume depletion or hypotension, the associated reduction in BP is sensed by the cardiac and arterial baroreceptors, resulting in a change in the rate of baroreceptor afferent discharge to the vasomotor centers in the brainstem.[63] These centers induce an increase in peripheral sympathetic outflow, initiating changes in arterial, venous, cardiac, and renal function that act to restore normal tissue perfusion (Fig. 10–10).

From these effects, it is apparent that an increase in sympathetic activity could induce hypertension by enhancing both cardiac output and SVR. Many examples of hyperadrenergic hypertension have been identified including pheochromocytoma and acute elevations in BP following cardiac bypass surgery, emotional stress, and traction to the femur in leg-lengthening operations in which stretching of the sciatic or femoral nerve is thought to be the initiating event.[64–67]

The role of the sympathetic nervous system in essential hypertension is less well established although it is clearly important in at least some patients.[68,69] As with renin secre-tion, sympathetic tone should be reduced by the elevation in BP. However, normal or mildly elevated plasma norepinephrine levels have been found in most patients with essential hypertension.[*,48,49,69–71] Furthermore, plasma levels may underestimate the total adrenergic effect since they may not detect (1) enhanced renal sympathetic tone, as evidenced by an elevation in the renal venous-arterial difference for norepinephrine or by a rise in urinary norepinephrine excretion,[68]

---

*The normal plasma norepinephrine concentration in many hypertensive patients may be a secondary response resulting from resetting of the arterial baroreceptors, so that the elevation in BP is not perceived by the central vasomotor centers. In this setting, some other factor may initiate the hypertension with the persistent sympathetic tone then contributing to its maintenance. Resetting has been repeatedly demonstrated in experimental forms of hypertension. It can develop within 48 h of the rise in BP[72] and appears to occur at the level of single carotid sinus fibers[73] with a possible contribution from central mechanisms.[74] Although maladaptive from the viewpoint of BP regulation, this response is not necessarily inappropriate since normal sympathetic tone permits the maintenance of a variety of other functions such as intestinal and sexual function and the defense against postural hypotension. Resetting is reversible with the restoration of normotension.[73]

(2) increased sensitivity to norepinephrine, an effect that may be mediated by an elevation in the cell calcium concentration (see "Dietary Factors: Calcium," below),[75] or (3) intermittent increments in sympathetic activity as might occur with emotional stress. As an example, patients with borderline hypertension or a positive family history in one or both parents frequently respond to stress differently from normals. When asked to perform intense mental tasks such as taking an IQ test, the "prehypertensive" subjects frequently develop an exaggerated sympathetic

response characterized by elevations in heart rate, BP, and plasma renin activity, and reductions in renal blood flow and urinary sodium excretion.[76-78] It is of interest that the spontaneously hypertensive rat also shows increased renal sympathetic nerve activity and a fall in sodium excretion with stress,[79] a response that appears to be centrally mediated by β_2-adrenergic receptors in the hypothalamus.[80] Furthermore, renal denervation attenuates the rise in BP in these animals.[79,81]

These findings suggest that genetically susceptible subjects may show an abnormal

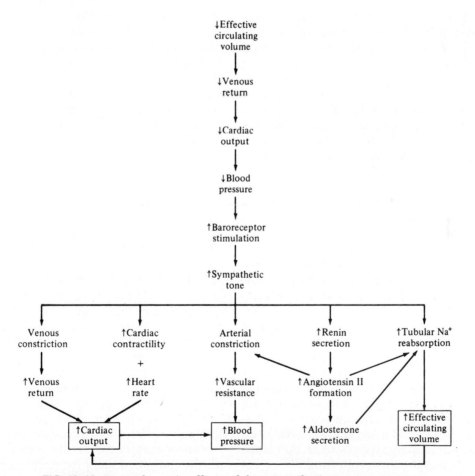

FIG. 10-10. Hemodynamic effects of the sympathetic nervous system.

sympathetic response to stress. It is possible that these intermittent elevations in BP could eventually become sustained. Epidemiologic studies have documented that hypertension is more prevalent with such stressful conditions as urban living and changing socioeconomic status.[82] Psychological studies of hypertensive patients have revealed conflicting data. However, evaluation of a small subgroup of patients with high plasma norepinephrine levels (when compared to those with normal levels) has shown an increased incidence of suppressed hostility, a behavior pattern linked to enhanced sympathetic activity.[49]

A contributory role of the sympathetic nervous system in the *maintenance* of essential hypertension is also suggested by the fall in BP toward normal that frequently follows the administration of sympathetic blockers.[83,84] These findings, however, do not necessarily imply that enhanced sympathetic activity is a primary event. Resetting of the baroreceptors to maintain normal sympathetic tone could explain the persistent adrenergic effect.

Increased sympathetic tone, however, may be important in the early stages of essential hypertension. In addition to the findings in "prehypertensive" subjects,[76-78] many patients with borderline hypertension have enhanced sympathetic activity (often leading to a high cardiac output)[19,22-24,85]; these hemodynamic abnormalities frequently return toward normal after the administration of a sympatholytic agent.[71,85]

Enhanced sympathetic activity also may play an important role in the association between obesity and hypertension.[86-88] In experimental animals, overfeeding enhances sympathetic tone, whereas fasting is capable of reversing this change and lowering the BP,[89] probably by decreasing central sympathetic outflow.[90] Similar results have been described in humans; weight reduction tends to ameliorate the hypertension,[87,88,91] a response that is associated with a fall in the plasma norepinephrine concentration.[91-93] These findings, however, do not necessarily prove a causal relationship, since elevated norepinephrine levels are also found in obese patients who are not hypertensive.[92]

ROLE OF THE KIDNEY

The kidney appears normal histologically in early essential hypertension. However, subtle alterations in renal function may play an important role in elevation in BP. Experimental support for this theory has come from studies of animals with hereditary hypertension. In both the Dahl rat (where the hypertension is exacerbated by a high sodium intake) and the spontaneously hypertensive rat, cross transplantation of kidneys from hypertension-prone to hypertension-resistant animals results in the development of hypertension.[94,95] Conversely, transplanting in the opposite direction protects against hypertension in previously susceptible rats.

There is suggestive evidence that a similar phenomenon may occur in humans.[96] Six patients with essential hypertension developed end-stage renal failure due to nephrosclerosis. They were then transplanted with kidneys from normotensive donors. At 4 to 5 years after transplantation, all the previously hypertensive patients had a normal BP. This finding is consistent with a central role for the kidney in the development of hypertension in these patients.

The importance of the kidney in hypertension can be best understood from consideration of the *pressure natriuresis* phenomenon.[97] In normal subjects, a small increase in BP produces a relatively large increment in urinary sodium excretion (Fig. 10–11). The mechanism by which this occurs is incompletely understood; decreased sodium reabsorption may occur in the proximal tubule of the juxtamedullary (or deep) nephrons or in the loop of Henle.[98,99] Transmission of the

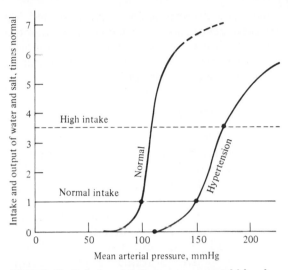

FIG. 10-11. Relationship between arterial blood pressure and urinary sodium chloride and water excretion in normal subjects and in patients with hypertension. (*From A. C. Guyton, T. G. Coleman, A. W. Cowley, Jr., K. W. Scheel, R. D. Manning, Jr., and R. A. Norman, Jr., Am. J. Med., 52:584, 1972.*)

increased arterial pressure to the medullary interstitium could, for example, reduce passive reabsorption out of the thin and thick ascending limbs of the loop of Henle.[99] Regardless of the mechanism, this relationship may be important in the maintenance of sodium balance. A rise in sodium intake sequentially increases the plasma volume, venous return to the heart, cardiac output, and BP. The last effect then promotes excretion of the excess sodium, returning circulatory hemodynamics to normal. The influence of other factors such as aldosterone will modify but not basically alter this process.[97]

The relationship between BP and sodium excretion must be altered in hypertension (Fig. 10-11). If sodium intake is equivalent, the patients with hypertension will excrete the same amount of sodium as a normal person but at a higher BP. This resetting

upward may be explained by different mechanisms in three forms of hypertension[97]: (1) in primary hyperaldosteronism, the elevation in distal sodium reabsorption will minimize the natriuresis induced by the high BP; (2) in renal failure, there are fewer functioning nephrons on which the BP can act; and (3) in essential hypertension, *renal vasoconstriction* with a 20 to 25 percent reduction in renal blood flow is an early finding in up to two-thirds of patients.[100,101] This abnormality may result in less of the systemic BP being transmitted to the kidney and therefore less efficient pressure natriuresis (as exemplified in the experiment in Fig. 10-9). The enhanced renal vascular resistance may be mediated by increased sympathetic tone or angiotensin II production, since renal perfusion can be improved with the use of sympathetic blockers or CEI.[101-103] (The mechanism by which the kidney might predispose to the development of hypertension in those patients whose renal blood flow is elevated, not reduced, is uncertain.[104])

The importance of intrarenal pressure in regulating the degree of hypertension is illustrated by the experiment in Fig. 10-12. If angiotensin II is chronically perfused at a uniform rate but the renal artery pressure is held constant by an arterial clamp, *severe and progressive* hypertension, sodium retention, and pulmonary edema occur. In comparison, releasing the arterial clamp raises the renal artery pressure, rapidly increasing sodium excretion and lowering the BP to a stable, only moderately elevated level. These results suggest that intrarenal hypertension is beneficial in this setting in that it limits sodium retention and therefore the rise in BP.

In addition to these primary changes in renal function, chronic hypertension can produce vascular damage that can contribute to the maintenance of the high BP (see p. 500). This could explain why as many as 25 percent of patients with primary hyperaldosteronism or Cushing's syndrome remain

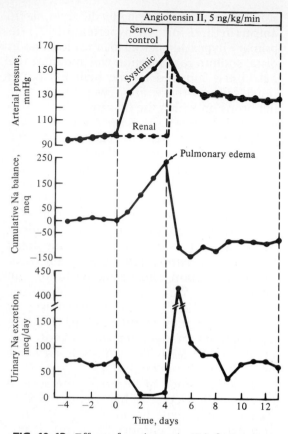

FIG. 10–12. Effect of angiotensin II infusion in a dog in which renal artery pressure was initially servo-controlled at the baseline level. Severe and progressive hypertension, sodium and water retention, and pulmonary edema developed by the fourth day of infusion. When the renal artery pressure was then allowed to rise to the systemic level, there was a rapid increase in sodium excretion and the blood pressure fell to a stable and less elevated value. (*From J. E. Hall, J. P. Granger, R. L. Hester, T. G. Coleman, M. J. Smith, Jr., and R. B. Cross, Am. J. Physiol., 246:F627, 1984.*)

hypertensive after cure of the endocrine abnormality.[105] Renal biopsy in these patients reveals arteriolar hyperplasia and glomerular sclerosis, alterations that are compatible with hypertensive injury. It is also possible, how-

ever, that underlying essential hypertension (which occurs in approximately 25 percent of the adult population) could contribute to the persistent elevation in BP and secondary renal damage in this setting.

REDUCED SECRETION OF VASODILATORS

The renal vasoconstriction that is present in many hypertensive patients could be due to reduced secretion of vasodilators, rather than enhanced release of angiotensin II or norepinephrine. The kidney normally produces a variety of vasodilators that could act as antihypertensive hormones including prostaglandins, bradykinin, and the renomedullary lipids.[106-109] The potential antihypertensive role of the medullary lipids is suggested by the following observations in experimental forms of hypertension: destruction of the renal medulla or administration of an antagonist of the renomedullary lipids exacerbates the hypertension[110,111]; in comparison, subcutaneous implantation of tissue from the renal medulla (but not the renal cortex) lowers the BP toward normal.[109,112]

The applicability of these findings to humans is uncertain. As many as one-third of patients with essential hypertension may have low urinary prostaglandin E_2 excretion,[106] a change that could contribute to renal vasoconstriction. In the majority of patients, however, it is likely that the secretion of vasodilator prostaglandins, perhaps induced by angiotensin II or norepinephrine,[113] appropriately minimizes the rise in BP. This possibility is suggested by the response to the administration of nonsteroidal anti-inflammatory drugs (NSAID), which diminish prostaglandin synthesis. These agents have no effect on BP in normals but can increase the BP in patients with hypertension.[106,114-117] It is of interest in this regard that sulindac, a NSAID that appears to be much less likely to reduce renal prostaglandin synthesis (see pp. 82, 83), also is less likely to raise the BP than other NSAID when given to hypertensive patients.[115-117] These findings are consistent with an appropriate antihypertensive effect of renal prostaglandins in most patients with essential hypertension.

Another potential abnormality is decreased release or effectiveness of atrial natriuretic peptide (ANP), a hormone that causes both renal vasodilation and an increase in sodium excretion. In one study of patients with essential hypertension, plasma ANP levels were elevated, a change that could represent an *appropriate* response to initial sodium retention.[118] The cause of this defect in sodium excretion remains unclear, however, as any of the factors described above (such as angiotensin II or norepinephrine) could contribute. Alternatively, the early sodium retention and rise in ANP could reflect reduced renal responsiveness to ANP, an abnormality that has been demonstrated in the salt-sensitive Dahl rat.[119]

DIETARY FACTORS

Dietary factors are thought to play an important role in the development of hypertension. Increased intake of sodium, calories (in obesity), and alcohol and reduced intake of calcium and potassium all may be important in selected patients.

SODIUM

There is a large body of evidence suggesting that sodium intake is a major factor in the production of hypertension in humans.[120,121] These data can be summarized by the following observations:

1. Epidemiologic studies of different societies suggest that the frequency of hypertension is directly related to sodium chloride intake, with virtually no hypertension being seen when daily salt intake is 3 g (50 meq) or less (Fig. 10–13).[120-122] A low sodium intake also appears to attenuate the rise in BP that normally occurs with aging.[121]

2. Forty to sixty percent of patients with essential hypertension show sodium sensitivity as evidenced by a rise in BP with sodium loading and/or a reduction in BP with dietary sodium restriction (see p. 522).[121,123-127] This pro-hypertensive effect of a high sodium intake may be demonstrable within the first few months of life. Newborns fed a high sodium diet had a small (2 to 2.5 mmHg) but statistically significant elevation in BP when compared to normally fed infants.[128]

FIG. 10–13. Correlation of average daily sodium intake (as estimated from 24-h urine sodium excretion) and prevalence of hypertension in different geographic areas. Hypertension is defined as a diastolic blood pressure greater than 90 mmHg and/or a systolic blood pressure greater than 140 mmHg. The different points for the United States are grouped according to sodium excretion. (*Adapted from G. A. MacGregor, Hypertension, 7:628, 1985. By permission of the American Heart Association, Inc.*)

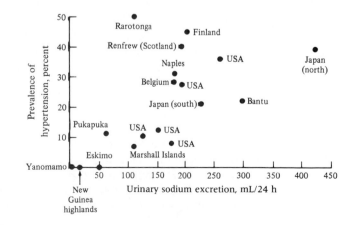

Despite these findings, it is essential to note that only a minority of patients become hypertensive. Therefore, *sodium intake contributes to the development of hypertension only in susceptible individuals.* In this setting, even "normal" levels of dietary sodium may be deleterious. This requirement for some genetic or acquired abnormality probably explains why dietary evaluation of hypertensive patients has not been able to demonstrate any increase in sodium intake when compared to normals.[129] On the other hand, the ingestion of extremely high levels of sodium (up to 1500 meq/day) produces only a minor elevation in BP in nonsusceptible subjects.[130]

Mechanism of Sodium Sensitivity. The mechanism by which sodium intake can cause hypertension is not well understood. One still theoretical possibility is outlined in Fig. 10–14.[131,132] As described above, there is evidence that a renal abnormality is responsible for the genetic tendency to hypertension. This is manifested in part by a relative defect in sodium excretion possibly due, for example, to an inability to appropriately suppress angiotensin II production or sympathetic tone.[34,62,124,127] In this setting, even a normal sodium intake will initially lead to sodium retention. The ensuing volume expansion will shut off the renin-angiotensin system (most sodium-sensitive patients have a relatively low plasma renin activity)[126,133] and can stimulate the release of a natriuretic hormone, perhaps from the hypothalamus, that is an endogenous digitalis-like compound (EDLC) in that it inhibits Na-K-ATPase activity. (This hormone is distinct from the atrial natriuretic peptides, which are vasodilators and do not affect Na-K-ATPase.[134]) The EDLC will have two effects: the natriuresis will restore euvolemia; and the decreased activity of the Na-K pump will result in an increase in the cell sodium concentration, since there is less sodium extrusion

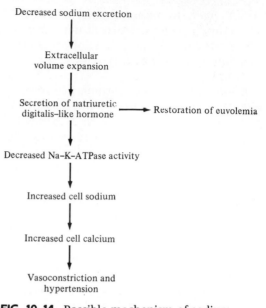

FIG. 10–14. Possible mechanism of sodium-sensitive hypertension in which impaired renal excretion of sodium is the primary abnormality and a natriuretic endogenous digitalis-like compound indirectly leads to systemic vasoconstriction.

from the cell. The elevation in cell sodium will diminish the gradient favoring passive sodium entry into the cell, thereby diminishing calcium efflux which normally occurs in part by passive sodium-calcium exchange. The subsequent rise in cell calcium can then cause vasoconstriction and hypertension, either by a direct effect or by increasing the responsiveness to vasoconstrictors such as angiotensin II and norepinephrine.

This model can also explain the antihypertensive effect of diuretics. The initial fall in BP with these agents is associated with plasma volume depletion and a decrease in cardiac output. With time, these parameters may return toward normal, with a reduction in SVR contributing to the fall in BP even though diuretics are not direct vasodilators.[135,136] It is possible that the initial volume depletion decreased the release of EDLC, resulting sequentially in enhanced activity of the Na-K pump, a fall in cell sodium, a fall in cell calcium, and vasodilatation.

There are a variety of mostly indirect findings that support this hypothesis. The cell sodium concentration (in circulating white cells and red cells) is elevated in many patients with hypertension, in association with a decrease in Na-K-ATPase activity.[131,132,137,138] An increase in cell sodium can also be demonstrated in many normotensive first-degree relatives of hypertensive patients[139] and can be at least partially reversed with the use of diuretics.[131,140] Assays for measurement of a circulating inhibitor of Na-K-ATPase are frequently positive,[138,141-143] particularly in patients with a low plasma renin activity.[143] Similar findings have been reported in experimental animals with sodium-sensitive forms of hypertension.[144] Finally, an elevation in the cell calcium concentration (as measured in platelets) is a common finding in essential hypertension and correlates closely both with the rise in BP in untreated patients (Fig. 10–15) and with the fall in BP that occurs

after the administration of antihypertensive medications (see Fig. 11–16).[145]

It must be emphasized, however, that this hypothesis remains unproven. In contrast to the enormous amount of information that has recently accumulated on the atrial natriuretic peptides,[146] the existence or site of origin of an EDLC has yet to be convincingly demonstrated. Furthermore, alternative explanations are possible for the impairment in cell transport. For example, insulin normally stimulates Na-K-ATPase activity. Obesity is common in hypertension[86-88]; this condition is typically associated with insulin resistance, which could be responsible for the reduction in Na-K-ATPase activity.[147]

In addition, decreased activity of the Na-K pump is not a universal finding in sodium-sensitive hypertension. Na-K-ATPase activity is actually increased in the Dahl rat and in some patients,[148,149] suggesting that a membrane abnormality favoring sodium entry into the cell may be a primary event, leading to a secondary rise in sodium extrusion by the pump. In this regard, enhanced sodium-lithium countertransport in red cells has

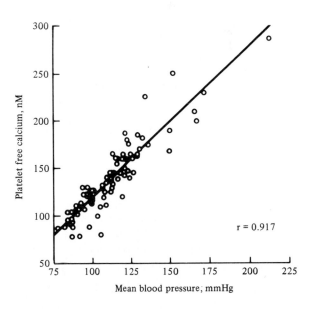

FIG. 10–15. Correlation between mean arterial pressure and intracellular free calcium concentration in platelets of 38 normotensive subjects, 9 patients with borderline hypertension, and 45 patients with established essential hypertension. (*From P. Erne, P. Bolli, E. Burgisser, and F. R. Buhler, N. Engl. J. Med., 310:1084, 1984. Reprinted by permission from the New England Journal of Medicine.*)

been found in many patients with essential hypertension and in many of their normotensive first-degree relatives,[150-152] some of whom show an elevation in BP with time.[153] It is as yet unclear if this change in red cell sodium transport is merely a marker for the development of hypertension or is of direct pathogenetic importance. It has been suggested that sodium-lithium countertransport might be similar to the sodium-hydrogen exchanger that is present in many cells, including those of the renal proximal tubule.[154] Increased sodium-hydrogen exchange theoretically could lead to hypertension by several mechanisms. Enhanced proximal sodium reabsorption, for example, could promote sodium retention and initiate the sequence illustrated in Fig. 10–14.[155] Alternatively, a transporter-mediated increment in sodium entry into vascular smooth muscle cells could raise the cell sodium and, secondarily, the cell calcium, producing vasoconstriction and hypertension.[154]

It may also be important to consider the role of *chloride* in sodium-sensitive hypertension. In both animals and humans with hypertension, the BP can be elevated by the administration of sodium with chloride but not with a nonhalide anion such as citrate or ascorbate.[156-158] This difference in BP response occurs despite the same degree of sodium retention and similar suppression of the renin-angiotensin system with both diets. However, the sodium chloride-treated group has a much larger increase in urinary calcium excretion, suggesting that changes in calcium metabolism might be responsible for the rise in BP.[158]

CALCIUM

It has recently been suggested that a defect in calcium handling (Table 10–2) may be of primary importance in many patients with essential hypertension, possibly exceeding the

TABLE 10–2. Abnormalities in Calcium Balance in Essential Hypertension

Decreased dietary intake
Urinary calcium leak (aggravated by sodium chloride intake)
Low plasma ionized calcium
Secondary hyperparathyroidism and elevated calcitriol levels
Elevated intracellular calcium (could account for vasoconstriction)
Impairment in cellular calcium metabolism

role of sodium.[159-161] The prevalence of essential hypertension appears to be inversely related to dietary calcium intake, with the risk rising two to three times as daily calcium intake falls from 1200 to less than 300 mg.[129] Many patients also have a high rate of urinary calcium excretion, a slightly decreased plasma ionized calcium concentration, and elevated levels of circulating parathyroid hormone and calcitriol.[159,161-163] These findings are compatible with a primary urinary calcium leak; they are most prominent in low-renin hypertension,[161] a setting in which salt sensitivity is more likely[126,133] and in which a high salt intake may promote calcium excretion.[158] There may, therefore, be a link between the roles of sodium and calcium in the development of hypertension. Calcium supplementation (1000 mg/day) can lower the BP by 10 mmHg or more in many of these patients.[164]

How these changes are related to the increase in the cell calcium concentration (see Fig. 10–15) that is presumed to be responsible for the rise in systemic vascular resistance is unclear. It seems paradoxical that reductions in dietary calcium intake and the plasma calcium concentration are associated with a rise in cell calcium. There is evidence, however, that calcium can inhibit its own flux across the cell membrane; as a result, hypocalcemia could promote calcium accumulation within the cells.[164]

It is also possible, however, that the elevated intracellular (particularly cytosolic) calcium concentration in essential hypertension is related to an impairment in cellular calcium metabolism. In this regard, defects in calmodulin binding and Ca-ATPase have been described.[159]

POTASSIUM

Dietary potassium intake is another potential influence on the systemic BP. In both animal models and patients with essential hypertension, potassium supplementation has been shown to produce a moderate fall in BP, averaging 5 to 6 mmHg in humans.[165-168] These findings have led to the suggestion that decreased potassium intake, as occurs in rural blacks, could be a contributing factor to the development of hypertension.[169]

How potassium affects the BP is not well understood.[166] It seems to be most effective in sodium-sensitive forms of hypertension and may act in part by enhancing urinary sodium excretion.[165,167] Potassium loading has been shown to reduce sodium reabsorption in the loop of Henle, an effect that may be appropriate for potassium homeostasis since the ensuing rise in sodium and water delivery to the distal nephron will promote secretion of the extra potassium.[170]

OBESITY

The incidence of hypertension is increased in obese patients.[88,171] Furthermore, when the National Health and Nutrition Examination Survey (NHANES) compared hypertensives to normals, higher body mass index was one of the major predictors of hypertension along with increasing age and, to a lesser degree, a positive family history.[172] A similar trend has been observed in children,

as obesity is almost 4 times as prevalent (53 versus 14 percent) in hypertensives.[173] The importance of obesity can also be illustrated by the reduction in BP that typically follows weight reduction, an effect that is independent of changes in sodium intake.[87,88,91]

The hypertension associated with obesity is characterized by elevations in plasma volume and cardiac output.[88,174] The SVR may be near normal but is higher than in normotensive obese patients.[174] Enhanced sympathetic activity,[92,93] perhaps induced by overeating,[89] is present in many obese patients and may play an important pathogenetic role. However, other factors are also likely to contribute to the rise in BP. For example, obesity is commonly associated with insulin resistance in peripheral tissues. The ensuing rise in insulin secretion could then augment renal sodium reabsorption (via a direct effect of insulin on the renal tubule),[175] leading to volume expansion and hypertension.[147] It is of interest that insulin also enhances Na-K-ATPase activity; consequently, insulin resistance could be responsible for the frequently observed reduction in activity of the Na-K pump.[147] This could raise the cell sodium and calcium concentrations, producing hypertension and vasoconstriction, as illustrated in Fig. 10–14.

ALCOHOL

Another potentially important factor in the development of hypertension is the excessive ingestion of alcohol.[176-178] Patients who have more than two drinks per day are 1.5 to 2 times as likely to become hypertensive[176]; lesser degrees of alcohol intake do not seem to produce this deleterious effect.

It is unclear how alcohol raises the BP. Intermittent withdrawal leading to enhanced sympathetic activity is one possibility, although this does not appear to be important in most patients. In general, the plasma volume, plasma levels of norepinephrine and renin, and urinary sodium excretion are normal in hypertensive patients with excessive alcohol intake.[179,180] Regardless of the mechanism, abstinence can lower the BP which, in one study of 16 patients, fell from 175/105 to 155/98.[179] On the other hand, restarting alcohol ingestion led to recurrent hypertension.

OTHER

Other dietary factors are less likely to play a role in the development of hypertension. Both smoking and caffeine have been shown to acutely raise the BP by as much as 10 to 12 mmHg.[181,182] However, this effect is acute, lasting less than 2 h, and is not seen with continuing use.[183] Thus, smoking does not appear to increase the incidence of hypertension,[178] although it does increase the risk of cardiovascular complications (see p. 500).

HEREDITY AND RACE

A genetic predisposition to becoming hypertensive appears to be important in many patients. Approximately 70 to 80 percent of patients with essential hypertension have a positive family history, in contrast to 40 percent or less for those with secondary hypertension due to renal artery stenosis.[184] If both parents are hypertensive, the risk of high BP in the offspring is roughly 2.5 times that if neither parent is hypertensive.[185] Furthermore, even normotensive relatives of hypertensive patients may have a somewhat higher BP than normotensive subjects with no family history of hypertension.[104,186]

This familial aggregation alone, however, does not necessarily distinguish between heredity and shared environmental factors. More convincing evidence has come from observations on *BP correlations within families:* this correlation is stronger between parents and children than between spouses[187]; is stronger between identical twins than between fraternal twins or siblings[187]; and does not exist between parents and adopted children.[188] Each of these findings is consistent with an important genetic influence in the development of hypertension.

Rather than being mediated by a single gene, the hereditary tendency to hypertension probably reflects the interaction of multiple genes.[187] These genes can affect many of the factors described above, including the vascular responsiveness to stress,[77,78] renal function,[96] and cellular sodium transport.[152,153]

Race is another consideration in hypertension. In particular, an elevation in BP is more common and more severe in blacks.[1,189,190] This is manifested by a threefold increase in overall mortality from hypertension, a six- to sevenfold increase in mortality in patients under the age of 50, and an eighteenfold rise in the incidence of end-stage renal failure from hypertensive nephrosclerosis.[189,191]

The factors responsible for the hypertension in blacks are incompletely understood. These patients frequently have a slight increase in plasma volume, a low plasma renin activity, and a more pronounced hypotensive response to diuretic therapy than whites.[189,190,192] This constellation of findings suggests that initial volume expansion due to retention of dietary sodium may play a primary role in this setting. Furthermore, the relatively low level of vasoconstrictors could lead to more of the systemic BP being transmitted to the kidney, an effect that could account for the markedly increased incidence of renal damage (see Chap. 4).

SUMMARY

Essential hypertension is a heterogeneous disorder in which multiple genetic, neurohumoral, and dietary factors can contribute to the elevation in BP (see Table 10–1). As will be seen in the next chapter, an understanding of these factors is frequently helpful in choosing an optimal antihypertensive regimen. For example, diuretics may be particularly effective in black patients in whom relative volume expansion appears to play an important role[192]; a sympathetic blocker is preferable in young patients with enhanced sympathetic activity and, frequently, an elevated cardiac output[19,71]; and a converting enzyme inhibitor can reverse the hemodynamic abnormalities induced by increased angiotensin II production.[46,53,62]

REFERENCES

1. Final Report of the Subcommittee on Definition and Prevalence of the 1984 Joint National Committee: Hypertension prevalence and the status of awareness, treatment and control in the United States, *Hypertension,* 7:457, 1985.

2. Veterans Administration Cooperative Study Group on Antihypertensive Agents: Effects of treatment on morbidity in hypertension: Results in patients with diastolic blood pressure averaging 115 through 129 mmHg, *J. Am. Med. Assoc.,* 202:1028, 1967.

3. Veterans Administration Cooperative Study Group on Antihypertensive Agents: Effects of treatment on morbidity in hypertension. II: Results in patients with diastolic blood pressure averaging 90 through 114 mmHg, *J. Am. Med. Assoc.,* 213:1143, 1970.

4. Hypertension Detection and Follow-up Program Cooperative Group: Five-year findings of the Hypertension Detection and Follow-up Program: I. Reduction in mortality of persons with high blood pressure, including mild hypertension; II. Mortality by race, sex, and age, *J. Am. Med. Assoc.,* 242: 2562, 2572, 1979.

5. Medical Research Council Working Party: MRC trial of treatment of mild hypertension: Principal results, *Br. Med. J.,* 291:97, 1985.

6. Narins, R. G.: Mild hypertension: A therapeutic dilemma, *Kidney Int.,* 26:881, 1984.

7. Pickering G.: Hypertension, *Am. J. Med.,* 52:570, 1972.

8. Lew, A.: High blood pressure, other risk factors and longevity: The insurance viewpoint, *Am. J. Med.,* 55:281, 1973.

9. Multiple Risk Factor Intervention Trial Research Group: MRFIT: Risk factor changes and mortality results, *J. Am. Med. Assoc.,* 248:1465, 1982.

10. Hyman, D., and N. M. Kaplan: Treatment of patients with mild hypertension, *Hypertension,* 7:165, 1985.

11. Kannel, W. B.: Role of blood pressure in cardiovascular morbidity and mortality, *Prog. Cardiovasc. Dis.,* 17:5, 1975.

12. Roberts, W. C.: The hypertensive diseases: Evidence that systolic hypertension is a greater risk factor to the development of other cardiovascular diseases than previously suspected, *Am. J. Med.,* 59:523, 1975.

13. Amery, A., W. Birkenhager, R. Brixko, et al.: Efficacy of antihypertensive drug treatment according to age, sex, blood pressure, and previous cardiovascular disease in patients over the age of 60, *Lancet,* 2:589, 1986.

14. Memorandum from the WHO/ISH Meeting: 1986 guidelines for the treatment of mild hypertension, *Hypertension,* 8:957, 1986.

15. The 1984 Report of the Joint National Committee on Detection, Evaluation, and Treatment of High Blood Pressure, *Arch. Intern. Med.,* 144:1045, 1984.

16. Lieberman, E.: Essential hypertension in children and youth: A pediatric perspective, *J. Pediatr.,* 85:1, 1974.

17. Page, E. W., and R. Christianson: The impact of mean arterial pressure in the middle trimester upon the outcome of pregnancy, *Am. J. Obstet. Gynecol.,* 125:740, 1976.

18. Koch-Weser, J.: Correlation of pathophysiology and pharmacotherapy in primary hypertension, *Am. J. Cardiol.,* 32:499, 1973.

19. Simon, A. C., M. A. Safar, J. A. Levenson, A. M. Kheder, and B. I. Levi: Systolic hypertension: Hemodynamic mechanism and choice of antihypertensive treatment, *Am. J. Cardiol.,* 44:505, 1979.

20. Bohlen, H. G.: Localization of vascular resistance changes during hypertension, *Hypertension,* 8:181, 1986.

21. Messerli, F. H., K. Sundgaard-Riise, H. O. Ventura, F. G. Dunn, L. B. Glade, and E. D. Frohlich: Essential hypertension in the elderly: Haemodynamics,

intravascular volume, plasma renin activity, and circulating catecholamine levels, *Lancet,* 2:983, 1983.

22. Eich, R. H., R. P. Cuddy, H. Smulyan, and R. H. Lyons: Hemodynamics in labile hypertension: A follow-up study, *Circulation,* 34:299, 1966.

23. Weiss, Y. A., M. E. Safar, G. M. London, A. C. Simon, J. A. Levenson, and P. M. Milliez: Repeat hemodynamic determinations in borderline hypertension, *Am. J. Med.,* 64:382, 1978.

24. Levenson, J. A., A. C. Simon, M. E. Safar, J. D. Bouthier, and G. M. London: Evaluation of brachial arterial blood velocity and volumic flow mediated by peripheral β-adrenoreceptors in patients with borderline hypertension, *Circulation,* 71:663, 1985.

25. Guyton, A. C.: *Arterial Pressure and Hypertension,* Saunders, Philadelphia, 1980, chap. 5.

26. Thomson, G. E.: Hypertension in the black population, *Cardiovasc. Rev. Rep.,* 2:351, 1981.

27. Messerli, F. H., K. Sundgaard-Riise, E. Reisin, G. Dreslinski, F. G. Dunn, and E. Frohlich: Disparate cardiovascular effects of obesity and arterial hypertension, *Am. J. Med.,* 74:808, 1983.

28. Dustan, H. P., R. C. Tarazi, E. L. Bravo, and R. A. Dart: Plasma and extracellular fluid volumes in hypertension, *Circ. Res.,* 32(suppl. 1):73, 1973.

29. London, G. M., J. A. Levenson, A. M. London, A. C. Simon, and M. E. Safar: Systemic compliance, renal hemodynamics, and sodium excretion in hypertension, *Kidney Int.,* 26:342, 1984.

30. Dustan, H. E., E. L. Bravo, and R. C. Tarazi: Volume-dependent essential and steroid hypertension, *Am. J. Cardiol.,* 31:606, 1973.

31. Finnerty, F. A., Jr.: Relationship of extracellular fluid volume to the development of drug resistance in the hypertensive patient, *Am. Heart J.,* 81:563, 1971.

32. Finnerty, F. A., Jr., M. Davidov, W. J. Mroczek, and L. Gavrilovich: Influence of extracellular fluid volume on response to antihypertensive drugs, *Circ. Res.,* 27(suppl. 1):71, 1970.

33. Frye, R. L., and E. Braunwald: Studies on Starling's law of the heart. I: The circulatory response to acute hypervolemia and its modification by ganglionic blockade, *J. Clin. Invest.,* 39:1043, 1960.

34. Campese, V. M., M. S. Romoff, D. Levitan, Y. Saglikes, R. M. Friedler, and S. G. Massry: Abnormal relationship between sodium intake and sympathetic nervous system activity in salt-sensitive patients with essential hypertension, *Kidney Int.,* 21:371, 1982.

35. Rose, B. D.: *Clinical Physiology of Acid-Base and Elec-*trolyte *Disorders,* 2d ed., McGraw-Hill, New York, 1984, chap. 3.

36. Inagami, T., M. Kawamura, K. Naruse, and T. Okamura: Localization of components of the renin-angiotensin system within the kidney, *Fed. Proc.,* 45:1414, 1986.

37. Hall, J. E.: Regulation of glomerular filtration rate and sodium excretion by angiotensin II, *Fed. Proc.,* 45:1431, 1986.

38. Malik, K. U., and A. Nasjletti: Facilitation of adrenergic transmission by locally generated angiotensin II in rat mesenteric arteries, *Circ. Res.,* 38:26, 1976.

39. Spertini, F., H. R. Brunner, B. Waeber, and H. Gavras: The opposing effects of chronic angiotensin converting enzyme blockade by captopril on the responses to exogenous angiotensin II and vasopressin vs. norepinephrine in rats, *Circ. Res.,* 48:612, 1981.

40. Gavras, H., H. R. Brunner, E. D. Vaughan, Jr., and J. H. Laragh: Angiotensin-sodium interaction in blood pressure maintenance of renal hypertensive and normotensive rats, *Science,* 180:1369, 1973.

41. Noth, R. H., S. Y. Jan, and P. J. Mulrow: Effects of angiotensin II blockade by saralasin in normal man, *J. Clin. Endocrinol. Metab.,* 45:10, 1977.

42. Watkins, L., Jr., J. A. Burton, E. Haber, J. R. Cant, F. W. Smith, and A. C. Barger: The renin-angiotensin-aldosterone system in congestive failure in conscious dogs, *J. Clin. Invest.,* 57:1606, 1976.

43. Francis, G. S., S. R. Goldsmith, T. B. Levine, M. T. Olivari, and J. N. Cohn: The neurohumoral axis in congestive heart failure, *Ann. Intern. Med.,* 101:370, 1984.

44. Schroeder, E. T., G. H. Anderson, S. H. Goldman, and D. H. P. Streeten: Effect of blockade of angiotensin II on blood pressure, renin and aldosterone in cirrhosis, *Kidney Int.,* 9:511, 1976.

45. Laragh, J. H., L. Baer, H. R. Brunner, F. R. Buhler, J. E. Sealey, and E. D. Vaughan, Jr.: Renin, angiotensin and aldosterone system in pathogenesis and management of hypertensive vascular disease, *Am. J. Med.,* 52:633, 1972.

46. Veterans Administration Cooperative Study on Antihypertensive Agents: Low-dose captopril for the treatment of mild to moderate hypertension, *Hypertension,* 5(suppl. III):III-139, 1983.

47. Hollenberg, N. K., S. L. Swartz, D. R. Passan, and G. H. Williams: Increased glomerular filtration rate after converting-enzyme inhibition in essential hypertension, *N. Engl. J. Med.,* 301:9, 1979.

48. Esler, M., A. Zweifler, O. Randall, S. Julius, and V. DeQuattro: The determinants of plasma renin ac-

tivity in essential hypertension, *Ann. Intern. Med.,* 88:746, 1978.

49. Esler, M., S. Julius, A. Zweifler, O. Randall, E. Garburg, H. Gardiner, and V. DeQuattro: Mild high-renin hypertension: Neurogenic human hypertension?, *N. Engl. J. Med.,* 296:405, 1977.

50. Buhler, F. R., J. H. Laragh, L. Baer, E. D. Vaughan, Jr., and H. R. Brunner: Propranolol inhibition of renin secretion, *N. Engl. J. Med.,* 287:1209, 1972.

51. Vaughan, E. D., Jr., R. M. Carey, M. J. Peach, J. A. Ackerly, and C. R. Ayers: The renin response to diuretic therapy: A limitation of anti-hypertensive potential, *Circ. Res.,* 42:376, 1978.

52. Pettinger, W. A., and K. Keeton: Altered renin release and propranolol potentiation of vasodilator drug hypotension, *J. Clin. Invest.,* 55:236, 1975.

53. Zusman, R. M.: Renin- and non-renin-mediated antihypertensive actions of converting enzyme inhibitors, *Kidney Int.,* 25:969, 1984.

54. Wenting, G. J., J. H. B. DeBruyn, A. J. Man in't Veld, A. J. J. Woittiez, F. H. M. Derkx, and M. A. D. H. Schalekamp: Hemodynamic effects of captopril in essential hypertension, renovascular hypertension and cardiac failure: Correlations with short- and long-term effects on plasma renin, *Am. J. Cardiol.,* 49:1453, 1982.

55. Wilkins, L. H., H. P. Dustan, J. F. Walker, and S. Oparil: Enalapril in low-renin essential hypertension, *Clin. Pharmacol. Therap.,* 34:297, 1983.

56. Man in't Veld, A. J., I. M. Schicht, F. H. Derkx, J. H. de Bruyn, and M. A. D. H. Schalekamp: Effects of an angiotensin-converting enzyme inhibitor (captopril) on blood pressure in anephric subjects, *Br. Med. J.,* 280:288, 1980.

57. Moore, T. J., F. R. Crantz, N. K. Hollenberg, R. J. Koletsky, M. S. Leboff, S. L. Swartz, L. Levine, S. Podolsky, R. G. Dluhy, and G. H. Williams: Contribution of prostaglandins to the antihypertensive action of captopril in essential hypertension, *Hypertension,* 3:168, 1981.

58. Genain, C. P., G. R. van Loon, and T. A. Kotchen: Distribution of renin activity and angiotensinogen in rat brain. Effects of dietary sodium chloride intake on brain renin, *J. Clin. Invest.,* 76:1939, 1985.

59. Oliver, J. A., and R. R. Sciacca: Local generation of angiotensin II as a mechanism of regulation of peripheral vascular tone in the rat, *J. Clin. Invest.,* 74:1247, 1984.

60. Dzau, V. J.: Significance of the vascular renin-angiotensin pathway, *Hypertension,* 8:553, 1986.

61. Doi, Y., K. Atarashi, R. Franco-Saenz, and P. J. Mulrow: Effect of changes in sodium or potassium balance, and nephrectomy, on adrenal renin and aldosterone concentrations, *Hypertension,* 6(suppl. I):I-124, 1984.

62. Redgrave, J., S. Rabinowe, N. K. Hollenberg, and G. H. Williams: Correction of abnormal renal blood flow response to angiotensin II by converting enzyme inhibition in essential hypertensives, *J. Clin. Invest.,* 75:1285, 1985.

63. Vick, R. L.: *Contemporary Medical Physiology,* Addison-Wesley, California, 1984, chap. 8.

64. Tarazi, R. C., F. G. Estafanous, and F. M. Fouad: Unilateral stellate block in the treatment of hypertension after coronary bypass surgery, *Am. J. Cardiol.,* 42:1013, 1978.

65. Fouad, F. M., F. G. Estafanous, E. L. Bravo, K. A. Iyer, J. H. Maydak, and R. C. Tarazi: Possible role of cardioaortic reflexes in postcoronary bypass hypertension, *Am. J. Cardiol.,* 44:866, 1979.

66. Kuchel, O.: Pseudopheochromocytoma, *Hypertension,* 7:151, 1985.

67. Yosipovitch, Z. H., and Y. Palti: Alterations in blood pressure during leg lengthening, *J. Bone Joint Surg.,* 49-A:1352, 1967.

68. Oparil, S.: The sympathetic nervous system in clinical and experimental hypertension, *Kidney Int.,* 30:437, 1986.

69. Goldstein, D. S.: Plasma catecholamines and essential hypertension. An analytical review. *Hypertension,* 5:86, 1983.

70. Brown, M. J., R. C. Causon, V. F. Barnes, P. Brennan, G. Barnes, and G. Greenberg: Urinary catecholamines in essential hypertension: Results of 24-hour urine catecholamine analyses from patients in the Medical Research Council trial for mild hypertension and from matched controls, *Q. J. Med.,* 57:637, 1985.

71. Julius, S., and M. Esler: Autonomic nervous cardiovascular regulation in borderline hypertension, *Am. J. Cardiol.,* 36:685, 1975.

72. Krieger, E. M.: Time course of baroreceptor resetting in acute hypertension, *Am. J. Physiol.,* 218:486, 1970.

73. Sleight, P., J. L. Robinson, D. E. Brooks, and P. M. Rees: Characteristics of single baroreceptor fibers and whole nerve activity in the normotensive and the renal hypertensive dog, *Circ. Res.,* 41:750, 1977.

74. Bunag, R. D., and E. Miyajima: Baroreflex impairment precedes hypertension during chronic cerebroventicular perfusion of hypertonic sodium chloride in rats, *J. Clin. Invest.,* 74:2065, 1984.

75. Vlachakis, N. D., R. Frederics, M. Velasquez, N. Alexander, F. Singer, and R. F. Maronde: Sympathetic system function and vascular reactivity in hypercalcemic patients, *Hypertension,* 4:452, 1982.

76. Hollenberg, N. K., G. H. Williams, and D. F. Adams: Essential hypertension: Abnormal renal vascular and endocrine responses to a mild psychological stimulus, *Hypertension,* 3:11, 1981.

77. Light, K. C., J. P. Koepke, P. A. Obrist, and P. W. Willis, IV: Psychological stress induces sodium and fluid retention in men at high risk for hypertension, *Science,* 220:429, 1983.

78. Falkner, B., G. Onesti, E. T. Angelakos, M. Fernandes, and C. Langman: Cardiovascular response to mental stress in normal adolescents with hypertensive parents. Hemodynamics and mental stress in adolescents, *Hypertension,* 1:23, 1979.

79. Koepke, J. P., and G. F. DiBona: High sodium intake enhances renal nerve and antinatriuretic responses to stress in spontaneously hypertensive rats, *Hypertension,* 7:357, 1985.

80. Koepke, J. P.: Hypothalamic β_2 adrenoceptor control of renal sympathetic nerve activity and urinary sodium excretion in conscious spontaneously hypertensive rats, *Circ. Res.,* 58:241, 1986.

81. Winternitz, S. R., R. E. Katholi, and S. Oparil: Role of the renal sympathetic nerves in the development and maintenance of hypertension in the spontaneously hypertensive rat, *J. Clin. Invest.,* 66:971, 1980.

82. Gutman, N. C., and H. Benson: Interaction of environmental factors and systemic arterial blood pressure: A review, *Medicine,* 50:543, 1971.

83. Louis, W. J., A. E. Doyle, and S. Anavekar: Plasma norepinephrine levels in essential hypertension, *N. Engl. J. Med.* 288:599, 1973.

84. Weinshilboum, R. M.: Antihypertensive drugs that alter adrenergic function, *Mayo Clin. Proc.,* 55:390, 1980.

85. Frohlich, E. D., V. H. Kozul, R. C. Tarazi, and H. P. Dustan: Physiological comparison of labile and essential hypertension, *Circ. Res.,* 27(suppl. 1):55, 1970.

86. Kannel, W. B., N. Brand, J. J. Skinner, Jr., T. R. Dawber, and P. M. McNamara: The relation of adiposity to blood pressure and development of hypertension, *Ann. Intern. Med.,* 67:48, 1967.

87. Reisin, E., R. Abel, M. Modan, D. S. Silverberg, H. E. Eliahou, and B. Modan: Effect of weight loss without salt restriction on the reduction of blood pressure in overweight hypertensive subjects, *N. Engl. J. Med.,* 298:1, 1978.

88. Reisin, E., E. D. Frohlich, F. H. Messerli, G. R. Dreslinski, F. G. Dunn, M. M. Jones, and H. M. Batson, Jr.: Cardiovascular changes after weight reduction in obesity hypertension, *Ann. Intern. Med.,* 98:315, 1983.

89. Landsberg, L., and J. B. Young: Fasting, feeding and regulation of the sympathetic nervous system, *N. Engl. J. Med.,* 298:1295, 1978.

90. Rappaport, E. B., J. B. Young, and L. Landsberg: Effects of 2-deoxy-D-glucose on the cardiac sympathetic nerves and the adrenal medulla in the rat: Further evidence for a dissociation of sympathetic nervous system and adrenal medullary responses, *Endocrinology,* 110:650, 1982.

91. Tuck, M. L., J. Sowers, L. Dornfeld, G. Kledzik, and M. H. Maxwell: The effect of weight reduction on blood pressure, plasma renin activity, and plasma aldosterone levels in obese patients, *N. Engl. J. Med.,* 304:930, 1981.

92. Sowers, J. R., L. A. Whitfield, R. A. Catania, N. Stern, M. L. Tuck, L. Dornfeld, and M. H. Maxwell: Role of the sympathetic nervous system in blood pressure maintenance in obesity, *J. Clin. Endocrinol. Metab.,* 54:1181, 1982.

93. Sowers, J. R., M. Nyby, N. Stern, F. Beck, S. Baron, R. Catania, and N. Vlachis: Blood pressure and hormone changes associated with weight reduction in the obese, *Hypertension,* 4:686, 1982.

94. Dahl, L. K., and M. Heine: Primary role of renal homografts in setting chronic blood pressure levels in rats, *Circ. Res.,* 36:692, 1975.

95. Bianchi, G., U. Fox, G. F. DiFrancesco, A. M. Giovanetti, and D. Pagetti: Blood pressure changes produced by kidney cross-transplantation between spontaneously hypertensive rats and normotensive rats, *Clin. Sci. Mol. Med.,* 47:435, 1974.

96. Curtis, J. J., R. G. Luke, H. P. Dustan, M. Kashgarian, J. D. Whelchel, P. Jones, and A. G. Diethelm: Remission of essential hypertension after renal transplantation, *N. Engl. J. Med.,* 309:1009, 1983.

97. Guyton, A. C., T. G. Coleman, A. W. Cowley, Jr., K. W. Scheel, R. D. Manning, Jr., and R. A. Norman, Jr.: Arterial pressure regulation: Overriding dominance of the kidneys in long-term regulation and in hypertension, *Am. J. Med.,* 52:584, 1972.

98. Haas, J. A., J. P. Granger, and F. G. Knox: Effect of renal perfusion pressure on sodium reabsorption from proximal tubules of superficial and deep nephrons, *Am. J. Physiol.,* 250:F425, 1986.

99. Knox, F. G., J. I. Mertz, J. C. Burnett, Jr., and A. Haramati: Role of hydrostatic and oncotic pressures in renal sodium reabsorption, *Circ. Res.,* 52:491, 1983.

100. London, G. M., J. A. Levenson, A. M. London, A. C. Simon, and M. E. Safar: Systemic compliance, renal hemodynamics, and sodium excretion in hypertension, *Kidney Int.,* 26:342, 1984.

101. Hollenberg, N. K., L. J. Borucki, and D. F. Adams: The renal vasculature in early essential hypertension, *Medicine,* 57:167, 1978.

102. London, G. M., M. E. Safar, J. E. Sassard, J. A. Levenson, and A. C. Simon: Renal and systemic hemodynamics in sustained essential hypertension, *Hypertension,* 6:743, 1984.

103. Hollenberg, N. K., L. G. Meggs, G. H. Williams, J. Katz, J. D. Garnic, and D. P. Harrington: Sodium intake and renal responses to captopril in normal man and in essential hypertension, *Kidney Int.,* 20: 240, 1981.

104. Bianchi, G., D. Cusi, C. Barlassina, G. P. Lupi, P. Ferrari, G. B. Picotti, M. Gatti, and E. Polli: Renal dysfunction as a possible cause of essential hypertension in predisposed subjects, *Kidney Int.,* 23:870, 1983.

105. O'Neil, L. W., J. M. Kissane, and P. M. Hartroft: The kidney in endocrine hypertension, *Arch. Surg.,* 100:498, 1970.

106. Smith, M. D., and M. J. Dunn: The role of prostaglandins in human hypertension, *Am. J. Kid. Dis.,* 5:A32, 1985.

107. O'Connor, D. T.: Response of the renal kallikrein-kinin system, intravascular volume and renal hemodynamics to sodium restriction and diuretic treatment in essential hypertension, *Hypertension,* 4(suppl. III):III-72, 1982.

108. Muirhead, E. E.: Renomedullary system of blood pressure control, *Hypertension,* 8(suppl. I):I-38, 1986.

109. Faber, J. E., K. W. Barron, A. C. Bonham, R. Lappe, E. E. Muirhead, and M. J. Brody: Regional hemodynamic effects of antihypertensive renomedullary lipids in conscious rats, *Hypertension,* 6:494, 1984.

110. Bing, R. F., G. I. Russell, H. Thurston, J. D. Swales, N. Godfrey, Y. Lazarus, and J. Jackson: Chemical renal medullectomy. Effect on urinary prostaglandin E_2 and plasma renin in response to variations in sodium intake and in relation to blood pressure, *Hypertension,* 5:951, 1983.

111. Masugi, F., T. Ogihara, S. Saeki, A. Otsuka, and Y. Kumahara: Role of acetyl glyceryl ether phosphorylcholine in blood pressure regulation in rats, *Hypertension,* 7:742, 1985.

112. Muirhead, E. E.: Antihypertensive function of the renal medulla, *Hosp. Prac.,* 10:99, 1975.

113. Rose, B. D.: *Clinical Physiology of Acid-Base and Electrolyte Disorders,* 2d ed., McGraw-Hill, New York, 1984, chap. 8.

114. Watkins, J., E. C. Abbott, C. N. Hensby, J. Webster, and C. T. Dollery: Attenuation of hypotensive effect of propranolol and thiazide diuretics by indomethacin, *Br. Med. J.,* 281:702, 1980.

115. Steiness, E., and S. Waldorff: Different interactions of indomethacin and sulindac with thiazides in hypertension, *Br. Med. J.,* 285:1702, 1982.

116. Wong, D. G., J. D. Spence, L. Lamki, D. Freeman, and J. W. D. McDonald: Effect of nonsteroidal anti-inflammatory drugs on control of hypertension by β-blockers and diuretics, *Lancet,* 1:997, 1986.

117. Puddey, I. E., L. J. Beilin, R. Vandongen, R. Banks, and I. Rouse: Differential effects of sulindac and indomethacin on blood pressure in treated essential hypertensive subjects, *Clin. Sci.,* 69:327, 1985.

118. Sagnella, G. A., N. K. Markandu, A. C. Shore, and G. A. MacGregor: Raised circulating levels of atrial natriuretic peptides in essential hypertension, *Lancet,* 1:179, 1986.

119. Hirata, Y., M. Ganguli, L. Tobian, and J. Iwai: Dahl S rats have increased natriuretic factor in atria but are markedly hyporesponsive to it, *Hypertension,* 6(suppl. I):I-148, 1984.

120. Freis, E. D.: Salt, volume and prevention of hypertension, *Circulation,* 53:589, 1976.

121. MacGregor, G. A.: Sodium is more important than calcium in essential hypertension, *Hypertension,* 7:628, 1985.

122. Page, L. B., A. Damen, and R. C. Moellering, Jr.: Antecedents of cardiovascular disease in six Solomon Islands studies, *Circulation,* 49:1132, 1974.

123. Kawasaki, T., C. S. Delea, F. C. Bartter, and H. Smith: The effect of high-sodium and low-sodium intakes on blood pressure and other related variables in human subjects with idiopathic hypertension, *Am. J. Med.,* 64:193, 1978.

124. Fujita, T., W. L. Henry, F. C. Bartter, C. R. Lake, C. S. Delea: Factors influencing blood pressure in salt-sensitive patients with hypertension, *Am. J. Med.,* 69:334, 1980.

125. Murphy, R. J. F.: The effect of "rice-diet" on plasma volume and extracellular fluid space in hypertensive subjects, *J. Clin. Invest.,* 29:912, 1950.

126. Longworth, D. L., J. I. Drayer, M. A. Weber, and J. H. Laragh: Divergent blood pressure responses during short-term sodium restriction in hypertension, *Clin. Pharmacol. Therap.,* 27:544, 1980.

127. Skrabal, F., H. Herholz, M. Neumayr, L. Hamberger, M. Ledochowski, H. Sporer, H. Hortnagl, S. Schwarz, and D. Schonitzer: Salt sensitivity in humans is linked to enhanced sympathetic responsiveness and to enhanced proximal tubular reabsorption, *Hypertension,* 6:152, 1984.

128. Hofman, A., A. Hazebroek, and H. A. Valkenburg: A randomized trial of sodium intake and blood pressure in newborn infants, *J. Am. Med. Assoc.,* 250:370, 1983.

129. McCarron, D. A., C. D. Morris, H. J. Henry, and J. L. Stanton: Blood pressure and nutrient intake in the United States, *Science,* 224:1392, 1984.

130. Luft, F. C., M. H. Weinberger, and C. E. Grim: Sodium sensitivity and resistance in normotensive humans, *Am. J. Med.,* 72:726, 1982.

131. de Wardener, H. E., and G. A. MacGregor: The relation of a circulating sodium transport inhibitor (the natriuretic hormone?) to hypertension, *Medicine,* 62:310, 1983.

132. Blaustein, J. P., and J. M. Hamlyn: Role of a natriuretic factor in essential hypertension: An hypothesis, *Ann. Intern. Med.,* 98:785, 1983.

133. Vaughan, E. D., Jr., J. H. Laragh, I. Gavras, F. R. Buhler, H. Gavras, H. R. Brunner, and L. Baer: Volume factor in low and normal renin essential hypertension, *Am. J. Cardiol.,* 32:523, 1973.

134. Grantham, J. J., and R. M. Edwards: Natriuretic hormones: At last, bottled in bond?, *J. Lab. Clin. Med.,* 103:333, 1984.

135. Shah, S., I. Khatri, and E. D. Freis: Mechanism of antihypertensive effect of thiazide diuretics, *Am. Ht. J.,* 95:611, 1978.

136. van Brummelen, P., A. J. Man in't Veld, and M. A. D. H. Schalekamp: Hemodynamic changes during long-term thiazide treatment of essential hypertension in responders and nonresponders, *Clin. Pharmacol. Therap.,* 27:328, 1980.

137. Lasker, N., L. Hopp, S. Grossman, R. Bamforth and A. Aviv: Race and sex differences in erythrocyte Na^+, K^+, and Na^+-K^+-adenosine triphosphatase, *J. Clin. Invest.,* 75:1813, 1985.

138. Poston, L., R. B. Sewell, S. P. Wilkinson, P. J. Richardson, R. Williams, E. M. Clarkson, G. A. MacGregor, and H. E. de Wardener: Evidence for a circulating sodium transport inhibitor in essential hypertension, *Br. Med. J.,* 282:847, 1981.

139. Meyer, P., R. P. Garay, C. Nazaret, G. Dagher, M. Bellet, M. Broyer, and J. Feingold: Inheritance of abnormal erythrocyte cation transport in essential hypertension, *Br. Med. J.,* 282:1114, 1981.

140. Thomas, R. D., R. P. S. Edmondson, P. H. Hilton, and N. F. Jones: Abnormal sodium transport from patients with essential hypertension and the effect of treatment, *Clin. Sci. Mol. Med.,* 48:169s, 1975.

141. MacGregor, G. A., S. Fenton, J. Alaghbaud-Zadeh, N. D. Markandu, J. E. Roulston, and H. E. de Wardener: Evidence for a raised concentration of a circulating sodium transport inhibitor in essential hypertension, *Br. Med. J.,* 283:1355, 1981.

142. Devynck, M. D., M. G. Pernollet, J. B. Rosenfeld, and P. Meyer: Measurement of digitalis-like compound in plasma: Application in studies of essential hypertension, *Br. Med. J.,* 287:631, 1983.

143. Hamlyn, J. M., P. D. Levinson, R. Ringel, P. A. Levin, B. P. Hamilton, M. P. Blaustein, and A. A. Kowarski: Relationships among endogenous digitalis-like factors in essential hypertension, *Fed. Proc.,* 44:2782, 1985.

144. Gruber, K. A., L. L. Rudel, and B. C. Bullock: Increased circulating levels of an endogenous digoxin-like factor in hypertensive monkeys, *Hypertension,* 4:348, 1982.

145. Erne, P., P. Bolli, E. Burgisser, and F. R. Buhler: Correlation of platelet calcium with blood pressure. Effect of antihypertensive therapy, *N. Engl. J. Med.,* 310:1084, 1984.

146. Ballerman, B. J., and B. M. Brenner: Biologically active atrial peptides, *J. Clin. Invest.,* 76:2041, 1985.

147. Modan, M., H. Halkin, S. Almog, A. Lusky, A. Eshkol, M. Shefi, A. Shitrit, and Z. Fuchs: Hyperinsulinemia. A link between hypertension obesity and glucose intolerance, *J. Clin. Invest.,* 75:809, 1985.

148. Pamnani, M. B., D. L. Clough, S. J. Huot, and F. J. Haddy: Vascular Na^+-K^+ pump activity in Dahl S and R rats, *Proc. Soc. Exp. Biol. Med.,* 165:440, 1980.

149. Cole, C. H.: Erythrocyte membrane sodium transport in patients with treated and untreated essential hypertension, *Circulation,* 68:17, 1983.

150. Canessa, M., N. Adragna, H. S. Solomon, T. M. Connolly, and D. C. Tosteson: Increased sodium-lithium countertransport in red cells of patients with essential hypertension, *N. Engl. J. Med.,* 302: 772, 1980.

151. Hilton, P. J.: Cellular sodium transport in essential hypertension, *N. Engl. J. Med.,* 314:222, 1986.

152. Woods, J. W., R. J. Falk, A. W. Pittman, P. J. Klemmer, B. S. Watson, and K. Naboodiri: Increased red-cell sodium-lithium countertransport in normotensive sons of hypertensive parents, *N. Engl. J. Med.,* 306:593, 1982.

153. Woods, J. W., and B. S. Watson: Red-cell sodium-lithium countertransport in sons of normotensive and hypertensive parents: A follow-up study, *N. Engl. J. Med.,* 310:1191, 1984.

154. Mahnensmith, R. L., and P. S. Aronson: The plasma membrane sodium-hydrogen exchanger and its role in physiological and pathophysiological processes, *Circ. Res.,* 56:773, 1985.

155. Weder, A. B.: Red cell lithium-sodium countertransport and renal lithium clearance in hypertension, *N. Engl. J. Med.,* 314:198, 1986.

156. Whitescarver, S. A., C. E. Ott, B. A. Jackson, G. P.

Guthrie, Jr., and T. A. Kotchen: Salt-sensitive hypertension: Contribution of chloride, *Science,* 223: 1430, 1984.

157. Passmore, J. C., S. A. Whitescarver, C. E. Ott, and T. A. Kotchen: Importance of chloride for deoxycorticosterone acetate-salt hypertension in the rat, *Hypertension,* 7(suppl. I):I-115, 1985.

158. Kurtz, T. W., and R. C. Morris, Jr: Halides as possible determinants of Na^+-dependent hypertension (abstract), *Kidney Int.,* 29:250, 1986.

159. McCarron, D. A.: Is calcium more important than sodium in the pathogenesis of essential hypertension?, *Hypertension,* 7:607, 1985.

160. Lau, K., and B. Eby: The role of calcium in genetic hypertension, *Hypertension,* 7:657, 1985.

161. Resnick, L. M., F. B. Müller, and J. H. Laragh: Calcium-regulating hormones in essential hypertension. Relation to plasma renin activity and sodium metabolism, *Ann. Intern. Med.,* 105:649, 1986.

162. Strazzullo, P., V. Nunziata, M. Cirillo, R. Giannattasio, L. A. Ferrara, P. L. Mattioli, and M. Mancini: Abnormalities of calcium metabolism in essential hypertension, *Clin. Sci.,* 65:137, 1983.

163. McCarron, D. A.: Low serum concentrations of ionized calcium in patients with hypertension, *N. Engl. J. Med.,* 307:226, 1982.

164. McCarron, D. A., and C. D. Morris: Blood pressure response to oral calcium in persons with mild to moderate hypertension. A randomized, double-blind, placebo-controlled, crossover trial, *Ann. Intern. Med.,* 103:825, 1985.

165. Fujita, T., and Y. Sato: Natriuretic and antihypertensive effects of potassium in DOCA-salt hypertensive rats, *Kidney Int.,* 24:731, 1983.

166. Workman, M. L., and M. S. Paller: Cardiovascular and endocrine effects of potassium in spontaneously hypertensive rats, *Am. J. Physiol.,* 249:H907, 1985.

167. MAcGregor, G. A., S. J. Smith, N. D. Markandu, R. A. Banks, and G. A. Sagnella: Moderate potassium supplementation in essential hypertension, *Lancet,* 2:567, 1982.

168. Kaplan, N. M., A. Carnegie, P. Raskin, J. A. Heller, and M. Simmons: Potassium supplementation in hypertensive patients with diuretic-induced hypokalemia, *N. Engl. J. Med.,* 312:746, 1985.

169. Langford, H. G.: Dietary potassium and hypertension: Epidemiologic data, *Ann. Intern. Med.,* 98:770, 1983.

170. Stokes, J. B.: Consequences of potassium recycling in the renal medulla. Effects on ion transport by the medullary thick ascending limb of Henle's loop, *J. Clin. Invest.,* 70:219, 1982.

171. Stamler, R., J. Stamler, W. F. Riedlinger, G. Algera, and R. H. Roberts: Weight and blood pressure, *J. Am. Med. Assoc.,* 240:1607, 1978.

172. Stanton, J. L., L. E. Braitman, A. M. Riley: C. S. Khoo, and J. L. Smith: Demographic, dietary, life style, and anthropomorphic correlates of blood pressure, *Hypertension,* 4(suppl. III):III-135, 1982.

173. Londe, S., J. J. Bourgognie, A. M. Robson, and D. Goldring: Hypertension in apparently normal children, *J. Pediatr.,* 78:569, 1971.

174. Messerli, F. H., K. Sundgaard-Riise, E. Reisin, G. Dreslinski, F. G. Dunn, and E. Frohlich: Disparate cardiovascular effects of obesity and arterial hypertension, *Am. J. Med.,* 74:808, 1983.

175. DeFronzo, R. A.: The effect of insulin on renal sodium metabolism, *Diabetologia,* 21:165, 1981.

176. Klatsky, A. L., G. D. Friedman, A. A. Siegelaub, and M. J. Gerard: Alcohol consumption and blood pressure. Kaiser-Permanente Multiphasic Health Examination data, *N. Engl. J. Med.,* 296:1194, 1977.

177. MacMahon, S. W., and R. N. Norton: Alcohol and hypertension: Implications for prevention and treatment, *Ann. Intern. Med.,* 105:124, 1986.

178. Friedman, G. D., A. L. Klatsky, and A. B. Siegelaub: Alcohol, tobacco, and hypertension, *Hypertension,* 4(suppl. III):III-143, 1982.

179. Potter, J. F., and D. G. Beevers: Pressor effect of alcohol in hypertension, *Lancet,* 1:119, 1984.

180. Arkwright, P. D., L. J. Beilin, R. Vandongen, I. A. Rouse, and C. Lalor: The pressor effect of moderate alcohol consumption in man: A search for mechanisms, *Circulation,* 66:515, 1982.

181. Freestone, S., and L. E. Ramsay: Effect of coffee and cigarette smoking on the blood pressure of untreated and diuretic-treated hypertensive patients, *Am. J. Med.,* 73:348, 1982.

182. Cryer, P. E., M. W. Haymond, J. V. Santiago, and S. D. Shah: Norepinephrine and epinephrine release and adrenergic mediation of smoking-associated hemodynamic and metabolic events, *N. Engl. J. Med.,* 295:573, 1976.

183. Curatolo, P. W., and D. Robertson: The health consequences of caffeine, *Ann. Intern. Med.,* 98:641, 1983.

184. Simon, N., S. S. Franklin, K. H. Bleifer, and M. H. Maxwell: Clinical characteristics of renovascular hypertension, *J. Am. Med. Assoc.,* 220:1209, 1972.

185. Deutscher, S., F. H. Epstein, and M. O. Kjelsberg: Familial aggregation of factors associated with coronary heart disease, *Circulation,* 33:911, 1966.

186. Grim, C. E., F. C. Luft, J. Z. Miller, P. L. Brown, M. A. Gannon, and M. H. Weinberger: Effects of sodium loading and depletion in normotensive first-degree relatives of essential hypertensives, *J. Lab. Clin. Med.,* 94:764, 1979.

187. Havlik, R. J., and M. Feinleib: Epidemiology and genetics of hypertension, *Hypertension,* 4(suppl. III): III-121, 1982.

188. Biron, P., J-G. Mongeau, and D. Bertrand: Familial aggregation of blood pressure in 558 adopted children, *Can. Med. Assoc. J.,* 115:773, 1976.

189. Thomson, G. E.: Hypertension in the black population, *Cardiovasc. Rev. Rep.,* 2:351, 1981.

190. Gillum, R. F.: Pathophysiology of hypertension in blacks and whites. A review of the basis of racial blood pressure differences, *Hypertension,* 1:468, 1979.

191. Rostand, S. G., K. A. Kirk, E. A. Rutsky, and B. A. Pate: Racial differences in the incidence of treatment for end-stage renal disease, *N. Engl. J. Med.,* 306:1276, 1982.

192. Veterans Administration Cooperative Study on Antihypertensive Agents: Comparison of propranolol and hydrochlorothiazide for the initial treatment of hypertension. II. Results of long-term therapy, *J. Am. Med. Assoc.,* 248:2004, 1982.

11

COURSE AND MANAGEMENT OF ESSENTIAL HYPERTENSION

Burton D. Rose

Natural History
  Tracking
  Course
Complications
  Arterial Disease
  Left Ventricular Hypertrophy and Heart Failure
  Nephrosclerosis
How and When to Take the Blood Pressure
  Office versus Ambulatory Blood Pressure
Diagnosis
Whom to Treat
  Adverse Effects of Therapy
  Indications for Therapy
How to Treat
  Nonpharmacologic Therapy
  Pharmacologic Therapy

Despite the prevalence of hypertension and the recognized benefits of antihypertensive therapy in many patients, several important management issues remain unsettled:

1. Which BP is more accurate—office versus ambulatory values?
2. Which patients should be evaluated for secondary hypertension?
3. What is the minimum level of BP that requires therapy?
4. Which antihypertensive agents should be used?

Before attempting to answer these questions, this chapter first reviews the natural history of essential hypertension and the cardiovascular and renal complications that can be induced by persistent elevations in BP.

NATURAL HISTORY

In most patients with essential hypertension, the BP reaches a level requiring therapy between the ages of 25 and 45. However, the onset of hypertension may occur before 20 or after 50 in approximately 20 percent of patients,[1] with adolescent hypertension being recognized with increasing frequency.[2]

TRACKING

Patients destined to develop persistent hypertension frequently have a BP that is higher than their peers (although still normal) as early as adolescence.[3-5] This relationship is illustrated in Table 11–1. Boys from the highest and lowest quintiles for BP were studied.

TABLE 11-1. Initial and 8-Year Follow-up Measurements of Blood Pressure and Weight in High and Low Blood Pressure Groups of 16- to 19-Year-Old Boys

	High (n = 32)		Low (n = 25)	
	Initial	8-year	Initial	8-year
BP	159/73	144/84	104/59	117/65
Weight, kg	90	95	59	77

Source: Adapted from J. M. Kotchen, H. E. McKean, and T. A. Kotchen, *Hypertension,* 4(suppl. III):III-128, 1982. Similar results were found in adolescent girls. By permission of the American Heart Association, Inc.

Three points deserve emphasis from these data:

1. The boys with higher pressures were heavier (90 versus 59 kg), confirming the association of BP with body weight.[6]
2. The BP tended to fall with time in the high group and rise in the low group, an example of the common phenomenon of regression toward the mean.
3. Group differences in BP persisted with time; the BP in the high group remained well above that in the low group. The former subjects were also much more likely to develop sustained hypertension during long-term follow-up.

This "tracking" of BP is not as easy to demonstrate in younger children.[3] For example, children in the lower fifteenth percentile for BP at age 7 tend to rise to the level of their peers by age 16. This finding is probably related to differences in growth. The children with an initially low BP were often smaller and had a delayed growth spurt. The eventual catch-up in size was presumably responsible for the equalization of BP.

COURSE

The BP in untreated essential hypertension usually rises slowly over many years,[7] al-though an accelerated phase with a rapid elevation in BP may occur in those patients with chronic severe hypertension (diastolic BP greater than 115 to 120 mmHg). If long-term follow-up is available, the gradual increase in BP can be seen to have three phases: labile or intermittent hypertension in which the mean BP is about 140/90 with spontaneous variations during the day into clearly normal or elevated values,[8] followed by borderline hypertension in which the BP is usually between 140/90 and 160/95 with occasional normal values[9] and, finally, sustained hypertension. As a result of this progressive elevation in BP, the incidence of sustained diastolic hypertension increases from about 10 percent at age 30 to about 30 percent at age 65.[10] Although a rise in BP with age also occurs in normotensive subjects, this effect is much less pronounced than in hypertensives, and the BP typically remains within the normal range—e.g., an elevation in BP from 120/70 at age 20 to 145/85 at age 60.[3,11]

The slow progression of essential hypertension is of potential diagnostic importance. In general, the diastolic BP does not exceed 120 mmHg before the age of 35 to 40, particularly in whites.[7] Thus, marked hypertension in a younger subject or an acute rise in BP over a previously stable baseline at any age is strongly suggestive of some form of secondary hypertension, such as renal artery stenosis (see "Diagnosis," below).[12]

COMPLICATIONS

Untreated hypertension is associated with a variety of cardiovascular complications (Table 11-2). The likelihood of developing these problems is related in part to the degree of BP elevation. In mild to moderate systolic or diastolic hypertension, for example, there is a two- to fourfold rise in myocardial infarction, stroke, heart failure, and overall mortality (Fig. 11-1).[13-17] The risk is even greater

TABLE 11-2. Cardiovascular and Renal Complications of Hypertension

Target Organ	Atherosclerotic	Hypertensive
Heart	Angina pectoris Myocardial infarction	Left ventricular hypertrophy Congestive heart failure
Brain	Transient ischemic attack Thrombotic stroke	Intracerebral or subarachnoid hemorrhage Lacunar infarcts Hypertensive encephalopathy
Kidney	Renal artery stenosis	Benign or malignant nephrosclerosis
Eye	Cholesterol emboli	Hemorrhages and exudates Papilledema
Peripheral arteries	Occlusion of the aorta or its branches Intermittent claudication	Aortic dissection

SOURCE: Adapted from R. W. Gifford, Jr., in M. Moser (ed.), *Hypertension: A Practical Approach*, Little, Brown, Boston, 1975.

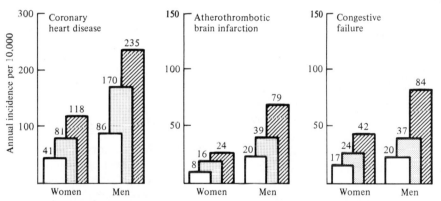

FIG. 11-1. Age-adjusted risk of cardiovascular morbidity in normotensive (≤140/90; open bars), borderline (stippled bars), and hypertensive (≥160/95; striped bars) men and women during 26-year follow-up in the Framingham Study. (*Adapted from W. B. Kannel, J. T. Doyle, A. M. Ostfeld, C. D. Jenkins, L. Kuller, R. N. Podell, and J. Stamler, Circulation, 70:155A, 1984. By permission of the American Heart Association, Inc.*)

with more severe hypertension as the incidence of cardiovascular events may be increased more than tenfold.[18]

In addition to the level of BP, *race, sex, and the presence of other risk factors for atherosclerosis* also influence the likelihood of developing cardiovascular complications. For reasons

that are incompletely understood, hypertension is a more serious disease in blacks. This is manifested (in comparison to whites) by a threefold increase in overall cardiovascular mortality, a six- to sevenfold increase in mortality under the age of 50, the earlier development of hypertensive nephrosclerosis, and an eighteenfold rise in the incidence of end-stage renal failure.[19-21] These findings can be partially but not totally explained by a higher prevalence of severe hypertension.[22]

Hypertensive complications are also about twice as common in men as in women (Fig. 11–1).[13,23,24] In addition to a lower prevalence of events, white women also appear to benefit less from antihypertensive therapy than men.[23,24] The reasons for these differences are not known.

The presence of other risk factors for coronary heart disease—particularly hypercholesterolemia and smoking—is also very important.[10] For example, the likelihood of dying from coronary heart disease is much higher in a patient with these risk factors and a systolic BP of 135 mmHg than it is in a normocholesterolemic, nonsmoker with an elevated systolic BP of 195 mmHg.[25] Comparative studies suggest that hypercholesterolemia is *as*[26] *or more important*[27] than hypertension as a risk factor for coronary disease. Furthermore, hypolipidemic therapy may significantly reverse this process: for every 1 percent reduction in the plasma cholesterol level there is approximately a 2 percent decrease in coronary risk, at least in men with an initial plasma cholesterol concentration above 265 mg/dL.[28] In comparison, *hypertension is the primary risk factor for cerebrovascular disease,* with the plasma cholesterol level and smoking playing a much smaller role (Fig. 11–2).[29,30] This difference in susceptibility probably explains why all studies of antihypertensive therapy have shown a reduced incidence of stroke,[31] while a beneficial effect on coronary disease has been more difficult to demonstrate (see "Whom to Treat," below). The fact that commonly used antihypertensive drugs either raise the circulating level of LDL-cholesterol (thiazides) or lower that of HDL-cholesterol (β-blockers) may also contribute to the relative inability to improve coronary risk.[32]

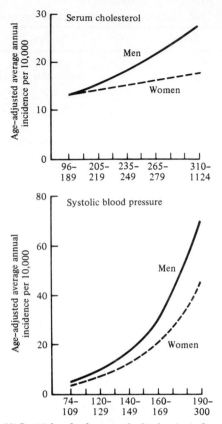

FIG. 11–2. Risk of atheroembolic brain infarction according to plasma cholesterol (in milligrams per deciliter) and systolic blood pressure (in millimeters of mercury) in men and women, 45 to 74, during 18-year follow-up in the Framingham Study. The effect of the plasma cholesterol is not significant in women and much less prominent than the blood pressure in men. [*Adapted from W. B. Kannel, in R. W. R. Russell (ed.): Cerebral Arterial Disease, Churchill Livingstone, Edinburgh, 1976.*]

ARTERIAL DISEASE

Most of the hypertensive complications in Table 11–2 are secondary to vascular damage. These changes may be due to atherosclerosis or to abnormalities directly induced by the elevation in BP: arteriolar and arterial hyperplasia and sclerosis, a dissecting aneurysm, and fibrinoid necrosis.[33,34]

Hypertension independently produces many vascular changes that are similar to those seen with hypercholesterolemia. These include adherence of circulating platelets to the endothelial surface, smooth muscle cell migration and proliferation in the media, and an increase in vascular permeability to macromolecules.[35] As a result, hypertension promotes the development of atherosclerotic lesions in susceptible subjects, an abnormality that can lead to a variety of clinical manifestations such as angina, myocardial infarction, thrombotic stroke, transient ischemic attacks, and intermittent claudication.[13,29]

Hyperplasia of the arterioles and small arteries is also common, representing a direct response of the small blood vessels to hypertension.[36] This change is initially beneficial in that the increase in arteriolar resistance protects the capillaries by preventing them from being exposed to the elevation in BP. With time, however, continued hyperplasia leads to diminished capillary perfusion. This sequence can be illustrated by the changes that occur in the retinal vessels.[37] In order of increasing severity, retinal arteriolar hyperplasia is manifested by enhanced prominence of the light reflex (as more of the light is reflected from the thickened arteriolar wall), vascular tortuosity, arteriovenous crossing changes (grades I and II), and then a copper-wire and silver-wire appearance of the arterioles (grades III and IV) as progressively less and eventually none of the blood can be visualized through the thickened vascular wall. In addition to these hyperplastic changes, hypertension can also directly induce focal or diffuse arteriolar spasm (which may in part reflect an autoregulatory response) and, with very severe disease, retinal hemorrhages and exudates and papilledema.[37]

The arterioles, in addition to hyperplasia, can also undergo hyaline thickening. This change, which is similar to that which occurs with aging, appears to be initiated by the deposition of inactive C3b (a complement protein), which nonspecifically binds to hyaluronic acid in the arteriolar wall.[38] Hypertension apparently accelerates this process by enhancing the permeability of the vascular wall to macromolecules.

In comparison to atherosclerosis and arteriolar hyperplasia which can occur with relatively mild hypertension, *fibrinoid necrosis* is usually seen only with marked elevations in BP (diastolic BP typically greater than 130 mmHg). This abnormality is associated with an increase in vascular permeability, leading to the insudation of plasma proteins (including fibrinoid material) into the vascular wall and a reduction in, or obliteration of, the vascular lumen.[33]

The development of fibrinoid necrosis may be related to the *failure of autoregulation*. With mild to moderate increases in BP, capillary blood flow and hydrostatic pressure are held relatively constant by constriction of the precapillary arterioles (autoregulation) and by the development of arteriolar hyperplasia (Fig. 11–3).[39,40] With more marked hypertension, however, further increments in arteriolar tone may not occur. The net result is enhanced intracapillary pressure (as more of the systemic pressure is now transmitted to the capillary), which can produce vascular damage and increase capillary permeability.

The level at which tissue perfusion is autoregulated and therefore the likelihood of developing fibrinoid necrosis is *dependent upon the baseline BP*. As illustrated in Fig. 11–3, patients with chronic hypertension autoregulate cerebral blood flow (as well as flow to other organs) at higher pressures than normal subjects. This change is probably due to arteriolar hyperplasia which protects the capillary from mild to moderate hypertension. The net effect is that autoregulation fails

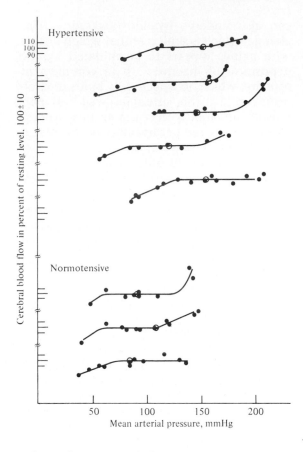

FIG. 11–3. Autoregulation of cerebral blood flow in five chronically hypertensive and three normotensive subjects. Some hypertensive patients show an upper limit of autoregulation at a mean arterial pressure of 150 to 175 mmHg, whereas others continue to autoregulate above 200 mmHg. This is in contrast to normal subjects who usually have an upper limit of autoregulation of less than 150 mmHg. Similarly, cerebral blood flow begins to decrease (lower limit of autoregulation) at higher pressures in hypertensive than normotensive subjects. These changes, which may be secondary to arteriolar hyperplasia, probably account for the observations that both ischemic symptoms (as the blood pressure is lowered) and malignant hypertension occur at higher pressures in patients with underlying hypertension. The blood pressure in these studies was elevated from the resting level (marked with an open circle on each curve) by an infusion of angiotensin II. [*Adapted from B. Johansson, S. Strandgaard, and N. A. Lassen, Circ. Res., 34 (suppl. 2): 167, 1984. By permission of the American Heart Association, Inc.*]

only with a marked elevation in BP. In contrast, previously normotensive patients lose the ability to autoregulate at a lower BP. For example, children and pregnant women typically have a diastolic BP between 60 and 70 mmHg. In these settings, acute hypertension due to glomerulonephritis or preeclampsia can cause fibrinoid necrosis at a diastolic BP as low as 100 mmHg.[41]

Clinically, these arteriolar and small arterial lesions can be lead to malignant nephrosclerosis (see "Nephrosclerosis," below), retinal hemorrhages and exudates (representing both ischemic damage and leakage of blood and plasma from abnormal vessels),[37,42] papilledema, and, in the brain, the development of small, miliary (Charcot-Bouchard) aneurysms, intracerebral or subarachnoid bleeding,

lacunar infarcts, or hypertensive encephalopathy.[31,34,43–46] Hypertensive encephalopathy is the least common neurologic complication of severe hypertension.[46] In this disorder, fibrinoid necrosis results in the exudation of plasma into the brain and in cerebral edema. The early clinical picture consists of headache, nausea, vomiting, apprehension, and confusion. Focal neurologic symptoms (which can wax and wane), marked retinal changes, twitching, seizures, coma, and death may then ensue over hours to days. These symptoms are usually reversible within 24 to 48 h with effective antihypertensive therapy,[46] although resolution of the retinal hemorrhages, exudates, and papilledema may take weeks to months.[47] The relatively indolent course before therapy and the rapid response to treatment distinguish hypertensive encephalopathy from thrombotic or hemorrhagic neurologic events in which there is typically a sudden onset of symptoms and, at best, slow recovery.

Hypertension-induced neurologic abnormalities must also be differentiated from the transient rise in BP that commonly follows any stroke.[48] The BP gradually falls toward normal in most of these patients, with a mean reduction of as much as 20/10 mmHg by 10 days. A similar response follows cerebral ischemia in animals, suggesting that the elevation in BP may be an appropriate attempt to maintain flow to poorly perfused areas of the brain. Thus, lowering the BP in this setting may be counterproductive, actually worsening the neurologic deficit. (The management of hypertension in patients with an acute cerebrovascular event will be discussed below.)

LEFT VENTRICULAR HYPERTROPHY AND HEART FAILURE

Left ventricular hypertrophy (LVH) that can progress to congestive heart failure is another frequent complication of chronic hypertension (Fig. 11–1).[13] As systemic vascular resistance rises, the left ventricle must contract more forcefully to maintain a normal cardiac output. This is initially achieved by hypertrophy of the ventricular muscle, a response that appears to be related both to the level of BP and to the activity of the sympathetic nervous system (which is increased, for example, during periods of stress).[49,50] This adrenergic contribution, which may be due to direct stimulation of cardiac hypertrophy by norepinephrine,[51] may have important implications in terms of antihypertensive therapy. In general, lowering the BP reduces the strain (or afterload) on the heart, resulting in regression of LVH.[49,52-55] This beneficial effect can be demonstrated with the sympathetic

blocking agents (such as methyldopa), converting enzyme inhibitors, and calcium channel blockers.[49,54,55] However, those drugs which lead to a reflex increase in sympathetic activity (diuretics, direct vasodilators, prazosin) may be less likely to reverse cardiac hypertrophy, even though the systemic BP has been substantially reduced.[49,56,57]

Left ventricular hypertrophy is best detected by cardiac ultrasound, a technique that is much more sensitive than the chest x-ray or the voltage or ST- and T-wave changes that may be seen on an electrocardiogram.[58-60] The use of ultrasonography has demonstrated that LVH is an early response, being demonstrable in some adolescents with only a high-normal BP (mean 137/87).[61]

If hypertension persists, LVH can ultimately progress to congestive heart failure. This may result from both *systolic and diastolic dysfunction.* The diastolic abnormality is related to increased stiffness of the ventricle, due to the enhanced muscle mass. Consequently, ventricular filling during diastole is impaired, leading to a reduction in cardiac output and, since compliance is decreased, an elevation in left heart filling pressures (and possibly pulmonary edema).[62-64]

The demonstration of a *normal ejection fraction* in a hypertensive patient with heart failure is indicative of diastolic dysfunction.[62-64] This is an important diagnosis to establish since management is different from that in heart failure due to impaired contractility. Inotropic agents such as digoxin are not likely to be beneficial if contractility is normal. Furthermore, decreasing venous return with a diuretic or reducing vascular resistance with a vasodilator (such as hydralazine or a converting enzyme inhibitor) can lead to marked hypotension in this setting.[63] Optimal therapy consists of a calcium channel blocker or a β-adrenergic blocker, either of which will produce ventricular relaxation and improve cardiac function.[63,64]

In addition to heart failure, LVH is associated with an increased incidence of ventricular premature beats[65] and up to a 3 times higher mortality rate following an acute myocardial infarction.[66] The latter effect may result from a decrease in coronary vascular reserve (induced by cardiac hypertrophy), producing a larger area of infarcted tissue.[67] Resolution of the hypertension postinfarction may also occur and is a paradoxically poor prognostic finding, since it reflects the loss of a relatively large fraction of the functioning myocardial mass.[66]

NEPHROSCLEROSIS

Hypertension can induce both vascular and glomerular damage in the kidney. These lesions can lead to progressive renal insufficiency, a disorder called *hypertensive nephrosclerosis.* The rate at which this occurs and the type of histologic changes that are seen are dependent upon the degree to which the BP is elevated. *Benign* nephrosclerosis occurs with mild to moderate hypertension and is associated with a slow decline in glomerular filtration rate (GFR) over many years. In comparison, severe hypertension can lead to *malignant* nephrosclerosis, which can produce acute and potentially irreversible renal failure. These disorders are not mutually exclusive since findings of both may be seen when an acute rise in BP is superimposed upon chronic hypertension, as occurs in the accelerated phase of essential hypertension.

BENIGN NEPHROSCLEROSIS

Vascular lesions are most prominent in this disorder, and the type of change varies with the size of the vessel.[68] Large arteries down to the size of the arcuate vessels may show arteriosclerotic changes characterized by fibrous thickening of the intima and narrowing of the lumen. Similar changes occur in the smaller interlobular arteries where there is also reduplication of the internal elastic lamina, resulting in a concentric layered appearance (Fig. 11–4). In contrast, hyaline, eosinophilic thickening occurs in the arterioles, due to the deposition of inactive C3b and other proteins into the damaged, more permeable arteriolar wall.[38,69]

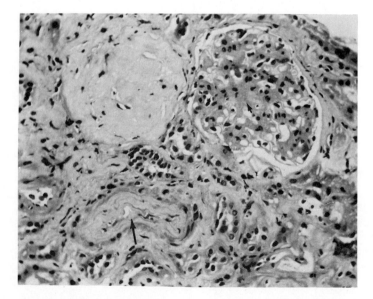

FIG. 11–4. Histologic changes in benign nephrosclerosis include thickening of the arterial wall with narrowing of the lumen (large arrow) and characteristic focal involvement of the glomeruli. Here one glomerulus is completely hyalinized, whereas the other glomerulus shows only moderate thickening of the mesangial areas (small arrow).

Glomerular involvement is typically focal with some glomeruli (particularly those in the outer cortex) being severely affected while others appear relatively normal. The earliest glomerular change is shrinkage of the tuft, followed by progressive collagen accumulation. The end result is a small, eosinophilic mass in which few or no cells can be seen (Fig. 11–4). Both kidneys are usually affected to roughly the same degree with similar pathologic and functional alterations.[70,71]

Pathogenesis. Both ischemia (due to the vascular lesions) and intraglomerular hypertension can contribute to the glomerular damage. In animal models of hypertension, the degree of glomerular sclerosis is dependent upon the degree to which the high systemic BP is transmitted to the glomeruli. The spontaneously hypertensive rat, for example, is characterized by vasoconstriction at the afferent (preglomerular) arteriole. As a result, the glomerular pressure is relatively normal and glomerular injury is a late finding.[72,73] In contrast, intraglomerular pressure rises and glomerular sclerosis is common in those animal models in which renal vascular resistance is normal or reduced.[74,75]

These findings may be applicable to essential hypertension in humans. Most patients have renal vasoconstriction and decreased renal blood flow early in the course of the disease.[76,77] This may explain why mild to moderate hypertension is usually associated with at most slowly progressive renal insufficiency.[78] In comparison, renal vasodilatation and increases in renal blood flow and GFR are present in some patients[76,79] who may be at higher risk for the development of glomerular sclerosis.

Even those patients with renal vasoconstriction and reduced renal perfusion may be susceptible to glomerular damage. If the increase in renal resistance is primarily at the *efferent* (postglomerular) arteriole (as can be produced by angiotensin II), the relative impairment of blood movement out of the glomerulus can raise the intraglomerular pressure[80] and predispose to glomerular injury even though renal blood flow is diminished (see Chap. 4). The observation that converting enzyme inhibitors can increase renal blood flow and, to a lesser degree, the GFR in some patients with essential hypertension is consistent with an important intrarenal role of angiotensin II in this setting.[81,82]

It should be noted that the vascular and glomerular changes of benign nephrosclerosis may also occur with aging, even in the absence of hypertension.[38,68,83] These abnormalities probably account for the progressive decline in GFR that normally is seen with increasing age, with the values in octogenarians being only one-half to two-thirds that of young adults.[84] It is possible, therefore, that even "normal" pressures are ultimately damaging to the kidney, with hypertension accelerating this process,[85] in part by enhancing vascular permeability.[38]

Clinical Presentation. Benign nephrosclerosis is not associated with any symptoms unless uremia is present. Consequently, this disorder is usually diagnosed when the plasma creatinine concentration is found to be elevated on routine laboratory testing in a hypertensive patient. Hyperuricemia (independent of diuretic therapy) is a relatively early finding that appears to reflect the reduction in renal blood flow induced by the arterial and arteriolar disease.[86] The urinalysis typically reveals a benign sediment with few cells or casts and no or mild proteinuria (generally less than 1 g/day). With advanced disease, however, protein excretion can increase, occasionally into the nephrotic range (up to 6.5 g/day).[87] Despite the relatively marked proteinuria, hypoalbuminemia and edema are unusual because the glomerular leak is less severe than that seen with the primary glomerular diseases (see p. 160).

Diagnosis. The diagnosis of benign nephrosclerosis is one of exclusion. Other disorders that can present with chronic renal insufficiency, hypertension, and a benign urinalysis include obstructive uropathy and tubulointerstitial diseases such as chronic pyelonephritis, analgesic abuse nephropathy, and polycystic kidney disease. The history and renal ultrasound usually allows these conditions to be distinguished from nephrosclerosis. Another disorder that can produce both hypertension and renal disease similar to benign nephrosclerosis is chronic lead intoxication.[88] If a history of lead exposure can be obtained, an ethylenediaminetetraacetic acid (EDTA) loading test should be performed to confirm the diagnosis.

Course and Treatment. Progressive renal insufficiency can be expected if the BP is not reduced. The rate at which this occurs is directly related to the severity of the hypertension.[89] On the other hand, the restoration of normotension usually results in stabilization of, or even improvement in, renal function.[89-91] It is possible that converting enzyme inhibitors may be particularly beneficial in this regard, since they appear to selectively dilate the efferent arteriole by reversing the angiotensin II-induced constriction at this site. This effect will directly lower the intraglomerular pressure and can minimize glomerular injury (see p. 123).[92]

It should be noted, however, that an abrupt decrease in BP in a patient with long-standing moderate to severe hypertension can initially lead to reductions in renal perfusion and GFR, since a high pressure is required to maintain perfusion in the presence of arteriolar hyperplasia.[93] Antihypertensive medications can be continued in this setting as long as the BP has not been excessively lowered (diastolic BP below 80 to 85 mmHg) and renal function is not markedly impaired. With time, persistent control of the BP will allow regression of the arteriolar hyperplasia and improvement in renal hemodynamics to or better than baseline values (see Fig. 3–7).[93]

MALIGNANT NEPHROSCLEROSIS

Both vascular and glomerular lesions are prominent in malignant nephrosclerosis, resulting in a histologic picture that may be difficult to distinguish from other vascular diseases such as scleroderma and the hemolytic-uremic syndrome. In the absence of underlying arteriosclerosis, the larger arteries may not be affected initially.[68,94] In contrast, damage to the endothelium of the interlobular arteries leads to migration of smooth muscle cells into the intima, within a mucoid or collagenous stroma.[33,95] The net effect is the development of a characteristic onionskin appearance in these vessels, similar to that seen in scleroderma (see Fig. 7–8a).

The distal interlobular arteries and afferent glomerular arterioles are also involved, although the histologic changes are different from those in the larger vessels. Fibrinoid necrosis is the primary finding (see Fig. 7–8b), with fibrin and platelet thrombi also being present in some cases.[68,95]

Marked ischemic changes are typically present in the glomeruli, including shrinkage of the glomerular tuft, wrinkling of the basement membrane, and focal areas of fibrinoid necrosis. Crescent formation similar to that in rapidly progressive glomerulonephritis also may occur in severe cases.[96]

With control of the BP, the acute vascular and glomerular lesions usually regress with residual scarring found in previously necrotic areas.[94,97] However, the larger arteries, which typically appear to be unaffected during the acute phase, frequently develop subintimal fibrous hyperplasia during the healing phase (Fig. 11–5). The resultant narrowing of the vascular lumen can contribute to a late decline in renal function.[94,97]

Pathogenesis. The primary event in malignant nephrosclerosis is thought to be dam-

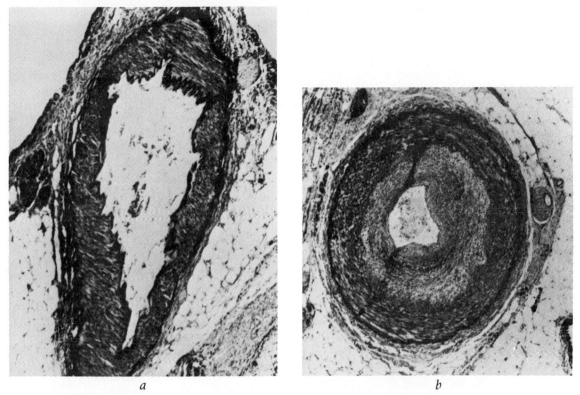

FIG. 11–5. Large renal artery involvement in malignant hypertension. (*a*) Minimal subintimal changes occur in patients who die within several months of the diagnosis of malignant nephrosclerosis. (*b*) In contrast, progressive subintimal fibrous hyperplasia, which may virtually occlude the vascular lumen, is commonly found in patients who survive for more than 1 year. (*From J. W. Woods, W. B. Blythe, and W. D. Huffines, N. Engl. J. Med. 291:10, 1974. Reprinted by permission from the New England Journal of Medicine.*)

age to the vascular wall induced by a rapid and marked rise in BP. The ensuing disruption of the vascular endothelium allows plasma constituents (including fibrinoid material) to enter the vascular wall, leading to luminal narrowing and vascular necrosis. Endothelial damage also can promote platelet activation, the formation of platelet and fibrin thrombi, and a further increase in vascular permeability due to the release by platelets of vasoasctive amines such as histamine and serotonin.[95] The mucoid thickening of the interlobular arteries could represent a reaction to, or organization of, the deposited fibrinoid material.

The vascular damage can also contribute to worsening of the hypertension. Luminal narrowing resulting in glomerular ischemia leads to activation of the renin-angiotensin system. The ensuing rise in angiotensin II can then initiate a vicious cycle in which a further elevation in BP produces more vascular damage and more renin release.[98]

As described above, the level of BP at which fibrinoid necrosis occurs depends upon the baseline BP. In patients with chronic essential hypertension, the associated arteriolar hyperplasia protects the distal blood vessels, and malignant nephrosclerosis is usually not seen unless the diastolic BP exceeds

130 mmHg. However, previously normotensive patients with an acute elevation in BP (as with acute glomerulonephritis) can develop vascular damage at lower pressures.

Clinical Presentation. Patients with malignant nephrosclerosis typically present with other findings of malignant hypertension including headache, blurred vision, dizziness, confusion, and, less commonly, hypertensive encephalopathy.[95,99,100] Retinal hemorrhages, exudates, and papilledema are frequently found on physical examination.

The renal findings consist of an elevated plasma creatinine concentration and a urinalysis similar to that in acute glomerulonephritis or vasculitis: hematuria, which may be macroscopic, red cell casts, and proteinuria which can reach the nephrotic range.[95,99] Anemia with a microangiopathic blood smear (see Fig. 7–12) is also frequently present, a finding which is probably due to traumatic hemolysis as the red cells move through the damaged vessels.[101] Another abnormality which may be seen is mild to moderate thrombocytopenia, presumably due to enhanced platelet consumption at the sites of platelet thrombus formation.[101]

Diagnosis. Two potential diagnostic problems can occur in the patient with malignant nephrosclerosis. First, the combination of hypertension and a nephritic urinary sediment can also be caused by acute glomerulonephritis or vasculitis. The associated hematologic findings also may suggest the hemolytic-uremic syndrome or thrombotic thrombocytopenic purpura (see p. 327). However, patients with any of these disorders usually have a less marked elevation in BP (diastolic BP less than 120 mmHg) without papilledema or a prior history of hypertension. Nevertheless, it many not be possible on clinical grounds alone to determine the correct diagnosis, and further diagnostic procedures, such as a renal biopsy, may be required.

Second, even if it is clear that hypertension is the initiating event, the cause of the elevation in BP should be ascertained. Although malignant nephrosclerosis can occur as part of an accelerated phase of essential hypertension, another disorder, particularly superimposed atherosclerotic renal artery stenosis, is responsible in many patients (see Chap. 12).[102]

Treatment and Course. Treatment of malignant hypertension consists of a rapid reduction in BP, usually initiated with parenteral drugs (such as nitroprusside or diazoxide) followed by chronic control of the BP with oral agents. Effective antihypertensive therapy has led to an improvement in the respective 1- and 5-year survival rates from 20 and 0 percent (untreated)[103] to 85 and 60 percent in treated patients without renal insufficiency.[103,104] The prognosis is not as good in patients who develop renal insufficiency during the acute episode, in whom the 1- and 5-year survival rates have, in the past, been only 55 and 25 percent.[97,104] It is possible, however, that a better outcome could now be achieved with current, more effective antihypertensive agents.

The major causes of death in patients with malignant nephrosclerosis are progressive renal failure and, less often, myocardial infarction or a cerebrovascular accident. The reason for the late loss of renal function is uncertain, but both inadequate control of hypertension and the development of large arterial lesions (Fig. 11–5) may be important.

Despite the possible late progression of the renal disease, control of the hypertension during the acute phase usually results in stabilization of, or improvement in, renal function,[93,100,105] particularly if the plasma creatinine concentration is below 5 mg/dL.[106] It should be noted, however, that antihypertensive therapy can initially lead to decline in renal function because a high BP is necessary for adequate renal perfusion. This response is typically transient since the arterial and arteriolar lesions will regress with persistent BP control.[93,105] Even patients who acutely require dialysis frequently recover enough function to discontinue dialysis within 3 to 6 months.[106-108] Bilateral nephrectomy, which had been advocated in the past for patients with refractory hypertension and renal failure,[109] should now be considered in only rare circumstances, given the possibility of a substantial improvement in renal function.

The decrease in tissue perfusion following initial antihypertensive therapy also occurs in the brain and other organs and can lead to potentially irreversible complications if the BP is lowered excessively. Cerebral infarction leading to blindness, coma, and death have been reported when the diastolic BP is rapidly reduced to less than 95 mmHg.[110,111] Thus, the first aim of treatment should be a diastolic BP of 100 to 105 mmHg. This level is usually sufficient both to maintain tissue perfusion and to allow regression of fibrinoid necrosis.

HOW AND WHEN TO TAKE THE BLOOD PRESSURE

Although measurement of the systemic BP is a simple procedure, a variety of factors can lead to erroneous results (Table 11–3). The following recommendations should be followed to minimize these problems:

1. The BP should be taken with the patient

TABLE 11–3. Pitfalls in Measurement of Blood Pressure

Apprehension in presence of physician
Blood pressure cuff too small
Pseudohypertension due to calcified vessels
Use of phase IV or V Korotkoff sounds
Auscultatory gap
Excessive pressure on stethoscope
Arm below level of heart
Disparity between two arms
Office versus ambulatory measurements

resting comfortably, preferably for at least 5 min. Even under optimal conditions, some patients are apprehensive when seeing the physician, and the resulting increase in sympathetic tone can raise the BP above its usual value. Figure 11–6 depicts the BP in hospitalized patients undergoing continuous BP monitoring with an intraarterial catheter. Arrival of the physician raised the BP by an average of 27/15 mmHg. This effect was largely dissipated within 5 to 10 min and was less prominent during a nurse's visit.[112]

2. It is important to use a proper-sized cuff. The length of the *bladder* should be 75 to 80 percent of the circumference of the upper arm; the width of the bladder should be more than 50 to 60 percent of the length of the upper arm.[113] If an inappropriately small cuff is used, the pressure produced by inflating the cuff may not penetrate to the brachial artery. As a result, a cuff pressure exceeding systolic is now required to shut off arterial flow. In extremely obese patients with large arms, the use of a normal-sized cuff can overestimate the BP by as much as 10 to 50 mmHg.[113,114] If a large cuff is not available, the BP can be taken in the forearm.

3. A similar problem leading to overestimation of the systemic BP (by as much as 50 mmHg) can occur in elderly patients with calcified blood vessels that are not readily compressed by the blood pressure cuff.[115,116] This problem should be suspected in an older patient with marked hypertension, particularly if there are no signs of end-organ damage. Soft tissue x-rays generally reveal vascular calcifications. In addition, a simple bedside maneuver may be helpful.[115] The cuff is inflated to a level above the systolic BP so that the arterial *pulse* is no longer palpable. If the pulseless radial or brachial artery can still be felt at this time, it is likely that a thickened vessel is present. Confirmation of the diagnosis of "pseudohypertension" can be made only by direct intraarterial measurement of the BP. This

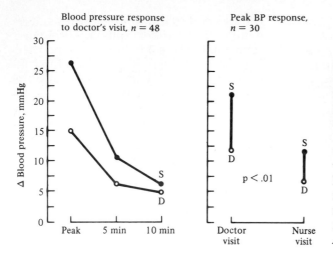

Blood pressure response to doctor's visit, n = 48

Peak BP response, n = 30

FIG. 11–6. Blood pressure response to doctor's or nurse's visit in patients undergoing continuous intraarterial blood pressure monitoring. The average peak rise in blood pressure to a doctor's visit was 27/15, an effect that was largely dissipated within 5 to 10 min (left panel). A nurse's visit produced a much less pronounced hemodynamic change (right panel). S and D refer to systolic and diastolic pressures, respectively. [*From G. Mancia, Hypertension, 5 (suppl. III):III-5, 1983. By permission of the American Heart Association, Inc.*]

is an important diagnosis to make since antihypertensive therapy based upon the cuff measurement may be inappropriate and can lead to potentially disabling symptoms.

4. When the BP is taken by auscultation, the cuff should be inflated to a pressure greater than systolic and then deflated slowly at a rate of 2 to 3 mmHg per heartbeat. The systolic pressure is equal to the pressure at which the pulse is first heard regularly (phase I). This sound is generated by blood flowing into the artery as the cuff pressure falls below systolic. The pulse continues to be heard (phases II and III) until there is an abrupt muffling (phase IV) and then, 8 to 10 mmHg later, the disappearance of sound (phase V).[117,118] Phase V is usually equated to the diastolic BP. However, the point of muffling should be used in the occasional patient in whom there is greater than a 10-mmHg difference between muffling and disappearance. This occurs most commonly in high-output states, such as anemia or aortic regurgitation, in which the turbulence induced by the high flow rate delays the disappearance of sound.

5. When taking the BP, the stethoscope should be applied lightly over the brachial artery. The use of excessive pressure can lower the diastolic reading by up to 10 to 15 mmHg.[119]

6. The systolic pressure should first be determined by palpation of the brachial or radial artery. This can avoid problems associated with an *auscultatory gap* (absent phase II). In this setting, the systolic pressure is heard followed by the absence of sound for 20 to 40 mmHg until the pulse can be detected again.[117] For example, the pulse may be heard at 180 mmHg in a patient with a BP of 180/100 and then become inaudible until the cuff pressure falls to 140 mmHg. If the cuff is initially inflated to only 170 mmHg, the pulse will first be heard at 140 mmHg, leading to marked underestimation of the systolic BP. The factors responsible for the auscultatory gap, which is an uncommon finding, are not well understood.

7. The BP should always be taken with the patient's arm at the level of the heart. If the arm is allowed to hang down when the BP is taken in the sitting or standing position, the brachial artery will be approximately 15 cm below the heart. As a result, the measured BP will be elevated

by 10 to 15 mmHg because of the added hydrostatic pressure induced by gravity.[120]

8. The BP should periodically be measured in both arms. If there is a disparity, e.g., due to atherosclerosis in the axillary artery, the arm with the higher pressure should be used. The BP should also be determined with the patient supine, sitting, and after standing for 1 to 3 min, looking for the presence of orthostatic hypotension.

With regard to the acute effect of stress on the measured BP, the initial visits to the physician's office represent another setting in which the BP can be falsely elevated. As depicted in Table 11-4, the process of acclimatization leads to a mean fall in systolic BP of 14 mmHg between the first and third visits with no further change on subsequent visits.[121] Thus, the decision to label a given patient as having mild or moderate hypertension should be delayed for several visits, when a more accurate assessment of the true BP can be made. However, some anxious patients will always have a higher BP in the physician's office than at home or in the workplace. In this setting, it may be desirable to make therapeutic decisions based upon ambulatory measurements.

OFFICE VERSUS AMBULATORY BLOOD PRESSURE

Every study to date which has evaluated the efficacy of treating essential hypertension has relied on the BP obtained in the physician's office (see below). However, recent studies involving the use of automatic or semiautomatic devices to monitor 24-h BP in the ambulatory setting have raised questions as to which BP most accurately reflects the risk of developing hypertensive complications.[122,123] The results of these studies can be summarized as follows:

1. The ambulatory BP varies during the day,

TABLE 11-4. Change in BP on Sequential Visits to Physician's Office in 110 Patients with Mild to Moderate Hypertension

	Change in Systolic BP	Change in Diastolic BP
1st to 2d visit	−10	−6
2d to 3d visit	−4	−1
3d to 5th visits	−1	0

SOURCE: Adapted from R. M. Hartley, R. Velez, R. W. Morris, M. F. D'Souza, and R. F. Heller, *Br. Med. J.*, 286:287, 1983.

increasing during periods of stress[50] and falling by as much as 20 to 40 mmHg systolic during sleep.[112]

2. The ambulatory BP is usually lower (mean about 15 mmHg systolic) than that measured in the physician's office.[124-126] An interesting corollary of this finding is that treatment with a placebo frequently lowers the BP taken by the physician but does not reduce the ambulatory measurements.[127] The effect of stress can also be appreciated from BP measurements obtained in the hospital. Removing the patient from the stresses of daily life often decreases the BP, even below ambulatory levels.[128]

3. In virtually every study, *the cardiovascular morbidity from hypertension correlates better with the ambulatory BP than with that obtained by the physician*.[50,124,125,129-131] As an example, when patients with the same office systolic BP are compared, the incidence of prior hypertensive events is lower in those patients with relatively normal mean 24-h ambulatory pressures (Fig. 11-7).

In the future, ambulatory BP monitoring may be generally used to determine the necessity for, and efficacy of, antihypertensive therapy. However, these devices are not widely available at the current time. A possible alternative is to base clinical decisions on casual (rather than continuous) values obtained by the patient at home or at work. In many patients, the casual ambulatory BP

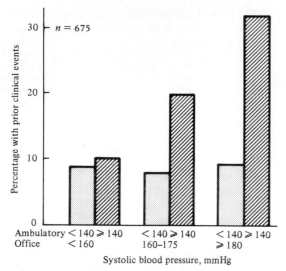

FIG. 11-7. Prevalence of prior cardiovascular events in patients with similar office blood pressures but with high or low ambulatory values. Patients with office hypertension (systolic BP ≥ 160 mmHg) but with normal ambulatory levels (systolic BP < 140 mmHg) have a much lower rate of complications. (*Adapted from M. Sokolow, D. Perloff, and R. Cowan, Cardiovasc. Rev. Rep., 1:295, 1980.*)

is closer to the 24-h mean value than that obtained by the physician.[126]

In summary, it seems reasonable to suggest that hypertensive patients measure their BP in the ambulatory setting. If this course is chosen, it is important for the physician to ascertain that the person taking the BP (such as the patient or spouse) is properly trained and that the machine used is accurate. It may be elected to withhold further therapy from those patients who are hypertensive in the physician's office but are repeatedly normotensive at work or at home. In this setting, it is essential that the patient be carefully followed for signs of end-organ damage. An increase in QRS voltage on the electrocardiogram, for example, suggests that left ventricular mass has increased and, therefore,

that the patient's BP is not under satisfactory control.[131]

DIAGNOSIS

Essential hypertension is by far the major cause of high BP and is even more common than generally appreciated. Although it had been thought that approximately 5 to 10 percent of patients had secondary, and therefore potentially correctible, hypertension, the true incidence may be under 1 percent, particularly with mild elevations in BP.[132,133]

Despite its frequency, essential hypertension can be diagnosed only by exclusion, since there is no specific test that is pathognomonic of this disorder. It is not feasible, however, to evaluate every patient for one of the major causes of secondary hypertension (Table 11-5). A rational approach to diagnosis is dependent upon understanding the typical characteristics of essential hypertension (see "Natural History," above): onset usually between the ages of 20 and 50, a slow increase in BP over many years if untreated, and frequently a positive family history of hypertension.[1,12] Only those patients who lack one or more of these findings (Table 11-6) or who have symptoms or signs typical of some secondary cause should undergo more than routine laboratory evaluation.[134] The latter consists of blood tests (urea nitrogen, creatinine, electrolytes, glucose, cholesterol, and

TABLE 11-5. Major Causes of Secondary Hypertension in Adults

Renal artery stenosis—unilateral or bilateral
Renal disease—volume- versus renin-mediated
Oral contraceptives
Pheochromocytoma
Primary mineralocorticoid excess
Cushing's syndrome
Pregnancy
Hypercalcemia

TABLE 11-6. Findings Suggestive of Secondary Hypertension

An acute rise in BP over a previously stable baseline

Severe or refractory hypertension including retinal hemorrhages or papilledema

Proven age of onset less than 20 (particularly if before puberty) or greater than 50

Unexplained hypokalemia

Negative family history

Systolic-diastolic abdominal bruit, especially in a young patient

---

calcium concentration), a urinalysis, and an electrocardiogram or cardiac ultrasound, looking for the possible presence of left ventricular hypertrophy.

The most common correctible cause of hypertension is renal artery stenosis, which frequently presents in a manner substantially different from essential hypertension. An abrupt rise in BP (from a previously stable baseline that may have been normal or even elevated), severe or refractory hypertension, an abdominal bruit, and unexplained hypokalemia (due to secondary hyperaldosteronism) all may be seen with renovascular disease.[12] Although renal artery stenosis is unusual in patients with mild, stable hypertension,[132,133] the incidence of this condition rises to 10 to 40 percent with acute or refractory hypertension.[102,132,135] Furthermore, *bilateral* renal arterial disease may be present in up to 40 percent of patients with the combination of marked hypertension and renal insufficiency (plasma creatinine concentration above 1.5 mg/dL) that is unexplained by any apparent primary renal disease.*[,135] Bilateral renal artery stenosis should also be suspected in those patients who develop acute renal failure following the administration of a con-

---

*These statistics do not apply to black patients in whom severe essential hypertension is more common[22] and renovascular disease is unusual.[102] The reason for this difference is not known.

verting enzyme inhibitor (see p. 83). This is an extremely important diagnosis to establish since restoration of normal perfusion can both lower the BP and improve renal function.[135] The sequential evaluation for renovascular hypertension is reviewed in the following chapter.

The physician should also be aware of the findings that are suggestive of one of the other causes of secondary hypertension:

1. An elevated blood urea nitrogen (BUN) and plasma creatinine concentration and an abnormal urinalysis are suggestive of *primary renal disease.* With acute glomerulonephritis, for example, the elevation in BP is primarily due to volume expansion resulting from a decrease in urine output.[136,137] In comparison, the absence of edema in a hypertensive patient with apparent acute glomerular disease (by history and urinalysis) raises the likelihood of a different diagnosis: renin-mediated hypertension due to a vascular disease such as vasculitis or scleroderma.[137-139]

2. Hypertension occurs in approximately 4 to 5 percent of women taking *oral contraceptives,* and a larger percentage have an elevation in BP that remains within the normal range.[140] Increasing age and duration of usage are the primary risk factors for this complication.[141] Although the mechanisms responsible for the hypertension are incompletely understood, the BP usually returns to the previous baseline within 2 to 12 months after the drug has been discontinued.[140,142]

3. *Pheochromocytoma* is a rare cause of hypertension. Paroxysmal elevations in BP or the triad of headache (usually pounding), palpitations, and diaphoresis should suggest the possible presence of this disorder.[143] Pheochromocytoma should also be considered in hypertensive patients with multiple endocrine neoplasia (type II or type III), von Hippel-Lindau disease, or neurofibromatosis.[144-147] A variety of tests have been used to initiate the evaluation for a

pheochromocytoma, including (*a*) measurement of urinary catecholamine and metabolite excretion (particularly metanephrines), (*b*) the plasma level of free norepinephrine and epinephrine both in the basal state and after the administration of clonidine (plasma catecholamines will be suppressed by clonidine in normal subjects but not in patients with a pheochromocytoma), and, if available, (*c*) radionuclide scanning with ^{131}I-metaiodobenzylguanidine, a compound resembling norepinephrine that is taken up by adrenergic tissue.[143,148] A CT scan of the adrenal glands and abdomen also may be useful, but there are too many false-positive results for this test to be considered conclusive in the absence of a proven increase in adrenergic activity.[143]

4. Hypokalemia with urinary potassium wasting (potassium excretion greater than 30 meq/day) is the only finding suggestive of one of the conditions that can cause *primary mineralocorticoid excess* (an adrenal adenoma being the most common).[149-151] Although the plasma potassium concentration may on occasion be normal in this disorder,[149] such patients are difficult to identify since not all patients with hypertension can be evaluated for hyperaldosteronism. If, however, the values are in the low-normal range (plasma potassium concentration 3.4 to 3.7 meq/L), it may be helpful to give the patient a high-sodium diet (200 meq/day) for several days. The ensuing increase in flow to the distal nephron will enhance potassium loss and induce overt hypokalemia in patients with nonsuppressible hyperaldosteronism but will be without effect in otherwise normal subjects who can shut off aldosterone secretion.[149,152]

Other causes of hypokalemia and hypertension include diuretic therapy and renal artery stenosis. However, the plasma renin activity is usually elevated in these settings, in contrast to the low values characteristic of primary hyperaldosteron-

ism. The latter diagnosis can be confirmed by demonstrating a nonsuppressible elevation in the plasma aldosterone level following sodium loading with or without the administration of exogenous mineralocorticoid.[149,150,153] A subsequent step is then required to distinguish an adrenal adenoma (which is treated surgically) from adrenal hyperplasia (which is generally unresponsive to surgery but can be treated with a potassium-sparing diuretic).[149,154,155] This distinction can be achieved most directly by a CT scan of the adrenal glands, a radionuclide iodocholesterol scan, or, if these tests do not demonstrate an adenoma, measurement of adrenal vein aldosterone levels, which will be unilaterally elevated with an adenoma but roughly equal on both sides with hyperplasia.[149,150]

5. The major findings suggestive of *Cushing's syndrome* are the classic cushingoid appearance (particularly central obesity, ecchymoses, and muscle weakness) or a history of chronic glucocorticoid therapy.[156,157] Hypokalemia may also occur and is thought to result from overproduction of hormones with mineralocorticoid activity such as deoxycosterone.[158]

Confirmation of the diagnosis requires the demonstration of excess cortisol production. This can be best achieved by the lack of adequate suppression of the plasma cortisol concentration after the administration of dexamethasone [1 mg at 11 p.m. the night before, followed, if suppression does not occur in an obese patient, by low-dose dexamethasone (0.5 mg every 6 h for 2 days) to exclude noncushingoid obesity] or by increased urinary free cortisol excretion in a 24-h collection.[159] If these tests are positive, excess ACTH production from a pituitary or ectopic tumor must be differentiated from an adrenal adenoma in which ACTH secretion is suppressed. The correct diagnosis can be established by CT scan of the adrenal glands,[160] measurement of plasma ACTH levels,[161] or use of the high-dose dexamethasone suppression test in which the plasma cortisol level will be substantially reduced only with a pituitary tumor.[156,161,162]

6. Hypertension in *pregnancy* is primarily due to preeclampsia or preexisting essential hypertension or renal disease. This topic is discussed in detail in Chap. 7.

7. An elevation in BP is also frequently found in patients with *hypercalcemia,* with or without primary hyperparathyroidism.[163-165] Correction of the hypercalcemia is usually associated with a reduction in BP toward normal unless irreversible renal insufficiency has occurred.

WHOM TO TREAT

Over the past 25 years, a series of studies have demonstrated that the treatment of hypertension reduces the incidence of cardiovascular complications. Nevertheless, the minimum level at which therapy should be begun remains unresolved. Before attempting to arrive at some recommendations, it is useful to first review the results of these studies.

The use of oral antihypertensive agents was initially evaluated in patients with malignant hypertension.[103,104] The efficacy of therapy in this setting is dependent upon the presence or absence of renal insufficiency. In those patients with well-preserved renal function, treatment improves the respective 1- and 5-year survival rates from 20 and 0 percent (untreated) to 85 and 60 percent (treated).[97,103,104] The substantial mortality that persists with lowering of the BP is probably due to end-organ damage from both prior hypertension and vascular injury during the acute episode.

Similar marked improvement was then demonstrated in patients with a diastolic BP between 115 and 129 mmHg.[166] At approximately 2 years, a cardiovascular complication developed in 27 of 70 untreated patients (mean BP 185/121) versus only 2 of 73 treated patients (mean BP 142/91), representing a reduction in total morbidity of greater than 90 percent.

A beneficial effect of therapy has also been shown in patients with moderate hypertension (diastolic BP between 105 and 114 mmHg).[167] At 5 years, cardiovascular morbidity and mortality are reduced by approximately 70 percent (Fig. 11–8). Thus, there seems to be little question that patients with a diastolic BP above 104 mmHg should be treated with antihypertensive agents.

The issue that remains is the necessity for therapy in patients with mild hypertension (diastolic BP between 90 and 104 mmHg). By 1980, five studies had evaluated this prob-

FIG. 11–8. Estimated cumulative incidence of all (nonfatal plus fatal) morbid events over a 5-year period in treated and untreated (control) patients with initial diastolic blood pressure between 105 and 114 mmHg. (*From Veterans Administration Cooperative Study on Antihypertensive Agents, J. Am. Med. Assoc., 213:1143, 1970. Copyright 1970, American Medical Association.*)

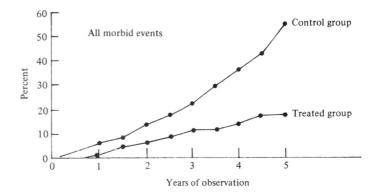

lem, the largest of which was the Hypertension Detection and Follow-up Program in the United States.[167-172] The results of these trials, which involved about 12,800 patients and had a duration of 3 to 7 years, are summarized in Table 11–7.[173] As can be seen, there is a substantial *percentage* reduction in cardiovascular mortality and morbidity. However, the *absolute* improvement is relatively small. For example, a 27 percent reduction in morbidity from 9.0 to 6.6 percent with therapy means that treating 100 patients for 3 to 7 years prevents a complication in 2 to 3 patients. The remaining patients experience

the expense and side effects of antihypertensive drugs with no benefit during this short-term follow-up. It should be noted that therapy is also effective in preventing the progression to more marked hypertension (diastolic BP above 110 mmHg), a change which occurs in about 15 percent of untreated patients.[23,171,172]

Since 1982, the results of two other large studies, the Multiple Risk Factor Intervention Trial (MRFIT) and the Medical Research Council (MRC) trial, have been published and have revealed less clear cut evidence of benefit.[23,174] As depicted in Table 11–8, there

TABLE 11–7. Cumulative Complications in Control and Treated Groups in the Five Initial Therapeutic Trials of Mild Hypertension

Complications	Control (*n* = 6400)		Treated (*n* = 6400)		Percent Improvement
	Number	Percent	Number	Percent	
Total morbid events	563	9.0	417	6.6	27
Total mortality	342	5.4	262	4.1	24
Cerebrovascular events: fatal and nonfatal	140	2.2	76	1.2	50
Fatal coronary events	79	1.2	46	0.7	42

Source: Adapted from R. G. Narins, *Kidney Int.,* 26:881, 1984. Reprinted by permission from Kidney International.

TABLE 11–8. Cumulative Complications in Control and Treated Groups in the MRFIT and MRC Trials of Mild Hypertension

Complications	Control (*n* = 12,640)		Treated (*n* = 12,720)		Percent Improvement
	Number	Percent	Number	Percent	
Total morbid events*	352	4.1	286	3.3	20
Total mortality	234	1.9	232	1.8	—
Cerebrovascular events: fatal and nonfatal*	109	1.3	60	0.7	46
Fatal coronary events	176	1.4	190	1.5	—

Source: Data from Refs. 23 and 174. By permission.
*The incidence of nonfatal events is derived only from the MRC trial (*n* = 8650 and 8700, respectively). MRFIT presented data only on fatal events.

was no decrease in total or coronary heart disease mortality although the incidence of total cardiovascular events was reduced, mostly due to fewer nonfatal strokes. This last finding is again consistent with the primary role of hypertension in the development of cerebrovascular disease (see Fig. 11–2).[29,30]

The reason that the absolute benefit is relatively small is that the *overall cardiovascular risk is much lower* in mild than in moderate hypertension. This can be appreciated by comparing Tables 11–7 and 11–8 to Fig. 11–8: the incidence of morbid events in the placebo or less treated groups at 5 years is only 4 to 9 percent with mild hypertension (Tables 11–7 and 11–8) versus approximately 55 percent in patients with moderate hypertension (Fig. 11–8).

The inability of MRFIT and the MRC trial to demonstrate a more pronounced beneficial effect of therapy also may have been related to different responses among subgroups of patients. For example, smoking is a determinant of both risk (a twofold increase) and the efficacy of therapy. In the MRC study (in which patients were randomly treated with a thiazide, propranolol, or placebo), propranolol produced a 38 percent reduction in coronary and cerebrovascular events in nonsmokers when compared to placebo, *a benefit that was entirely lost in smokers*.[23] This effect may have been related to a smoking-induced increment in the hepatic metabolism of propranolol.[175] In contrast, the efficacy of thiazide therapy was not influenced by smoking. However, the pattern of response was different from that with propranolol. Although thiazides lowered the frequency of stroke, there was *no decrease in coronary morbidity* as was seen with propranolol in nonsmokers. These findings suggest that it may be desirable to avoid propranolol in smokers (it is uncertain if this also applies to other β-blockers) and that thiazides may have a *deleterious* effect on coronary heart disease.

ADVERSE EFFECTS OF THERAPY

The concept that antihypertensive therapy can have adverse cardiovascular effects was first suggested by the Australian trial of mild hypertension. Figure 11–9 depicts the relationship between the average diastolic BP during the study and the incidence of trial end points (morbidity and mortality). More of the actively treated patients had a diastolic BP below 90 mmHg, reflecting the effect of antihypertensive therapy. However, *when patients with the same BP* were compared, the cardiovascular morbidity was actually higher with treatment. At an average diastolic BP of 90 to 94 mmHg, for example, total morbidity was almost twice as high in patients who

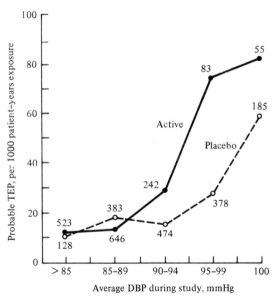

FIG. 11–9. Relationship between average diastolic BP and the incidence of trial end points (cardiovascular morbidity and mortality) during the 3 years of the Australian trial on mild hypertension. The number of patients in the actively treated and placebo groups at each level of BP is given. (*From A. P. Doyle, Clin. Sci., 63:431s, 1982.*)

achieved this BP with active therapy rather than placebo.

The MRFIT also suggested that treatment might be harmful in at least some patients.[174] Those patients who began with an *abnormal resting electrocardiogram* (tall R waves, ST- and T-wave changes, arrhythmias, conduction defects) had a *65 percent increase in coronary mortality* over 7 years with treatment (special intervention) when compared to similar patients who received less or no therapy (usual care) (Fig. 11–10). In contrast, coronary mortality was appropriately reduced in treated patients whose electrocardiogram was initially normal (Table 11–9).

TABLE 11-9. Coronary Heart Disease Deaths (per 1000 Patient Years) in Patients with Mild Hypertension according to the Resting Electrocardiogram*

	Normal EKG		Abnormal EKG	
MRFIT	SI	UC	SI	UC
	2.3	3.0	4.2	2.5
HDFP	SC	RC	SC	RC
	2.0	3.1	4.3	3.5

SOURCE: Data from Refs. 174 and 176.
* Abbreviations: SI = special intervention; UC = usual care; SC = stepped care; RC = referred care.

The findings of the MRFIT have been criticized because it was designed to assess the efficacy of reversing a variety of cardiac risk factors (including hypercholesterolemia and smoking), not specifically the treatment of hypertension. Consequently, the subgroup data may lack statistical power. However, data from the Hypertension Detection and Follow-up Program (HDFP) and the Oslo Hypertension Study also suggest that therapy can increase coronary risk in at least some patients.[176-178] In the HDFP, for example, patients in the stepped (intensive) care group who began with a normal electrocardiogram had reduced coronary mortality when compared to the referred care group who generally received less or no therapy (Table 11–9). In contrast, those patients in the stepped care group who began with an abnormal electrocardiogram had a slightly, although not statistically significant, higher coronary mortality. These patients, however, continued to have a net benefit from therapy since cerebrovascular deaths were reduced.

The MRFIT also found that the increase in coronary deaths was entirely due to sudden death (consistent with an arrhythmic event) and that the *enhanced risk was limited to those patients receiving a diuretic.*[174] This seemingly deleterious effect of diuretics may have been dose-related: the percentage of patients receiving more than 50 mg of hydrochlorothia-

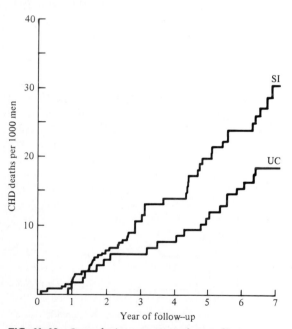

FIG. 11-10. Cumulative coronary heart disease (CHD) mortality rates for hypertensive men with an abnormal resting electrocardiogram in the special intervention (SI) and usual care (UC) groups at seven years in the Multiple Risk Factor Intervention Trial. Mortality was 65 percent *higher* in the treated (SI) group. (*Adapted from Multiple Risk Factor Intervention Trial Research Group, Am. J. Cardiol. 55:1, 1985.*)

zide or chlorthalidone was 51 percent in the special intervention group but only 15 percent in the usual care group. As described above, the MRC trial also suggested an adverse effect of diuretic therapy: in nonsmokers, coronary events were reduced by one-third in patients treated with propranolol (versus placebo); this beneficial response was lost in those receiving a thiazide.[23]

The mechanism by which diuretics may be harmful to some patients with mild hypertension is uncertain, as hypokalemia, hypomagnesemia, hypercholesterolemia, and mild hyperglycemia all could contribute (see "How to Treat: Diuretics," below). The inability to demonstrate these findings in earlier studies may have been related to the severity of the hypertension. The *benefit of lowering the BP may outweigh any unfavorable effect of therapy* in patients with more than mild hypertension. In the MRFIT, for example, the effect of antihypertensive therapy was dependent upon the diastolic BP as well as the electrocardiogram.[174] In patients with a *normal* electrocardiogram, cardiovascular mortality was improved if the diastolic BP were greater than or equal to 95 mmHg; in contrast, there seemed to be a small increase in coronary deaths between 90 and 94 mmHg. These findings, however, have not been found in all studies; antihypertensive therapy was as effective between 90 and 94 mmHg as it was between 95 and 104 mmHg in the HDFP.[170]

INDICATIONS FOR THERAPY

The data presented above demonstrate the need for flexibility in deciding which patients with mild hypertension should be treated.[179] The potential benefits of therapy must be weighed against the deleterious effects of the drugs. In addition to the possible increase in mortality in certain patients treated with diuretics, each of the antihypertensive agents that are currently in use has side effects (such as fatigue, depression, and impotence) that can interfere with normal daily life. In the MRC trial, for example, symptoms severe enough to lead to discontinuation of therapy developed in 15 to 25 percent of patients taking either a thiazide or propranolol versus less than 5 percent with placebo.[23] Furthermore, the incidence of side effects may be *even higher than suspected from questioning the patient.* In one study of 74 patients, only 9 percent claimed to feel worse after the institution of antihypertensive therapy with a β-blocker, methyldopa, or a diuretic.[180] However, spouses or other close relatives noted changes (decreased energy, diminished libido, altered mood) in almost all patients. As is discussed below, it is possible that the incidence of side effects would have been substantially lower if a converting enzyme inhibitor or calcium channel blocker had been used.

At the least, no decision concerning therapy should be made until the BP has been measured on three separate occasions. As shown in Table 11–4, acclimatization to the physician can lead to a mean fall in BP of 14/7 between the first and third visits. Even hypertension persisting after three visits may disappear spontaneously with continued follow-up in some patients. Eighteen percent of placebo-treated patients in the MRC trial had a diastolic BP that was persistently under 90 mmHg at 1 to 3 years.[23] The incidence of spontaneous cure is even higher if 95 mmHg is used as the dividing point: 48 percent of placebo-treated patients in the Australian study had an initial, repeatedly measured diastolic BP between 95 and 109 mmHg that fell below 95 mmHg during the ensuing 3 years.[181] Thus, in the patient with an initial diastolic BP between 90 and 100 mmHg who is not at any acute risk, the three measurements of BP should be made over at least 6 months.

It is also advisable to arrange for measurement of the patient's BP in the ambulatory setting at this time. In addition to possibly providing a more accurate assessment of the BP, continued involvement of the patient in his or her care may improve compliance with subsequent dietary or medical therapy.

With these considerations in mind, the following recommendations can be made concerning the use of antihypertensive agents (Table 11-10)[182,183]:

1. Patients with a diastolic BP persistently above 94 mmHg should be treated. Nonpharmacologic therapies (such as dietary sodium restriction, weight reduction, and avoidance of excess alcohol, as indicated) can be tried initially since these modalities can minimize the need for drug treatment.

2. The necessity to treat a diastolic BP of 90 to 94 mmHg remains controversial.[173] At the least, all patients in this group should be tried on nonpharmacologic therapy and, if this is ineffective, antihypertensive agents added if there is end-organ damage, a positive family history of serious hypertensive complications, other risk factors for coronary disease such as hypercholesterolemia or smoking, or an increase in the diastolic BP to 95 mmHg or above. Drug therapy can also be tried in the absence of these indications, particularly

if control can be achieved with one medication and no side effects (such as a once-daily converting enzyme inhibitor or, in blacks, a low dose of a diuretic; see p. 535). The use of multiple agents, especially if associated with side effects, should probably be avoided when one considers the relatively small *absolute* benefit that is likely to be attained in this setting (see Table 11-8).

3. The necessity for therapy is uncertain in patients with hypertension in the physician's office but a diastolic BP below 90 mmHg in the ambulatory setting. Assuming that the accuracy of the ambulatory values has been documented, antihypertensive agents can be withheld and the patient carefully monitored for signs of end-organ damage, such as an increase in QRS voltage on the electrocardiogram[131] or an increase in left ventricular mass on cardiac ultrasound.[58-60]

These recommendations have not considered the necessity for therapy in the elderly or in patients with isolated systolic hypertension.

HYPERTENSION IN THE ELDERLY

Several unique problems must be addressed when approaching the older patient (>60 years old) with hypertension. The development of arterial calcification can lead to overestimation of the true BP by as much as 50 mmHg, since the BP cuff will be less able to compress the brachial artery. As described above, this problem can be suspected at the bedside. The cuff should be inflated to a level above the systolic BP so that the arterial *pulse* is no longer palpable; if the brachial or radial artery can still be felt at this time, it is likely that a thickened vessel is present.[115] The presence of "pseudohypertension" can be confirmed only by direct, intraarterial measurement of the BP, which will also serve as a guide for the necessity for antihypertensive therapy.

Antihypertensive agents also must be used

TABLE 11-10. Indications for Medical Treatment in Mild Hypertension

Decision should be based upon measurement of BP on at least 3 separate visits.

Nonpharmacologic therapy can be used initially.

Medical treatment should be begun if
 1. Diastolic BP of 95 mmHg or above
 2. Diastolic BP between 90 and 94 if
  a. Evidence of end-organ damage
  b. Family history of complications
  c. Other risk factors for coronary disease
 3. Systolic BP above 160 mmHg, independent of diastolic BP
 4. The same considerations apply to older patients

Therapy may be withheld if ambulatory BP is normal, although careful monitoring for end-organ damage is essential.

more carefully in older patients. Side effects tend to be more common because aging frequently leads to decreases in hepatic and renal function and in baroreceptor responsiveness (the baroreceptors are the major protection against orthostatic hypotension). As a result, therapy should be begun with lower doses than generally used, e.g., 25 mg of hydrochlorothiazide or 250 mg of methyldopa per day.

Three trials have evaluated the effectiveness of treating hypertension in the elderly. In small numbers of patients, both the Veterans Administration and HDFP studies suggested that older hypertensive patients benefit from lowering of the BP.[169,184] This issue has been more definitively examined by the European Working Party on Hypertension in the Elderly (EWPHE); 850 patients over the age of 60 with a mean BP of 183/101 (range of diastolic BP between 90 and 119 mmHg) were studied.[185] As in younger patients, decreasing the BP (mean BP 19/5 lower than in placebo-treated patients) resulted in a 35 to 45 percent reduction in cardiovascular morbidity and mortality. However, the *absolute* benefit was much greater than in younger patients because the number of events in the absence of treatment was much higher. In the MRC trial (patient age 35 to 64), for example, the incidence of stroke in the placebo group was 2.6 per 1000 patient years; a 45 percent reduction with therapy represented only 1.2 fewer strokes per 1000 patient years.[23] The comparable value in the elderly was 37 strokes per 1000 patient years with placebo; a 43 percent reduction in this setting represented 16 (versus 1.2) fewer strokes per 1000 patient years.[185] Similarly, the decrease in the total number of cardiovascular events (per 1000 patient years) with therapy was 43 in older patients versus only 1.5 in the MRC trial. Thus, the *data in favor of therapy are actually more compelling in the elderly* in that many more patients will directly benefit from reduction of the BP (except perhaps

patients over the age of 80).[17] To be fair, some of this difference could reflect the higher range of diastolic BP (90 to 119 mmHg) in the EWPHE than in the MRC (90 to 109 mmHg). However, even older patients with mild hypertension showed substantial improvement with therapy in the EWPHE.

ISOLATED SYSTOLIC HYPERTENSION

Each of the above studies grouped patients according to the level of diastolic BP. However, the systolic BP is a separate and perhaps greater risk factor for hypertensive complications,[14-17] causing a two- to fourfold increase in myocardial infarction, stroke, and mortality even at a normal diastolic pressure (see Fig. 10-3).[16,186] This relationship has, in the past, been ascribed in part to systolic hypertension (BP>160/<90) being due to decreased vascular compliance (see p. 472) and therefore merely being a marker for underlying vascular disease. The Framingham Study examined this issue by using loss of the dicrotic notch in the carotid tracing as a sign of decreased vascular compliance.[186] It was concluded that the systolic BP influences the risk of cardiovascular disease independent of vascular stiffness.

Isolated systolic hypertension is primarily a finding in older patients, increasing in incidence from less than 4 percent under the age of 55 to 20 to 40 percent over the age of 75.[16,186] The pathogenesis is also age-dependent. Although reduced vascular compliance is usually the primary problem, a sympathetically mediated increase in the rate of ventricular ejection is generally responsible for an elevated systolic BP in younger subjects.[187]

There is as yet no proof that treating isolated systolic hypertension is beneficial.[188] Nevertheless, it seems reasonable to attempt to lower the systolic BP to 140 to 150 mmHg,[16,189] given the marked increase in risk.[17] The induction of diastolic *hypotension* is generally not a problem (unless the baseline diastolic BP is below 75 to 80 mmHg), since antihypertensive therapy usually produces a preferential reduction in the systolic pressure in this setting.[190]

HYPERTENSION POST-CVA

Although the treatment of hypertensive emergencies is beyond the scope of this chapter, it is important to consider the acute management of hypertension in the patient with a cerebrovascular accident. Although hypertension is a major risk factor for the development of a transient ischemic attack or thrombotic stroke, it is essential to recognize that the elevation in BP is not having any deleterious effect at the time of the stroke. To the contrary, hypertension may be beneficial by helping to maintain flow to borderline ischemic areas.[31,48,191] For example, the BP frequently rises spontaneously (and transiently) with cerebral ischemia, presumably reflecting an attempt to maximize cerebral perfusion.[48] As a result, antihypertensive therapy should be withheld for several weeks unless the patient has heart failure, a diastolic BP above 120 to 130 mmHg, or evidence of hypertensive encephalopathy.[31,191] If the BP is lowered, a slow infusion of nitroprusside is preferable, since the short half-life of this drug minimizes the risk of inducing cerebral hypoperfusion.

Management of the BP is different in the hypertensive patient with a subarachnoid hemorrhage. In this setting, an elevation in BP increases the risk of rebleeding, and nitroprusside should be used to maintain the systolic pressure between 140 and 160 mmHg.[191] Lowering the BP further may be deleterious by inducing ischemia in areas of arterial vasospasm. It is possible that calcium channel blockers may also be safe to use since they seem to preferentially reverse the cerebral vasospasm.[192]

Similar considerations apply to the patient with an intracerebral hemorrhage, a complication that is usually directly induced by severe hypertension.[34,43] Reducing the BP may decrease further bleeding and minimize brain swelling, but it can also produce ischemia in the surrounding brain tissue and worsen the neurologic deficit.[191] If necessary, nitroprusside can be carefully administered, pending the preferred therapy of surgical decompression.

HOW TO TREAT

Blood pressure reduction can be achieved by alterations in diet or lifestyle (Table 11–11) or by the administration of medications. The first two modalities are usually preferable since the cost and side effects associated with drug therapy can be avoided. Furthermore, many of these changes are also beneficial from a general health viewpoint, independent of any reduction in the systemic BP.

NONPHARMACOLOGIC THERAPY

The mechanisms by which dietary factors contribute to the genesis of essential hypertension is discussed in detail in Chap. 10. This section will review the findings that suggest that modifying the diet and lifestyle can lower the BP in selected patients.[193]

SODIUM RESTRICTION

Forty to sixty percent of patients with essential hypertension show sodium sensitivity as

TABLE 11–11. Nonpharmacologic Therapy of Hypertension

Dietary changes
   Moderate sodium restriction
   Weight reduction if obese
   Calcium supplementation (?)
   Restrict alcohol ingestion
   Increase potassium intake (?)
   High fiber, low saturated fat, or vegetarian diet
Aerobic exercise
Relaxation techniques

evidenced by a rise in BP with sodium loading and a reduction in BP with sodium restriction.[194-199] Perhaps the best controlled study is illustrated in Fig. 11–11. Nineteen patients with mild essential hypertension (mean BP 156/98) decreased their sodium intake from 190 to 86 meq/day. They were then randomly given either sodium chloride or placebo tablets in a double-blind, crossover fashion; the former was sufficient to raise net sodium intake to about 162 meq/day. The mean BP rose by an average of 12/6 mmHg during the period of high sodium intake but remained at the baseline level with the placebo tablets. These changes in BP, which reflected in part changes in the plasma volume, occurred in only 12 of the 19 patients, indicating that only some patients are sodium-sensitive.[195]

In general, restricting sodium intake is most effective in patients with a low plasma renin activity in whom volume factors may be of greater importance.[197] This blunting of the renin response[194,200] allows the effect of volume depletion on the BP to be more fully expressed since it is not counteracted by increased production of the vasoconstrictor angiotensin II.

Two further points regarding the response to sodium restriction deserve emphasis. First, the relationship between sodium intake and the systemic BP appears to be steepest between 70 and 120 meq per day.[198,201] Thus, a daily sodium intake of 70 to 80 mcq is probably optimal. More marked sodium restriction is relatively unpalatable and frequently produces little further change in BP, because increased activity of the renin-angiotensin system counteracts the effect of continued volume depletion.[194] Similar considerations apply to diuretic therapy, the efficacy of which can also be minimized by enhanced renin release.[202]

Second, the efficacy of sodium restriction increases with the severity of the elevation in BP (Fig. 11–12).[194,200] Thus, limiting sodium in-

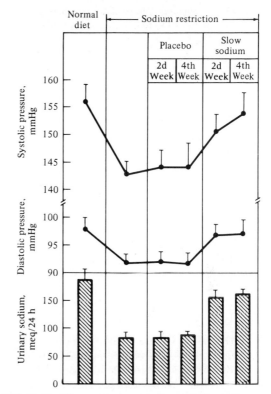

FIG. 11–11. The average systolic and diastolic blood pressure and urinary sodium excretion in 19 hypertensive subjects on a normal diet 2 weeks after dietary sodium restriction and at 2-week intervals during the randomized crossover trial of placebo or sodium chloride ("slow sodium") tablets. (*From G. A. MacGregor, N. D. Markandu, F. E. Best, D. M. Elder, J. M. Cam, G. A. Sagnella, and M. Squires, Lancet, 1:351, 1982.*)

take is most important in patients with moderate to advanced hypertension. The mechanism responsible for this relationship is incompletely understood, but impaired renin responsiveness (perhaps reflecting acquired renal damage) again appears to be important.

In addition to lowering the BP, sodium restriction also may be beneficial by *minimizing potassium losses* in those patients concomitantly being treated with a diuretic.[203] At a

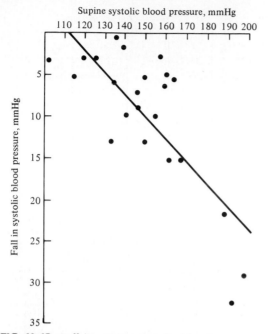

FIG. 11–12. Fall in supine systolic blood pressure with sodium restriction plotted against pretreatment supine systolic blood pressure in 19 different trials. (*Adapted from G. A. MacGregor, Hypertension, 7:628, 1985. By permission of the American Heart Association, Inc.*)

sodium intake of 72 meq per day, for example, the potassium deficit is only about one-half that seen with 195 meq per day.[203] This effect is probably related to decreased flow to the distal nephron with sodium restriction, thereby diminishing distal potassium secretion.

Patient compliance with sodium restriction can be assessed by a 24-h or overnight urine collection or by having the patient test his or her urine with a chloride-sensitive dipstick.[204] Estimation of sodium chloride excretion remains effective even in patients being treated with a diuretic. Although diuretics increase sodium excretion, the associated volume loss activates sodium-retaining mechanisms such as the renin-angiotensin-aldosterone system.

A new steady state is soon achieved, in which the sodium-retaining and diuretic effects balance out and intake is again equal to excretion. What is not generally appreciated is that this response occurs very quickly, usually within 3 to 7 days.[205]

Finally, sodium restriction may be beneficial even in those patients who do not have a reduction in BP. To the degree that a hypotensive response is limited by an increase in renin release, the patient will become more sensitive to those antihypertensive agents that act in part by diminishing either renin secretion (β-adrenergic blockers) or the production of angiotensin II (converting enzyme inhibitors).

WEIGHT REDUCTION

In obese patients, weight reduction can lower the BP, independent of any associated decrease in sodium intake.[206-210] This is generally a dose-dependent effect as the BP can fall by an average of about 1 mmHg for every 1 kg of weight lost (Fig. 11–13).[207-209] Reduc-

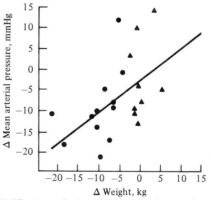

FIG. 11–13. Correlation between change in mean arterial pressure and change in weight in patients who did (circles) or who did not (triangles) lose weight. (*From E. Reisin, E. D. Frohlich, F. H. Messerli, G. R. Dreslinksy, F. G. Dunn, M. M. Jones, and H. M. Batson, Ann. Intern. Med., 98:315, 1983.*)

tions in plasma volume, cardiac output, and plasma norepinephrine level all may contribute to the hypotensive response.[208-210]

Weight reduction is also beneficial because of its favorable effect on plasma lipids: in one study, total cholesterol fell by about 6 percent.[211] This is in contrast to the potentially deleterious changes that can be induced by commonly used antihypertensive agents: a 5 to 15 mg/dL rise in total cholesterol with thiazide diuretics and a marked rise in triglycerides and a 10 percent fall in HDL-cholesterol with β-blockers.[32,211]

CALCIUM SUPPLEMENTATION

Abnormal calcium metabolism, as manifested by a decrease in both calcium intake and the plasma concentration of ionized calcium, appears to be present in many patients with essential hypertension (see p. 486).[212,213] Correcting these defects with calcium supplementation (1000 mg/day) can lower the BP by 10 mmHg or more in almost 45 percent of patients as well as almost 20 percent of normotensive subjects.[214] The long-term safety of this regimen remains unproven, however; calcium can *raise* the BP in some patients,[214] and constipation and, in susceptible subjects, hypercalcemia or kidney stones may be a problem.[215]

ALCOHOL INTAKE

The ingestion of more than two drinks per day can increase the risk of hypertension.[216,217] Conversely, decreasing alcohol intake below this level can reduce the BP; in one study of 16 patients, the mean BP fell from 175/105 to 155/98 with abstinence.[218] Thus, control of alcohol ingestion may be of primary importance in selected patients.

POTASSIUM SUPPLEMENTATION

Low dietary potassium intake may be another factor predisposing to the development of hypertension.[219] On the other hand, the ad-

ministration of about 60 meq of supplemental potassium per day can produce a modest (4 percent) reduction in BP[220]; a similar response can occur with correction of diuretic-induced hypokalemia.[221] However, the role of extra potassium is at present uncertain considering the relatively small antihypertensive effect and the possible risk of hyperkalemia in patients with impaired renal function.

OTHER DIETARY MODIFICATIONS

Increasing dietary fiber, consuming a vegetarian diet, and enhancing the intake of polyunsaturated fatty acids all have been shown to produce a small reduction in BP in hypertensive patients.[222-224] Although their mechanism of action and their role in the treatment of hypertension is undefined, they may all be desirable from the viewpoint of the patient's overall health.

AEROBIC EXERCISE

Aerobic exercise appears to have a beneficial effect on the systemic BP. Patients with a low level of fitness have an increased risk of hypertension.[225] On the other hand, a 5 to 15 mmHg reduction in BP can be achieved in many hypertensive patients following the institution of regular exercise, such as jogging 2 miles per day.[193,226-228] This response, which is lost with the resumption of a sedentary lifestyle,[226] is frequently associated with a fall in circulating norepinephrine levels, a change that could account for the decrease in BP.[227,228] The mechanism by which sympathetic tone is diminished by exercise is not known.

RELAXATION TECHNIQUES

A variety of relaxation or biofeedback techniques have been tried in hypertensive patients. In general, a small reduction in BP of 5 to 10 mmHg can be achieved in many patients.[229] This beneficial response is thought to be mediated by decreased sympathetic activity, presumably induced by diminished stress.

SUMMARY

Nonpharmacologic therapies offer the possibility of substantially reducing the BP without the cost or side effects of antihypertensive medications. The benefit, at least in selected patients, of sodium restriction, weight reduction, limitation of alcohol intake, and aerobic exercise appear to be well established. It is also possible that the use of calcium or potassium supplements will prove to be important, although the risk/benefit ratio for these modalities is uncertain at this time.

PHARMACOLOGIC THERAPY

Antihypertensive medications are required if the above modalities are ineffective. In the stepped-care approach that has generally been in use, medical therapy begins with a thiazide diuretic or a β-adrenergic blocker. Several large studies have attempted to clarify this issue further by specifically comparing the efficacy of these two classes of drugs in the initial management of essential hypertension.[23,230,231] However, recent findings have questioned this approach, in terms of both safety and drug-induced side effects. The remainder of this chapter will review the problems with diuretics and β-blockers and consider possible newer alternatives to these drugs, particularly the converting enzyme inhibitors and calcium channel blockers. A complete discussion of all of the different antihypertensive agents that are available is beyond the scope of this chapter.

DIURETICS

Thiazide diuretics have traditionally been the mainstay of antihypertensive therapy. The loop diuretics, such as furosemide, are more potent diuretics but are less effective in lowering the BP.[203] This apparently paradoxical finding may be related to the short duration of action of these drugs in comparison to the relatively long-acting thiazides. Although the initial natriuresis with furosemide is relatively large, it lasts for only 6 h. The ensuing volume depletion activates volume-regulatory mechanisms (such as the renin-angiotensin-aldosterone and sympathetic nervous systems) that promote sodium retention during the remaining 18 h of the day, thereby minimizing the net diuretic effect.[232]

The antihypertensive action of a thiazide diuretic is initially mediated by a fall in cardiac output induced by the diuresis. With time, however, the plasma volume and cardiac output may rise toward normal, but the decline in BP is in part sustained by a decrease in systemic vascular resistance.[233,234] The mechanism by which diuretics lead to vasodilatation is not well understood, since the associated increase in renin release would be expected to raise vascular resistance. One possible explanation (which could also explain the hypotensive effect of sodium restriction) involves the role of an endogenous, digitalis-like natriuretic hormone in the genesis of the vasoconstriction that is responsible for maintenance of the hypertension (see p. 484).[235,236] Diuretic-induced hypovolemia would reduce the secretion of this hormone, thereby allowing cell Na-K-ATPase activity to rise. The ensuing reduction in cell sodium and calcium concentrations would then lower vascular tone toward normal. The observation that volume depletion is essential for a reduction in BP following diuretic therapy is compatible with this hypothesis. If hypovolemia does not occur because the diuretic is ineffective or sodium intake is not restricted, the decreases in vascular resistance and systemic BP are attenuated or prevented.[203,237]

Despite the efficacy of diuretics, the data presented above from the MRFIT, MRC, and HDFP studies (see Table 11–9) suggest that the thiazides can lead to coronary morbidity and mortality (particularly sudden death) in at least some patients.[23,174,176,177] Diuretic therapy has been shown to increase the incidence of ventricular arrhythmias,[238] a complication that could result from one or more metabolic changes induced by these agents including hypokalemia,[238,239] hypomagnesemia,[240] hyperglycemia,[241,242] and hyperlipidemia.[32,243]

The role of any one of these factors is, of course, difficult to prove. Hypokalemia (defined as a plasma potassium concentration below 3.5 meq/L), for example, occurs in up to 50 percent of patients treated with 50 to 100 mg of hydrochlorothiazide (or its equivalent).[239] It has been argued that this relatively small change in potassium balance is too mild to pose a serious cardiac risk.[244] However, mild hypokalemia can become severe hypokalemia during a stress response. This effect is probably mediated by epinephrine which, acting via the β_2-adrenergic receptors, drives potassium from the extracellular fluid into the cells.[245,246] Figure 11–14 illustrates the effect of infusing epinephrine to achieve a plasma concentration similar to that occurring during an acute myocardial infarction. In the basal state, epinephrine lowered the plasma potassium concentration from 3.8 to 3.2 meq/L. If, however, these normal subjects were pretreated with a thiazide diuretic, the baseline plasma potassium concentration fell to about 3.3 meq/L and epinephrine now lowered the plasma potassium level to below 2.5 meq/L in some subjects.

It is possible that marked diuretic- and epinephrine-induced hypokalemia could predispose to ventricular arrhythmias during an episode of coronary ischemia, particularly if superimposed upon underlying hypomagnesemia. There is some evidence in support of this hypothesis, as an increased incidence of both ventricular fibrillation and ventricular tachycardia has been described in patients with an acute myocardial infarction who were initially hypokalemic, especially if the plasma

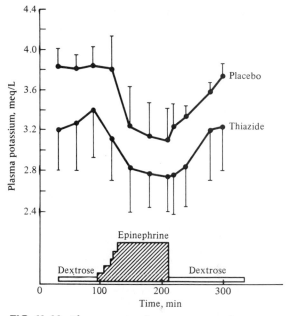

FIG. 11–14. Plasma potassium concentration during an infusion of epinephrine in six patients pretreated with a placebo or a thiazide for 7 days. (*From A. Struthers, R. Whitesmith, and J. L. Reid, Lancet, 1:1358, 1983.*)

potassium concentration were below 3.0 meq/L (a measurement that includes a possible acute epinephrine effect) (Fig. 11–15).[247,248] It may be relevant to note in this regard, that the increased risk in the MRFIT occurred entirely in treated patients who had an abnormal electrocardiogram, a marker for underlying cardiac disease.[174] The MRFIT also suggested a possible dose-dependent effect: the percentage of patients receiving more than 50 mg per day of hydrochlorothiazide or chlorthalidone was 51 percent in the special intervention group versus only 15 percent in the usual care group.[174]

At present, it is uncertain what conclusions should be drawn concerning the safety of chronic diuretic therapy. One could choose to treat all hypokalemic patients with potassium chloride or a potassium-sparing diu-

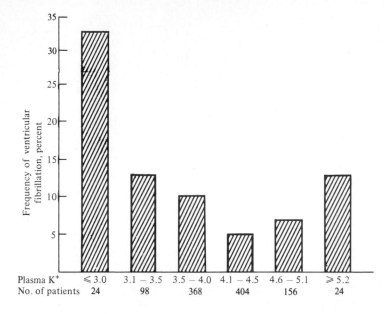

FIG. 11–15. Number and percentage of patients with acute myocardial infarction who developed ventricular fibrillation as a function of the plasma potassium concentration (in milliequivalents per liter) obtained within 3 h of admission. (*From J. E. Nordrehaug and G. von der Lippe, Br. Ht. J., 50:525, 1983.*)

retic. It is not proven, however, that this would make diuretics safer to use. In the MRC trial, for example, raising the plasma potassium concentration toward normal did not reverse the increased incidence of ventricular arrhythmias in patients receiving a diuretic.[249] This finding suggests that other factors, such as hypomagnesemia, may also be important in enhancing cardiac irritability.

In summary, it seems prudent to consider alternative antihypertensive agents for first-line therapy, using drugs that lack the metabolic complications* and, it is hoped, lack the increased coronary risk that may be associated with diuretic therapy. One exception may be in black patients who generally respond much better to diuretics (by a mean of 7 to up to 20 mmHg) than they do to other drugs such as β-blockers or converting enzyme inhibitors.[188,230,231,251] Thiazides may also be particularly effective in patients already being treated with a converting enzyme

inhibitor; the rise in angiotensin II that normally limits the effectiveness of the diuretic[202] is now prevented by converting enzyme inhibition.[252,253] In these settings, the thiazide should be used in the lowest effective dose: 25 or 50 mg of hydrochlorothiazide or chlorthalidone per day.[230,254]

Diuretics also continue to be important in those conditions in which *volume expansion* is an important determinant of the rise in BP, both by a direct effect and by limiting the antihypertensive action of other drugs.[255,256] Examples include refractory essential hypertension,[255-257] acute glomerulonephritis,[258] and chronic renal failure.[259] In these settings, there is frequently a strong stimulus to sodium retention, and a loop diuretic may be required to produce an adequate diuresis.

β-ADRENERGIC BLOCKERS

The problem with the use of β-adrenergic blockers (such as propranolol, atenolol, or metoprolol) is more related to symptoms than to safety. In the MRC trial, for example, 20 to 25 percent of patients discontinued propranolol within 5 years because of suspected adverse effects (versus less than 5 percent

*It is not generally appreciated that thiazides also cause impotence in approximately 6 to 7 percent of men, a frequency that is higher than that seen with β-blockers.[23,250] The mechanism by which this occurs is not known.

withdrawal from placebo therapy).[23] It is likely that many other patients also became symptomatic but were willing to continue therapy.[180]

The side effects that occur with β-blockers (and with other sympatholytic agents such as methyldopa, clonidine, prazosin, and reserpine) are a *direct reflection of interference with normal sympathetic functioning.* The most prominent complaints include lethargy, fatigue, impotence, Raynaud's phenomenon (due to unopposed α-adrenergic vasoconstriction), bradycardia, dyspnea, and decreased exercise capacity.[23,230,260,261] Mental depression also may be an important problem. In one study of Medicaid patients, almost 30 percent of young hypertensives (age 20 to 44) treated with a β-blocker also required an antidepressant, an incidence 2 to 3 times greater than that of patients treated with different antihypertensive drugs.[262] In addition, other problems that can occur in susceptible patients include heart failure, exacerbation of obstructive lung or peripheral vascular disease, and masking of the early symptoms of, and delayed recovery from, hypoglycemia.[263-265]

There are also two acute and potentially fatal problems that can arise from the use of β-blockers. First, abrupt discontinuance of therapy can lead to a withdrawal syndrome which, in patients with coronary artery disease, can be manifested by accelerated angina, myocardial infarction, or sudden death.[266-268] Enhanced sensitivity to β-adrenergic stimuli, presumably due to up-regulation of β-receptors in response to chronic β-blockade, is thought to be primarily responsible for these symptoms.[267,268] This state can persist for up to 2 weeks, so slow tapering is essential if treatment is to be withdrawn.[267]

Second, a marked elevation in BP (of as much as 90 mmHg) due to unopposed α-adrenergic vasoconstriction can occur when sympathetic tone is increased due to an underlying pheochromocytoma or severe hypoglycemia.[269-272]

To some degree, the use of a β_1-selective, hydrophilic (which should limit movement across the blood-brain barrier) agent such as atenolol can minimize these side effects.[264,265] However, this protection is only relative. Marked hypertension can still occur during hypoglycemia,[271,272] although it may be less prominent than that seen with a nonselective drug such as propranolol.[272] Similarly, atenolol can reduce sleep disturbances produced by *lipophilic* agents such as propranolol or metoprolol[273] but has not been shown to diminish the more common neurologic symptoms of lethargy and fatigue.

In summary, the β-blockers are effective drugs that can reduce cerebrovascular and coronary morbidity, at least in nonsmokers.[23] However, these agents appear to have too many side effects that are a *predictable result of their mechanism of action* to be considered optimal first-line agents.* Nevertheless, there are patients who may particularly benefit from treatment with β-blockers. Included in this group are patients who have angina, a recent myocardial infarction, heart failure with a normal ejection fraction (which is indicative of diastolic dysfunction),[63] or evidence of increased sympathetic tone such as resting tachycardia or systolic hypertension in a young patient in whom reduced vascular compliance would not be expected to be responsible for the rise in systolic BP.[187]

THE IDEAL ANTIHYPERTENSIVE AGENT

Considering the problems with diuretics and β-blockers, it is useful to consider the properties that an ideal antihypertensive agent should have. These include the following:

1. Effective in most patients as a single agent

---

*Similar considerations apply to other sympatholytic agents. The α_1-blocker prazosin, for example, has been advocated for initial therapy because it is effective and modestly lowers both LDL-cholesterol and triglycerides, in comparison to the hyperlipidemic effects of thiazides and β-blockers.[32,274] However, headache, fatigue, mood changes, and dizziness are prominent symptoms in many patients.[274]

2. No interference with sympathetic function
3. No reflex activation of sympathetic function
4. No sodium retention (a common problem with direct vasodilators)
5. Minimum side effects
6. Once-daily dosage
7. Proven long-term safety

The efficacy of any of the available antihypertensive drugs is variable, with the reduction in BP ranging from 0 to 25 mmHg in different patients.[275-277] One way to maximize the effectiveness of therapy (and to minimize the incidence of side effects) is to identify those patients who are most likely to respond to a given agent. As described above, blacks appear to be particularly sensitive to diuretic therapy.[188,230,231,251] In other patients, it has been suggested that the hypotensive response can be predicted with a reasonable degree of accuracy by measurement of the plasma renin activity: high renin responding best to β-blockers and low renin best to diuretics.[275,276,278] More recent studies, however, suggest that the *plasma renin activity is of limited value* in predicting the effect of therapy, with the difference in response between low and high renin groups being only a few mmHg.[279,280] This finding appears to be true even with converting enzyme inhibitors, as patients with low plasma renin (and presumably low angiotensin II) levels may have a substantial reduction in BP, although the change tends to be somewhat less than that seen in patients with a normal or elevated plasma renin activity.[281-285]

The patient's age may be somewhat more helpful than the plasma renin activity in choosing an antihypertensive regimen. β-blockers are most effective in patients under the age of 40, but produce little change in BP when given alone to patients over the age of 60.[286,287] This relationship could reflect the higher plasma renin levels found in younger patients, since the efficacy of β-blockers appears to

vary directly with the plasma renin activity.[276,286] In comparison, calcium channel blockers have the opposite age distribution, being most effective in older patients.[287] It had been thought that converting enzyme inhibitors would, like β-blockers, be of greatest use in young patients with high renin and angiotensin II levels. However, these agents may also be beneficial in the elderly.[288,289]

In summary, there is a certain amount of trial and error involved in finding the optimal therapeutic regimen for a given patient. In the past, this process generally began with a diuretic or β-blocker. However, these agents may be replaced as first-line drugs by converting enzyme inhibitors and calcium channel blockers, which appear to have a more favorable side effect profile. Although their efficacy is well established, it is important to note that the experience with these drugs is relatively limited and their long-term safety is not yet proven.

CONVERTING ENZYME INHIBITORS

There are currently two converting enzyme inhibitors (CEI) available in the United States: captopril and enalapril. These drugs lower the BP by reducing systemic vascular resistance.[290] Although they inhibit converting enzyme and, therefore, the conversion of angiotensin I into angiotensin II, the mechanism by which they produce vasodilation is incompletely understood. The observation that CEI may have a hypotensive effect even in patients with a low plasma renin activity[281-285] suggests that factors other than reduced angiotensin II formation may also be important.[291] For example, CEI may, in some patients, increase the plasma levels of both bradykinin (converting enzyme is also a kininase) and prostaglandins (by an unknown mechanism).[291-294] These vasodilator hormones could contribute to the decreases in vascular resistance and BP.

Alternatively, the efficacy of CEI in patients with low plasma renin levels could still be explained by reduced angiotensin II production, if the plasma levels did not reflect the *local activity* of the renin-angiotensin system. Complete renin-angiotensin systems have been identified in a variety of extrarenal tissues, including vascular endothelium and the brain.[295,296] Inhibition of angiotensin II production at these sites could explain the antihypertensive response to CEI in low-renin states, including bilaterally nephrectomized patients who have no renal renin.[285]

It is also possible that *intrarenal* angiotensin II may be physiologically important at a time when circulating levels are low. Approximately 40 percent of patients with essential hypertension do not normally increase renal blood flow or urinary sodium excretion after a sodium load, resulting in a larger rise in BP than seen in those with normal vascular and urinary responses.[297] These "nonmodulators" appropriately suppress plasma renin, angiotensin II, and aldosterone levels after volume expansion. Nevertheless, the response to a sodium load in this low-renin setting can be normalized by CEI, suggesting that intrarenal angiotensin II might be responsible for the inability to increase renal blood flow or urinary sodium excretion

Converting enzyme inhibitors are very effective first-line drugs. When captopril was administered to patients with mild to moderate hypertension, 65 to 70 percent became normotensive; this value was increased to 85 to 90 percent by the addition of a diuretic.[252,253] This combination is particularly useful because CEI have three beneficial effects in this setting: they prevent the rise in angiotensin II that normally limits the hypotensive action of the diuretic[202]; they minimize the degree of diuretic-induced hypokalemia (due to the associated reduction in aldosterone release); and they prevent the diuretic-induced rise in cholesterol levels by an unknown mechanism.[32,298]

Converting enzyme inhibitors are attractive antihypertensive agents because they *lack the predictable side effects associated with other drugs*. The major physiologic role of angiotensin II is BP and volume regulation. Thus, inhibiting the formation of this hormone does not produce the symptoms commonly seen with β-blockers (fatigue, lethargy, depression, impotence, Raynaud's phenomenon) or other sympatholytic agents such as methyldopa (fatigue, dry mouth, impotence, orthostatic hypotension).[253] The metabolic effects associated with diuretic therapy also do not occur, and there is no reflex activation of the sympathetic nervous system (potentially producing tachycardia and angina) as frequently follows the use of direct vasodilators such as hydralazine, minoxidil, or nifedipine. This lack of sympathetic activation may be related to prevention of the normal facilitory role of angiotensin II on both norepinephrine release and its vasoconstrictive effect.[299,300] Finally, CEI do not lead to fluid retention because of the reductions in angiotensin II and aldosterone levels, both of which normally promote sodium reabsorption.[301,302] The net effect is that CEI tend to lead to a better "quality of life" than other antihypertensive agents.[303,304]

Side effects, however, do occur and can be divided into two general groups: those that are due to the decrease in angiotensin II formation and those that represent a toxic or idiosyncratic reaction to the drug (Table 11–12).

TABLE 11–12. Side Effects Associated with Converting Enzyme Inhibitors

Related to decreased angiotensin II levels
  1. Hypotension—especially first dose on diuretic therapy
  2. Hyperkalemia—primarily with renal insufficiency
  3. Acute renal failure—primarily with bilateral renal artery stenosis
  4. Contraindicated in pregnancy
Toxic or idiosyncratic side effects
  1. Neutropenia—dose-related, highest risk in collagen disease with renal insufficiency
  2. Rash
  3. Abnormal taste
  4. Proteinuria

Fortunately, *most of these complications can be prevented or their incidence minimized by appropriate use of the drug.* Hypotension, particularly following the first dose, is a potentially serious problem. Some patients have an acute reduction in BP exceeding 50 mmHg, a change that can occasionally produce symptoms of cerebral ischemia.[305] The magnitude of the fall in BP is proportional to the baseline plasma renin activity (in contrast to the chronic response)[284,305] and is most prominent in hypovolemic, diuretic-treated patients. As a result, any patient started on a CEI optimally should discontinue diuretics for 3 to 5 days. The patient should then be instructed to take the first dose (6.25 mg of captopril or 2.5 mg of enalapril) only after he or she is in bed for the night. This regimen should minimize the risk to almost all patients. The acute decrease in BP is progressively attenuated with subsequent doses, and hypotension is a problem only when excessive doses are given.

A rise in the plasma potassium concentration is a relatively common finding with the use of CEI.[306] Decreased aldosterone secretion, due to the fall in angiotensin II levels, is responsible for this problem. In general, the increase in the plasma potassium concentration is less than 0.5 meq/L.[306] However, more pronounced hyperkalemia can occur in patients with renal insufficiency or those concurrently treated with a potassium supplements or a potassium-sparing diuretic, both of which should be avoided when a CEI is used.[306,307]

Acute renal failure due to angiotensin II inhibition can be seen in two clinical settings. Prerenal azotemia or postischemic acute tubular necrosis can occur if the systemic BP is excessively reduced,[308] a problem that can follow the use of almost any antihypertensive agent. A different mechanism is involved in patients with bilateral renal artery stenosis or unilateral stenosis in a solitary functioning kidney (see p. 83). In these conditions, lowering the systemic BP toward normal reduces the *intrarenal* pressure *below normal* because of the pressure gradient across the stenotic lesion. Maintenance of the GFR in the presence of intrarenal hypotension can normally be achieved by autoregulation, a process that involves in part angiotensin II-induced constriction of the efferent arteriole. Therefore, blocking angiotensin II formation with a CEI can impair the autoregulatory response and lead to an acute decline in renal function. Awareness of this complication is important since the development of acute renal failure following the institution of therapy with a CEI should lead to evaluation for bilateral renal artery stenosis, assuming that there has not been a marked reduction in BP (see Chap. 12). A similar decrease in renal function can also occur in some patients with severe heart failure and a low baseline BP after the administration of a CEI to diminish afterload.[309]

In contrast to these deleterious effects when intrarenal pressure is reduced, CEI usually have a favorable effect on renal hemodynamics when given to uncomplicated patients with essential hypertension. In this setting, renal blood flow and, occasionally, the GFR are increased as the vasoconstrictive actions of angiotensin II (including a decrease in glomerular capillary permeability) are reversed.[81,82]

Converting enzyme inhibitors are contraindicated in pregnancy. Although angiotensin II is a systemic vasoconstrictor, it appears to act as a vasodilator in the uterus by increasing the uterine production of prostaglandins. In pregnant rabbits, the adminsitration of a CEI leads to a decrease in uterine flow (due to diminished prostaglandin release) and marked fetal wastage.[310]

The major toxic or idiosyncratic side effects associated with captopril have been rash, neutropenia, abnormalities in taste, and, less often, proteinuria (which can be in the nephrotic range due to membranous nephropathy).[311,312]

The incidence of these complications is in part dose-related. As a result, initial studies with captopril utilizing up to 450 mg/day showed a relatively high frequency of side effects. However, recent trials have demonstrated that 100 to at most 150 mg/day is the maximum effective dose in most patients.[252,253] At these lower doses, captopril is much better tolerated; the incidence of rash has fallen from 11 to 6 percent; that of abnormal taste from 6 to 2.4 percent.[313]

The development of reversible and potentially fatal neutropenia is uncommon, although certain patients are at higher risk. The incidence of this complication, which almost always occurs within the first 3 months of therapy, rises from the negligible value of 0.02 percent in otherwise normal patients, to 0.4 percent in patients with a plasma creatinine concentration above 2 mg/dL, and then to 7.2 percent in patients with both renal insufficiency and either lupus or scleroderma.[314] Patients in the last group should probably be treated with enalapril (if a CEI is to be used), since this drug may have less bone marrow toxicity.

There is reason to believe that enalapril might have fewer toxic side effects than captopril. The complications seen with captopril are similar to those with penicillamine,[315] which also has a sulfhydryl group. Enalapril lacks a sulfhydryl group and appears to have a lower incidence of rash, taste abnormalities, and possibly bone marrow suppression.[316] Furthermore, there seems to be little cross-reactivity between these drugs; some patients who have developed a rash on captopril have not had the same problem when switched to enalapril.[317] It is not yet clear if there is any increased risk of bone marrow toxicity with the use of enalapril (as there is with captopril) in patients with renal failure. This is an important issue since CEI appear to be uniquely beneficial in minimizing the rate of progression of underlying renal disease (see p. 123). These drugs can reduce hemodynamic injury by directly lowering the intraglomerular pressure, an effect that is achieved by reversal of the angiotensin II-induced constriction of the efferent (postglomerular) arteriole.

Enalapril also has other advantages. It needs to be taken only once or, at low doses, twice a day as opposed to 2 or 3 times a day with captopril.[252,318] In addition, the intestinal absorption of captopril is reduced 30 to 40 percent if taken with meals,[290] an effect that does not appear to occur with enalapril. It should be emphasized, however, that the clinical experience with enalapril is relatively limited at this time, and its long-term safety is even less certain than that of captopril.

In summary, converting enzyme inhibitors offer tremendous potential as first-line drugs in the treatment of hypertension: they are generally well tolerated if used appropriately; they do not interfere with sympathetic function; they do not produce the metabolic changes seen with diuretic therapy; and they are broadly effective in patients of all ages.[252,253,288,289] Even black patients, who generally do not respond very well to a CEI alone,[251] may have a marked reduction in BP with the combination of a CEI and a diuretic.[319]

CALCIUM CHANNEL BLOCKERS

Calcium channel blockers represent another class of useful antihypertensive agents. Their effectiveness seems to be based upon their ability to reverse the elevation in cell calcium concentration that, when present in smooth muscle cells, can lead to vasoconstriction and hypertension. For example, the cell calcium concentration in platelets (which have α-adrenergic receptors and contractile elements similar to smooth muscle cells) appears to correlate directly with the systemic BP, being elevated in untreated patients in proportion to the severity of the hypertension (see Fig. 10–15) and falling toward normal following effective antihypertensive therapy with a diuretic, β-blocker, or calcium channel blocker (Fig. 11–16).[320] The reduction in cell calcium with these agents could, for example, reflect reversal of the effects of angiotensin II, norepinephrine, or a digitalis-like natriuretic hormone on cell composition (see p. 484).[321]

Nifedipine, verapamil, and diltiazem are the calcium channel blockers that are currently available. These drugs lower the BP

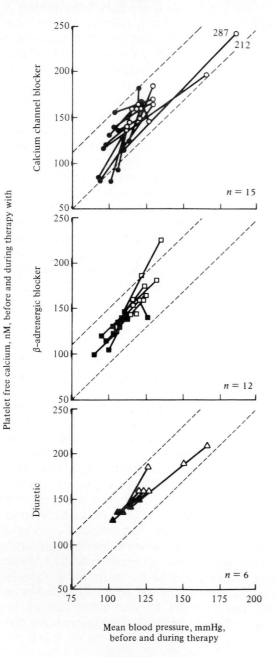

FIG. 11–16. Relationship between intracellular free calcium concentration in platelets and the mean blood pressure before (open symbols) and after (closed symbols) antihypertensive therapy with a calcium channel blocker, β-blocker, or diuretic. The broken lines depict the 95 percent confidence limits of this relationship in untreated patients. (*From P. Erne, P. Bolli, E. Burgisser, and F. R. Buhler, N. Engl. J. Med., 310:1084, 1984. Reprinted by permission from the New England Journal of Medicine.*)

primarily by reducing vascular resistance (particularly nifedipine), although verapamil and to a lesser degree diltiazem also may reduce the cardiac output because of their negative inotropic effects.[322-324] They are most effective in older patients and share some of the advantages of the converting enzyme inhibitors in that they do not reduce sympathetic function and, with the exception of nifedipine, do not usually produce fluid retention[325,326] as do other direct vasodilators such as minoxidil and hydralazine.[327] The latter effect could be due to partial suppression of aldosterone release, since the stimulatory effect of angiotensin II on the adrenal zona glomerulosa cells is mediated by an increase in cell calcium.[328]

Unfortunately, none of the current calcium channel blockers is optimal for first-line therapy. Verapamil is probably the best tolerated, with constipation being the most common side effect.[322,323,329] However, it has to be given 2 or usually 3 times a day and should not be used with a β-blocker because of the combined risk from their negative inotropic and chronotropic effects. The problems with nifedipine are different, being primarily related to the acute vasodilatation induced by this relatively short-acting drug* which must

---

*Although not desirable for chronic therapy, the rapid reduction in vascular resistance makes sublingual or chewed nifedipine capsules (10 to 20 mg) very effective in the treatment of hypertensive "urgencies" in which the diastolic BP is above 120 to 130 mmHg but there are no signs of malignant hypertension or other life-threatening condition requiring parenteral antihypertensive agents.[330-332] In this setting, the aim of therapy is an *acute but controlled* reduction in BP, which can be achieved by nifedipine without a significant risk of hypotension. Clonidine (0.2 mg followed by 0.1 mg every 1 to 2 h to a maximum of 0.7 mg),[332,333] atenolol (100 mg),[334] the triad of furosemide, propranolol, and minoxidil,[335] and captopril[336] have also been effectively used in these patients. Captopril is probably least desirable because of the possibility of an excessive reduction in BP, since the hypotensive response cannot be controlled.[305] Before beginning therapy, however, it is important to note that almost 30 percent of patients with a hypertensive urgency will have a marked reduction in BP to a safe level with 1 h of rest in a quiet, dark room.[337]

be taken 3 or 4 times a day. Headache, flushing, a feeling of hot limbs, and reflex tachycardia are common complaints,[322,323,338] leading to a rate of discontinuation that may exceed 20 percent.[322] Edema may also occur. This problem appears to be primarily related to the redistribution of fluid between the vascular space and the interstitium, rather than renal sodium retention.[339] Vasodilatation at the precapillary arteriole could be responsible by raising the intracapillary pressure, thereby favoring the movement of fluid into the interstitium.

Despite these limitations, future calcium channel blockers will have more desirable characteristics (including once-daily dosage) that will allow them to be used more effectively. For example, a long-acting nifedipine preparation and nitrendipine (a compound related to nifedipine) are as effective antihypertensive agents as regular nifedipine, but are much less likely to produce the above side effects, presumably due to their slower onset of action.[340,341]

RECOMMENDATIONS FOR MEDICAL THERAPY

There is at this time no clear consensus regarding the optimal means by which antihypertensive therapy should be begun. Considering the common problems with patient compliance,[342] it is obviously desirable to choose drugs that are effective, that can be given once or at most twice a day, and that have few side effects. For the reasons outlined above, converting enzyme inhibitors, particularly enalapril if its apparently low incidence of toxic side effects is confirmed, seem to come closest to meeting these criteria. If the antihypertensive response to a CEI is inadequate, a low dose of a thiazide-type diuretic (25 to 50 mg of hydrochlorothiazide per day) can be added. This combination has a synergistic effect,[252,253,319] since the rise in angiotensin II that normally limits the effect of the diuretic[202] is now prevented by converting enzyme inhibition. The sequence of administration should be reversed in blacks, who respond much better to a diuretic than to other antihypertensive drugs.[188,230,231,251] Although a CEI has a relatively small effect when given alone to black patients, a substantial fall in BP frequently occurs in patients already taking a diuretic.[252,319] The net effect is that the CEI-diuretic combination is equally effective in blacks and whites.[252]

The safest way to use a thiazide is uncertain. Coronary mortality may be increased with these drugs,[174,177,178] particularly in patients with an abnormal resting electrocardiogram (Table 11-9). It is possible that limiting the dose to a maximum of 50 mg of hydrochlorothiazide (or its equivalent) can diminish this risk.[174] In addition, hypokalemia should probably be treated if it occurs.[343] A potassium-sparing diuretic, such as amiloride, may be preferable to potassium chloride supplements since the former also minimizes magnesium wasting.[344]

The general aim of therapy is to lower the diastolic BP to 80 to 85 mmHg.[182] A lesser reduction in diastolic BP (to 90 to 95 mmHg) is also beneficial but offers less complete protection against hypertensive complications.[345] If this BP goal is not achieved with a CEI and a diuretic, a calcium channel blocker can be added. These drugs are likely to become even more useful when long-acting preparations that produce fewer side effects and can be taken only once or twice a day become available.

Patients who are resistant to this regimen can be empirically treated with other antihypertensive agents. Included in this group are β-blockers, centrally or peripherally acting sympatholytic agents (methyldopa, guanabenz, clonidine, prazosin), and direct vasodilators (hydralazine and the more potent minoxidil). Truly refractory hypertension is most often due to a secondary cause such as renal artery stenosis, poor compliance with dietary and medical therapy, or volume expansion.[257] To test for the last possibility, the patient should be diuresed with a loop diuretic to "dry weight." This is defined as the point at which the BP becomes normal or the patient develops signs (an overwise unexplained rise in the BUN) or symptoms (cramps, weakness, orthostatic dizziness) of hypovolemia. Many "refractory" hypertensives will have a beneficial response to this regimen, with recurrent volume expansion then being prevented by maintenance diuretic therapy.[255,257] The fall in BP is presumably related to volume loss. In addition to this direct effect the associated increase in renin release will make the patient more responsive to a CEI.[256]

These recommendations apply to uncomplicated patients with essential hypertension. A different regimen may be preferable in selected patients with underlying cardiac disease. Patients with angina pectoris, for example, can be started on a β-blocker or calcium channel blocker, thereby treating both the coronary ischemia and hypertension. Optimal therapy in congestive heart failure, on the other hand, is dependent upon whether systolic or diastolic dysfunction is the primary abnormality. When decreased diastolic filling is the major problem, as evidenced by a normal ejection fraction, treatment with a β-blocker or calcium channel blocker can produce ventricular relaxation and improve cardiac function.[63,64] Decreasing venous return with a diuretic or lowering vascular resistance with a vasodilator (such as a CEI) in this setting can lead to marked hypotension.[63] In contrast, diminishing vascular resistance with a CEI is desirable in patients with impaired cardiac contractility (abnormal ejection fraction), since the reduction in afterload can enhance cardiac performance.[346]

Finally, a β-blocker is the preferred initial therapy when there are signs of a primary increase in β-adrenergic tone. This can be manifested by resting tachycardia or by isolated systolic hypertension in a young patient.

The preferential rise in systolic BP in this setting is due to a sympathetically mediated increase in the rate of ventricular contraction, rather than a decrease in vascular compliance as is commonly present in older patients.[187]

CAN MEDICAL THERAPY BE DISCONTINUED?

Patients started on antihypertensive agents for essential hypertension are generally told that there will be a lifelong need for medical therapy. A variety of studies, however, have evaluated the possibility that therapy can be discontinued after a period of good BP control. In two of these studies, for example, antihypertensive medications were withdrawn from patients whose diastolic BP had been maintained below 90 mmHg for at least 1 to 2 years.[347,348] At 12 to 18 months, only 15 to 20 percent were still normotensive. These relatively discouraging findings are even less impressive when a possible placebo effect is considered. In the Medical Research Council trial described above, approximately 20 percent of initially hypertensive patients who were treated with a placebo had a spontaneous and persistent reduction in diastolic BP to below 90 mmHg.[23]

More encouraging results were obtained from the Hypertension Detection and Follow-up Program.[349] In this study, 50 percent of patients from whom therapy was withdrawn were still normotensive at 1 year. The improved outcome may have been related in part to patient selection; only those patients who had been *normotensive for 5 years* (as opposed to 1 to 2 years in the previous studies) were included. Furthermore, the HDFP was able to identify subgroups that were more likely to remain normotensive:

1. Patients with initially mild hypertension (diastolic BP under 104 mmHg) had a higher success rate than those with more marked elevations in BP.
2. Patients whose BP was controlled with only one drug were about twice as likely to maintain a normal BP as those who were treated with 2 or more drugs.
3. The overall 50 percent success rate at 1 year could be increased to 70 to 80 percent by the addition of dietary therapy: weight reduction in obese patients and sodium restriction in those who were not overweight (Fig. 11–17).

These findings suggest that it may be reasonable to attempt to withdraw antihypertensive therapy from patients who are willing to modify their diet and who have mild hypertension that has been controlled for a period of years by one drug. It is important to note, however, that this effect may be transient since the percent of patients remaining normotensive seems to continue to decline with time. It is possible, therefore, that the number of patients in whom the hypertension does not recur may be similar to what would be seen with placebo therapy. A recent study of 2800 patients in the MRC trial seems to confirm this possibility.[350] Discontinuation of placebo tablets had no effect on BP; in comparison, cessation of active therapy with a thiazide or propranolol resulted in a rise in BP that reached the mean level of the placebo group by 9 to 12 months. Although about 45 percent of previously treated patients remained normotensive at 24 months, similar findings were found in the placebo group. Thus, discontinuation of therapy can be tried since many patients are not really hypertensive. However, careful follow-up is essential.

A somewhat separate issue is whether the *intensity* of therapy can be reduced, thereby diminishing the incidence of drug-induced side effects and improving patient compliance. One study, for example, evaluated 51 patients whose BP was controlled (diastolic BP under 90 mmHg) for 6 months with two or three drugs.[351] Most patients were able to decrease total drug dosage and many were able to discontinue one drug. This change in regimen was accompanied by a reduction in or cessation of side effects in 80 percent of

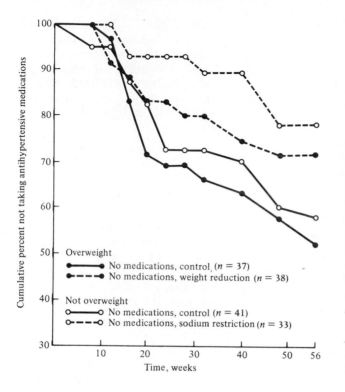

FIG. 11–17. Cumulative percent of well-controlled patients with initially mild hypertension who are able to remain off antihypertensive medications. Overweight patients who lost weight and nonoverweight patients treated with sodium restriction had about a 20 percent higher success rate than similar patients who did not make these dietary modifications. (*Adapted from H. G. Langford, M. D. Blaufox, A. Oberman, C. M. Hawkins, J. D. Curb, G. R. Cutter, S. Wassertheil-Smoller, S. Pressel, C. Babcock, J. D. Abernethy, J. Hotchkiss, and M. Tyler, J. Am. Med. Assoc., 253:657, 1985. Copyright 1985, American Medical Association.*)

patients. Similar results have been reported in 67 patients whose BP had been controlled (mean posttreatment diastolic BP, 83 mmHg) only with chlorthalidone.[352] All patients remained normotensive when the diuretic dose was lowered from 50 to 25 mg/day; only 8 had a rise in BP at 12.5 mg per day, whereas 31 developed recurrent hypertension at 1 year after the drug had been discontinued. Although these findings are compatible with the hypertensive process being ameliorated by effective treatment, a placebo effect or initially excessive drug therapy could also be responsible. For example, 12.5 or 25 mg of chlorthalidone frequently produces a substantial fall in BP even though many patients are routinely treated with higher doses.[254] Despite the uncertain mechanism and efficacy, it seems prudent to try to taper drug therapy at least in those chronically well controlled

patients who are on a multiple drug regimen or who have drug-induced side effects.

EFFECT OF NONSTEROIDAL ANTI-INFLAMMATORY DRUGS

Nonsteroidal anti-inflammatory drugs (NSAID) are widely used in the treatment of rheumatic disorders and act primarily by inhibiting the synthesis of prostaglandins. Although they generally produce few hemodynamic changes in otherwise normal subjects, the associated reduction in vasodilator prostaglandins can raise the BP by 5 to 10 mmHg in patients with hypertension.[294,353-356] Thus, these drugs should be used with care in this setting. There is some evidence, however, that one NSAID, sulindac, may be safer to use since it has less or no effect on renal prostaglandin synthesis and therefore is less likely to increase the BP (see p. 83).[354-356]

REFERENCES

1. Simon, N., S. S. Franklin, K. H. Bleifer, and M. H. Maxwell: Clinical characteristics of renovascular hypertension, *J. Am. Med. Assoc.,* 220:1209, 1972.
2. Kilcoyne, M.: Adolescent hypertension, *Am. J. Med.,* 58:735, 1975.
3. Kotchen, J. M., H. E. McKean, and T. A. Kotchen: Blood pressure trends with aging, *Hypertension,* 4(suppl. III):III-128, 1982.
4. Froom, P., M. Bar-David, J. Ribak, D. Van Dyk, B. Kallner, and J. Benbassat: Predictive value of systolic blood pressure in young men for elevated systolic blood pressure 12 to 15 years later, *Circulation,* 68:467, 1983.
5. Rabkin, S. W., F. A. Mathewson, and R. B. Tate: Relationship of blood pressure in 20- to 39-year-old men to subsequent blood pressure and incidence of hypertension over a 30-year observation period, *Circulation,* 65:291, 1982.
6. Stanton, J. L., L. E. Braitman, A. M. Riley, C. S. Khoo, and J. L. Smith: Demographic, dietary, life style, and anthropomorphic correlates of blood pressure, *Hypertension,* 4(suppl. III):III-135, 1982.
7. Platt, R.: Heredity in hypertension, *Lancet,* 1:899, 1963.
8. Horgan, M. J., H. L. Kennedy, and N. E. Padgett: Do borderline hypertensive patients have labile blood pressure?, *Ann. Intern. Med.,* 94:466, 1981.
9. Julius, S.: Borderline hypertension: An overview, *Med. Clin. N. Am.,* 61:495, 1977.
10. Castelli, W. P., and K. Anderson: A population at risk: Prevalence of high cholesterol levels in hypertensive patients in the Framingham Study, *Am. J. Med.,* 80(suppl. 2A):23, 1986.
11. Miall, W. E., and H. G. Lovell: Relation between change of blood pressure and age, *Br. Med. J.,* 2:660, 1967.
12. Vaughan, E. D., Jr.: Renovascular hypertension, *Kidney Int.,* 27:811, 1985.
13. Kannel, W. B., J. T. Doyle, A. M. Ostfeld, C. D. Jenkins, L. Kuller, R. N. Podell, and J. Stamler: Optimal resources for primary prevention of atherosclerotic diseases. Atherosclerosis study group, *Circulation,* 70:155A, 1984.
14. Kannel, W. B., W. P. Castelli, O. M. McNamara, P. A. McKee, and M. Feinleib: Role of blood pressure in the development of congestive heart failure: The Framingham Study, *N. Engl. J. Med.,* 287:781, 1972.
15. Roberts, W. C.: The hypertensive diseases: Evidence that systolic hypertension is a greater risk factor to the development of other cardiovascular diseases than previously suspected, *Am. J. Med.,* 59:523, 1975.
16. Gifford, R. W., Jr: Isolated systolic hypertension in the elderly. Some controversial issues, *J. Am. Med. Assoc.,* 247:781, 1982.
17. Amery, A., W. Birkenhager, R. Brixko, et al: Efficacy of antihypertensive drug treatment according to age, sex, blood pressure, and previous cardiovascular disease in patients over the age of 60, *Lancet,* 2:589, 1986.
18. Veterans Administration Cooperative Study Group on Antihypertensive Agents: Effects of treatment on morbidity in hypertension: Results in patients with diastolic blood pressure averaging 115 through 129 mmHg, *J. Am. Med. Assoc.,* 202:1028, 1967.
19. Thomson, G. G.: Hypertension in the black population, *Cardiovasc. Rev. Rep.,* 2:351, 1981.
20. Levy, S. B., L. B. Talner, M. N. Coel, R. Holle, and R. A. Stone: Renal vasculature in essential hypertension: Racial differences, *Ann. Intern. Med.,* 88:12, 1978.
21. Rostand, S. G., K. A. Kirk, E. A. Rutsky, and B. A. Pate: Racial differences in the incidence of treatment for end-stage renal disease, *N. Engl. J. Med.,* 306:1276, 1982.
22. Final Report of the Subcommittee on Definition and Prevalence of the 1984 Joint National Committee: Hypertension prevalence and the status of awareness, treatment and control in the United States, *Hypertension,* 7:457, 1985.
23. Medical Research Council Working Party: MRC trial of treatment of mild hypertension: Principal results, *Br. Med. J.,* 291:97, 1985.
24. Hypertension Detection and Follow-up Program Cooperative Group: Five-year findings of the Hypertension Detection and Follow-up Program: I. Reduction in mortality of persons with high blood pressure, including mild hypertension; II. Mortality by race, sex, and age, *J. Am. Med. Assoc.,* 242:2562, 2572, 1979.
25. Madhavan, S., and M. H. Alderman: The potential effect of blood pressure reduction on cardiovascular disease. A cautionary note, *Arch. Intern. Med.,* 141:1583, 1981.
26. Martin, M. J., S. B. Hulley, W. S. Browner, L. H. Kuller, and D. Wentworth: Serum cholesterol, blood pressure, and mortality: Implications from a cohort of 361,662 men, *Lancet,* 2:933, 1986.

27. Campeau, L., M. Enjalbert, J. Lesperance, M. G. Bourassa, P. Kwiterovich, Jr., S. Wacholder, and A. Sniderman: The relation of risk factors to the development of atherosclerosis in saphenous-vein bypass grafts and the progression of disease in the native circulation. A study 10 years after aorto-coronary bypass surgery, *N. Engl. J. Med.,* 311:1329, 1984.

28. Lipid Research Clinics Program: The Lipid Research Clinics Coronary Primary Prevention Trial results, I. Reduction in incidence of coronary heart disease; II. The relationship of reduction in incidence of coronary heart disease to cholesterol lowering, *J. Am. Med. Assoc.,* 251:351, 365, 1984.

29. Dauber, T. R.: *The Framingham Study. The Epidemiology of Atherosclerotic Disease,* Harvard, Cambridge, 1980, chaps. 7 and 8.

30. Havlik, R. J., and M. Feinleib: Epidemiology and genetics of hypertension, *Hypertension,* 4(suppl. III): III-121, 1982.

31. Gifford, R. A.: Hypertension and stroke, *J. Am. Coll. Cardiol.,* 1:521, 1983.

32. Weinberger, M. H.: Antihypertensive therapy and lipids: Paradoxical influences on cardiovascular disease risk, *Am. J. Med.,* 80 (suppl. 2A):64, 1986.

33. Kashgarian, M.: Pathology of small blood vessel disease in hypertension, *Am. J. Kid. Dis.,* 5:A104, 1985.

34. Sandok, B. A., and J. P. Whisnant: Hypertension and the brain, *Arch. Intern. Med.,* 133:947, 1974.

35. Chobanian, A. V., P. I. Brecker, and C. C. Haudenschild: Effects of hypertension and of antihypertensive therapy on atherosclerosis, *Hypertension,* 8(suppl. I):I–15, 1986.

36. Folkow, B.: Structural factors: The vascular wall. Consequences of treatment, *Hypertension,* 5(suppl. III):III-58, 1983.

37. Dollery, C. T.: Hypertensive retinopathy, in J. Genest, O. Kuchel, P. Hamet, and M. Cantin (eds.), *Hypertension,* 2d ed., McGraw-Hill, New York, 1983.

38. Gamble, C. N.: The pathogenesis of hyaline arteriolosclerosis, *Am. J. Pathol.,* 122:410, 1986.

39. Johansson, B., S. Strandgaard, and N. A. Lassen: On the pathogenesis of hypertensive encephalopathy: The hypertensive "breakthrough" of autoregulation of cerebral blood flow with forced vasodilatation, flow increase, and blood-brain-barrier damage, *Circ. Res.,* 34:167, 1974.

40. Harper, S. L., and H. G. Bohlen: Microvascular adaptation in the cerebral cortex of adult spontaneously hypertensive rats, *Hypertension,* 6:408, 1984.

41. Koch-Weser, J.: Hypertensive emergencies, *N. Engl. J. Med.,* 290:211, 1974.

42. Kohner, E. M., and C. Dollery: Hypertensive retinopathy, in J. Genest, E. Koiw, and O. Kuchel (eds.), *Hypertension: Physiopathology and Treatment,* McGraw-Hill, New York, 1977.

43. Prineas, J., and J. Marshall: Hypertension and cerebral infarction, *Br. Med. J.,* 1:14, 1966.

44. Fisher, C. M.: Lacunar strokes and infarcts: A review, *Neurology,* 32:871, 1982.

45. Mohr, J. P.: Lacunar stroke, *Hypertension,* 8:349, 1986.

46. Finnerty, F. A., Jr.: Hypertensive encephalopathy, *Am. J. Med.,* 52:672, 1972.

47. Bock, K. D.: Regression of retinal vascular changes by antihypertensive therapy, *Hypertension,* 6(suppl. III):III-158, 1984.

48. Wallace, J. D., and L. L. Levy: Blood pressure after stroke, *J. Am. Med. Assoc.,* 246:2177, 1981.

49. Tarazi, R. C.: The progression from hypertrophy to heart failure, *Hosp. Pract.,* 18(8):101, 1983.

50. Devereux, R. B., T. G. Pickering, G. A. Harshfield, H. D. Kleinert, L. Denby, L. Clark, D. Pregibon, M. Jason, B. Kleiner, J. S. Borer, and J. H. Laragh: Left ventricular hypertrophy in patients with hypertension: Importance of blood pressure response to regularly recurring stress, *Circulation,* 68:470, 1983.

51. Simpson, P.: Norepinephrine-stimulated hypertrophy of cultured rat myocardial cells is an alpha$_1$ adrenergic response, *J. Clin. Invest.,* 72:732, 1983.

52. Kannel, W. B., T. Gordon, and D. Offutt: Left ventricular hypertrophy by electrocardiogram: Prevalence, incidence and mortality in the Framingham Study, *Ann. Intern. Med.,* 71:89, 1969.

53. Hypertension Detection and Follow-up Program Cooperative Group: Five-year findings of the Hypertension Detection and Follow-up Program, *Hypertension,* 7:105, 1985.

54. Fouad, F. M., Y. Nakashima, R. C. Tarazi, and E. E. Salcedo: Reversal of left ventricular hypertrophy in hypertensive patients treated with methyldopa. Lack of association with blood pressure control, *Am. J. Cardiol.,* 49:795, 1982.

55. Ventura, H. O., E. D. Frohlich, F. H. Messerli, I. Kobrin, and B. B. Kardon: Cardiovascular effects and regional blood flow distribution associated with angiotensin converting enzyme inhibition (captopril) in essential hypertension, *Am. J. Cardiol.,* 55:1023, 1985.

56. Sen, S., R. C. Tarazi, P. A. Khairallah, and F. M. Bumpus: Cardiac hypertrophy in spontaneously

hypertensive rats, *Circ. Res.,* 35:775, 1974.

57. Drayer, J. I., J. M. Gardin, M. A. Weber, and W. S. Aronow: Cardiac muscle mass during vasodilation therapy of hypertension, *Clin. Pharmacol. Therap.,* 33:727, 1983.

58. Savage, D. D., J. I. Drayer, W. L. Henry, E. C. Mathews, Jr., J. H. Ware, J. M. Gardin, E. R. Cohen, S. E. Epstein, and J. H. Laragh: Echocardiographic assessment of cardiac anatomy and function in hypertensive subjects, *Circulation,* 59:623, 1979.

59. Cohen, A., A. D. Hagan, J. Watkin, J. J. Mitas, J. Schvartzman, A. Mazzoleni, I. M. Cohen, S. E. Warren and W. V. Vieweg: Clinical correlates in hypertensive patients with left ventricular hypertrophy diagnosed with echocardiography, *Am. J. Cardiol.,* 47:335, 1981.

60. Rowlands, D. B., D. R. Glover, M. A. Ireland, R. A. McLeay, T. J. Stallard, R. D. Watson, and W. A. Littler: Assessment of left-ventricular mass and its response to antihypertensive treatment, *Lancet,* 1: 467, 1982.

61. Culpepper, W. S., III, P. C. Sodt, F. H. Messerli, D. G. Ruschhaupt, and R. A. Arcilla: Cardiac status in juvenile borderline hypertension, *Ann. Intern. Med.,* 98:1, 1983.

62. Soufer, R., D. Wohlgelernter, N. A. Vita, M. Amuchestegui, H. D. Sostman, H. J. Berger, and B. L. Zaret: Intact systolic left ventricular function in clinical congestive heart failure, *Am. J. Cardiol.,* 55: 1032, 1985.

63. Topol, E. J., T. A. Traill, and N. J. Fortuin: Hypertensive hypertrophic cardiomyopathy of the elderly, *N. Engl. J. Med.,* 312:277, 1985.

64. Given, B. D., T. H. Lee, P. H. Stone, and V. J. Dzau: Nifedipine in severely hypertensive patients with congestive heart failure and preserved ventricular systolic function, *Arch. Intern. Med.,* 145:281, 1985.

65. Messerli, F. H., H. O. Ventura, D. J. Elizardi, F. G. Dunn, and E. D. Frohlich: Hypertension and sudden death. Increased ventricular ectopic activity in left ventricular hypertrophy, *Am. J. Med.,* 77:18, 1984.

66. Kannel, W. B., P. Sorlie, W. P. Castelli, and D. McGee: Blood pressure and survival after myocardial infarction: The Framingham study, *Am. J. Cardiol.,* 45:326, 1980.

67. Koyanagi, S., C. Eastham, and M. L. Marcus: Effects of chronic hypertension and left ventricular hypertrophy on the incidence of sudden cardiac death after coronary artery occlusion in conscious dogs, *Circulation,* 65:1192, 1982.

68. Heptinstall, R. H.: *Pathology of the Kidney,* 3d ed., Little, Brown, Boston, 1983, chap. 5.

69. Wiener, J., R. G. Lattes, B. G. Meltzer, and D. Spiro: The cellular pathology of experimental hypertension, IV: Evidence for increased vascular permeability, *Am. J. Pathol.,* 54:187, 1969.

70. Dustan, H. P., E. F. Poutasse, A. C. Corcoran, and I. H. Page: Separated renal functions in patients with renal arterial disease, pyelonephritis, and essential hypertension, *Circulation,* 23:34, 1961.

71. Hunt, J. C., F. T. Maher, L. F. Greene, and S. G. Sheps: Functional characteristics of the separate kidneys in hypertensive man, *Am. J. Cardiol.,* 17:493, 1966.

72. Arendshorst, W. J., and W. H. Beierwaltes: Renal and nephron hemodynamics in spontaneously hypertensive rats, *Am. J. Physiol.,* 236:F246, 1979.

73. Feld, L. G., J. B. van Liew, R. G. Galaske, and J. W. Boylan: Selectivity of renal injury and progression in the spontaneously hypertensive rat, *Kidney Int.,* 12:332, 1977.

74. Azar, S., M. A. Johnson, B. Hertel, and L. Tobian: Single-nephron pressures, flows and resistances in hypertensive kidneys with nephrosclerosis, *Kidney Int.,* 12:28, 1977.

75. Dworkin, L. D., T. H. Hostetter, H. G. Rennke, and B. M. Brenner: Hemodynamic basis for glomerular injury in rats with desoxycorticosterone-salt hypertension, *J. Clin. Invest.,* 73:1448, 1984.

76. London, G. M., J. A. Levenson, A. M. London, A. C. Simon, and M. E. Safar: Systemic compliance, renal hemodynamics, and sodium excretion in hypertension, *Kidney Int.,* 26:342, 1984.

77. Hollenberg, N. K., L. J. Borucki, and D. F. Adams: The renal vasculature in early essential hypertension, *Medicine,* 57:167, 1978.

78. Baldwin, D. S., and J. Neugarten: Treatment of hypertension in renal disease, *Hypertension,* 5:A57, 1985.

79. Bianchi, G., D. Cusi, C. Barlassina, G. P. Lupi, P. Ferrari, G. B. Picotti, M. Gatti, and T. Polli: Renal dysfunction as a possible cause of essential hypertension in predisposed subjects, *Kidney Int.,* 23:870, 1983.

80. Myers, B. D., W. M. Deen, and B. M. Brenner: Effects of norepinephrine and angiotensin II on the determinants of glomerular ultrafiltration and proximal tubular reabsorption in the rat, *Circ. Res.,* 37:101, 1975.

81. Hollenberg, N. K., S. L. Swartz, D. R. Passan, and G. H. Williams: Increased glomerular filtration rate

after converting-enzyme inhibition in essential hypertension, *N. Engl. J. Med.,* 301:9, 1979.

82. Hollenberg, N. K., L. G. Meggs, G. H. Williams, J. Katz, J. D. Garnic, and D. P. Harrington: Sodium intake and renal responses to captopril in normal man and in essential hypertension, *Kidney Int.,* 20: 240, 1981.

83. Kaplan, C., B. Pasternack, H. Shah, and G. Gallo: Age-related incidence of sclerotic glomeruli in human kidneys, *Am. J. Pathol.,* 80:227, 1975.

84. Rowe, J. W., R. Andres, J. D. Tobin, A. H. Norris, and N. W. Shock: The effect of age on creatinine clearance in man: A cross sectional and longitudinal study, *J. Gerontol.,* 31:155, 1976.

85. Lindeman, R. D., J. D. Tobin, and N. W. Shock: Association between blood pressure and rate of decline in renal function with age, *Kidney Int.,* 26:861, 1984.

86. Messerli, F. H., E. D. Frohlich, and G. R. Dreslinski: Serum uric acid in essential hypertension: An indicator of renal vascular involvement, *Ann. Intern. Med.,* 93:817, 1980.

87. Mujais, S. K., D. S. Emmanouel, B. S. Kasinath, and B. H. Spargo: Marked proteinuria in hypertensive nephrosclerosis, *Am. J. Nephrol.,* 5:190, 1985.

88. Batuman, V., E. Landy, J. K. Maesaka, and R. P. Wedeen: Contribution of lead to hypertension with renal impairment, *N. Engl. J. Med.,* 309:17, 1983.

89. Moyer, J. H., C. Heider, K. Pevey, and R. V. Ford: The effect of treatment on the vascular deterioration associated with hypertension, with particular emphasis on renal function, *Am. J. Med.,* 24:177, 1958.

90. Mitchell, H. C., R. M. Graham, and W. A. Pettinger: Renal function during long-term treatment of hypertension with minoxidil: Comparison of benign and malignant hypertension, *Ann. Intern. Med.,* 93: 676, 1980.

91. Nabel, E. G., A. Kugelmass, G. Zins, E. Phipps, and V. J. Dzau: Does blood pressure control alter renal function in refractory hypertension, *Circulation,* 70: II-213, 1984.

92. Anderson, S., H. G. Rennke, and B. M. Brenner: Therapeutic advantage of converting enzyme inhibitors in arresting progressive renal disease associated with systemic hypertension in the rat, *J. Clin. Invest.,* 77:1993, 1986.

93. Mroczek, W. J., M. Davidov, L. Gavrilovich, and F. A. Finnerty, Jr.: The value of aggressive therapy in the hypertensive patient with azotemia, *Circulation,* 40:893, 1969.

94. McCormack, L. J., J. E. Beland, R. E. Schneckloth, and A. C. Corcoran: Effects of antihypertensive

treatment on the evolution of the renal lesions in malignant nephrosclerosis, *Am. J. Pathol.,* 34:1011, 1958.

95. Ramos, O.: Malignant hypertension: The Brazilian experience, *Kidney Int.,* 26:209, 1984.

96. Spargo, B. H., N. G. Ordonez, and J. C. Ringus: The differential diagnosis of crescentic glomerulonephritis: The pathology of specific lesions with prognostic implications, *Hum. Pathol.,* 8:187, 1977.

97. Woods, J. W., W. B. Blythe, and W. D. Huffines: Management of malignant hypertension complicated by renal insufficiency: A follow-up study, *N. Engl. J. Med.,* 291:10, 1974.

98. Laragh, J. H., L. Baer, H. R. Brunner, F. R. Buhler, J. E. Sealey, and E. D. Vaughan, Jr.: Renin, angiotensin and aldosterone system in the pathogenesis and management of hypertensive vascular disease, *Am. J. Med.,* 52:633, 1972.

99. Kincaid-Smith, P., J. McMichael, and E. A. Murphy: The clinical course and pathology of hypertension with papilloedema, *Q. J. Med.,* 27:117, 1958.

100. Sevitt, L. H., D. J. Evans, and O. M. Wrong: Acute oliguric renal failure due to accelerated (malignant) hypertension, *Q. J. Med.,* 40:127, 1971.

101. Gavras, H., W. C. Brown, J. J. Brown, A. F. Lever, A. L. Linton, R. F. MacAdam, G. P. McNicol, J. I. S. Robertson, and C. Wardrop: Microangiopathic hemolytic anemia and the development of the malignant phase of hyperfusion, *Circ. Res.,* 28/29 (suppl. II):II-127, 1971.

102. Davis, B. A., J. E. Crook, R. E. Vestal, and J. A. Oakes: Prevalence of renovascular hypertension in patients with grade III or IV hypertensive retinopathy, *N. Engl. J. Med.,* 301:1273, 1979.

103. Harrington, M., P. Kincaid-Smith, and J. McMichael: Results of treatment in malignant hypertension: A seven-year experience in 94 cases, *Br. Med. J.,* 2:969, 1959.

104. Perry, H. M., Jr., H. S. Schroeder, F. S. Catanzaro, D. Moore-Jones, and G. H. Camel: Studies on the control of hypertension, VIII: Mortality, morbidity and remissions during twelve years of intensive therapy, *Circulation,* 33:958, 1966.

105. Woods, J. W., and W. B. Blythe: Management of malignant hypertension complicated by renal insufficiency, *N. Engl. J. Med.,* 277:57, 1967.

106. Lawton, W. J.: The short-term course of renal function in malignant hypertensives with renal insufficiency, *Clin. Nephrol.,* 17:277, 1982.

107. Cordingley F. T., N. F. Jones, A. J. Wing, and P. J. Hilton: Reversible renal failure in malignant hypertension, *Clin. Nephrol.,* 14:98, 1980.

108. Isles, C. G., A. McLay, and J. M. Jones: Recovery

in malignant hypertension presenting as acute renal failure, *Q. J. Med.,* 53:439, 1984.

109. Mahoney, J. F., G. R. Gibson, G. R. Sheil, B. G. Storey, G. S. Stokes, and J. H. Stewart: Bilateral nephrectomy for malignant hypertension, *Lancet,* 1:1036, 1972.

110. Ledingham, J. G. G., and B. Rajagopalan: Cerebral complications in the treatment of accelerated hypertension, *Q. J. Med.,* 48:25, 1979.

111. Haas, D. C., D. H. P. Streeten, R. C. Kim, A. N. Naalbandian, and A. I. Obeid: Death from cerebral hypoperfusion during nitroprusside treatment of acute angiotensin-dependent hypertension, *Am. J. Med.,* 75:1071, 1983.

112. Mancia, G.: Methods for assessing blood pressure values in humans, *Hypertension,* 5 (suppl. III):III-5, 1983.

113. Kirkendall, W. M., M. Feinleib, E. D. Freis, and A. L. Mark: Recommendations for human blood pressure determination by sphygmomanometers, *Circulation,* 62:1146A, 1980.

114. Berliner, K., H. Fujiy, D. H. Lee, M. Yildiz, and B. Barnier: Blood pressure measurements in obese persons: Comparisons of intra-arterial and auscultatory measurements, *Am. J. Cardiol.,* 8:10, 1961.

115. Messerli, F. H., H. O. Ventura, and C. Amodeo: Osler's maneuver and pseudohypertension, *N. Engl. J. Med.,* 312:1548, 1985.

116. Spence, J. D., W. J. Sibbald, and R. D. Cape: Pseudohypertension in the elderly, *Clin. Sci. Mol. Med.,* 55:399s, 1978.

117. Kirkendall, W. M., A. C. Burton, F. H. Epstein, and E. D. Freis: Recommendations for human blood pressure determination by sphygmomanometers, *Circulation,* 36:980, 1967.

118. Maurer, A. H., and A. Noordergraaf: Korotkoff sound filtering for automated three phase measurement of blood pressure, *Am. Ht. J.,* 91:584, 1976.

119. Londe, S., and T. S. Klitzner: Ausculatory blood pressure measurement—Effect of pressure on the head of the stethoscope, *West. J. Med.,* 141:193, 1984.

120. Mitchell, P. L., W. Parlin, and H. Blackburn: Effect of vertical displacement of the arm on indirect blood-pressure measurement, *N. Engl. J. Med.,* 271:72, 1964.

121. Hartley, R. M., R. Velez, R. W. Morris, M. F. DeSouza, and R. F. Heller: Confirming the diagnosis of mild hypertension, *Br. Med. J.,* 286:287, 1983.

122. Pickering, T. G., G. A. Harshfield, R. B. Devereux, and J. H. Laragh: What is the role of ambulatory

blood pressure monitoring in the management of hypertensive patients?, *Hypertension,* 7:171, 1985.

123. Brunner, H. R., B. Waeber, and J. Nussberger: Blood pressure recording in the ambulatory patient and evaluation of cardiovascular risk, *Clin. Sci.,* 68:485, 1985.

124. Sokolow, M., D. Perloff, and R. Cowan: Contribution of ambulatory blood pressure to assessment of patients with mild to moderate elevation of office blood pressure, *Cardiovasc. Rev. Rep.,* 1:295, 1980.

125. Perloff, D., M. Sokolow, and R. Cowan: The prognostic value of ambulatory blood pressures, *J. Am. Med. Assoc.,* 249:2792, 1983.

126. Kleinert, H. D., G. A. Harshfield, T. G. Pickering, R. B. Devereux, P. A. Sullivan, R. M. Marion, W. K. Mallory, and J. H. Laragh: What is the value of home blood pressure measurement in patients with mild hypertension?, *Hypertension,* 6:574, 1984.

127. Gould, B. A., S. Mann, A. B. Davies, D. G. Altman, and E. B. Raftery: Does placebo lower blood pressure?, *Lancet,* 2:1377, 1981.

128. Young, M. A., D. B. Rowlands, T. J. Stallard, R. D. Watson, and W. A. Littler: Effect of environment on blood pressure: Home versus hospital, *Br. Med. J.,* 286:1235, 1983.

129. Floras, J. S., J. V. Jones, M. D. Hassan, B. Osikowska, P. S. Sever, and P. Sleight: Cuff and ambulatory blood pressure in subjects with essential hypertension, *Lancet,* 2:107, 1981.

130. Sokolow, M., D. Werdegar, H. K. Kain, and A. T. Hinman: Relationships between level of blood pressure measured casually and by portable recorders and severity of complications in essential hypertension, *Circulation,* 34:279, 1966.

131. Ibrahim, M. M., R. C. Tarazi, H. P. Dustan, and R. W. Gifford, Jr.: Electrocardiogram in evaluation of resistance to antihypertensive therapy, *Arch. Intern. Med.,* 137:1125, 1977.

132. Levin, A., M. D. Blaufox, H. Castle, G. Entwisle, and H. Langford: Apparent prevalence of curable hypertension in Hypertension Detection and Follow-up Program, *Arch. Intern. Med.,* 145:424, 1985.

133. Tucker, R. M., and D. R. Labarthe: Frequency of surgical treatment for hypertension in adults at the Mayo Clinic from 1973 through 1975, *Mayo Clin. Proc.,* 52:549, 1977.

134. Report of the Joint National Committee on Detection, Evaluation, and Treatment of High Blood Pressure. A Cooperative Study, *J. Am. Med. Assoc.,* 237:255, 1977.

135. Ying, C. Y., C. P. Tifft, H. Gavras, and A. V. Chobanian: Renal revascularization in the azotemic

hypertensive patient resistant to therapy, *N. Engl. J. Med.,* 311:1070, 1984.

136. Rodriguez-Iturbe, B., B. Baggio, J. Colina-Chourio, S. Favaro, R. Garcia, F. Sussana, L. Castillo, and A. Borsatti: Studies on the renin-aldosterone system in the acute nephritic syndrome, *Kidney Int.,* 19:445, 1981.

137. Powell, H. R., R. Rotenberg, A. L. Williams, and D. A. McCredie: Plasma renin activity in acute post-streptococcal glomerulonephritis and the hemolytic-uraemic syndrome, *Arch. Dis. Child.,* 49:802, 1974.

138. Stockigt, J. R., D. J. Topliss, and M. J. Hewett: High-renin hypertension in necrotizing vasculitis, *N. Engl. J. Med.,* 300:1218, 1979.

139. Traub, Y. M., A. P. Shapiro, G. P. Rodnan, T. A. Medsger, R. H. McDonald, V. D. Steen, T. A. Osial, Jr., and S. F. Tolchin: Hypertension and renal failure (scleroderma renal crisis) in progressive systemic sclerosis. Review of a 25-year experience with 68 cases, *Medicine,* 62:335, 1983.

140. Laragh, J. H.: Oral contraceptive-induced hypertension—Nine years later, *Am. J. Obstet. Gynecol.,* 126:141, 1976.

141. Goldhaber, S. Z., C. H. Hennekens, R. F. Spark, D. A. Evans, B. Rosner, J. D. Taylor, and E. H. Kass: Plasma renin substrate, renin activity, and aldosterone levels in a sample of oral contraceptive users from a community survey, *Am. Ht. J.,* 107:119, 1984.

142. Crane, M. G., J. J. Harris, and W. Winsor, III: Hypertension, oral contraceptive agents, and conjugated estrogens, *Ann. Intern. Med.,* 74:13, 1971.

143. Bravo, E. L., and R. W. Gifford, Jr.: Pheochromocytoma: Diagnosis, localization and management, *N. Engl. J. Med.,* 311:1298, 1984.

144. Hamilton, B. P., L. Landsberg, and R. J. Levine: Measurement of urinary epinephrine in screening for pheochromocytoma in multiple endocrine neoplasia type II, *Am. J. Med.,* 65:1027, 1978.

145. Khairi, M. R., R. N. Dexter, N. J. Burzynski, and C. C. Johnston, Jr.: Mucosal neuroma, pheochromocytoma and medullary thyroid carcinoma: Multiple endocrine neoplasia type 3, *Medicine,* 54:89, 1975.

146. Clinicopathologic Conference: Renal mass in a man with von Hippel-Lindau disease, *Am. J. Med.,* 71:287, 1981.

147. Kalff, V., B. Shapiro, R. Lloyd, J. C. Sisson, K. Holland, M. Nakajo, and W. H. Beierwaltes: The spectrum of pheochromocytoma in hypertensive patients with neurofibromatosis, *Arch. Intern. Med.,* 142:2092, 1982.

148. Sisson, J. C., M. S. Frager, T. W. Valk, M. D. Gross, D. P. Swanson, D. M. Wieland, M. C. Tobes, W. H. Beierwaltes, and N. W. Thompson: Scintigraphic localization of pheochromocytoma, *N. Engl. J. Med.,* 305:12, 1981.

149. Bravo, E. L., R. C. Tarazi, H. P. Dustan, F. M. Fouad, S. C. Textor, R. W. Gifford, and D. G. Vidt: The changing clinical spectrum of primary aldosteronism, *Am. J. Med.,* 74:641, 1983.

150. Melby, J. C.: Primary aldosteronism, *Kidney Int.,* 26:769, 1984.

151. Rose, B. D.: *Clinical Physiology of Acid-Base and Electrolyte Disorders,* 2d ed., McGraw-Hill, New York, 1984, chap. 27.

152. George, J. M., L. Wright, N. Bell, and F. C. Bartter: The syndrome of primary aldosteronism, *Am. J. Med.,* 48:343, 1970.

153. Holland, O. B., H. Brown, L. Kuhnert, C. Fairchild, M. Risk, and C. E. Gomez-Sanchez: Further evaluation of saline infusion for the diagnosis of primary aldosteronism, *Hypertension,* 6:717, 1984.

154. Biglieri, E. G.: Adrenocortical components in hypertension, *Cardiovasc. Rev. Rep.,* 3:734, 1982.

155. Griffing, G. T., A. G. Cole, S. A. Aurecchia, B. H. Sindler, P. Komanicky, and J. C. Melby: Amiloride in primary hyperaldosteronism, *Clin. Pharmacol. Therap.,* 31:57, 1982.

156. Gold, E. M.: The Cushing's syndromes: Changing views of diagnosis and treatment, *Ann. Intern. Med.,* 90:829, 1979.

157. Nugent, C. A., H. R. Warner, J. T. Dunn, and F. H. Tyler: Probability theory in the diagnosis of Cushing's syndrome, *J. Clin. Endocrinol. Metab.,* 24:621, 1964.

158. Christy, N. P., and J. H. Laragh: Pathogenesis of hypokalemic alkalosis in Cushing's syndrome, *N. Engl. J. Med.,* 265:1083, 1961.

159. Eddy, R. L., A. L. Jones, P. F. Gilliland, J. D. Ibarra, Jr., J. Q. Thompson, and J. F. McMurry, Jr.: Cushing's syndrome. A prospective study of diagnostic methods, *Am. J. Med.,* 55:621, 1973.

160. White, F. E., M. C. White, P. L. Drury, I. K. Fry, and G. M. Besser: Value of computed tomography of the abdomen and chest in investigation of Cushing's syndrome, *Br. Med. J.,* 284:771, 1982.

161. Aron, D. C., J. B. Tyrrell, P. A. Fitzgerald, J. W. Finding, and P. H. Forsham: Cushing's syndrome: Problems in diagnosis, *Medicine,* 60:25, 1981.

162. Tyrrell, J. B., J. W. Findling, D. C. Aron, P. A. Fitzgerald, and P. H. Forsham: An overnight high-dose dexamethasone suppression test for rapid differential diagnosis of Cushing's syndrome, *Ann. Intern. Med.,* 104:180, 1986.

163. Rosenthal, F. D., and S. Roy: Hypertension and hyperparathyroidism, *Br. Med. J.,* 4:396, 1972.

164. Sangal, A. K., and D. G. Beevers: Parathyroid hypertension, *Br. Med. J.,* 286:498, 1983.

165. Weidmann, P., S. G. Massry, J. W. Coburn, M. H. Maxwell, J. Atleson, and C. R. Kleeman: Blood pressure effects of acute hypercalcemia: Studies in patients with chronic renal failure, *Ann. Intern. Med.,* 76:741, 1972.

166. Veterans Administration Cooperative Study Group on Antihypertensive Agents: Effects of treatment on morbidity in hypertension: Results in patients with diastolic blood pressure averaging 115 through 129 mm Hg, *J. Am. Med. Assoc.,* 202:1028, 1967.

167. Veterans Administration Cooperative Study Group on Antihypertensive Agents: Effects of treatment on morbidity in hypertension, II: Results in patients with diastolic blood pressure averaging 90 through 114 mmHg, *J. Am. Med. Assoc.,* 213:1143, 1970.

168. Smith, McF. W.: Public Health Service Hospitals Cooperative Study Group: Treatment of mild hypertension. Results of a 10 year intervention trial, *Circ. Res.,* 40:98, 1977.

169. Hypertension Detection and Follow-up Program Cooperative Group: Five-year findings of the Hypertension Detection and Follow-up Program: I. Reduction in mortality of persons with high blood pressure, including mild hypertension; II. Mortality by race, sex, and age, *J. Am. Med. Assoc.,* 242:2562, 2572, 1979.

170. Hypertension Detection and Follow-up Program Cooperative Group: The effect of treatment on mortality in "mild" hypertension, *N. Engl. J. Med.,* 307:976, 1982.

171. Management Committee: The Australian therapeutic trial in mild hypertension, *Lancet,* 1:1261, 1980.

172. Helgeland A.: Treatment of mild hypertension: A five-year controlled drug trial. The Oslo study, *Am. J. Med.,* 69:725, 1980.

173. Narins, R. G.: Mild hypertension: A therapeutic dilemma, *Kidney Int.,* 26:881, 1984.

174. Multiple Risk Factor Intervention Trial Research Group: Baseline resting electrocardiographic abnormalities, antihypertensive treatment, and mortality in Multiple Risk Factor Intervention Trial, *Am. J. Cardiol.,* 55:1, 1985.

175. Walle, T., R. P. Byington, C. D. Furberg, K. M. McIntyre, and P. S. Vokonas: Biologic determinants of propranolol disposition: Results from 1308 patients in the Beta-blocker Heart Attack Trial, *Clin. Pharmacol. Therap.,* 38:509, 1985.

176. Hypertension Detection and Follow-up Program Cooperative Research Group: The effect of antihypertensive drug treatment on mortality in the presence of resting electrocardiographic abnormalities at baseline: The HDFP experience, *Circulation,* 70:996, 1984.

177. Leren, P., and A. Helgeland: Coronary heart disease and treatment of hypertension: Some Oslo study data, *Am. J. Med.,* 80(suppl. 2A):3, 1986.

178. Kuller, L. H., S. B. Hulley, J. D. Cohen, and J. Neaton: Unexpected effects of treating hypertension in men with electrocardiographic abnormalities: A critical analysis, *Circulation,* 73:114, 1986.

179. Hyman, D., and N. M. Kaplan: Treatment of patients with mild hypertension, *Hypertension,* 7:165, 1985.

180. Jachuck, S. J., H. Brierley, S. Jachuck, and P. M. Willcox: The effect of hypotensive drugs on the quality of life, *J. R. Coll. Gen. Pract.,* 32:103, 1982.

181. Management Committee: The Australian therapeutic trial in mild hypertension: Untreated mild hypertension, *Lancet,* 1:185, 1982.

182. Memorandum from the WHO/ISH Meeting: 1986 guidelines for the treatment of mild hypertension, *Hypertension,* 8:957, 1986.

183. The 1984 Report of the Joint National Committee on Detection, Evaluation, and Treatment of High Blood Pressure, *Arch. Intern. Med.,* 144:1045, 1984.

184. Veterans Administration Study Group on Antihypertensive Agents: Effect of treatment on mortality in hypertension: III. Influence of age, diastolic pressure, and prior cardiovascular disease: Further analysis of side effects, *Circulation,* 45:991, 1972.

185. Amery, A., W. Birkenhager, P. Brixko, C. Bulpitt, D. Clement, M. Deruyttere, A. De Schaepdryver, C. Dollery, R. Fagard, and F. Forette: Mortality and morbidity results from the European Working Party on High Blood Pressure in the Elderly trial, *Lancet,* 1:1349, 1985.

186. Kannel, W. B., P. A. Wolf, D. L. McGee, T. R. Dawber, P. McNamara, and W. P. Castelli: Systolic blood pressure, arterial rigidity, and risk of stroke. The Framingham Study, *J. Am. Med. Assoc.,* 245:1225, 1981.

187. Simon, A. C., M. A. Safar, J. A. Levenson, A. M. Kheder, and B. I. Levi: Systolic hypertension: Hemodynamic mechanism and choice of antihypertensive treatment, *Am. J. Cardiol.,* 44:505, 1979.

188. Hulley, S. B., C. D. Furberg, B. Gurland, R. McDonald, H. M. Perry, H. W. Schnapper, J. A. Schoenberger, W. M. Smith, and T. M. Vogt: Systolic hypertension in the elderly program (SHEP): Antihypertensive efficacy of chlorthalidone, *Am. J. Cardiol.,* 56:913, 1985.

189. Rowe, J. W.: Systolic hypertension in the elderly, *N. Engl. J. Med.,* 309:1246, 1983.
190. Koch-Weser, J.: Correlation of pathophysiology and pharmacotherapy in primary hypertension, *Am. J. Cardiol.,* 32:499, 1973.
191. Lavin, P.: Management of hypertension in patients with acute stroke, *Arch. Intern. Med.,* 146:66, 1986.
192. Allen, G. S., H. S. Ahn, T. J. Preziosi, R. Battye, S. C. Boone, S. N. Chou, D. L. Kelly, B. K. Weir, R. A. Crabbe, P. J. Lavik, S. B. Rosenbloom, F. C. Dorsey, C. R. Ingram, D. E. Mellits, L. A. Bertsch, D. P. Boisvert, M. B. Hundley, R. K. Johnson, J. A. Strom, and C. R. Transou: Cerebral arterial spasm— A controlled trial of nimodipine in patients with subarachnoid hemorrhage, *N. Engl. J. Med.,* 308:619, 1983.
193. Kaplan, N. M.: Non-drug treatment of hypertension, *Ann. Intern. Med.,* 102:359, 1985.
194. MacGregor, G. A.: Sodium is more important than calcium in essential hypertension, *Hypertension,* 7: 628, 1985.
195. MacGregor, G. A., N. D. Markandu, F. E. Best, D. M. Elder, J. M. Cam, G. A. Sagnella, and M. Squires: Double-blind randomised crossover trial of moderate sodium restriction in essential hypertension, *Lancet,* 1:351, 1982.
196. Fujita, T., W. L. Henry, F. C. Bartter, C. R. Lake, and C. S. Delea: Factors influencing blood pressure in salt-sensitive patients with hypertension, *Am. J. Med.,* 69:334, 1980.
197. Longworth, D. L., J. I. Drayer, M. A. Weber, and J. H. Laragh: Divergent blood pressure responses during short-term sodium restriction in hypertension, *Clin. Pharmacol. Therap.,* 27:544, 1980.
198. Houston, M. C.: Sodium and hypertension. A review, *Arch. Intern. Med.,* 146:179, 1986.
199. Redgrave, J., S. Rabinowe, N. K. Hollenberg, and G. H. Williams: Correction of abnormal renal blood flow response to angiotensin II by converting enzyme inhibition in essential hypertensives, *J. Clin. Invest.,* 75:1285, 1985.
200. Parfrey, P. S., N. D. Markandu, J. E. Roulston, B. E. Jones, J. C. Jones, and G. A. MacGregor: Relation between arterial pressure, dietary sodium intake, and renin system in essential hypertension, *Br. Med. J.,* 283:94, 1981.
201. Kawasaki, T., C. S. Delea, F. C. Bartter, and H. Smith: The effect of high-sodium and low-sodium intakes on blood pressure and other related variables in human subjects with idiopathic hypertension, *Am. J. Med.,* 64:193, 1978.
202. Vaughan, E. D., Jr., R. M. Carey, M. J. Peach, J. A. Ackerly, and C. R. Ayers: The renin response to diuretic therapy: A limitation of antihypertensive potential, *Circ. Res.,* 42:376, 1978.
203. Ram, C. V. S., B. N. Garrett, and N. M. Kaplan: Moderate sodium restriction and various diuretics in the treatment of hypertension. Effects on potassium wastage and blood pressure control, *Arch. Intern. Med.,* 141:1015, 1981.
204. Kaplan, N. M., M. Simmons, C. McPhee, A. Carnegie, C. Stefanu, and S. Cade: Two techniques to improve adherence to dietary sodium restriction in the treatment of hypertension, *Arch. Intern. Med.,* 142:1638, 1982.
205. Maronde, R. F., M. Milgrom, N. D. Vlachakis, and L. Chan: Response of thiazide-induced hypokalemia to amiloride, *J. Am. Med. Assoc.,* 249:237, 1983.
206. Reisin, E., R. Abel, M. Modan, D. S. Silverberg, H. E. Eliahou, and B. Modan: Effect of weight loss without salt restriction on the reduction of blood pressure in overweight hypertensive subjects, *N. Engl. J. Med.,* 298:1, 1978.
207. Maxwell, M. H., T. Kushiro, L. P. Dornfeld, M. L. Tuck, and A. U. Waks: BP changes in obese hypertensive subjects during rapid weight loss. Comparison of restricted v unchanged salt intake, *Arch. Intern. Med.,* 144:1581, 1984.
208. Hovell, M. F.: The experimental evidence for weight-loss treatment of essential hypertension: A critical review, *Am. J. Public Health,* 72:359, 1982.
209. Tuck, M. L., J. Sowers, L. Dornfeld, G. Kledzik, and M. H. Maxwell: The effect of weight reduction on blood pressure, plasma renin activity and plasma aldosterone levels in obese patients, *N. Engl. J. Med.,* 304:930, 1981.
210. Sowers, J. R., M. Nyby, N. Stern, F. Beck, S. Baron, R. Catania, and N. Vlachis: Blood pressure and hormone changes associated with weight reduction in the obese, *Hypertension,* 4:686, 1982.
211. MacMahon, S. W., G. J. MacDonald, L. Bernstein, G. Andrews, and R. B. Blacket: Comparison of weight reduction with metoprolol in treatment of hypertension in young overweight patients, *Lancet,* 1:1233, 1985.
212. McCarron, D. A.: Is calcium more important than sodium in the pathogenesis of essential hypertension?, *Hypertension,* 7:607, 1985.
213. Resnick, L. M., F. B. Müller, and J. H. Laragh: Calcium regulatory hormones in essential hypertension. Relation to plasma renin activity and sodium metabolism, *Ann. Intern. Med.,* 105:649, 1986.
214. McCarron, D. A., and C. D. Morris: Blood pressure response to oral calcium in persons with mild to

moderate hypertension. A randomized, double-blind, placebo-controlled, crossover trial, *Ann. Intern. Med.,* 103:825, 1985.

215. Heath, H., III, and C. W. Callaway: Calcium tablets for hypertension?, *Ann. Intern. Med.,* 103:946, 1985.

216. Klatsky, A. L., G. D. Friedman, A. A. Siegelaub, and M. J. Gerard: Alcohol consumption and blood pressure. Kaiser-Permanente Multiphasic Health Examination data, *N. Engl. J. Med.,* 296:1194, 1977.

217. MacMahon, S. W., and R. N. Norton: Alcohol and hypertension: Implications for prevention and treatment, *Ann. Intern. Med.,* 105:124, 1986.

218. Potter, J. F., and D. G. Beevers: Pressor effect of alcohol in hypertension, *Lancet,* 1:119, 1984.

219. Langford, H. G.: Dietary potassium and hypertension: Epidemiologic data, *Ann. Intern. Med.,* 98:770, 1983.

220. MacGregor, G. A., S. J. Smith, N. D. Markandu, R. A. Banks, and G. A. Sagnella: Moderate potassium supplementation in essential hypertension, *Lancet,* 2:567, 1982.

221. Kaplan, N. M., A. Carnegie, P. Raskin, J. A. Heller, and M. Simmons: Potassium supplementation in hypertensive patients with diuretic-induced hypokalemia, *N. Engl. J. Med.,* 312:746, 1985.

222. Anderson, J. W.: Plant fiber and blood pressure, *Ann. Intern. Med.,* 98:842, 1983.

223. Rouse, I. L., L. J. Beilin, B. K. Armstrong, and R. Vandongen: Blood-pressure lowering effect of a vegetarian diet: Controlled trial in normotensive subjects, *Lancet,* 1:5, 1983.

224. Puska, P., J. M. Iacono, A. Nissinen, H. J. Korhonen, E. Vartianen, P. Pietineu, R. Dougherty, U. Leino, M. Mutanen, S. Moisio, and J. Huttunen: Controlled, randomized trial on the effect of dietary fat on blood pressure, *Lancet,* 1:1, 1983.

225. Blair, S. N., N. N. Goodyear, L. W. Gibbons, and K. H. Cooper: Physical fitness and incidence of hypertension in healthy normotensive men and women, *J. Am. Med. Assoc.,* 252:487, 1984.

226. Cade, R., D. Mars, H. Wagemaker, C. Zauner, D. Packer, M. Privette, M. Cade, J. Peterson, and D. Hood-Lewis: Effect of aerobic exercise training on patients with systemic arterial hypertension, *Am. J. Med.,* 77:785, 1984.

227. Duncan, J. J., J. E. Farr, S. J. Upton, R. D. Hagan, M. E. Oglesby, and S. N. Blair: The effects of aerobic exercise on plasma catecholamines and blood pressure in patients with mild essential hypertension, *J. Am. Med. Assoc.,* 254:2609, 1985.

228. Nelson, L., G. L. Jennings, M. D. Esler, and P. I. Korner: Effect of changing levels of physical exercise on blood pressure and haemodynamics in essential hypertension, *Lancet,* 2:473, 1986.

229. Health and Public Policy Committee, American College of Physicians: Biofeedback for hypertension, *Ann. Intern. Med.,* 102:709, 1985.

230. Veterans Administration Cooperative Study Group on Antihypertensive Agents: Comparison of propranolol and hydrochlorothiazide for the initial treatment of hypertension. II. Results of long-term therapy, *J. Am. Med. Assoc.,* 248:2004, 1982.

231. Veterans Administration Cooperative Study Group on Antihypertensive Agents: Efficacy of nadolol alone and combined with bendroflumethiazide and hydralazine for systemic hypertension, *Am. J. Cardiol.,* 52:1230, 1983.

232. Kelly, R. A., C. S. Wilcox, W. E. Mitch, T. W. Meyer, P. F. Souney, C..M. Rayment, P. A. Friedman, and S. L. Swartz: Response of the kidney to furosemide. II. Effect of captopril on sodium balance, *Kidney Int.,* 24:233, 1983.

233. Shah, S., I. Khatri, and E. D. Freis: Mechanism of antihypertensive effect of thiazide diuretics, *Am. Ht. J.,* 95:611, 1978.

234. van Brummelen, P., A. J. Man in't Veld, and M. A. D. H. Schalekamp: Hemodynamic changes during long-term thiazide treatment of essential hypertension in responders and nonresponders, *Clin. Pharmacol. Therap.,* 27:328, 1980.

235. Blaustein, M. P., and J. M. Hamlyn: Role of a natriuretic factor in essential hypertension: An hypothesis, *Ann. Intern. Med.,* 98:785, 1983.

236. deWardener, H. E., and G. A. MacGregor: The relation of a circulating sodium transport inhibitor (the natriuretic hormone?) to hypertension, *Medicine,* 62:310, 1983.

237. deCarvalho, J. G. R., F. G. Dunn, G. Lohmoller, and E. D. Frohlich: Hemodynamic correlates of prolonged thiazide therapy: Comparison of responders and nonresponders, *Clin. Pharmacol. Therap.,* 22:875, 1977.

238. Medical Research Council Working Party on Mild to Moderate Hypertension: Ventricular extrasystoles during thiazide treatment: Substudy of MRC mild hypertension trial, *Br. Med. J.,* 287:1249, 1983.

239. Morgan, D. B., and C. Davidson: Hypokalemia and diuretics: An analysis of publications, *Br. Med. J.,* 1:905, 1980.

240. Swales, J. D.: Magnesium deficiency and diuretics, *Br. Med. J.,* 285:1377, 1982.

241. Veterans Administration Cooperative Study Group on Antihypertensive Agents: Propranolol or hydrochlorothiazide alone for the initial treatment of

hypertension. IV. Effect on plasma glucose and glucose tolerance, *Hypertension,* 7:1008, 1985.

242. Struthers, A. D., M. B. Murphy, and C. T. Dollery: Glucose tolerance during antihypertensive therapy in patients with diabetes mellitus, *Hypertension,* 7 (suppl. II):II-95, 1985.

243. Weidmann, P., A. Gerber, and R. Mordasini: Effects of antihypertensive therapy on serum lipoproteins, *Hypertension,* 5(suppl. III):III-120, 1983.

244. Harrington, J. T., J. M. Isner, and J. P. Kassirer: Our national obsession with potassium, *Am. J. Med.,* 73:155, 1982.

245. Brown, M. J., D. C. Brown, and M. B. Murphy: Hypokalemia from beta$_2$-receptor stimulation by circulating epinephrine, *N. Engl. J. Med.,* 309:1414, 1983.

246. Struthers, A., R. Whitesmith, and J. L. Reid: Prior thiazide diuretic treatment increases adrenaline-induced hypokalaemia, *Lancet,* 1:1358, 1983.

247. Nordrehaug, J. E., and G. von der Lippe: Hypokalemia and ventricular fibrillation in acute myocardial infarction, *Br. Ht. J.,* 50:525, 1983.

248. Nordrehaug, J. E., K. A. Johannessen, and G. von der Lippe: Serum potassium concentration as a risk factor of ventricular arrhythmias early in acute myocardial infarction, *Circulation,* 71:645, 1985.

249. Medical Research Council Working Party on Mild to Moderate Hypertension: Adverse reactions to bendrofluazide and propranolol for the treatment of mild hypertension, *Lancet,* 2:539, 1981.

250. Curb, J. D., N. O. Borhani, T. P. Blaszkowski, N. Zimbaldi, S. Fotiu, and W. Williams: Long-term surveillance for adverse effects of antihypertensive drugs, *J. Am. Med. Assoc,* 253:3263, 1985.

251. Moser, M., and J. Lunn: Responses to captopril and hydrochlorothiazide in black patients with hypertension, *Clin. Pharmacol. Therap.,* 32:307, 1982.

252. Veterans Administration Cooperative Study Group on Antihypertensive Agents: Captopril: Evaluation of low doses, twice-daily doses, and the addition of diuretic for the treatment of mild to moderate hypertension, *Clin. Sci.,* 63(suppl. 8):443s, 1982.

253. Veterans Administration Cooperative Study Group on Antihypertensive Agents: Low-dose captopril for the treatment of mild to moderate hypertension. I. Results of a 14-week trial, *Arch. Intern. Med.,* 144:1947, 1984.

254. Materson, B. J., J. R. Oster, U. F. Michael, S. M. Bolton, Z. C. Burton, J. E. Stambaugh, and J. Morledge: Dose response to chlorthalidone in patients with mild hypertension: Efficacy of a lower dose, *Clin. Pharmacol. Therap.,* 24:192, 1978.

255. Dustan, H. P., R. C. Tarazi, and E. L. Bravo: Depen-dence of arterial pressure on intravascular volume in treated hypertensive patients, *N. Engl. J. Med.,* 286:861, 1972.

256. Gavras, H., B. Waeber, G. R. Kershaw, C. S. Liang, S. C. Textor, H. R. Brunner, C. P. Tifft, and I. Gavras: Role of reactive hyperreninemia in blood pressure changes induced by sodium depletion in patients with refractory hypertension, *Hypertension,* 3:441, 1981.

257. Gifford, R. W., Jr, and R. C. Tarazi: Resistant hypertension: Diagnosis and management, *Ann. Intern. Med.,* 88:661, 1978.

258. Rodriguez-Iturbe, B., B. Baggio, J. Colina-Chourio, S. Favaro, R. Garcia, F. Sussana, L. Castillo, and A. Borsatti: Studies on the renin-aldosterone system in the acute nephritic syndrome, *Kidney Int.,* 19:445, 1981.

259. Stokes, G. S., M. K. Mani, and J. H. Stewart: Relevance of salt, water and renin to hypertension in chronic renal failure, *Br. Med. J.,* 3:126, 1970.

260. Veterans Administration Cooperative Study Group on Antihypertensive Agents: Propranolol in the treatment of essential hypertension, *J. Am. Med. Assoc.,* 237:2303, 1977.

261. Feit, A., R. Holtzman, M. Cohen, and N. el-Sherif: Effect of labetalol on exercise tolerance and double product in mild to moderate essential hypertension, *Am. J. Med.,* 78:937, 1985.

262. Avorn, J., D. E. Everitt, and S. Weiss: Increased antidepressant use in patients prescribed β-blockers, *J. Am. Med. Assoc.,* 255:357, 1986.

263. Koch-Weser, J.: Metoprolol, *N. Engl. J. Med.,* 301: 698, 1979.

264. Frishman, W. H.: Drug therapy: Atenolol and timolol, two new systemic beta-adrenoceptor antagonists, *N. Engl. J. Med.,* 306:1456, 1982.

265. McLeod, A. A., and D. G. Shand: Atenolol: A long-acting beta$_1$-adrenoceptor antagonist, *Ann. Intern. Med.,* 96:244, 1982.

266. Miller, R. R., H. G. Olson, E. A. Amsterdam, and D. T. Mason: Propanolol withdrawal rebound phenomenon: Exacerbation of coronary events after abrupt cessation of antianginal therapy, *N. Engl. J. Med.,* 293:416, 1975.

267. Rangno, R. E., S. Nattel, and A. Lutterodt: Prevention of propranolol withdrawal mechanism by prolonged small dose propranolol schedule, *Am. J. Cardiol.,* 49:828, 1982.

268. Lefkowitz, R. J., M. G. Caron, and G. L. Stiles: Mechanisms of membrane-receptor regulation. Biochemical, physiological, and clinical insights derived from studies of the adrenergic receptors, *N. Engl. J. Med.,* 310:1570, 1984.

269. Pritchard, B. N. C., and E. J. Ross: Use of propranolol in conjuction with alpha-receptor blocking drugs in pheochromocytoma, *Am. J. Cardiol.,* 18: 394, 1966.

270. Lager, I., G. Blohme, and U. Smith: Effect of cardioselective and nonselective β-blockade on the hypoglycaemic response in insulin-dependent diabetics, *Lancet,* 1:458, 1979.

271. Ryan, J. R., W. LaCorte, A. Jain, and F. G. McMahon: Hypertension in hypoglycemic diabetics treated with beta-adrenergic antagonists, *Hypertension,* 7:443, 1985.

272. Shepherd, A. M. M., M. S. Lin, and T. K. Keeton: Hypoglycemia-induced hypertension in a diabetic patient on metoprolol, *Ann. Intern. Med.,* 94:357, 1981.

273. Westerlund, A.: Atenolol and timolol (letter), *N. Engl. J. Med.,* 307:1343, 1982.

274. Stamler, R., J. Stamler, F. C. Gosch, D. K. Berkson, A. Dyer, and P. Hershinow: Initial antihypertensive drug therapy: Alpha blocker or diuretic. Initial report of a randomized controlled trial, *Am. J. Med.,* 80(suppl. 2A):90, 1986.

275. Vaughan, E. D., Jr., J. H. Laragh, I. Gavras, F. R. Buhler, H. Gavras, H. R. Brunner, and L. Baer: Volume factor in low and normal renin essential hypertension, *Am. J. Cardiol.,* 32:523, 1973.

276. Buhler, F. R., J. H. Laragh, L. Baer, E. D. Vaughan, Jr., and H. R. Brunner: Propranolol inhibition of renin secretion, *N. Engl. J. Med.,* 287:1209, 1972.

277. Weidmann, P., D. Hirsch, M. H. Maxwell, and R. Okun. Plasma renin and blood pressure during treatment with methyldopa, *Am. J. Cardiol.,* 34:671, 1974.

278. Laragh, J. H., R. L. Letcher, and T. G. Pickering: Renin profiling for diagnosis and treatment of hypertension, *J. Am. Med. Assoc.,* 241:151, 1979.

279. Freis, E. D., B. J. Materson, and W. Flamenbaum: Comparison of propranolol or hydrochlorothiazide alone for treatment of hypertension. II. Evaluation of the renin-angiotensin system, *Am. J. Med.,* 74:1029, 1983.

280. Weber, M. A., and J. I. Drayer: Single-agent and combination therapy of essential hypertension, *Am. Ht. J.,* 108:311, 1984.

281. Brunner, H. R., H. Gavras, B. Waeber, G. R. Kershaw, G. A. Turini, R. A. Vukovich, D. N. McKinstry, and I. Gavras: Oral angiotensin-converting enzyme inhibitor in long-term treatment of hypertensive patients, *Ann. Intern. Med.,* 90:19, 1979.

282. Wilkins, L. H., H. P. Dustan, J. F. Walker, and S. Oparil: Enalapril in low-renin essential hypertension, *Clin. Pharmacol. Therap.,* 34:297, 1983.

283. Gavras, H., J. Biollaz, B. Waeber, H. R. Brunner, I. Gavras, and R. O. Davies: Antihypertensive effect of the new oral angiotensin converting enzyme inhibitor "MK-421," *Lancet,* 2:543, 1981.

284. Wenting, G. J., J. H. B. de Bruyn, A. J. Man in't Veld, A. J. J. Woittiez, F. H. M. Derkx, and M. A. D. H. Schalekamp: Hemodynamic effects of captopril in essential hypertension, renovascular hypertension and cardiac failure: Correlations with short and long-term effects on plasma renin, *Am. J. Cardiol.,* 49:1453, 1982.

285. Man in't Veld, A. J., I. M. Schicht, F. H. Derkx, J. H. de Bruyn, and M. A. D. H. Schalekamp: Effects of an angiotensin-converting enzyme inhibitor (captopril) on blood pressure in anephric subjects, *Br. Med. J.,* 280:288, 1980.

286. Buhler, F. R., F. Burkhart, B. E. Lutold, M. Kung, G. Marbet, and M. Pfister: Antihypertensive beta blocking action as related to renin and age: A pharmacologic tool to identify pathogenic mechanisms in essential hypertension, *Am. J. Cardiol.,* 36: 653, 1975.

287. Muller, F. B., P. Bolli, P. Erne, W. Kiowski, and F. R. Buhler: Use of calcium antagonists as monotherapy in the management of hypertension, *Am. J. Med.,* 77(suppl. 2B):11, 1984.

288. Jenkins, A. C., J. R. Knill, and G. R. Dreslinski: Captopril in the treatment of the elderly hypertensive patient, *Arch. Intern. Med.,* 145:2029, 1985.

289. Liberatore, S. M., and G. Botta: Treatment of essential arterial hypertension with captopril: Outpatient drug-supervision study with particular reference to elderly patients, *Cardiovasc. Rev. Rep.,* 7:29, 1986.

290. Bravo, E. L., D. G. Vidt, and F. M. Fouad: Captopril, *N. Engl. J. Med.,* 306:214, 1982.

291. Zusman, R. M.: Renin- and non-renin-mediated antihypertensive actions of converting enzyme inhibitors, *Kidney Int.,* 25:969, 1984.

292. Swartz, S. L., G. H. Williams, N. K. Hollenberg, T. J. Moore, and R. G. Dluhy: Converting enzyme inhibition in essential hypertension: The hypotensive response does not reflect only reduced angiotensin II formation, *Hypertension,* 1:106, 1979.

293. Swartz, S. L., G. H. Williams, N. K. Hollenberg, L. Levine, R. G. Dluhy, and T. J. Moore: Captopril-induced changes in prostaglandin production. Relationship to vascular responses in normal man, *J. Clin. Invest.,* 65:1257, 1980.

294. Moore, T. J., F. R. Crantz, N. K. Hollenberg, R. J. Koletsky, M. S. Le Boff, S. L. Swartz, L. Levine, S. Podolsky, R. G. Dluhy, and G. H. Williams: Contributions of prostaglandins to the antihypertensive

action of captopril in essential hypertension, *Hypertension*, 3:168, 1981.

295. Oliver, J. A., and R. R. Sciacca: Local generation of angiotensin II as a mechanism of regulation of peripheral vascular tone in the rat, *J. Clin. Invest.*, 74:1247, 1984.

296. Genain, C. P., G. R. van Loon, and T. A. Kotchen: Distribution of renin activity and angiotensinogen in rat brain. Effects of dietary sodium chloride intake on brain renin, *J. Clin. Invest.*, 76:1939, 1985.

297. Redgrave, J., S. Rabinowe, N. K. Hollenberg, and G. H. Williams: Correction of abnormal renal blood flow response to angiotensin II by converting enzyme inhibition in essential hypertensives, *J. Clin. Invest.*, 75:1285, 1985.

298. Weinberger, M. H.: Influence of an angiotensin converting-enzyme inhibitor on diuretic induced metabolic effects in hypertension, *Hypertension*, 5(suppl. III):III-132, 1983.

299. Clough, D. P., M. G. Collis, J. Conway, R. Hatton, and J. R. Keddie: Interaction of angiotensin converting enzyme inhibitors with the function of the sympathetic nervous system, *Am. J. Cardiol.*, 49:1410, 1982.

300. Imai, Y., K. Abe, M. Seino, T. Haruyama, J. Tajima, M. Sato, T. Goto, M. Hiwatari, V. Kasai, K. Yoshinaga, and H. Sekino: Attenuation of pressor responses to norepinephrine and Pitressin and potentiation of pressor response to angiotensin II by captopril in human subjects, *Hypertension*, 4:444, 1982.

301. Hall, J. E.: Regulation of glomerular filtration rate and sodium excretion by angiotensin II. *Fed. Proc.*, 45:1414, 1986.

302. Kokko, J. P.: Primary acquired hypoaldosteronism, *Kidney Int.*, 27:690, 1985.

303. Croog, S. H., S. Levine, M. A. Testa, B. Brown, C. J. Bulpitt, C. D. Jenkins, G. L. Klerman, and G. H. Williams: The effects of anithypertensive therapy on the quality of life, *N. Engl. J. Med.*, 314:1657, 1986.

304. Helgeland, A., R. Strommen, C. H. Hageland, and S. S. Tretli: Enalapril, atenolol, and hydrochlorothiazide in mild to moderate hypertension. A comparative multicentre study in general practice in Norway, *Lancet*, 1:872, 1986.

305. Hodsman, G. P., C. G. Isles, G. D. Murray, T. P. Usherwood, D. J. Webb, and J. I. S. Robertson: Factors related to first dose hypotensive effect of captopril: Prediction and treatment, *Br. Med. J.*, 286:832, 1983.

306. Textor, S. C., E. L. Bravo, F. M. Fouad, and R. C. Tarazi: Hyperkalemia in azotemic patients during

angiotensin-converting enzyme inhibition and aldosterone reduction with captopril, *Am. J. Med.*, 73:719, 1982.

307. Burnakis, T. G., and H. J. Mioduch: Combined therapy with captopril and potassium supplementation. A potential for hyperkalemia, *Arch. Intern. Med.*, 144:2371, 1984.

308. Steinman, T. I., and P. Silva: Acute renal failure, skin rash, and eosinophilia associated with captopril therapy, *Am. J. Med.*, 75:154, 1983.

309. Packer, M., W. H. Lee, and P. D. Kessler: Preservation of glomerular filtration rate in human heart failure by activation of the renin-angiotensin system, *Circulation*, 74:766, 1986.

310. Ferris, T. F., and E. K. Weir: Effect of captopril on uterine blood flow and prostaglandin E synthesis in the pregnant rabbit, *J. Clin. Invest.*, 71:809, 1983.

311. Case, D. B., S. A. Atlas, J. A. Mouradian, R. A. Fishman, R. L. Sherman, and J. H. Laragh: Proteinuria during long-term captopril therapy, *J. Am. Med. Assoc.*, 244:346, 1980.

312. Textor, S. C., G. N. Gephardt, E. L. Bravo, R. C. Tarazi, F. M. Fouad, R. Tubbs, and J. T. McMahon: Membranous glomerulopathy associated with captopril therapy, *Am. J. Med.*, 74:705, 1983.

313. Dombey, S.: Optimal dose of captopril in hypertension (letter), *Lancet*, 1:529, 1983.

314. Cooper, R. A.: Captopril-associated neutropenia. Who is at risk?, *Arch. Intern. Med.*, 143:659, 1983.

315. Jaffe, I. A.: Adverse effects profile of sulfhydryl compounds in man, *Am. J. Med.*, 80:471, 1986.

316. Stumpe, K. O., R. Kolloch, and A. Overlack: Captopril and enalapril: Evaluation of therapeutic efficacy and safety, *Pract. Cardiol.*, 10(7):111, 1984.

317. Navis, G. J., P. E. de Jong, C. G. M. Kallenberg, J. De Monchy, and D. De Zeeuw: Absence of cross-reactivity between captopril and enalapril, *Lancet*, 1:1017, 1984.

318. Veterans Administration Cooperative Study Group on Antihypertensive Agents: Time course of antihypertensive effect of low-dose captopril in mild to moderate hypertension, *Clin. Pharmacol. Therap.*, 36:307, 1984.

319. Freier, P. A., G. L. Wollam, W. D. Hall, D. J. Unger, M. B. Douglas, and R. P. Bain: Blood pressure, plasma volume, and catecholamine levels during enalapril therapy in blacks with hypertension, *Clin. Pharmacol. Therap.*, 36:731, 1984.

320. Erne, P., P. Bolli, E. Burgisser, and F. R. Buhler: Correlation of platelet calcium with blood pressure. Effect of antihypertensive therapy, *N. Engl. J. Med.*, 310:1084, 1984.

321. Huelsemann, J. L., R. B. Sterzel, D. E. McKenzie,

and C. S. Wilcox: Effects of a calcium entry blocker on blood pressure and renal function during angiotensin-induced hypertension, *Hypertension,* 7:374, 1984.

322. Massie, B. M., A. T. Hirsch, I. K. Inouye, and J. F. Tubau: Calcium channel blockers as antihypertensive agents, *Am. J. Med.,* 77(suppl. 4A):135, 1984.

323. Klein, W. W.: Treatment of hypertension with calcium channel blockers: European data, *Am. J. Med.,* 77(suppl. 4A):143, 1984.

324. Halperin, A. K., and L. X. Cubeddu: The role of calcium channel blockers in the treatment of hypertension, *Am. Ht. J.,* 111:363, 1986.

325. Luft, F. C., G. R. Aronoff, R. S. Sloan, N. S. Fineberg, and M. H. Weinberger: Calcium channel blockade with nitrendipine, *Hypertension,* 7:438, 1985.

326. Zanchetti, A., and G. L. Leonetti: Natriuretic effect of calcium antagonists, *J. Cardiovasc. Pharmacol.,* 7(suppl. 4):S-533, 1985.

327. Markham, R. V., Jr., A. Gilmore, W. A. Pettinger, D. C. Brater, J. R. Corbett, and B. G. Firth: Central and regional hemodynamic effects and neurohumoral consequences of minoxidil in severe congestive heart failure and comparison to hydralazine and nitroprusside, *Am. J. Cardiol.,* 52:774, 1983.

328. Aguilera, G., and K. J. Catt: Participation of voltage-dependent calcium channels in the regulation of adrenal zona glomerulosa function by angiotensin II and potassium, *Endocrinology,* 118:112, 1986.

329. Halperin, A. K., K. M. Gross, J. F. Rogers, and L. X. Cubeddu: Verapamil and propranolol in essential hypertension, *Clin. Pharmacol. Therap.,* 36:750, 1984.

330. Haft, J. I., and W. E. Litterer: Chewing nifedipine to rapidly treat hypertension, *Arch. Intern. Med.,* 144:2357, 1984.

331. Ellrodt, A. T., M. J. Ault, M. S. Riedinger, and G. H. Murata: Efficacy and safety of sublingual nifedipine in hypertensive emergencies, *Am. J. Med.,* 79 (suppl. 4A):19, 1985.

332. Anderson, R. J.: Current concepts in treatment of hypertensive urgencies, *Am. Ht. J.,* 111:211, 1986.

333. Anderson, R. J., G. R. Hart, C. P. Crumpler, W. G. Reed, and C. A. Matthews: Oral clonidine loading in hypertensive urgencies, *J. Am. Med. Assoc.,* 246: 848, 1981.

334. Bannan, L. T., and D. G. Beevers: Emergency treatment of high blood pressure with oral atenolol, *Br. Med. J.,* 282:1757, 1981.

335. Alpert, M. A., and J. H. Bauer: Rapid control of severe hypertension with minoxidil, *Arch. Intern. Med.,* 142:2099, 1982.

336. Tschollar, W., and G. G. Belz: Sublingual captopril in hypertensive crisis, *Lancet,* 2:34, 1985.

337. Nielsen, P. E., A. Krogsgaard, A. McNair, and T. Hilden: Emergency treatment of severe hypertension emulated in a randomized study: Effect of rest and furosemide and a randomized evaluation of chlorpromazine, dihydralazine, and diazoxide, *Acta Med. Scand.,* 208:473, 1980.

338. McLeay, R. A. B., T. J. Stallard, R. D. S. Watson, and W. A. Littler: The effect of nifedipine on arterial pressure and reflex cardiac control, *Circulation,* 67:1084, 1983.

339. Marone, C., S. Luisoli, F. Bomio, C. Beretta-Piccoli, M. G. Bianchetti, and P. Weidmann: Blood sodium-blood volume state, aldosterone, and cardiovascular responsiveness after calcium entry blockade with nifedipine, *Kidney Int.,* 28:658, 1985.

340. Lund-Johansen, P.: Hemodynamic effects of calcium channel blockers at rest and during exercise in essential hypertension, *Am. J. Med.,* 79(suppl. 4A):11, 1985.

341. Moser, M., J. Lunn, D. T. Nash, J. F. Burris, N. Winer, G. Simon, and N. Vlachakis: Nitrendipine in the treatment of mild to moderate hypertension, *J. Cardiovasc. Pharmacol.,* 6(suppl. 7):S-1085, 1984.

342. Haynes, R. B., M. E. Mattson, A. V. Chobanian, J. M. Dunbar, T. O. Engebretson, Jr., T. F. Garrity, H. Leventhal, R. J. Levine, and R. L. Levy: Management of patient compliance in the treatment of hypertension, *Hypertension,* 4:415, 1982.

343. Rose, B. D., and L. A. Turka: Diuretics and hypertension, in N. H. Kaplan, J. H. Laragh, and B. M. Brenner (eds.), *Perspectives in Hypertension, Vol. 1, The Kidney in Hypertension,* Raven, New York, 1987.

344. Lau, K., D. Thomas, and B. Eby: Effects of amiloride on renal Mg handling: Evidence for enhanced transport in the distal tubule (abstract), *Kidney Int.,* 29:163, 1986.

345. Taguchi, J., and E. D. Freis: Partial reduction of blood pressure and prevention of complications in hypertension, *N. Engl. J. Med.,* 291:329, 1974.

346. Packer, M., W. H. Lee, N. Medina, and M. Yushak: Influence of renal function on the hemodynamic and clinical responses to long-term captopril therapy in severe chronic heart failure, *Ann. Intern. Med.,* 104:147, 1986.

347. Veterans Administration Cooperative Study Group on Antihypertensive Agents: Return of elevated blood pressure after withdrawal of antihypertensive drugs, *Circulation,* 51:1107, 1975.

348. Levinson, P. D., I. M. Khatri, and E. D. Freis: Persistence of normal BP after withdrawal of drug

treatment in mild hypertension, *Arch. Intern. Med.,* 142:2265, 1982.

349. Lanford, H. G., M. D. Blaufox, A. Oberman, C. M. Hawkins, J. D. Curb, G. R. Cutter, S. Wassertheil-Smoller, S. Pressel, C. Babcock, J. D. Abernethy, J. Hotchkiss, and M. Tyler: Dietary therapy slows return of hypertension after stopping prolonged medication, *J. Am. Med. Assoc.,* 253:657, 1985.

350. Medical Research Council Working Party on Mild Hypertension: Course of blood pressure in mild hypertensives after withdrawal of long-term anti-hypertensive treatment, *Br. Med. J.,* 293:988, 1986.

351. Finnerty, F. A., Jr.: Step-down therapy in hypertension. Importance in long-term management, *J. Am. Med. Assoc.,* 246:2593, 1981.

352. Finnerty, F. A., Jr.: Step-down treatment of mild systemic hypertension, *Am. J. Cardiol.,* 53:1304, 1984.

353. Watkins, J., E. C. Abbott, C. N. Hensby, J. Webster, and C. T. Dollery: Attenuation of hypotensive effect of propranolol and thiazide diuretics by indomethacin, *Br. Med. J.,* 281:702, 1980.

354. Steiness, E., and S. Waldorff: Different interactions of indomethacin and sulindac with thiazides in hypertension, *Br. Med. J.,* 285:1702, 1982.

355. Puddey, I. F., L. J. Beilin, R. Vandongen, R. Banks, and I. Rouse: Differential effects of sulindac and indomethacin on blood pressure in treated essential hypertensive subjects, *Clin. Sci.,* 69:327, 1985.

356. Wong, D. G., J. D. Spence, L. Lamki, D. Freeman, and J. W. D. McDonald: Effect of non-steroidal anti-inflammatory drugs on control of hypertension by β-blockers and diuretics, *Lancet,* 1:997, 1986.

12

RENOVASCULAR HYPERTENSION

Burton D. Rose

Pathogenesis
    Renin and the Degree of Arterial Stenosis
    Unilateral Renal Artery Stenosis
    Bilateral Renal Artery Stenosis
Diagnosis
    Radiologic Evaluation
    Medical Evaluation
    Renal Vein Renin Levels
Treatment
    Natural History
    Medical Therapy
    Surgical Therapy
    Percutaneous Transluminal Angioplasty
    Recommendations

The classic experiments by Goldblatt in 1934 demonstrated that persistent hypertension can be produced by constricting one or both renal arteries.[1] A similar sequence has clearly been demonstrated in humans, with the renal artery narrowing most often being due to atherosclerosis or fibromuscular dysplasia, conditions with different clinical characteristics (Table 12–1). Fibromuscular dysplasia is primarily a disease of females (about 80 percent) who are usually under the age of 40.[2,3] It is characterized by multiple areas of dysplasia within the vascular wall, particularly the media.[4] The most common sites of involvement are the *distal* two-thirds of the main renal artery and the proximal intrarenal branches. Similar changes also may be found in the celiac, hepatic, and iliac arteries.[5]

In comparison, atherosclerosis primarily affects men over the age of 45.[*,2,3,6] The area of stenosis is usually at the aortic orifice or in the proximal one-third of the main renal artery, not more distally as with fibromuscu-

lar dysplasia. In addition, evidence of extrarenal atherosclerotic vascular disease is frequently present.

A variety of other vascular lesions are less common causes of renovascular hypertension. These include renal artery thrombosis or dissection (occurring after trauma or superimposed upon an underlying vascular lesion), segmental renal infarcts, multiple atheroemboli, vasculitis, scleroderma, neurofibromatosis (which can also be associated with pheochromocytoma), and the hemolytic-uremic syndrome.[9-18] Renin-mediated hypertension can also occur in nonvascular

*Hypercholesterolemia, hypertension, smoking, and diabetes mellitus are the major risk factors for the development of atherosclerosis (see p. 500). However, *premature* atherosclerosis, occurring under the age of 45 in nondiabetics, may be due to heterozygous homocystinuria in as many as 30 percent of cases.[7] Establishing the diagnosis by methionine loading may be important since the administration of folic acid and pyridoxine may lessen the severity of the disease.[8]

TABLE 12-1. Clinical Characteristics of Fibromuscular Dysplasia and Atherosclerotic Renal Artery Stenosis

Characteristic	Fibromuscular Dysplasia	Atherosclerosis
Typical age at onset	<40	>45
Gender	80 percent female	Primarily males
Distribution of lesions	Distal main renal artery and intrarenal branches	Aortic orifice and proximal main renal artery
Progression of lesions	Uncommon	Common, may progress to complete occlusion

diseases such as unilateral ureteral obstruction, solitary or multiple renal masses (cysts or tumors), and posttraumatic subcapsular hematoma.[19-22] In these conditions, alterations in the normal renal architecture can promote renin secretion by producing focal areas of glomerular ischemia.

PATHOGENESIS

RENIN AND THE DEGREE OF ARTERIAL STENOSIS

Activation of the renin-angiotensin system is the primary event in renovascular hypertension. In general, the systemic blood pressure (BP) does not begin to rise until there has been more than a 70 to 80 percent narrowing of the renal artery.[23-25] Two factors contribute to this phenomenon. First, the major renal arteries are very large in relation to the arterioles, which are the primary site of vascular resistance. As a result, a marked reduction in the diameter of the vascular lumen is required in the large vessels before there is a significant reduction in the pressure perfusing the juxtaglomerular apparatus in the afferent arteriole,[23] the site of renin release.

Second, the arterial and glomerular pressures in the stenotic kidney are not only dependent upon the systemic BP and the resistance across the stenosis: they also vary with the more distal glomerular resistances at the afferent and efferent arterioles (Fig. 12-1). As the renal artery stenosis initially lowers the pressure perfusing the afferent

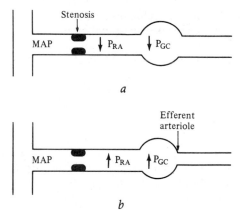

a

b

FIG. 12-1. The effect of renal artery stenosis on intrarenal pressures. Initially, the increased resistance across the stenosis [arrow, panel (*a*)] reduces the pressure both in the poststenotic renal artery (P_{RA}) and in the glomerular capillary (P_{GC}). This afferent arteriolar hypotension promotes the secretion of renin, leading to the local formation of angiotensin II, which preferentially constricts the efferent arteriole [arrow, panel (*b*)]. This increase in distal resistance returns the P_{RA} and P_{GC} toward normal without requiring an elevation in the systemic mean arterial pressure (MAP).

arteriole, the cells of the juxtaglomerular apparatus secrete renin. This leads to the local formation of angiotensin II, which preferentially constricts the efferent arteriole. The ensuing increase in distal vascular resistance raises the pressure in the more proximal segments of the renal artery (Fig. 12–1). As a result, afferent arteriolar pressure returns toward normal, thereby removing the stimulus to further renin secretion *without requiring an elevation in the systemic BP* (Fig. 12–2).[25] This predominant intrarenal effect is related to the much higher concentration of angiotensin II within the kidney (its site of formation) as compared with that in the systemic circulation where it mixes with blood from other organs.

Systemic hypertension occurs when the renal artery stenosis is sufficiently severe

that this intrarenal compensation becomes inadequate. In the experiment depicted in Fig. 12–2, creating a stenosis that initially lowers the intrarenal pressure from 100 down to 40 mmHg does not produce an elevation in the systemic BP. In comparison, producing a more marked reduction in intrarenal pressure (to, for example, 20 mmHg) with a tighter stenosis leads to a further increment in renin release and an 18-mmHg increase in BP.[25] The greater stimulus to renin secretion in this setting results in circulating angiotensin II levels that are now high enough to produce systemic hypertension.[25] It is only by raising the systemic BP that the distal intrarenal pressure can be increased toward normal.

In addition to maintaining the renal arterial pressure, the efferent arteriolar constric-

FIG. 12–2. Effect of inducing moderate renal artery stenosis (distal renal artery pressure reduced to 40 mmHg) on the mean arterial pressure (MAP), renal blood flow (RBF), renal vascular resistance (RVR), and the plasma renin activity (PRA) in normal dogs ($n = 15$). Left: Renal artery pressure and renal blood flow (measured as the Doppler shift in kilohertz) initially fall owing to the stenosis, leading to a reduction in RVR as part of the autoregulatory response and a rise in RBF. Within 30 min, the renal artery pressure has returned toward normal, in association with a small elevation in PRA, an increase in RVR due to arteriolar constriction, and no change in mean arterial pressure. Right: The prior administration of a converting enzyme inhibitor prevents the rise in RVR and renal artery pressure, suggesting that these responses were mediated by the intrarenal effect of angiotensin II. (*From W. P. Anderson, P. I. Korner, and C. I. Johnston, Hypertension, 1:292, 1979. By permission of the American Heart Association, Inc.*)

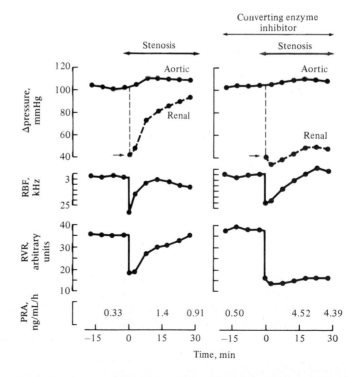

tion induced by angiotensin II also maintains the intraglomerular pressure and, therefore, the GFR (Fig. 12–1). This effect, which is part of the autoregulatory response, has important clinical implications. Interfering with the formation of angiotensin II with a converting enzyme inhibitor can lower the GFR and lead to renal failure in patients with bilateral renal artery stenosis or unilateral stenosis in a solitary functioning kidney (see "Treatment: Medical Therapy," below).

UNILATERAL RENAL ARTERY STENOSIS

The increase in angiotensin II production induced by unilateral renal artery stenosis can raise the systemic BP both by causing arteriolar vasoconstriction and by several indirect effects such as volume expansion (both angiotensin II and the associated rise in aldosterone secretion promote renal sodium retention)[26] and facilitation of the release and efficacy of norepinephrine.[27–29] The sympathetic nervous system may also be involved via direct activation of the renal afferent nerves by renal ischemia.[30,31]

Several observations in humans support a potentially important contributory role for norepinephrine in the genesis of hypertension in this setting. The administration of a converting enzyme inhibitor, for example, lowers both angiotensin II production and urinary norepinephrine excretion in patients with unilateral renal artery stenosis at the same time as it lowers the BP.[27] This finding suggests that the increase in sympathetic activity is in some way linked to activation of the renin-angiotensin system. Patients (and animals) with unilateral renovascular disease also tend to have an exaggerated fall in BP following the administration of a centrally acting sympatholytic agent such as clonidine,[27] pointing toward either a central effect of angiotensin II[29] or a reflex role for renal ischemia.[30,31]

In theory, the rise in BP in unilateral renal artery stenosis should be *limited by the pressure natriuresis phenomenon* (see p. 480).[32,33] In normal kidneys, a small elevation in BP enhances sodium and water excretion, thereby returning the BP toward normal. However, this protective response, which may be mediated by an elevation in pressure in the vasa recta capillaries in the renal medulla,[33] is impaired in unilateral renal artery stenosis because of the *effect of the increased circulating angiotensin II on the nonstenotic kidney.* Angiotensin II produces both renal vasoconstriction, which minimizes the degree to which the rise in pressure is transmitted to the medulla, and sodium retention.[34,35] As a result, the *pressure natriuresis relationship is reset* in the nonstenotic kidney in that a higher than normal BP is required before sodium excretion is enhanced (see Fig. 10–9).[35]

The importance of these changes can be illustrated by the response to the administration of an angiotensin II antagonist or a converting enzyme inhibitor (CEI). The GFR, sodium excretion, and the urine volume *all increase markedly* in the nonstenotic kidney despite the reduction in the systemic BP.[36,37] In comparison, there is no change or a reduction in the GFR in the stenotic kidney in which the intrarenal pressure is substantially lower (Fig. 12–3).

EFFECT OF RELEASING THE STENOSIS

Reversing the stenosis in experimental animals (usually by releasing an arterial clamp) leads to a rapid decrease in BP that begins within 1 h but is not complete for 12 h.[34,38] In addition to the reduction in angiotensin II production, enhanced release of vasodilator medullary lipids by the postischemic kidney also may contribute to the initial hypotensive response.[39]

These findings are not always replicable in humans, however, because chronic exposure of the nonstenotic kidney to hypertension

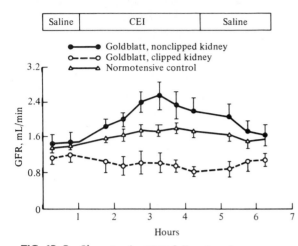

FIG. 12–3. Changes in GFR following the administration of a converting enzyme inhibitor in control rats and in the clipped (stenotic) and unclipped kidneys of rats with unilateral renal artery stenosis. The GFR rose in the unclipped kidney but fell in the clipped kidney due to interference with autoregulation. (*From W. C. Huang, D. W. Ploth, P. D. Bell, J. Work, and L. G. Navar, Hypertension, 3:285, 1981. By permission of the American Heart Association, Inc.*)

can lead to the development of nephrosclerosis (see "Treatment," below).[40,41] These vascular lesions, which increase in severity with time, can then maintain the hypertension even if the stenosis in the other kidney is corrected.[40] Thus, patients who have had hypertension due to unilateral renal artery stenosis for more than 5 years have a much lower success rate following correction of the stenosis than patients whose disease has been of shorter duration.[41] The mechanism responsible for the persistent elevation in BP in this setting is not understood, although enhanced renin release by the nephrosclerotic kidney may be involved.

BILATERAL RENAL ARTERY STENOSIS

The factors responsible for maintenance of the hypertension are somewhat different in patients with bilateral renal artery stenosis (or unilateral stenosis in a solitary functioning kidney). In this condition, the total renal mass is relatively hypoperfused. Thus, the angiotensin II- and aldosterone-induced increases in sodium reabsorption lead to volume expansion that is less likely to be limited by pressure natriuresis, since the rise in BP is not fully transmitted to either kidney. As sodium retention occurs, the increase in volume enhances renal perfusion, thereby decreasing the stimulus to renin secretion. At this time, the plasma renin activity may return to the normal range, as renal perfusion and the elevation in BP are maintained by volume expansion (Fig. 12–4).[42–44] If the ex-

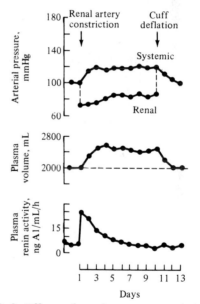

FIG. 12–4. Effects of renal artery stenosis in a solitary kidney on systemic and renal arterial pressure, plasma volume, and plasma renin activity. The secondary volume expansion maintains the hypertension, allowing the plasma renin activity to return toward normal. [*Adapted from V. J. Dzau, L. G. Siwek, S. Rosen, E. R. Farhi, H. Mizoguchi, and A. C. Barger, Hypertension, 3 (suppl. I):I-63, 1981. By permission of the American Heart Association, Inc.*]

cess volume is removed, however, there will be no fall in BP since renin release will increase. Thus, patients with this disorder are persistently hypertensive, although varying between renin- and volume-mediated mechanisms.[43,44]

DIAGNOSIS

Establishing the diagnosis of renal artery stenosis is particularly important because it is potentially curable by surgery or percutaneous angioplasty (see "Treatment," below). However, the incidence of renovascular disease may be under 1 percent if all hypertensives are included.[45-47] In one study, for example, renal arteriography was performed prospectively in 490 hypertensive patients.[47] Of 152 low-risk patients with no clinical clues suggestive of secondary hypertension, renal artery stenosis was found in only one.

The low overall incidence of renovascular hypertension makes it unrealistic to evaluate every hypertensive patient for this disorder. As a result, it is important to be aware of those findings that suggest the possible presence of renal artery stenosis (or some other less common cause of secondary hypertension) (Table 12–2). For example, the incidence of renal artery stenosis rises to 10 to 40 percent in patients with an acute eleva-

TABLE 12-2. Clinical Findings Suggestive of Renovascular Hypertension

An acute elevation in BP above a previously stable level
Severe or refractory hypertension
    With renal insufficiency, suggestive of bilateral disease
Retinal hemorrhages, exudates, or papilledema
Systolic-diastolic bruit (systolic bruit alone is less meaningful)
Proven age of onset less than 20 (especially if before puberty) or greater than 50
Negative family history of hypertension
Unexplained hypokalemia

tion in BP, marked hypertensive retinopathy (hemorrhages, exudates, or papilledema), or severe or refractory hypertension.[46-49] Furthermore, the combination of marked hypertension and otherwise unexplained renal insufficiency (plasma creatinine concentration above 1.5 mg/dL) suggests that the patient may have *bilateral* renal artery stenosis.[49]

Other findings that may also be helpful are a negative family history of hypertension, proven age of onset less than 20 (especially if before puberty) or greater than 50, the presence of a systolic and diastolic abdominal bruit (particularly in a young patient in whom diffuse atherosclerosis would be unlikely), and hypokalemia with urinary potassium wasting (due to the renin-induced secondary hyperaldosteronism).[50,51] The last finding also can occur with *primary* hyperaldosteronism, a disorder in which the plasma renin activity is typically low, not elevated as in renovascular disease.[52] For reasons that are not well understood, renal artery stenosis is uncommon in blacks, even in patients with severe hypertension.[3,48,53]

RADIOLOGIC EVALUATION

When the history or physical examination are suggestive, the diagnosis of renal artery stenosis can be established by renal arteriography (Fig. 12–5c and d).[54] However, the invasive nature of this test and its potential complications (acute renal failure due to the radiocontrast media or to atheroembolic disease) has led to a search for a simpler screening procedure (Table 12–3). A rapid-sequence intravenous pyelogram (IVP) (looking for a unilateral decrease in kidney size and/or delayed calyceal appearance time) has probably been the most widely used (Fig. 12–5a and b). Unfortunately, this test is normal in approximately 20 to 25 percent of patients with unilateral renal artery stenosis.[50,54,55] As a result, a negative IVP can not

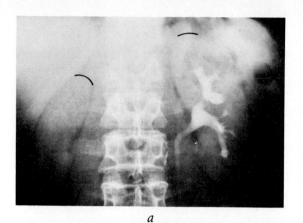 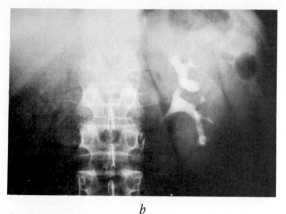

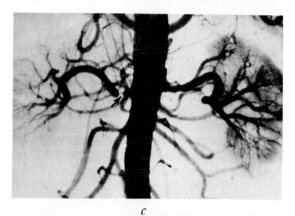 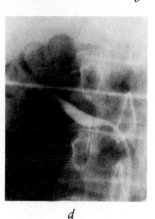

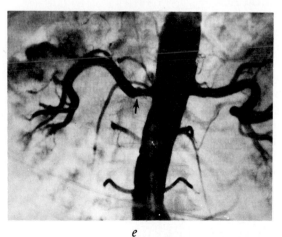

FIG. 12-5. Radiologic findings in unilateral renal artery stenosis. (*a*) Rapid-sequence intravenous pyelogram at 2 min demonstrates radiocontrast media in the calyces of the left kidney and a smaller, nonvisualized right kidney. (*b*) At 5 min, some calyceal visualization is now present in the right kidney. (*c*) An aortogram in this patient shows a 90 percent occlusion of the right renal artery (arrow), presumably due to an atheromatous plaque. (*d*) A balloon-tipped catheter is passed into the stenoic segment and then inflated in an attempt to dilate the vessel by percutaneous angioplasty. (*e*) Repeat aortogram after the angioplasty catheter is removed reveals almost complete reversal of the stenosis.

TABLE 12-3. Screening Tests for Renovascular Hypertension

Radiologic evaluation
 Rapid-sequence intravenous pyelogram
 Intravenous digital subtraction angiogram
 Sequential radioisotope scan
 Renal arteriogram—the definitive test
Medical evaluation
 Plasma renin activity
   Basal and after converting enzyme inhibition
 Hypotensive response to saralasin or converting
   enzyme inhibition

exclude the presence of renovascular disease when there is a high clinical index of suspicion. Furthermore, an IVP is even less likely to be positive in bilateral renal artery stenosis, since there may be a smaller difference in function between the two kidneys (unless one renal artery is totally occluded, leading to unilateral nonvisualization).

It had been hoped that intravenous digital subtraction angiography (DSA), which allows the main renal arteries to be visualized, would be a better screening procedure. However, the false-negative rate is still about 10 to 12 percent, and another 7 percent of patients will have a study which is not interpretable because the renal vessels are not well seen.[55,56] Ostial lesions at the aortic orifice and intrarenal lesions are most likely to be missed with this procedure. Thus an apparently normal intravenous DSA may be of limited value in young patients since fibromuscular dysplasia can primarily involve the intrarenal vessels.

Sequential radioisotope scanning has also been evaluated in a relatively small number of patients. This simple, noninvasive procedure can, depending upon the isotope that is used, detect a unilateral reduction in blood flow or filtration rate in the stenotic kidney. This test has a false-negative rate of 6 to 14 percent, and a predictive value of about 90 percent when the history suggests a 50 percent likelihood of disease.[55,57]

It is possible that the false-negative rate

with renal scanning can be reduced to an even lower level by the prior administration of 12.5 to 25 mg of the converting enzyme inhibitor captopril.[58] Diminishing the formation of angiotensin II can increase the likelihood of a lateralizing scan by enhancing the *difference in filtration* between the two kidneys (Fig. 12-3): the GFR tends to rise in the nonstenotic kidney because flow is enhanced, whereas the GFR frequently falls in the stenotic kidney (despite a rise in flow) because maintenance of the intrarenal and intraglomerular pressures requires angiotensin II (Fig. 12-2).[36,37]

Although preliminary results suggest that the captopril GFR scan may be an excellent screening test,[58] there is a potential risk of first-dose hypotension, particularly in volume-depleted patients on diuretic therapy in whom plasma renin levels may be very high.[59] This problem can usually be minimized by discontinuing the diuretic for 3 to 5 days.

MEDICAL EVALUATION

Measurement of the plasma renin activity (PRA) and the BP response to saralasin (an angiotensin II antagonist) or converting enzyme inhibition have also been used in an attempt to identify patients with renal artery stenosis. Accurate assessment of the PRA requires that it be measured under conditions which can control for the many factors that can affect renin secretion.[50,60] For example, the PRA is increased by standing, by a low sodium intake, and by antihypertensive medications that lead to volume depletion (diuretics), direct vasodilation (hydralazine, minoxidil, nifedipine), or reduced angiotensin II formation (captopril, enalapril),[43,50,61-63] which removes the feedback inhibition of angiotensin II on renin release.[50] On the other hand, renin secretion is reduced by a high sodium intake or by a β-blocker or other sympatholytic agent (methyldopa, clonidine) which blocks the sympathetic stimulation to renin release.[62-66]

As a result, the PRA can be accurately assessed only when all these factors are taken into consideration. Thus, the PRA should be correlated with a 24-h urine collection for sodium (an estimate of sodium intake) and, optimally, all antihypertensive medications should be discontinued for 2 weeks. Unfortunately, these requirements limit the usefulness of the PRA. It may be difficult to discontinue therapy, particularly in patients with marked hypertension who are most likely to have renovascular disease. Even when performed under ideal conditions, however, both false-positive and false-negative results may be obtained: a high or high-normal PRA is seen in 10 to 15 percent of patients with essential hypertension, and a normal or even reduced PRA may be found in up to 20 percent of patients with renal artery stenosis, especially those with volume-mediated hypertension due to bilateral disease (Fig. 12–4).[43,44,50,60]

These problems also limit the usefulness of measuring the hypotensive response to saralasin or a converting enzyme inhibitor. The acute fall in BP with these drugs is directly related to the baseline PRA,[67,68] which is not strongly predictive of the presence or absence of renovascular hypertension. Thus, a relatively high incidence (15 to 25 percent) or both false-positive and false-negative tests is seen, even when performed under optimal conditions.[69-71]

An alternative test involves measurement of the change in the PRA 1 h after the administration of intravenous saralasin or 25 mg of captopril. Patients with renal artery stenosis show a marked rise in the PRA versus a relatively small elevation in patients with essential hypertension.[72,73] This difference may be related to increased sensitivity of the ischemic kidney to a fall in the systemic BP. However, the accuracy of this test is impaired by a low-sodium diet or diuretic therapy, both of which must be discontinued for 1 to 2 weeks. Furthermore, some risk may be involved since the acute reduction in BP can exceed 50 mmHg, particularly in patients with residual volume depletion.[59,69]

In summary, there is as yet no noninvasive radiologic or serologic screening test with sufficient accuracy and safety that, if negative, can reliably exclude the diagnosis of renovascular hypertension.[69] Thus, *the clinical index of suspicion remains of primary importance,* although it should be emphasized that evaluation for renal artery stenosis with an invasive procedure such as a renal arteriogram should be undertaken only if the patient is a candidate for correction by surgery or percutaneous angioplasty. A radioisotope scan (perhaps with prior captopril administration)[58] or an intravenous DSA can be used if the history is only moderately suggestive, and further workup performed if a positive result is obtained. On the other hand, a renal arteriogram or an intra*arterial* DSA (in which a much lower dose of radiocontrast material is administered) should be the initial test when the clinical suspicion is very high, since these are the only procedures that can reliably establish or exclude the diagnosis. Consider, for example, the following case history.

Case History 12–1. A 49-year-old man presents with severe hypertension. He has a history of smoking and mild hypertension that has been well controlled for 10 years (BP averaging 145/90) on a diuretic. One month prior to admission, he begins to complain of headaches, and his BP is noted to be 190/140 (after having been at his baseline level 2 months previously). Other than the rise in BP, his physical examination is unremarkable. Laboratory data reveal only the new appearance of moderate hypokalemia. A renal arteriogram is then performed and demonstrates a 90 percent stenosis due to an atherosclerotic lesion

1.5 cm from the origin of the right renal artery (as in Fig. 12–5*c*).

Comment. The relatively common course of events in this patient began with chronic mild hypertension and smoking, leading sequentially to an atherosclerotic plaque in the right renal artery, increased renin secretion, an acute elevation in BP, and hypokalemia due to secondary hyperaldosteronism. The history so strongly suggests renovascular hypertension that a renal arteriogram was performed before any less invasive screening procedures. Although primary hyperaldosteronism also can cause hypertension and hypokalemia, this rare disorder usually leads to a slow rise in BP over a prolonged period, not acute, severe hypertension.

RENAL VEIN RENIN LEVELS

Documenting the presence of renal artery stenosis does not prove that the stenosis is responsible for the hypertension. The physiologic significance of a stenotic lesion is best assessed by simultaneous measurement of the PRA in blood from each of the renal veins. Renin secretion should be increased in the ischemic kidney and, due to the elevation in BP, suppressed in the normally perfused kidney. Thus, the major criteria for a positive test are as follows (Fig. 12–6):[43,69,74]

1. The renal venous renin activity in the stenotic kidney is more than 1.5 times that in the contralateral kidney.
2. The venous-arterial difference in the non-stenotic kidney is close to zero, indicating suppression of renin release. Arterial renin activity can be estimated from that in the inferior vena cava below the kidney, since the extrarenal circulations do not secrete or metabolize renin, i.e., venous renin activity is the same as arterial. Contralateral suppression is considered to be

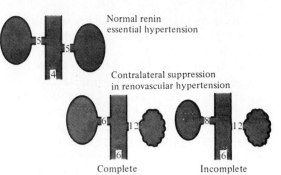

FIG. 12–6. Typical renal vein renin activities in essential and unilateral renovascular hypertension. In essential hypertension, both renal vein renins are the same and slightly greater than arterial renin (estimated from the infrarenal inferior vena cava) owing to renal renin secretion. In a positive test in renal artery stenosis, there is hypersecretion of renin from the affected side with relatively complete contralateral suppression (see text). Incomplete contralateral suppression (renal vein renin exceeding 1.2 times that in the inferior vena cava) is suggestive of bilateral disease or secondary nephrosclerosis and may be associated with a lower rate of surgical success. (*From J. H. Laragh, J. E. Sealey, F. R. Buhler, E D. Vaughan, Jr., H. R. Brunner, H. Gavras, and L. Baer, Am. J. Med., 58:4, 1975.*)

present if the ratio of the renal vein to inferior vena cava renin activity is 1.2 or less.

In patients with segmental renal arterial lesions, segmental renal venous samples should be obtained, if possible, since these samples may give a more positive result than those from the major renal veins.[75]

The incidence of true positive renal vein renin measurements can be enhanced by maneuvers that increase renin secretion in the underperfused stenotic kidney. These include tilting the patient during the procedure or the prior administration of a diuretic, vasodilator, or converting enzyme inhibitor.[43,50,76] On the other hand, false-negative tests may be obtained if renin secretion is impaired by the use of a β-blocker or other sympatholytic agent.

The frequency of normalization or marked reduction in BP following correction of unilateral renal artery stenosis is over 90 percent if the renal vein renins lateralize to the stenotic kidney.[43,50,69,74] In a variety of studies, however, a positive response to surgery or angioplasty also occurs in 50 to 75 percent of patients with *nonlateralizing* renal vein renins.[40,69,77] To some degree, the latter findings reflect a selection bias, since it is likely that only those patients with a strong clinical history for renovascular hypertension underwent surgery. Nevertheless, the basic observation remains unchanged: a physiologically significant stenosis may be present even if the renal vein renins do not lateralize. Multiple factors can contribute to a false-negative test, including catheter malposition, nonsimultaneous sampling, errors in the assay, segmental lesions, renin suppression by volume expansion (Fig. 12–4) or antihypertensive therapy, and loss of lateralization due to the development of nephrosclerosis in the contralateral kidney.[69]

Thus, interpretation of renal vein renins (as with many of the screening tests described above) must be made in concert with the clinical history. Correction of the stenosis should be attempted *regardless of the renal vein renin results* in a young patient with fibromuscular dysplasia, a patient with an otherwise unexplained acute elevation in BP (as in Case history 12–1), or a patient with poorly controlled hypertension due to drug resistance or unacceptable side effects. Conversely, surgery or angioplasty may be withheld if the renal vein renins do not lateralize in a patient with stable, well controlled hypertension, who is more likely to have a physiologically insignificant stenosis, or a patient who has been hypertensive for more than 5 years, since there is a lesser likelihood of a positive response to correction of the stenosis, pre-sumably due to nephrosclerosis in the contralateral kidney.[41,77]

Renal vein renin measurements also may be helpful in patients with *bilateral* renovascular disease. The kidney with the higher renal vein renin concentration is probably more ischemic and should be corrected first (see "Treatment," below).

It has also been suggested that the response to surgery or angioplasty can be predicted from the BP response to the chronic administration of a converting enzyme inhibitor.[78] When 27 patients were evaluated, the BP on therapy was almost identical with that obtained postoperatively on no medications. These results, however, represent a mean response, and substantial interpatient variation was present. Thus, approximately one-fifth of patients had more than a 20 mmHg difference between the pre- and postoperative BP measurements. Even patients with no reduction in BP may still have renovascular hypertension in which the BP is maintained by volume expansion at the time of study, not angiotensin II (Fig. 12–4).[44,79] Consequently, the response to converting enzyme inhibition cannot reliably predict the likelihood of a positive response to surgery or angioplasty.

TREATMENT

There are three therapeutic modalities that can be used in renovascular hypertension: antihypertensive medications and correction of the stenosis by either surgery or percutaneous angioplasty. The choice between these modalities is dependent upon a variety of factors including the patient's age and overall health, the cause of the stenosis (atherosclerosis versus fibromuscular dysplasia), the duration of hypertension, the presence of unilateral or bilateral disease, and the ability of medical therapy to control the BP with minimal side effects. It is also important to understand the natural history of the disease since there is a variable incidence of progressive vascular damage.

NATURAL HISTORY

The clinical course of atherosclerotic renal artery stenosis is different from that of fibromuscular dysplasia. Serial evaluation of patients with atherosclerotic disease has demonstrated progressive stenosis in 45 to 60 percent (within 4 to 7 years), with total occlusion developing in 10 to 15 percent of all stenotic arteries, and up to 40 percent in those vessels in which there is greater than a 75 percent narrowing of the vascular lumen.[6,80,81] These changes, which can occur even if the BP is well controlled,[80,81] are frequently accompanied by a decrease in renal size and, particularly with bilateral renal artery stenosis, a rise in the plasma creatinine concentration.[81,82]

In comparison, fibromuscular dysplasia is a much more benign disease. Progressive stenosis may occur in about one-third of patients, but total occlusion, decreasing renal size, and renal insufficiency are not seen.[80] Thus, the choice of therapy in fibromuscular disease is based largely upon BP control and whether surgery or angioplasty is preferable in young patients to avoid the need for lifelong antihypertensive therapy. Correction of the stenosis to preserve renal function is an issue only with atherosclerotic disease.

MEDICAL THERAPY

Antihypertensive medications are frequently effective in renovascular hypertension and may normalize the BP in many patients. Converting enzyme inhibitors (CEI: captopril or enalapril) appear to be particularly effective,[83,84] a finding that is consistent with the primary role of angiotensin II in this disorder. Thus, the combination of a CEI with a diuretic (to control the volume component as in Fig. 12–4) can control the BP in up to 90 percent of patients.[83,84]

Despite its antihypertensive efficacy, the use of a CEI in renovascular hypertension is occasionally limited by the development of acute renal failure (Fig. 12–7).[83–86] As described above, efferent arteriolar constriction by intrarenal angiotensin II helps to maintain the glomerular capillary pressure and, therefore, the GFR when the renal artery pressure is reduced (see Fig. 12–1).[87,88] Consequently, the GFR may fall if this autoregulatory response is impaired by the administration of a CEI. This is most likely to occur in bilateral renal artery stenosis (or unilateral stenosis in a solitary functioning kidney) since the total renal mass is underperfused. In these conditions, an acute (and often mild) decline in renal function following the use of a CEI has

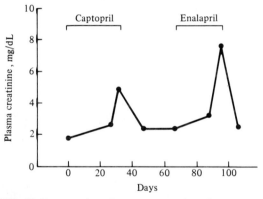

FIG. 12–7. Transient increases in the plasma creatinine concentration following the administration of captopril or enalapril to a patient with bilateral renal artery stenosis. This decline in renal function was not due to an excessive fall in blood pressure and was not seen with the use of other antihypertensive agents. (*From D. E. Hricik, P. J. Browning, R. Kopelman, W. E. Goorno, N. E. Madias, and V. J. Dzau, N. Engl. J. Med., 308:373, 1983. By permission from the New England Journal of Medicine.*)

been observed in 30 to 60 percent of patients.[84,86] Discontinuation of therapy rapidly returns the GFR to its baseline value.

Diuretic-induced hypovolemia may be an important additional risk factor for the development of acute renal failure after the administration of a CEI. Volume depletion increases renin secretion and makes maintenance of the GFR more angiotensin II-dependent. This can be illustrated by the following observations in experimental animals in which the renal perfusion pressure is reduced: the ability to maintain the GFR by autoregulation is impaired by a CEI; this impairment is *more pronounced with concurrent hypovolemia,* resulting in a greater fall in GFR.[88] There is suggestive evidence that these findings are applicable to humans. Almost all patients with bilateral renal artery stenosis and CEI-induced acute renal failure were also taking diuretics.[83,85] In some of these patients, stopping the diuretic and liberalizing sodium intake led to an improvement in GFR (as manifested by a fall in the plasma creatinine concentration) even though the CEI was continued.[89,90]

The potential risk of inducing acute renal failure, however, does *not* mean that CEI therapy should be routinely avoided in the presence of bilateral renovascular disease. Many patients will have an excellent antihypertensive response in this setting without a major decline in GFR, particularly if diuretics are used carefully and/or one of the kidneys has a relatively mild stenosis.[83,84] Careful monitoring of renal function after the institution of therapy is essential, since it is not possible to identify in advance those patients who can be safely treated.

Other antihypertensive drugs that do not interfere with angiotensin II formation generally do not diminish renal function in bilateral renal artery stenosis.[85,91] It is important to note, however, that autoregulation can protect the GFR only over a limited pressure range (see p. 74). If the intrarenal pressure is low enough, the GFR and renal blood flow ultimately begin to fall.[88] Thus, reducing the BP with *any antihypertensive drug* can lead to renal failure if marked intrarenal hypotension is produced. This can occur when both stenoses are very severe or when there has been an excessive antihypertensive response (Fig. 12–8).[24,49] Surgery or angioplasty is usually required for the former problem since medical therapy cannot adequately control the BP without lowering the GFR.[24,49]

UNILATERAL RENAL ARTERY STENOSIS

The possible deleterious effect of a CEI in unilateral renal artery stenosis has received less attention. In general, there is no important decline in GFR (Fig. 12–8)[24,84] because reversal of angiotensin II-induced vasoconstriction can substantially increase the GFR in the *nonstenotic* kidney (Fig. 12–3).[36,37] Some degree of renal insufficiency may occur, however, if prolonged hypertension has produced nephrosclerosis in the nonstenotic kidney.[83,84]

These findings do not address the issue of function in the ischemic kidney. In one study of 14 patients with unilateral renal artery stenosis, the administration of a CEI led to *complete cessation of GFR* in the affected kidney as assessed by radioisotope scanning.[92] This change will generally be missed on routine clinical examination since there is little fall in total GFR.[92] The long-term implication of this finding is uncertain. Prolonged hypofiltration could lead to irreversible atrophy, a possibility that has been demonstrated in animals with unilateral renal artery stenosis.[95] Tubular atrophy and interstitial fibrosis and a reduction in kidney weight were found in the stenotic kidney of animals treated with a CEI. These changes were not seen or appeared to be less prominent when different antihypertensive agents were administered.

In summary, medical therapy in renovas-

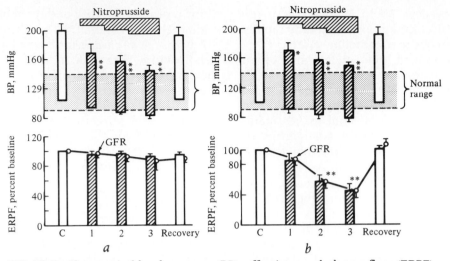

FIG. 12–8. Changes in blood pressure (BP), effective renal plasma flow (ERPF), and glomerular filtration rate (GFR) during intravenous infusion of nitroprusside to patients with renal artery stenosis. (*a*) Renal perfusion and GFR were relatively constant despite a substantial fall in BP in eight patients with unilateral renal artery stenosis. (*b*) In comparison, lowering the BP produced progressive reductions in ERPF and GFR in eight patients with marked bilateral renal artery stenosis. Double asterisks indicated p < 0.01; single asterisk indicates p < 0.05. (*From S. C. Textor, A. C. Novick, R. C. Tarazi, V. Klimas, D. G. Vidt, and M. Pohl, Ann. Intern. Med., 102:308, 1985.*)

cular hypertension is frequently effective but does not correct the underlying problem. As a result, progression of atherosclerotic lesions may occur and antihypertensive medications can lead to a further impairment in GFR, particularly if a CEI is used. Although surgery or percutaneous angioplasty can correct the stenotic lesion, these procedures have their own risks, and recurrent stenosis is not uncommon in patients with atherosclerotic disease.

SURGICAL THERAPY

Bypassing the stenotic lesion can usually be achieved by surgery. An aortorenal bypass is most common, but an ileorenal, splenorenal, or hepatorenal bypass may be required in the presence of marked aortic atherosclerosis.[77,94] In addition, in situ branch surgery has been performed in selected patients for intrarenal fibromuscular dysplasia.[77]

In patients with *bilateral* renal artery stenosis, only the more ischemic kidney (as identified from the IVP, renal vein renins, or renal arteriogram)[95] is usually corrected at the initial operation.[77,94] This regimen minimizes the duration of surgery and therefore the operative risk. An exception, in which total surgical correction can be attempted at a single operation, occurs in patients in whom one kidney is markedly atrophic owing to a totally occluded renal artery. In this setting, a unilateral nephrectomy plus bypass on the contralateral side can be performed.[94] Total occlusion, however, does not necessarily imply that the kidney is not viable. Kidney size above 8 to 9 cm, visualization during the pyelographic phase of the arteriogram or IVP, or the demonstration of viable glomeruli and tubules on a specimen taken during surgery all suggest that bypass of the occluding lesion can lead to return of at least some kidney function.[94]

Two questions need to be addressed when considering surgical correction of renal artery stenosis:

1. What is the long-term efficacy?
2. What is the morbidity and mortality of the procedure?

EFFICACY

Most studies have shown that the hypertension is cured or improved by surgery in 65 to 90 percent of patients.[40,41,96-99] These general statistics are of limited value, however, since it is possible to identify subgroups that are likely to do substantially better or worse than these overall results (Table 12-4). The prognosis is best in those patients with a unilateral lesion, hypertension of less than 5 years duration, fibromuscular dysplasia, and lateralizing renal vein renins.[41,69,96-99] When these criteria are met in a young patient with fibromuscular dysplasia, the likelihood of surgical success is about 95 percent.[41,98] In comparison, the success rate following surgery is much less in an older patient with atherosclerosis and hypertension for more than 5 years.[41,77] The deleterious effect of prolonged hypertension is probably related to the development of nephrosclerosis in the non-stenotic kidney[40,41] and is frequently associated with renal insufficiency.[100]

Bilateral Renal Artery Stenosis. The fall in BP when one side is corrected in bilateral renal artery stenosis is related in part to the degree of stenosis in the *less involved* kidney. Bypassing the more severely affected lesion will lower the BP until intrarenal hypotension develops in the still stenotic contralateral kidney. At this time, increased angiotensin II production by the now ischemic kidney will prevent any further hypotensive response.

Surgery in bilateral renal artery stenosis also may be performed for a second reason, the *preservation of renal function*. Patients with bilateral disease may develop progressive renal failure due to worsening of the stenoses[81,82,101] or to a fall in renal perfusion pressure following antihypertensive therapy.[24,84-86] In these patients, renal function can be stabilized or improved by correction of the stenotic lesions.[24,49,81,82,101-104] Even patients who progress to end-stage renal failure and dialysis may recover enough function to allow dialysis to be discontinued.[103,104]

MORTALITY

The risk of surgery is dependent upon the patient's age and the presence or absence of other cardiovascular disease. Healthy, young patients with fibromuscular dysplasia have very little operative morbidity.[98] In comparison, older patients with diffuse atherosclerosis are clearly at higher risk, with a mortality rate between 2 and 9 percent.[97,98,100,105] It has been suggested that the outcome can be improved by identifying high-risk patients with symptomatic coronary or cerebral atherosclerosis. In one study of 100 patients,

TABLE 12-4. Factors Affecting Response to Correction of Renal Artery Stenosis

	Favorable	Unfavorable
Cause	Fibromuscular dysplasia	Atherosclerosis
Duration of hypertension	Less than 5 years	Greater than 5 years
Renal vein renins	Lateralizing	Nonlateralizing
Degree of involvement	Unilateral	Bilateral
Severity of stenosis	Partial	Complete

correction of these lesions *before* renovascular surgery was associated with a net mortality of only 2 percent.[96]

PERCUTANEOUS TRANSLUMINAL ANGIOPLASTY

Percutaneous transluminal angioplasty (PTA) represents a nonsurgical means of dilating a stenotic renal artery.[106] This procedure involves the insertion of a balloon-tipped catheter into the narrowed vessel. As the balloon is transiently inflated (see Fig. 12–5d), controlled intimal and medial injury is induced, resulting in an increase in the vessel diameter.[107,108] The endothelial damage also promotes platelet deposition, which can lead to thrombus formation.[107,108] Consequently, aspirin and dipyridamole are given for 3 months after angioplasty to prevent recurrent stenosis.[109]

Several reviews of the efficacy of PTA in renovascular hypertension have appeared in the past few years. The following conclusions can be drawn from these studies:

1. PTA is as effective as surgery in fibromuscular dysplasia, curing the hypertension in 50 to 80 percent, and lowering the BP in most of the remaining patients.[109–112]
2. PTA is substantially less effective in atherosclerotic disease, with less than 30 percent of patients being cured and up to 50 percent having no reduction in BP.[110–112] The response is strongly determined by whether or not the vessel can be dilated (the success rate being 55 to 60 percent).[111] More than 80 percent of patients are cured or improved following a successful dilation, whereas few patients benefit when there is no change in vessel diameter.[111]

The type and location of the lesion are important determinants of success with PTA in patients with atherosclerotic disease. The optimal lesion is partially occluding, noncalcified, and located in the renal artery, rather than at the ostium which usually reflects aortic disease. On the other hand, PTA probably should not be attempted with calcified, ostial, or totally occluding lesions.

3. PTA should probably also be avoided in patients with bilateral atherosclerotic disease. A substantial reduction in BP is unusual in this setting,[110,111] and there is an appreciable risk of inducing a permanent decline in renal function (occasionally requiring dialysis) due to atheroembolic disease.[113]
4. Even when initially successful, recurrent stenosis occurs in 5 to 50 percent of patients with atherosclerosis.[110,111,114,115] This is typically manifested by recurrent hypertension and can be treated with repeat angioplasty, if necessary.

Complications associated with PTA include radiocontrast media-induced renal failure, atheroemboli, renal artery dissection or thrombus formation, or rarely rupture of the vessel or the balloon.[110,115] These problems occur in 5 to 15 percent of patients with unilateral disease but are usually not serious.[110,111,115] However, surgery may be required if renal artery dissection or thrombosis leads to total occlusion of the vessel.

RECOMMENDATIONS

Optimal therapy for renal artery stenosis is frequently uncertain because of the potential complications associated with each of the available therapies. Furthermore, there are no satisfactory studies comparing the long-term efficacy of medical treatment versus surgery or angioplasty. Although early studies did show approximately a 50 percent reduction in long-term cardiovascular mortality with surgery, the BP was not as well controlled in the medically treated patients, in part because of the lack of availability of newer antihypertensive medications.[116] Even if surgery were somewhat more effective, however, the long-term benefit would still have to be weighed against the 2 to 9 percent operative mortality rate in those patients who are most likely to have an indication for surgery: older patients with diffuse atherosclerosis.[96-98,100,105]

At the present time, the preferred therapy varies with the cause and extent of the renovascular disease:

1. Patients with *fibromuscular dysplasia* should be treated with PTA. This procedure is as effective as surgery in this setting, without the associated morbidity.[110-112] Although medical therapy also may be effective, a potentially curative procedure (assuming that the lesion is correctible) is desirable since these patients are usually young.

2. Patients with *bilateral atherosclerotic disease* and progressive renal insufficiency should have corrective surgery (if they are operative candidates) to preserve renal function.[24,49,81,82,101-104] Angioplasty should generally be avoided in this setting (unless both lesions are nonostial and nonoccluding), because of the low success rate and the risk of inducing renal failure due to atheroembolic disease.[111,113]

   Patients with bilateral atherosclerotic involvement and *stable* renal function can be tried on medical therapy. However, these patients should be carefully monitored, given the frequent progression of the atherosclerotic lesions[6,80,81] and the possible development of renal failure as the systemic BP is lowered (Figs. 12–7 and 12–8).[24,84-86] Surgery is indicated if the BP cannot be controlled or the plasma creatinine concentration rises.

3. Treatment of atherosclerotic *unilateral* renal artery stenosis depends in part upon the patient's age, preference for medical or corrective therapy, and the location and severity of the lesion. Medical therapy, particularly with a converting enzyme inhibitor and a diuretic, is usually able to control the BP.[83,84] It is uncertain, however, what to do when the GFR markedly deteriorates on the stenotic side following the administration of a converting enzyme inhibitor. This complication can be detected noninvasively by performing a radioisotope scan once the patient is stable.[92] Possible loss of the stenotic kidney due to ischemic atrophy[93] is not desirable, particularly in view of the potential for atherosclerosis to ultimately involve the contralateral kidney. Therefore, persistent loss of GFR by scan should probably lead to discontinuation of the converting enzyme inhibitor, although other medications can produce the same result if the stenosis is sufficiently severe.[24]

   Indications for corrective therapy include inability to control the BP, inability to maintain renal function in the stenotic kidney with antihypertensive medications, and patient preference to attempt to cure the hypertension. PTA is most effective in atherosclerotic renal artery stenosis when it succeeds in dilating the affected artery.[111] This is most likely to occur with partially occluding, noncalcified lesions that are in the renal artery, not at the ostium. Thus, PTA can be tried if these criteria are met. If not, surgery is preferred if the patient is a good operative candidate.

REFERENCES

1. Goldblatt, H., J. Lynch, R. F. Hanzal, and W. W. Summerville: Studies on experimental hypertension, I: The production of persistent elevation of systolic blood pressure by means of renal ischemia, *J. Exp. Med.,* 59:347, 1934.

2. Simon, N., S. S. Franklin, K. H. Bleifer, and M. H. Maxwell: Clinical characteristics of renovascular hypertension, *J. Am. Med. Assoc.,* 220:1209, 1972.

3. Final Report of the Subcommittee on Definition and Prevalence of the 1984 Joint National Com-

mittee: Hypertension prevalence and the status of awareness, treatment and control in the United States, *Hypertension*, 7:457, 1985.

4. Ratliff, N. B.: Renal vascular disease: Pathology of large blood vessel disease, *Am. J. Kid. Dis.*, 5:A93, 1985.

5. Sheps, S. G., O. W. Kincaid, and J. C. Hunt: Serial renal function and angiographic observations in idiopathic fibrous and fibromuscular stenosis of the renal arteries, *Am. J. Cardiol.*, 30:55, 1972.

6. Wollenwever, J., S. G. Sheps, and G. D. Davis: Clinical course of atherosclerotic renovascular disease, *Am. J. Cardiol.*, 21:60, 1968.

7. Boers, G. H. J., A. G. H. Smals, F. J. M. Trijbels, B. Fowler, J. A. J. M. Bakkeren, H. L. Schoonderwaldt, W. J. Kleijer, and P. W. C. Kloppenborg: Heterozygosity for homocystinuria in premature peripheral and cerebral occlusive arterial disease, *N. Engl. J. Med.*, 313:709, 1985.

8. Mudd, S. H.: Vascular disease and homocysteine metabolism, *N. Engl. J. Med.*, 313:751, 1985.

9. Sheil, A. G., G. S. Stokes, D. J. Tiller, J. May, J. R. Johnson, and J. H. Stewart: Reversal of renal failure by revascularization of kidneys with thrombosed renal arteries, *Lancet*, 2:865:1973.

10. Spark, R. F.: Renal trauma and hypertension, *Arch. Intern. Med.*, 136:1097, 1976.

11. Edwards, B. S., A. W. Stanson, K. E. Holley, and S. G. Sheps: Isolated renal artery dissection. Presentation, evaluation, management, and pathology, *Mayo Clin. Proc.*, 57:564, 1982.

12. Schambelan, M., M. Glickman, J. R. Stockigt, and E. G. Biglieri: Selective renal-vein renin sampling in hypertensive patients with segmental renal lesions, *N. Engl. J. Med.*, 290:1153, 1974.

13. Dalakos, T. G., D. H. P. Streeten, D. Jones, and A. Obeid: "Malignant" hypertension resulting from atheromatous embolization predominantly in one kidney, *Am. J. Med.*, 57:135, 1974.

14. Stockigt, J. R., D. J. Topliss, and M. J. Hewett: High-renin hypertension in necrotizing vasculitis, *N. Engl. J. Med.*, 300:1218, 1979.

15. Lagneau, P., and J. B. Michel: Renovascular hypertension and Takayasu's disease, *J. Urol.*, 134: 876, 1985.

16. Lopez-Ovejero, J. A., S. D. Saal, W. A. D'Angelo, J. S. Cheigh, K. H. Stenzel, and J. H. Laragh: Reversal of vascular and renal crises of scleroderma by oral angiotensin-converting-enzyme blockade, *N. Engl. J. Med.*, 300:1417, 1979.

17. Riccardi, V. M.: Von Recklinghausen neurofibromatosis, *N. Engl. J. Med.*, 305:1617, 1981.

18. Powell, H. R., R. Rotenberg, A. L. Williams, and D. A. McCredie: Plasma renin activity in acute poststreptococcal glomerulonephritis and the hemolytic-uraemic syndrome, *Arch. Dis. Child.*, 49:802, 1974.

19. Weidmann, P., C. Beretta-Piccoli, D. Hirsh, F. C. Reubi, and S. G. Massry: Curable hypertension with unilateral hydronephrosis, *Ann. Intern. Med.*, 87:437, 1977.

20. Babka, J. C., M. S. Cohen, and J. Sode: Solitary intrarenal cyst causing hypertension, *N. Engl. J. Med.*, 291:343, 1974.

21. Nash, D. A., Jr.: Hypertension in polycystic kidney disease without renal failure, *Arch. Intern. Med.*, 137: 1571, 1977.

22. Grim, C. E., M. F. Mullins, J. P. Nison, and G. Ross, Jr.: Unilateral "Page kidney" hypertension in man, *J. Am. Med. Assoc.*, 213:42, 1975.

23. Young, D. F., N. R. Cholvin, and A. C. Roth: Pressure drop across artificially induced stenoses in femoral arteries of dogs, *Circ. Res.*, 36:735, 1975.

24. Textor, S. C., A. C. Novick, R. C. Tarazi, V. Klimas, D. G. Vidt, and M. Pohl: Critical perfusion pressure for renal function in patients with bilateral atherosclerotic renal vascular disease, *Ann. Intern. Med.*, 102:308, 1985.

25. Anderson, W. P., P. I. Korner, and C. I. Johnston: Acute angiotensin II-mediated restoration of distal renal artery pressure in renal artery stenosis and its relationship to the development of sustained one-kidney hypertension in conscious dogs, *Hypertension*, 1:292, 1979.

26. Hall, J. E.: Regulation of glomerular filtration rate and sodium excretion by angiotensin II, *Fed. Proc.*, 45:1431, 1986.

27. Oparil, S.: The sympathetic nervous system in clinical and experimental hypertension, *Kidney Int.*, 30:437, 1986.

28. Imai, Y., K. Abe, M. Seino, T. Haruyama, J. Tajima, M. Sato, T. Goto, M. Hiwatari, V. Kasai, K. Yoshinaga, and H. Sekino: Attenuation of pressor responses to norepinephrine and Pitressin and potentiation of pressor response to angiotensin II by captopril in human subjects, *Hypertension*, 4:444, 1982.

29. Faber, J. E., and M. J. Brody: Central nervous system action of angiotensin during onset of renal hypertension in awake rats, *Am. J. Physiol.*, 247: H349, 1984.

30. Katholi, R. E., S. R. Winternitz, and S. Oparil: Decrease in peripheral sympathetic nervous sys-

tem activity following renal denervation or un-clipping in the one-kidney one-clip Goldblatt hypertensive rat, *J. Clin. Invest.*, 69:55, 1982.

31. Katholi, R. E.: Renal nerves in the pathogenesis of hypertension in experimental animals and humans, *Am. J. Physiol.*, 245:F1, 1983.

32. Guyton, A. C., T. G. Coleman, A. W. Cowley, Jr., K. W. Scheel, R. D. Manning, Jr., and R. A. Norman, Jr.: Arterial pressure regulation: Overriding dominance of the kidneys in long-term regulation and in hypertension, *Am. J. Med.*, 52:584, 1972.

33. Knox, F. G., J. I. Mertz, J. C. Burnett, Jr., and A. Haramati: Role of hydrostatic and oncotic pressures in renal sodium reabsorption, *Circ. Res.*, 52:491, 1983.

34. Ploth, D. W.: Angiotensin-dependent renal mechanisms in two-kidney, one-clip renal vascular hypertension, *Am. J. Physiol.*, 245:F131, 1983.

35. Hall, J. E., A. C. Guyton, M. J. Smith, Jr., and T. G. Coleman: Blood pressure and renal function during chronic changes in sodium intake: Role of angiotensin, *Am. J. Physiol.*, 239:F271, 1980.

36. Huang, W. C., C. A. Jackson, and L. G. Navar: Nephron responses to converting enzyme inhibition in non-clipped kidney of Goldblatt hypertensive rat at normotensive pressures, *Kidney Int.*, 28:128, 1985.

37. Huang, W. C., and L. G. Navar: Effects of unclipping and converting enzyme inhibition on bilateral renal function in Goldblatt hypertensive rats, *Kidney Int.*, 23:816, 1983.

38. Kumar, A., R. F. Bing, J. D. Swales, and H. Thurston: Delayed reversal of Goldblatt hypertension by angiotensin II infusion in the rat, *Am. J. Physiol.*, 246:H811, 1984.

39. Muirhead, E. E.: Antihypertensive functions of the kidney, *Hypertension*, 2:444, 1980.

40. MacKay, A., P. Boyle, J. J. Brown, A. M. M. Cumming, H. Forrest, A. G. Graham, A. F. Lever, J. I. S. Robertson, and P. F. Semple: The decision on surgery in renal artery stenosis, *Q. J. Med.*, 52:363, 1983.

41. Hughes, J. S., H. G. Dove, R. W. Gifford, Jr., and A. F. Feinstein: Duration of blood pressure elevation in accurately predicting surgical cure of renovascular hypertension, *Am. Ht. J.*, 101:408, 1981.

42. Nabel, E. G., G. H. Gibbons, and V. J. Dzau: Pathophysiology of experimental renovascular hypertension, *Am. J. Kid. Dis.*, 5:A111, 1985.

43. Laragh, J. H., J. E. Sealey, F. R. Buhler, E. D. Vaughan, Jr., H. R. Brunner, H. Gavras, and L. Baer: The renin axis and vasoconstriction-volume analysis for understanding and treating renovascular and renal hypertension, *Am. J. Med.*, 58:4, 1975.

44. Kurtzman, N. A., V. K. G. Pillay, P. W. Rogers, and D. Nash, Jr.: Renal vascular hypertension and low plasma renin activity: Interrelationship of volume and renin in pathogenesis of hypertension, *Arch. Intern. Med.*, 133:195, 1974.

45. Tucker, R. M., and D. R. Labarthe: Frequency of surgical treatment for hypertension in adults at the Mayo Clinic from 1973 through 1975, *Mayo Clin. Proc.*, 52:549, 1977.

46. Levin, A., M. D. Blaufox, H. Castle, G. Entwisle, and H. Langford: Apparent prevalence of curable hypertension in Hypertension Detection and Follow-up Program, *Arch. Intern. Med.*, 145:424, 1985.

47. Horvath, J. S., R. C. Waugh, D. J. Tiller, and G. G. Duggin: The detection of renovascular hypertension: A study of 490 patients by renal angiography, *Q. J. Med.*, 51:139, 1982.

48. Davis, B. A., J. E. Crook, R. E. Vestal, and J. A. Oakes: Prevalence of renovascular hypertension in patients with grade III or IV hypertensive retinopathy, *N. Engl. J. Med.*, 301:1273, 1979.

49. Ying, C. Y., C. P. Tifft, H. Gavras, and A. V. Chobanian: Renal revascularization in the azotemic hypertensive patient resistant to therapy, *N. Engl. J. Med.*, 311:1070, 1984.

50. Vaughan, E. D., Jr.: Renovascular hypertension, *Kidney Int.*, 27:811, 1985.

51. Grim, C. E., F. C. Luft, M. H. Weinberger, and C. M. Grim: Sensitivity and specificity of screening tests for renovascular hypertension, *Ann. Intern. Med.*, 91:617, 1979.

52. Bravo, E. L., R. C. Tarazi, H. P. Dustan, F. M. Fouad, S. C. Textor, R. W. Gifford, and D. G. Vidt: The changing clinical spectrum of primary aldosteronism, *Am. J. Med.*, 74:641, 1983.

53. Keith, T. A., III: Renovascular hypertension in black patients, *Hypertension*, 4:438, 1983.

54. Bookstein, J. J., H. L. Abrams, R. E. Buenger, J. Lecky, S. S. Franklin, M. D. Reiss, K. H. Bleifer, E. C. Klatte, P. D. Varady, and M. H. Maxwell: Radiologic aspects of renovascular hypertension, *J. Am. Med. Assoc.*, 220:1225, 1972.

55. Havey, R. J., F. Krumlovsky, F. del Greco, and H. G. Martin: Screening for renovascular hypertension. Is renal digital-substraction angiography the preferred noninvasive test?, *J. Am. Med. Assoc.*, 254:388, 1985.

56. Osborne, R. W., Jr., J. Goldstone, B. J. Hillman, T. W. Ovitt, J. M. Malone, and S. Nudelman: Digital video subtraction angiography: Screening tech-

nique for renovascular hypertension, *Surgery,* 90: 932, 1981.

57. Chiarini, C., E. D. Esposti, F. Losinno, N. Monetti, P. Pavlica, A. Santoro, A. Sturani, F. Vecchi, A. Zuccala, and P. Zucchelli: Renal scintigraphy versus renal vein renin activity for identifying and treating renovascular hypertension, *Nephron,* 32:8, 1982.

58. Nally, J. V., B. Gupta, H. S. Clarke, M. L. Gross, W. J. Potvin, and J. T. Higgins: Captopril-enhanced renal flow studies in detecting renovascular hypertension (abstract), *Kidney Int.,* 29:254, 1986.

59. Hodsman, G. P., C. G. Isles, G. D. Murray, T. P. Usherwood, D. J. Webb, and J. I. S. Robertson: Factors related to first dose hypotensive effect of captopril: Prediction and treatment, *Br. Med. J.,* 286:832, 1983.

60. Pickering, T. G., T. A. Sos, E. D. Vaughan, Jr., D. B. Case, J. E. Sealey, G. A. Harshfield, and J. H. Laragh: Predictive value and changes of renin secretion in patients undergoing successful renal angioplasty, *Am. J. Med.,* 76:398, 1984.

61. Vaughan, E. D., Jr., R. M. Carey, M. J. Peach, J. A. Ackerly, and C. R. Ayers: The renin response to diuretic therapy: A limitation of antihypertensive potential, *Circ. Res.,* 42:376, 1978.

62. Pettinger, W. A., and H. C. Mitchell: Renin release, saralasin and the vasodilator-beta-blocker drug interaction in man, *N. Engl. J. Med.,* 292:1214, 1975.

63. Zacest, R., E. Gilmore, and J. Koch-Weser: Treatment of essential hypertension with combined vasodilation and beta-adrenergic blockade, *N. Engl. J. Med.,* 286:617, 1972.

64. Hollifield, J. W., K. Sherman, R. V. Zwagg, and D. G. Shand: Proposed mechanisms of propranolol's antihypertensive effect in essential hypertension, *N. Engl. J. Med.,* 295:68, 1976.

65. Weidmann, P., D. Hirsch, M. H. Maxwell, and R. Okun: Plasma renin and blood pressure during treatment with methyldopa, *Am. J. Cardiol.,* 34:671, 1974.

66. Niarchos, A. P., L. Baer, and I. Radichevich: Role of renin and aldosterone suppression in the antihypertensive mechanisms of clonidine, *Am. J. Med.,* 65:614, 1978.

67. Laragh, J. H., R. L. Soffer, and D. B. Case: Converting enzyme, angiotensin II and hypertensive disease, *Am. J. Med.,* 64:147, 1978.

68. Wenting, G. J., J. H. B. de Bruyn, A. J. Man in't Veld, A. J. J. Woittiez, F. H. M. Derkx, and M. A. D. H. Schalekamp: Hemodynamic effects of captopril in essential hypertension, renovascular hypertension and cardiac failure: Correlations with

short and long-term effects on plasma renin, *Am. J. Cardiol.,* 49:1453, 1982.

69. Rudnick, M. R., and M. H. Maxwell: Diagnosis of renovascular hypertension: Limitations of renin assays, in R. G. Narins (ed.), *Controversies in Nephrology and Hypertension,* Churchill Livingstone, New York, 1984.

70. Horne, M. L., V. M. Conklin, R. E. Keenan, P. D. Varady, and J. DiNardo: Angiotensin II profiling with saralasin: Summary of Eaton collaborative study, *Kidney Int.,* 15(suppl.):S-115, 1979.

71. Hollenberg, N. K., G. H. Williams, D. F. Adams, T. Moore, C. Brown, L. J. Borucki, F. Leung, S. Bavli, H. S. Solomon, D. Passan, and R. Dluhy: Response to saralasin and angiotensin's role in essential and renal hypertension, *Medicine,* 58:115, 1978.

72. Case, D. B., and J. H. Laragh: Reactive hyperreninemia following angiotensin blockade with either saralasin or converting enzyme inhibitor: A new approach to screen for renovascular hypertension, *Ann. Intern. Med.,* 91:153, 1979.

73. Muller, F. B., J. E. Sealey, D. B. Case, S. A. Atlas, T. G. Pickering, M. S. Pecker, J. J. Preibisz, and J. H. Laragh: The captopril test for identifying renovascular disease in hypertensive patients. *Am. J. Med.,* 80:633, 1986.

74. Maxwell, M. H., L. S. Marks, A. N. Lupu, P. J. Cahill, S. S. Franklin, and J. J. Kaufman: Predictive value of renin determinations in renal artery stenosis, *J. Am. Med. Assoc.,* 238:2617, 1977.

75. Schambelan, M., M. Glickman, J. R. Stockigt, and E. G. Biglieri: Selective renal-vein renin sampling in hypertensive patients with segmental renal lesions, *N. Engl. J. Med.,* 290:1153, 1974.

76. Re, R., R. Novelline, M-T. Escourrou, C. Athanasoulis, J. Burton, and E. Haber: Inhibition of angiotensin-converting enzyme for diagnosis of renal artery stenosis, *N. Engl. J. Med.,* 298:582, 1978.

77. Novick, A. C., and R. A. Straffon: The current status of surgical therapy for renal artery disease, *Am. J. Kid. Dis.,* 1:188, 1981.

78. Staessen, J., C. Bulpitt, R. Fagard, P. Lijnen, and A. Amery: Long-term converting-enzyme inhibition as a guide to surgical curability of hypertension associated with renovascular disease, *Am. J. Cardiol.,* 51:1317, 1983.

79. Gavras, H., H. R. Brunner, E. D. Vaughan, Jr., and J. H. Laragh: Angiotensin-sodium interaction in blood pressure maintenance of renal hypertensive and normotensive rats, *Science,* 180:1369, 1973.

80. Pohl, M. A., and A. C. Novick: Natural history of atherosclerotic and fibrous renal artery disease: Clinical implications, *Am. J. Kid. Dis.,* 5:A120, 1985.

81. Dean, R. H., R. W. Keiffer, B. M. Smith, J. A. Oates, J. H. J. Nadeau, J. W. Hollifield, and W. D. Dupont: Renovascular hypertension: Anatomic and renal function changes during drug therapy, *Arch. Surg.,* 116:1408, 1981.

82. Besarab, A., R. S. Brown, N. T. Rubin, E. Salzman, L. Wirthlin, T. Steinman, R. R. Atlia, and J. Skillman: Reversible renal failure following bilateral renal occlusive disease: Clinical features, pathology and the role of surgical revascularization, *J. Am. Med. Assoc.,* 235:2838, 1976.

83. Franklin, S. S., and R. D. Smith: Comparison of effects of enalapril plus hydrochlorothiazide versus standard triple therapy on renal function in renovascular hypertension, *Am. J. Med.,* 79(suppl. 3C):14, 1985.

84. Hollifield, J. W., L. C. Moore, S. D. Winn, M. A. Marshall, C. McCombs, M. G. Frazer, and V. Goncharenko: Angiotensin converting enzyme inhibition in renovascular hypertension, *Cardiovasc. Rev. Rep.,* 3:673, 1982.

85. Hricik, D. E., P. J. Browning, R. Kopelman, W. E. Goorno, N. G. Madias, and V. J. Dzau: Captopril-induced functional renal insufficiency in patients with bilateral renal-artery stenoses or renal artery stenosis in a solitary kidney, *N. Engl. J. Med.,* 308:373, 1983.

86. Jackson, B., P. G. Matthews, B. P. McGrath, and C. I. Johnston: Angiotensin converting enzyme inhibition in renovascular hypertension: Frequency of reversible renal failure, *Lancet,* 1:225, 1984.

87. Schnermann, J., J. P. Briggs, and P. C. Weber: Tubuloglomerular feedback, prostaglandins, and angiotensin in the autoregulation of glomerular filtration rate, *Kidney Int.,* 25:53, 1984.

88. Hall, J. E., A. C. Guyton, T. E. Jackson, T. G. Coleman, T. E. Lohmeier, and N. C. Trippodo: Control of glomerular filtration rate by renin-angiotensin system, *Am. J. Physiol.,* 233:F366, 1977.

89. Hricik, D. E.: Captopril induced renal insufficiency and the role of sodium balance, *Ann. Intern. Med.,* 103:222, 1985.

90. Watson, M. L., G. M. Bell, A. L. Muir, T. A. Buist, R. J. Kellet, and P. L. Padfield: Captopril/diuretic combination in severe renovascular disease: A cautionary note (letter), *Lancet,* 2:404, 1983.

91. Helmchen, U., H. J. Grone, G. J. Kirchertz, H. Bader, R. M. Bohle, U. Kneissler, and M. C. Khosla: Contrasting renal effects of different antihypertensive agents in hypertensive rats with bilaterally constricted renal arteries, *Kidney Int.,* 22(suppl. 12): S-198, 1982.

92. Wenting, G. J., H. L. Tan-Tjiong, F. H. M. Derkx, J. H. B. de Bruyn, and A. J. Man in't Veld: Split renal function after captopril in unilateral renal artery stenosis, *Br. Med. J.,* 288:886, 1984.

93. Michel, J-B., J-C. Dussaule, L. Choudat, C. Auzan, D. Nochy, P. Corvol, and J. Menard: Effect of antihypertensive treatment in one-clip, two kidney hypertension in rats, *Kidney Int.,* 29:1011, 1986.

94. Novick, A. C.: Atherosclerotic renovascular disease, *J. Urol.,* 126:567, 1982.

95. Bookstein, J. J., M. H. Maxwell, H. L. Abrams, R. E. Buenger, J. Lecky, and S. S. Franklin: Cooperative study of radiologic aspects of renovascular hypertension. Bilateral renovascular disease, *J. Am. Med. Assoc.,* 237:1706, 1978.

96. Novick, A. C., R. A. Straffon, B. H. Steward, R. W. Gifford, and D. Vidt: Diminished operative morbidity and mortality in renal revascularization, *J. Am. Med. Assoc.,* 246:749, 1981.

97. Foster, J. H., M. H. Maxwell, S. S. Franklin, K. H. Bleifer, O. H. Trippel, O. C. Julian, P. T. DeCamp, and P. D. Varady: Renovascular occlusive disease. Results of operative treatment, *J. Am. Med. Assoc.,* 231:1043, 1975.

98. Stanley, J. C., and W. J. Fry: Surgical treatment of renovascular hypertension, *Arch. Surg.,* 112:1291, 1977.

99. Lawrie, G. M., G. C. Morris, Jr., I. D. Soussou, D. S. Starr, A. Silvers, D. H. Glaeser, and M. E. DeBakey: Late results of reconstructive surgery for renovascular disease, *Ann. Surg.,* 191:528, 1980.

100. Shapiro, A. P., R. H. McDonald, Jr., and E. Scheib: Renal artery stenosis and hypertension, II: Current criteria for surgery, *Am. J. Cardiol.,* 37:1065, 1976.

101. Morris, G. C., Jr., M. E. DeBakey, and D. A. Cooley: Surgical treatment of renal failure of renovascular origin, *J. Am. Med. Assoc.,* 182:609, 1962.

102. Novick, A. C., M. A. Pohl, M. Schreiber, R. W. Gifford, Jr., and D. G. Vidt: Revascularization for preservation of renal function in patients with atherosclerotic renovascular disease, *J. Urol.,* 129: 907, 1982.

103. Novick, A. C., S. C. Textor, B. Bodie, and R. B. Khauli: Revascularization to preserve renal function in patients with atherosclerotic renovascular disease, *Urol. Clin. N. Am.,* 11:477, 1984.

104. Wasser, W. G., L. R. Krakoff, M. Haimov, S. Glabman, and H. A. Mitty: Restoration of renal function after bilateral renal artery occlusion. *Arch. Intern. Med.,* 141:1647, 1981.

105. Franklin, S. S., J. D. Young, Jr., M. H. Maxwell, J. H. Foster, J. M. Palmer, J. Cerny, and P. D. Varady: Operative morbidity and mortality in renovascular disease, *J. Am. Med. Assoc.,* 231:1148, 1975.

106. Kuhlmann, U., W. Vetter, J. Furrer, U. Lutolf, W. S. Siegenthaler, and A. Gruntzig: Renovascular hypertension: Treatment by percutaneous transluminal dilatation, *Ann. Intern. Med.,* 92:1, 1980.

107. Block, P. C., R. K. Myler, S. Stertzer, and J. T. Fallon: Morphology after transluminal angioplasty in human beings, *N. Engl. J. Med.,* 305:382, 1981.

108. Steele, P. M., J. H. Chesebro, A. W. Stanson, D. R. Holmes, Jr., M. K. Dewanjee, L. Baldimon, and V. Fuster: Balloon angioplasty. Natural history of the pathophysiological response to injury in a pig model, *Circ. Res.,* 57:105, 1985.

109. Madias, N. E., and V. G. Millan: PTRA in the treatment of renovascular hypertension, *Hosp. Pract.,* 16(8):105, 1981.

110. Sos, T. A., T. G. Pickering, S. Saddekni, M. Srur, D. B. Case, M. F. Silane, E. D. Vaughan, Jr., and J. H. Laragh: The current role of angioplasty in the treatment of renovascular hypertension, *Urol. Clin. N. Am.,* 11:503, 1984.

111. Sos, T. A., T. G. Pickering, K. Sniderman, S. Saddekni, D. B. Case, M. F. Silane, E. D. Vaughan, Jr., and J. H. Laragh: Percutaneous transluminal renal angioplasty in renovascular hypertension due to atheroma or fibromuscular dysplasia, *N. Engl. J. Med.,* 309:274, 1983.

112. Council on Scientific Affairs: Percutaneous transluminal angioplasty, *J. Am. Med. Assoc.,* 251:764, 1984.

113. Luft, F. C., C. E. Grim, and M. H. Weinberger: Intervention in patients with renovascular hypertension and renal insufficiency, *J. Urol.,* 130:564, 1983.

114. Health and Public Policy Committee, American College of Physicians: Percutaneous transluminal angioplasty, *Ann. Intern. Med.,* 99:864, 1983.

115. Levin, D. C.: Percutaneous transluminal angioplasty of the renal arteries, *J. Am. Med. Assoc.,* 251:759, 1984.

116. Hunt, J. C., S. G. Sheps, E. G. Harrison, Jr., C. G. Strong, and P. E. Bernatz: Renal and renovascular hypertension, *Arch. Intern. Med.,* 133:988, 1974.

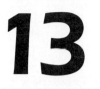

13

USE OF DRUGS IN THE PATIENT WITH RENAL INSUFFICIENCY

William M. Bennett

Patients with renal dysfunction, due to primary renal disease or the decline in GFR that frequently occurs with aging, commonly receive medications for both the underlying disorder and intercurrent illnesses. Because of the important role of the kidney as a pathway for drug elimination, an increased incidence of adverse reactions can occur if drug dosage is not reduced. Retention of the drug or its active or toxic metabolites and, less commonly, increased sensitivity to the drug due to the uremic milieu all may contribute to the enhanced drug toxicity. In addition, fluid and electrolyte disorders (edema, hyperkalemia, hypermagnesemia) and increased azotemia may be induced by the metabolic load associated with drug usage.

This chapter reviews dose modifications for patients with renal disease.[1-3] General principles are set forth, followed by specific guidelines for dosage adjustment. This information is largely presented in tabular form, but some classes of drugs are discussed in more detail.

PRESCRIBING FOR THE PATIENT WITH RENAL DYSFUNCTION

GENERAL PRINCIPLES

Many drugs and their metabolites are excreted in the urine. This may occur by glomerular filtration and/or tubular secretion by the organic acid and base secretory pathways in the proximal tubule. Tubular secretion is particularly important with drugs which are highly protein-bound (as with many penicillins and diuretics) since they circulate in too large a form to be filtered across the glomerulus.

A decline in renal function can have a major impact on the circulating drug concentration of those drugs that are metabolized or excreted by the kidney. In general, when a drug is given at regular intervals, the plasma level rises until a steady-state concentration is achieved. The time to reach 90 percent of this steady-state concentration is approximately equal to 3.3 times the half-life of the drug (50 percent at the first half-life, 75 percent at the second half-life, 87.5 percent at the third half-life, etc.).

The prolongation of drug half-life that can occur with renal failure has two consequences: the time required to reach the steady state is prolonged; and, if the dose is unchanged, the plasma concentration in the steady state will be higher than normal. Although the latter can be prevented by lowering the net drug dose, this change can delay attainment of a therapeutic plasma level of the drug. As a result, an initial loading dose may be necessary. With most drugs, the loading dose is the same as that in patients with normal renal function. With some drugs such as the cardiac glycosides, however, the volume of distribution of the drug is reduced by renal failure (by an unknown mechanism).[4] Thus, the loading dose of digoxin should only be 50 to 75 percent of normal.

There are two major strategies that are used to adjust the maintenance dose: the constant dose-varying interval method and the varying dose-constant interval method. The former varies the interval between doses, leaving the individual dose the same as that in patients without kidney disease. The interval is based upon the percent reduction in renal function and can be calculated from the following formula:

$$\text{Dose interval} = \text{normal interval} \times \frac{\text{normal } C_{cr}}{\text{patient's } C_{cr}}$$

where the C_{cr} represents the creatinine clearance, a measure of the GFR.

The alternative is to decrease the size of individual doses. The appropriate dose can be calculated from a formula similar to that for the dose interval:

$$\text{Dose} = \text{normal dose} \times \frac{\text{patient's } C_{cr}}{\text{normal } C_{cr}}$$

This regimen leads to more constant plasma drug concentrations, but often necessitates impractical fractions of usual doses.

In practice, both methods can be used with equal efficacy. Suppose, for example, that a drug which is excreted entirely in unchanged form by the kidney (such as an aminoglycoside antibiotic or vancomycin) is administered to a patient whose creatinine clearance is 50 percent of normal. In this setting, the individual dose can be reduced by one-half or the interval between doses can be doubled.

However, alterations in drug dosage are usually not this simple, since a variety of other pharmacokinetic variables may be present. These include partial or total metabolism to inactive metabolites by the liver, the presence of genetic factors such as rapid or slow hepatic acetylation of drugs such as hydralazine or procainamide,[5] drug-drug interactions, and changes in the volume of distribution or protein binding by the uremic milieu. These factors have led to the common use of drug level monitoring in an attempt to optimize therapy.

Even plasma drug levels, however, require proper interpretation to avoid incorrect dosing. For example, the exact time interval from the last dose must be known. In addition, the possible effects of renal failure also must be taken into account. This is particularly important for drugs that are protein-bound, since protein binding can be diminished by hypoalbuminemia (due to the nephrotic syndrome) or by the retention of uremic toxins (especially organic anions such as hippurate) that can displace the drug from its binding site.[6-9]

These problems can be illustrated by the changes that typically occur in the metabolism of phenytoin.[6,7,10] Protein binding of this drug is reduced by renal failure. As a result, more free (or unbound) drug is available to be metabolized, leading to a reduction in the *total* drug concentration. In contrast, the plasma level of the *physiologically active* free drug is relatively unchanged since the opposing effects of more rapid metabolism and less protein binding tend to balance. Thus, the dosage schedule for phenytoin does not need to be altered in renal failure (or with hypoalbuminemia). However, the therapeutic plasma level of this drug in renal failure is only 4 to 8 μg/mL.[7] This is lower than the level of 10 to 20 μg/mL in patients with relatively normal renal function because of the decrease in the fraction that is protein-bound.

Another potential problem with drug levels is that they may not reflect the presence of pharmacologically active metabolites. Examples of such compounds include normeperidine, a metabolite of meperidine that can accumulate in renal failure and produce seizures,[11] and N-acetylprocainamide, a long-lasting active metabolite of procainamide which has antiarrhythmic properties.[12]

USE OF TABLES

Tables 13–1 through 13–5 present a guide to drug use in patients with renal insufficiency. These tables have been modified from data available in the literature, and some key references are provided.[13–86] A more extensive bibliography is presented elsewhere.[1,2]

These tables list drugs in alphabetic order by generic name in several major classes. The primary routes of elimination are indicated as are minor, but significant pathways of drug metabolism or excretion (in parentheses), the usual biologic half-life, and the change in half-life in end-stage renal disease (ESRD). ESRD is considered to be present when the glomerular filtration rate (GFR) is less than 10 mL/min or the plasma creatinine concentration is greater than 7 mg/dL. It is assumed that liver function is normal and that drugs which alter hepatic metabolism are not being concurrently used.

An "adjustment factor" is given for each drug as a rough guide to modify the dosage or dosage interval in severe renal failure. Either the interval between doses can be multiplied or the individual dose divided by this number to estimate the proper dosage

regimen. It should be emphasized again that these calculations can only be used as rough guidelines and should not replace measurement of plasma drug levels when potentially toxic agents are being administered. The word "avoid" in the adjustment factor column indicates that the danger of side effects is likely to outweigh any therapeutic benefit. There may, of course, be some patients for whom this conclusion is not appropriate, and clinical judgment must be used in the individual case.

The adjustment factor in ESRD is based upon there being nearly complete loss of glomerular filtration. In patients with lesser degrees of renal insufficiency (creatinine clearance of 20 to 70 mL/min), the adjustment factor will be smaller since it should be multiplied by the *fractional decrease* in GFR. For example, a creatinine clearance of 35 mL/min represents approximately a two-thirds reduction in GFR. Therefore, the adjustment factor for gentamicin, which is 4 to 6 in ESRD, will be only 2.5 to 4 in this setting (4 to 6 times two-thirds equals 2.5 to 4).

In many patients, the creatinine clearance can be estimated relatively accurately from the plasma creatinine concentration (see p. 5). Since the plasma creatinine concentration is determined by muscle mass as well as the GFR, factors that affect the muscle mass such as age, sex, and lean body weight (LBW) also must be considered. The following formula has been useful in estimating the creatinine clearance from the plasma creatinine concentration (P_{cr}) in adult men[87]:

$$C_{cr} \text{ (in mL/min)} = \frac{(140 - age) \times LBW \text{ (in kg)}}{P_{cr} \times 72}$$

This value should be multiplied by 0.85 in women in whom a lower fraction of body weight is composed of muscle.

The value of this formula can be illustrated by the meaning of a plasma creatinine concentration of 1.4 mg/dL. This will represent a

TABLE 13-1. Antimicrobial Agents*

Drug	Major Excretion Routes	t½, h Normal	t½, h ESRD	Adjustment Factor†	Dialysis	Toxic Effects and Remarks
Antifungal Drugs						
Amphotericin	Nonrenal	24	24	1.5	No (H,P)	Nephrotoxic; renal tubular acidosis, hypokalemia.
Flucytosine	Renal	3–6	75–200	4–8	Yes (H,P)	Hepatic dysfunction, bone marrow suppression more common in azotemic patients.
Ketoconazole	Hepatic	1.5–3.3	1.8	Unchanged	No (H)	Interferes with cyclosporine metabolism and enhances its nephrotoxicity.
Miconazole	Hepatic	20–24	20–24	Unchanged	No (H,P)	Hyponatremia.
Antituberculous Drugs						
Ethambutol	Renal	4	7–15	2	Yes (H,P)	Decreased visual acuity, peripheral neuritis.
Isoniazid	Hepatic	0.7–4[a]	17[a]	1.5	Yes (H,P)	[a]Genetic slow acetylators have more renal excretion of unchanged drug, and t½ is prolonged in renal failure. This subgroup should have dosage adjusted in ESRD.
Rifampicin	Hepatic	1.5–5	1.8–3.1	Unchanged	No (H)	May cause acute renal failure, potassium wasting, and renal tubular defects.
Antiviral Agents						
Acyclovir	Renal	2.1–3.8	20	4–6	Yes (H)	Neurotoxic in renal failure; may cause acute renal failure when given rapidly by intravenous route.
Amantadine	Renal	12	500	4–6	No (H,P)	—
Aminoglycoside Antibiotics[b]						[b]Agents in this group are nephrotoxic and ototoxic and cause rare respiratory paralysis; serum levels useful to ensure efficacy. Need usual loading dose in renal failure.
Amikacin	Renal	2–2.5	30	4–6	Yes (H,P)	Group toxicity; may add 15 mg/L to peritoneal dialysis solutions.
Gentamicin	Renal	2	24–28	4–6	Yes (H,P)	Group toxicity; may add 5 mg/L to peritoneal dialysis solutions.
Netilmicin	Renal	2.2–2.7	40	4–6	Yes (H,P)	Group toxicity; may add 5 mg/L to peritoneal dialysis solutions.
Streptomycin	Renal	2.5	100	6–8	Yes (H,P)	Minimal nephrotoxicity.
Tobramycin	Renal	2.5	50–60	4–6	Yes (H,P)	Group toxicity; may add 5 mg/L to peritoneal dialysis solutions.

TABLE 13-1. *Antimicrobial Agents* * (Continued)

Drug	Major Excretion Routes	t½, h Normal	t½, h ESRD	Adjustment Factor†	Dialysis	Toxic Effects and Remarks
Cephalosporins [c,d]						[c] Agents in this group cause rare allergic interstitial nephritis; may cause bleeding in ESRD patients. [d] Absorbed well when given intraperitoneally.
Cefaclor	Renal	1	3	3	Yes (H,P)	Group toxicity.
Cefamandole	Renal	1	11	1.5	Yes (H)	Group toxicity.
Cefazolin	Renal	1.8–2	40–70	3–4	Yes (H) No (P)	Group toxicity; Ineffective for urinary infections in ESRD.
Cefoperazone	Hepatic	1.6–2.4	2.1	Unchanged	Yes (H)	Group toxicity.
Cefotaxime	Renal (hepatic)	1	2.6	2–3	Yes (H)	Group toxicity.
Cefoxitin	Renal	1	13–20	3–4	Yes (H)	May raise plasma creatinine by interfering with the drug assay; group toxicity.
Ceftazidime	Renal (hepatic)	1.2	13	6–8	Yes (H) No (P)	Group toxicity.
Ceftizoxime	Renal	1.4	30	6–8	Yes (H)	Group toxicity.
Ceftriaxone	Hepatic	7–9	12–24	Unchanged	No (H)	Group toxicity.
Cephalexin	Renal	0.9	20–40	1.5–2	Yes (H,P)	Need usual doses to treat urinary infections in ESRD; group toxicity.
Cephalothin	Renal (hepatic)	0.5–1	3–18	1.5–2	Yes (H)	Convulsions in high doses; group toxicity.
Cephapirin	Renal (hepatic)	0.6–0.8	2.4–2.7	1–2	Yes (H)	Group toxicity.
Cephradine	Renal	1.3	6–15	4	Yes (H,P)	Group toxicity.
Moxalactam	Renal (hepatic)	2.3	18–23	2–3	Yes (H)	Group toxicity.
Penicillins [e]						[e] Agents in this group cause allergic interstitial nephritis; seizures and coagulopathy at high blood levels.
Amoxicillin	Renal	0.9–2.3	5–20	2	Yes (H)	Group toxicity; need usual doses to treat urinary infection in ESRD.
Ampicillin	Renal	0.8–1.5	7–20	2	Yes (H)	Group toxicity; high doses needed for urinary infection in ESRD.
Azlocillin	Renal (hepatic)	0.8–1.5	5–6	1.5	Yes (H)	Group toxicity.
Carbenicillin	Renal	1.5	10–20	3–4	Yes (H)	Group toxicity; 4.7 meq of sodium per gram.
Cloxacillin	Hepatic (renal)	0.5	1	Unchanged	No (H)	Group toxicity.
Dicloxacillin	Hepatic (renal)	0.7	1–2	Unchanged	No (H)	Group toxicity.
Methicillin	Renal (hepatic)	0.5–1	4	1.5–2	No (H,P)	Group toxicity.

TABLE 13-1. Antimicrobial Agents* (Continued)

Drug	Major Excretion Routes	t½, h Normal	t½, h ESRD	Adjustment Factor†	Dialysis	Toxic Effects and Remarks
Mezlocillin	Renal (hepatic)	0.6–1.2	2.6–5.4	1.5	Yes (H)	Group toxicity.
Nafcillin	Hepatic	0.5	1.2	Unchanged	No (H)	Group toxicity.
Penicillin G	Renal (hepatic)	0.5	6–20	2–2.5	Yes (H) No (P)	Group toxicity; potassium salt has 1.7 meq/million units.
Ticarcillin	Renal	1.2	16	3–4	Yes (H) No (P)	Group toxicity; same as carbenicillin.
Miscellaneous Antimicrobials						
Azthreonam	Renal (hepatic)	1.7–2.4	6–8	3–4	Yes (H,P)	—
Chloramphenicol	Hepatic (renal)	1.6–3.3	3–7	Unchanged	No (H,P)	—
Clavulanic acid	Renal	1	3–4	1.5	Yes (H)	Combined with amoxicillin or ticarcillin for clinical use.
Clindamycin	Hepatic	2–4	3–5	Unchanged	No (H,P)	
Erythromycin	Hepatic	1.4	5–6	1.5	No (H,P)	Ototoxic in large doses.
Metronidazole	Hepatic	6–14	8–15	1.5–2	Yes (H)	Neurotoxic and gastrointestinal symptoms may mimic uremia.
Nitrofurantoin	Renal	0.3–0.6	1	Avoid	Yes (H)	Peripheral sensory neuropathy due to metabolite accumulation.
Pentamidine	?	Extensive tissue uptake	?	2	?	Nephrotoxic.
Sulfisoxazole	Renal	3–7	6–12	2–3	Yes (H,P)	Need usual doses to treat urinary infections in ESRD.
Sulfamethoxazole	Renal	9–11	20–50	2	Yes (H)	Need usual doses to treat urinary infections in ESRD.
Trimethoprim	Renal	9–13	20–49	2	Yes (H)	Antifolate activity; may increase plasma creatinine due to competition for secretion.
Vancomycin	Renal	6–8	200–250	8–10	No (H,P)	Ototoxic at levels >50 µg/mL.
Tetracyclines[f]						[f]Agents in this group potentiate acidosis, raise BUN and phosphorus, and potentiate tissue catabolism.
Doxycycline	Renal (hepatic)	15–24	18–25	1.5	No (H,P)	Group drug of choice in uremia for extrarenal infection.
Minocycline	Hepatic	12–16	12–18	Unchanged	No (H,P)	Group toxicity.
Tetracycline	Renal	6–10	50–100	3[g]	No (H,P)	Group toxicity; [g]Avoid if possible.

* Abbreviations: ESRD = end-stage renal disease; H = hemodialysis; P = peritoneal dialysis; t½ = elimination half-life.
† In severe renal failure (creatinine clearance < 10 mL/min), divide usual dose size or multiply usual dose interval by the adjustment factor shown.

TABLE 13–2. Cardiovascular, Antihypertensive, and Diuretic Agents*

Drug	Major Excretion Routes	t½, h Normal	t½, h ESRD	Adjustment Factor†	Dialysis	Toxic Effects and Remarks
Antiarrhythmic Drugs						
Amiodarone	Hepatic	3–100 days	?	Unchanged	No (H)	Thyroid dysfunction, peripheral neuropathy; increases plasma digoxin.
Disopyramide	Hepatic	5–8	10–18	4	Yes (H)	Pharmacologically active metabolite; urinary retention.
Lidocaine	Hepatic	1.2–2.2	1.3–3.0	Unchanged	No (H)	t½ dependent on hepatic blood flow.
Procainamide	Renal	2.5–4.9	5.3–5.9	3–4	Yes (H)	Renal excretion of pharmacologically active metabolite; lupus syndrome.
Quinidine	Renal (nonrenal)	3–16	3–16	Unchanged	Yes (H,P)	Rare lupus syndrome; increases plasma digoxin.
Antihypertensive Drugs[a]						[a]Blood pressure best guide to dosage.
Captopril	Renal	1.9	21–32	2	Yes (H)	Proteinuria, leukopenia; acute renal failure may occur with bilateral renal artery stenosis.
Clonidine	Renal (nonrenal)	6–23	39–42	Unchanged	No (H)	Excessive sedation.
Enalapril	Hepatic	24–36	40–60	2	Yes (H)	Active moiety enaprilat formed by hepatic ester hydrolysis; acute renal failure may occur with bilateral renal artery stenosis.
Guanethidine	Renal	120–240	?	Unchanged	?	Tricyclic antidepressants reduce efficacy; orthostatic hypotension.
Guanabenz	Hepatic	12–14	?	Unchanged	?	—
Hydralazine	Hepatic (gastrointestinal)	2–2.5	7–16	Unchanged	No (H,P)	Slow acetylators may have enhanced effects; lupus syndrome.
Methyldopa	Renal (hepatic)	8	7–16	2–3	Yes (H,P)	Excessive sedation; retention of active metabolites.
Minoxidil	Nonrenal	2.8–4.2	2.8–4.2	Unchanged	Yes (H)	Fluid retention; pericardial effusion.
Nitroprusside	Nonrenal	<10 min	<10 min	Unchanged	No (H,P)	Toxic metabolite thiocyanate should be monitored if infusions are >24–48 h.
Prazosin	Hepatic	1.8–4.6	?	Unchanged	No (H,P)	Marked hypotension with first dose in 1–2 percent of patients.
Reserpine	Hepatic	46–170	87–300	Avoid	No (H,P)	Excessive sedation; gastrointestinal bleeding; depression.
β-Adrenergic Blockers						
Acebutolol	Renal (hepatic)	8–9	7	3	No (H)	—
Atenolol	Renal	6–9	15–35	3–4	Yes (H)	Accumulates in ESRD.
Labetalol	Hepatic	3–8	3–8	Unchanged	No (H)	—
Metoprolol	Hepatic	2.5–4.5	2.5–4.5	Unchanged	Yes (H)	—
Nadolol	Renal	14–24	45	3	Yes (H)	Accumulates in ESRD.
Pindolol	Hepatic	3–4	3–4	Unchanged	?	—
Propranolol	Hepatic	2–6	1–6	Unchanged	No (H)	Decreased hepatic extraction in ESRD.
Timolol	Hepatic	3–4	4	Unchanged	No (H)	—

TABLE 13-2. Cardiovascular, Antihypertensive, and Diuretic Agents* (Continued)

Drug	Major Excretion Routes	t½, h Normal	t½, h ESRD	Adjustment Factor†	Dialysis	Toxic Effects and Remarks
Calcium Channel Blockers						
Diltiazem	Hepatic	2–8	3.5	Unchanged	No (H, P)	Active metabolites.
Nifedipine	Hepatic	4–5.5	5–7	Unchanged	No (H,P)	Active metabolites; edema; acute renal dysfunction reported.
Verapamil	Hepatic	3–7	2.4–4	Unchanged	No (H,P)	Active metabolites; acute renal dysfunction reported.
Cardiac Glycosides[b]						[b] Can add to uremic gastrointestinal symptoms; serum levels good guide to dosage; loading dose 50–75 percent of normal in ESRD; toxicity enhanced by dialysis removal of potassium and magnesium.
Digitoxin	Hepatic	160–190	240	1.5–2	No (H,P)	8–10 percent converted to digoxin.
Digoxin	Renal	30–40	87–100	3–4	No (H,P)	Radioimmunoassay may overestimate serum levels in ESRD. Serum levels rise with quinidine therapy.
Diuretics[c]						[c] Agents in this group produce extracellular fluid volume depletion.
Acetazolamide	Renal	2.4–5.8	?	Avoid	?	Ineffective; may potentiate acidosis; produce urolithiasis.
Amiloride	Renal (hepatic)	6–9.5	8–140	Avoid	?	Hyperkalemia when GFR <30 mL/min.
Bumetanide	Renal (nonrenal)	1.2–1.5	1.5	Unchanged	?	Muscle weakness; cramps; ototoxicity (may be less than other loop diuretics).
Chlorthalidone	Renal (nonrenal)	50–80	?	2	?	Ineffective in ESRD.
Ethacrynic acid	Hepatic (renal)	2–4	?	Unchanged	No (H)	Ototoxic, particularly in combination with aminoglycoside antibiotics.
Furosemide	Renal	0.3–1.6	1.3–14	Unchanged	No (H)	Ototoxic, particularly in combination with aminoglycoside antibiotics; allergic interstitial nephritis. High doses useful in ESRD.
Metolazone	Renal	4	?	Unchanged	No (H)	Very high doses may be useful in ESRD.
Spironolactone	Hepatic	10–35	10–35	Avoid	?	Hyperkalemia with GFR <30 mL/min; active metabolite (canrenone).
Thiazides	Renal	1–2	4–6	Avoid	?	Ineffective in ESRD; hyperuricemia.
Triamterene	Hepatic	1.5–2.5	10	Avoid	?	Hyperkalemia with GFR <30 mL/min; rare calculi; folate antagonist.

*Abbreviations ESRD = end-stage renal disease; H = hemodialysis; P = peritoneal dialysis; t½ = elimination half-life.
†In severe renal failure (creatinine clearance <10 mL/min), divide usual dose size or multiply usual dose interval by the adjustment factor shown.

TABLE 13-3. Sedatives, Hypnotics, and Drugs Used in Psychiatry*

Drug	Major Excretion Routes	t½, h Normal	t½, h ESRD	Adjustment Factor†	Dialysis	Toxic Effects and Remarks
Barbiturates[a]						[a] Agents in this group may increase osteomalacia in ESRD patients; excessive sedation.
Phenobarbital	Hepatic (renal)	60–150	117–160	1.5–2	Yes (H,P)	Group toxicity.
Secobarbital	Hepatic	20–35	?	Unchanged	No (H,P)	Group toxicity.
Benzodiazepines[b]						[b] Agents in this group may cause excessive sedation or encephalopathy in dialysis patients.
Chlordiazepoxide	Hepatic	5–30	5–30	1.5–2	No (H)	Active metabolite; group toxicity.
Clonazepam	Hepatic	5–30	5–30	Unchanged	?	Group toxicity.
Diazepam	Hepatic	20–90	20–90	Unchanged	No (H)	Active metabolites; group toxicity.
Flurazepam	Hepatic	47–100	47–100	Unchanged	No (H)	Active metabolite; group toxicity.
Haloperidol	Hepatic (gastrointestinal)	10–36	?	Unchanged	No (H,P)	Excessive sedation; hypotension.
Lithium carbonate	Renal	14–28	Prolonged	2–3	Yes (H,P)	Nephrogenic diabetes insipidus, renal tubular acidosis, chronic interstitial fibrosis. Toxicity when serum levels > 1.2 meq/L; toxicity enhanced by volume depletion, diuretics, and nonsteroidal anti-inflammatory drugs.
Meprobamate	Hepatic	6–17	6–17	2–3	Yes (H,P)	Excessive sedation.
Phenothiazines[c]						[c] Prototype chlorpromazine; agents in this group anticholinergic; cause urinary retention, orthostatic hypotension.
Chlorpromazine	Hepatic	11–42	11–42	Unchanged	No (H,P)	Group remarks, excessive sedation.
Tricyclic Antidepressants[d]						[d] Agents in this group are anticholinergic; urinary retention; may decrease antihypertensive effect of clonidine, methyldopa guanabenz, guanethidine; excessive sedation.
Amitriptyline	Hepatic	32–40	?	Unchanged	No (H,P)	Group remarks.
Desipramine	Hepatic	12–54	?	Unchanged	No (H,P)	Group remarks.
Doxepin	Hepatic	8–25	10–18	Unchanged	No (H,P)	Group remarks.
Imipramine	Hepatic	6–20	?	Unchanged	No (H,P)	Group remarks.
Nortriptyline	Hepatic	18–93	15–66	Unchanged	No (H,P)	Group remarks.
Protriptyline	Hepatic	54–98	?	Unchanged	No (H,P)	Group remarks.

* Abbreviations: ESRD = end-stage renal disease; H = hemodialysis; P = peritoneal dialysis; t½ = elimination half-life.
† In severe renal failure (creatinine clearance <10 mL/min), divide usual dose size or multiply usual dose interval by the adjustment factor shown.

TABLE 13-4. Analgesics*

Drug	Major Excretion Routes	t½, h Normal	t½, h ESRD	Adjustment Factor†	Dialysis	Toxic Effects and Remarks
Acetaminophen	Hepatic	2	2	1.5	Yes (H) No (P)	Nephrotoxic in massive overdose.
Acetylsalicylic acid	Hepatic	2–19	2–19	1.5	Yes (H,P)	Adds to uremic gastrointestinal and hematologic abnormalities; may decrease GFR when renal blood flow is prostaglandin dependent.
Codeine	Hepatic	2.5–3.5	?	Unchanged	?	Excessive sedation; respiratory depression.
Meperidine	Hepatic	2.4–4.4	2.4–4.4	1.5	No (H)	Excessive sedation; respiratory depression; active metabolite accumulates and can cause seizures.
Methadone	Gastrointestinal	18–97	13–55	1.5	No (H,P)	Excessive sedation; respiratory depression.
Morphine	Hepatic (renal)	2.3	?	1.5	No (H,P)	Excessive sedation; respiratory depression; ESRD patients may have increased sensitivity to small doses.
Pentazocine	Hepatic	2	?	Unchanged	Yes (H)	Excessive sedation; respiratory depression.
Propoxyphene	Hepatic	12	12–20	3	No (H,P)	Active metabolite; excessive sedation.

*Abbreviations: ESRD = end-stage renal disease; H = hemodialysis; P = peritoneal dialysis; t½ = elimination half-life.
†In severe renal failure (creatinine clearance <10 mL/min), divide usual dose size or multiply usual dose interval by the adjustment factor shown.

creatinine clearance of approximately 101 mL/min in an 85-kg, 20-year-old man:

$$C_{cr} = \frac{(140 - 20) \times 85}{1.4 \times 72} = 101 \text{ mL/min}$$

In contrast, the same plasma creatinine concentration in a 40-kg, 80 year-old woman corresponds to a creatinine clearance of only about 20 mL/min:

$$C_{cr} = \frac{(140 - 80) \times 40 \times 0.85}{1.4 \times 72} = 20 \text{ mL/min}$$

These findings call attention to the danger of overdosing elderly, malnourished, or cirrhotic patients who have a markedly impaired GFR, despite a normal or near-normal plasma creatinine concentration (see p. 79). Even with these considerations in mind, however, it is important to remember that the creatinine clearance can overestimate the GFR by 40 percent or more in advanced renal disease due to the tubular secretion of creatinine (see Chap. 1). Thus careful monitoring is still essential.

Use of the plasma creatinine concentration in the above formula is dependent upon the patient being in the *steady state*. The plasma creatinine concentration is not an

TABLE 13-5. Miscellaneous Drugs*

Drug	Major Excretion Routes	t½, h Normal	t½, h ESRD	Adjustment Factor†	Dialysis	Toxic Effects and Remarks
Anticoagulants						
Heparin	Nonrenal	1–2	0.5–3	Unchanged	No (H,P)	May potentiate uremic bleeding.
Warfarin	Hepatic	42	30	Unchanged	No (P)	Active metabolites excreted by the kidney; may potentiate uremic bleeding.
Antidiabetic Drugs						
Acetohexamide	Hepatic	6–8	31	Avoid	No (P)	Accumulation of metabolite with hypoglycemic properties.
Chlorpropamide	Renal (nonrenal)	24–42	50–200	Avoid	No (P)	Prolonged hypoglycemia in azotemic patients; impairs renal water excretion.
Glipizide	Hepatic	3–7	?	Unchanged	?	—
Glyburide	Hepatic	10–16	?	Unchanged	?	—
Insulin (regular)	Hepatic (renal)	2–3	Prolonged	2	?	—
Tolbutamide	Hepatic (nonrenal)	4–5	4–5	Unchanged	No (H)	May impair renal water excretion.
Antihistamines						
Chlorpheniramine	Hepatic	12–15	Prolonged	Unchanged	Yes (H) No (P)	Excessive sedation.
Diphenhydramine	Hepatic	4–7	?	2–3	?	Excessive sedation; anticholinergic; may cause urinary retention.
Antineoplastic and Immunosuppressive Drugs[a]						[a] Most agents in this group cause narrow depression which may add to uremic bleeding and infection.
Azathioprine	Hepatic	0.2–1	Slightly prolonged	1.5	Yes (H)	Allopurinol increases drug activity by slowing rate of metabolism.
Bleomycin	Renal (hepatic)	1.3–9	2–30	2	No (H)	Pulmonary toxicity enhanced in renal failure.
Busulfan	Hepatic	2.6	?	Unchanged	?	May cause hemorrhagic cystitis.
Cisplatin	Nonrenal (renal)	2–72	1–240	2	Yes (H)[b]	Nephrotoxic, toxicity modified by hydration; renal magnesium wasting. [b] Dialysis only effective within 3 h of a dose.
Cyclophosphamide	Hepatic (nonrenal)	5–6	4–12	Unchanged	No (H,P)	Hemorrhagic cystitis, bladder fibrosis, bladder carcinoma; sterility; alopecia; inappropriate ADH secretion.
Cyclosporine	Hepatic	12–24	12–24	Unchanged	No (H,P)	Nephrotoxic; hypertension; hyperkalemia; seizures; hirsutism.
Doxorubicin	Hepatic	16–24	16–24	1.3–1.5	?	Cardiotoxicity; rare acute renal failure, nephrotic syndrome.

TABLE 13-5. Miscellaneous Drugs* (Continued)

Drug	Major Excretion Routes	t½, h Normal	t½, h ESRD	Adjustment Factor†	Dialysis	Toxic Effects and Remarks
Melphalan	Nonrenal	2	4–6	1.5	?	Group remarks.
Methotrexate	Renal (hepatic)	3.5–60	Prolonged	Unchanged	Yes (H)	Folate deficiency; high doses nephrotoxic because of tubular precipitation of metabolite.
Vincristine	Renal (hepatic)	0.1–3	0.1–3	Unchanged	?	Neurotoxic, inappropriate ADH secretion.
Agents Used for Arthritis and Gout[c]						[c] Most agents in this group can add to uremic bleeding and gastrointestinal symptoms; nonsteroidal anti-inflammatory drugs may reduce renal function as well as cause interstitial nephritis, nephrotic syndrome, and hyperkalemia.
Allopurinol	Renal (nonrenal)	0.7	Prolonged	2–3	?	Oxypurinol metabolite associated with fever, eosinophilia, skin desquamation, and decreased renal function. Rare xanthine stones.
Auranofin	Nonrenal	17–35	?	Unchanged	?	Nephrotoxic; proteinuria and rare nephrotic syndrome.
Colchicine	Hepatic	0.3	0.7	2	No (H)	Aggravates gastrointestinal symptoms.
Fenoprofen	Hepatic	2–3	?	Unchanged	No (H)	Group toxicity.
Ibuprofen	Hepatic	2.5	2.5	Unchanged	No (H)	Group toxicity.
Indomethacin	Hepatic	4–12	4–12	Unchanged	No (H)	Group toxicity.
Naproxen	Hepatic	17	15	Unchanged	No (H)	Group toxicity.
Probenecid	Nonrenal (renal)	4–12	?	Unchanged	?	Ineffective as low GFR: may precipitate urolithiasis.
Sulfinpyrazone	Renal (nonrenal)	3–5	3–5	Unchanged	?	May precipitate urolithiasis; rare renal failure; ineffective at low GFR.
Sulindac	Hepatic	8–16	?	Unchanged	?	May be less likely to reduce renal blood flow and GFR than other congeners.
Agents Used in Neurology						
Bromocriptine	Hepatic	3	?	Unchanged	?	Orthostatic hypotension.
Carbamazepine	Hepatic	20–35	?	1.3	No (H)	May cause inappropriate ADH secretion.
Levodopa	Nonrenal	0.8–1.6	?	Unchanged	?	Active metabolite with long t½.
Phenytoin	Hepatic	24	8	Unchanged	No (H,P)	Decreased protein binding and low total plasma concentration (see text).
Primidone	Renal (hepatic)	8	12	2–3	Yes (H)	Excessive sedation; folic acid deficiency; partially converted to phenobarbital.

TABLE 13-5. Miscellaneous Drugs* (Continued)

Drug	Major Excretion Routes	t½, h Normal	t½, h ESRD	Adjustment Factor†	Dialysis	Toxic Effects and Remarks
Trimethadione	Hepatic	12–24	?	2–3	?	Nephrotic syndrome; active metabolites.
Valproic Acid	Hepatic	1–12	10	Unchanged	No (H,P)	Hepatotoxicity.
Neuromuscular Agents[d]						[d] Aminoglycosides, hypokalemia, acidosis, hypermagnesemia enhance neuromuscular blocking effects.
Atracrurium	Nonrenal	20 min	20 min	Unchanged	?	Can be used safely in renal failure.
Gallamine	Renal	2–3	9	Avoid	Yes (H,P)	Prolonged apnea.
Pancuronium	Renal (hepatic)	2.2	4.3	Avoid	?	Active metabolites accumulate in ESRD; duration of action prolonged.
Pyridostigmine	Renal (nonrenal)	1.5–2	6	Unchanged	?	ESRD patients may have prolonged action.
Succinylcholine	Nonrenal	3	?	Unchanged	?	Prolonged apnea; hyperkalemia after large doses in ESRD.
Tubocurarine	Renal (hepatic)	0.1–2	5	Unchanged	?	Group remarks.
Vercuronium	Hepatic	1	1.5	Unchanged	?	Can be used safely in renal failure.
Other Drugs						
Cimetidine	Renal (hepatic)	2	5	1.5–2	No (H,P)	May increase plasma creatinine due to competition for renal secretion; confusion; rare acute interstitial nephritis.
Clofibrate	Hepatic (gastrointestinal)	6–25	110	4	No (H)	Myopathy; reduce dose for nephrotic syndrome.
Metoclopramide	Hepatic	14–18	7–20	4	No (H)	Extrapyramidal movements, dyskinesis.
Propylthiouracil	Renal (hepatic)	1–2	8.5	2	?	Cardiotoxicity; leukopenia.
Ranitidine	Renal	1.5–3	6–9	2	Yes (H)	—
Theophylline	Hepatic	3–12	5–9	1.5	Yes (H,P)	May add to uremic gastrointestinal symptoms; seizures at high blood concentrations.

* Abbreviations: ESRD = end-stage renal disease; H = hemodialysis; P = peritoneal dialysis; t½ = elimination half-life.
† In severe renal failure (creatinine clearance <10 mL/min), divide usual dose size or multiply usual dose interval by the adjustment factor shown.

accurate reflection of the GFR in the presence of acute renal failure. Suppose, for example, that a patient with a plasma creatinine concentration of 1 mg/dL suddenly develops severe renal failure. In this setting, the plasma creatinine concentration will still be close to 1 mg/dL on day 1 (despite a marked reduction in GFR) but will rise progressively on successive days as creatinine is retained. In such a patient, it may be simplest to assume that ESRD is present and to use the appropriate adjustment factor. Alternatively, the creatinine clearance can be estimated from a 24-h urine collection according to the following formula:

$$C_{cr} = \frac{U_{cr} \times V}{P_{cr}}$$

where V represents the urine volume in milliliters per minute or liters per day. Since the plasma creatinine concentration is not stable, the average value for the two days of the collection should be used.

A similar problem can occur during the recovery phase from acute renal failure, as the fall in the plasma creatinine concentration lags behind the increase in GFR by the time required to excrete the excess creatinine. As a result, inadequate plasma levels can occur if drug dosage is not increased above that when renal function was impaired.

The tables also include information on drug removal by hemodialysis or peritoneal dialysis. "Yes" indicates sufficient removal of the drug by dialysis to require an additional maintenance dose or, with peritoneal dialysis, addition of the drug to the dialysis fluid to achieve an adequate plasma level. The latter approach is widely used in the treatment of peritonitis since drug absorption through the peritoneum is usually excellent. In general, the most dialyzable drugs are those with a low molecular weight that are not highly protein bound or lipid-soluble (the latter favoring a large extravascular volume of distribution).

On the other hand, "No" means that one dialysis day removes less than a usual dose. This designation, however, does not preclude the use of dialysis or hemoperfusion in the treatment of a drug overdose.

Finally, the toxic effects and remarks are those that the author deems appropriate for many patients with renal insufficiency. These comments are meant to make the reader aware of issues that may be important in a given patient; they are not meant to imply that each side effect occurs in every patient with renal disease who is treated with the drug.

SPECIFIC CONSIDERATIONS FOR COMMONLY USED DRUGS IN RENAL FAILURE

ANALGESIC AND NARCOTIC DRUGS

Care must be taken with the administration of narcotic agents to patients with renal failure. As mentioned above, the use of repeated doses of meperidine can lead to the accumulation of normeperidine, a polar metabolite produced in the liver.[11] This can produce neurotoxicity and seizures in selected patients. Uremic patients are also more sensitive to the respiratory depressant effects of morphine, perhaps due to reduced renal metabolism of this drug.[54] As a result, morphine must be given with caution in this setting. Individual patients also may have enhanced sensitivity to other narcotics, although these agents are generally safe in the presence of renal failure. Narcotics are not significantly removed by dialysis.

Acetaminophen is the minor analgesic of choice in patients with renal disease. Although metabolites can accumulate, they have no known pharmacologic activity or toxic effects.[52] The use of aspirin and nonsteroidal anti-inflammatory drugs should be minimized since their effects on platelet function and the gastrointestinal tract can enhance already present uremic abnormalities.

PSYCHOTHERAPEUTIC DRUGS

Patients with advanced renal disease are frequently subjected to a great deal of emotional stress, possibly leading to anxiety or depression. Benzodiazepines, which are converted in the liver to inactive metabolites, can be used safely for mild to moderate symptoms.[46,47] Insomnia is another frequent complaint that can also be managed by this class of drugs. However, excessive sedation can occur. Sedation can also result from the use of antihistamines to treat uremic pruritus.

Tricyclic antidepressants, which are the mainstay of therapy for severe depression, generally have no unique side effects in patients with renal failure. There are, however, problems that can occur. These include orthostatic hypotension following extracellular fluid removal by dialysis, interference with the antihypertensive action of guanethidine (by preventing its uptake by the peripheral neuron) and clonidine (by an unknown mechanism),[88,89] and urinary retention because of anticholinergic effects. Imipramine is probably the drug of choice for the depressed patient with psychomotor retardation whereas amytriptyline may be more appropriate for agitation.

Major psychoses are handled pharmacologically in the same way as they are in patients with normal renal function. Both the phenothiazines and lithium can be safely used in selected patients. However, careful monitoring of the drug level is essential with lithium, as the plasma concentration should be maintained between 0.6 and 1.0 meq/L.[49]

CARDIAC AND ANTIHYPERTENSIVE DRUGS

Cardiac and antihypertensive drugs are frequently required in patients with renal failure. Beta-blockers, for example, are used extensively to treat hypertension, angina, and arrhythmias. With propranolol, two counterbalancing effects tend to occur: decreased hepatic extraction and hepatic enzyme induction. As a result, the overall half-life of elimination is relatively normal, and the dose does not need to be altered. Dose reduction, however, is required with longer acting con-

geners (such as atenolol and nadolol) which are largely eliminated by the kidney.[31]

Dosage adjustments are also variable with anti-arrhythmic agents.[12] Procainamide is N-acetylated to a pharmacologically active metabolite, N-acetylprocainamide, that has anti-arrhythmic effects similar to the parent compound. This metabolite has a long half-life and is eliminated almost entirely by the kidney. As a result, the interval between doses of procainamide should be increased in advanced renal failure. Lidocaine undergoes hepatic extraction and metabolism similar to propranolol, but the pharmacologically active metabolites do not produce central nervous system or other toxicity. Therefore, no dosage adjustment is necessary for lidocaine or for quinidine, the metabolism of which is not significantly affected by renal disease. In comparison, disopyramide can accumulate in renal failure, and a lower net dose should be given.

The dosage of cardiac glycosides generally has to be reduced in patients with renal failure. The initial digitalizing dose is 50 to 75 percent of normal because of a diminished volume of distribution of the drug.[1] With digoxin, the net maintenance dose also should be decreased, since its half-life is prolonged to 4 days due to a marked reduction in urinary excretion. Thus, the maintenance dose is primarily determined by the rate of non-renal losses; in most patients, a therapeutic plasma digoxin concentration can be achieved with 0.125 mg given 3 to 5 times per week. Dialysis does not lower digoxin levels, but sudden shifts in potassium can provoke cardiac arrhythmias. For this reason, it is recommended that the dialysate potassium concentration be 3 meq/L in digitalized patients.

Patients treated with digoxin should be monitored for toxicity by following the electrocardiogram and plasma digoxin levels (by radioimmunoassay). The latter may, however, overestimate the digoxin concentration since substances retained or produced in renal failure can be measured as digoxin by the radio-immunoassay.[90]

In comparison to digoxin, digitoxin is eliminated from the body primarily by nonrenal routes. As a result, renal failure has little effect on digitoxin pharmacokinetics.[45] The half-life of digitoxin is about 6 days when renal function is normal and is only prolonged to 8.5 days with anuria. Thus, the dosage regimen needs only minor alterations with this drug. Nevertheless, the long half-life frequently limits the use of digitoxin because it delays recovery from toxic arrhythmias.

Diuretics are often less effective or ineffective in patients with advanced renal disease, because less drug reaches the luminal site of action.[34] Furosemide, bumetanide, and ethacrynic acid act in the thick ascending limb of the loop of Henle and can produce a natriuresis in patients with a GFR as low as 5 to 10 mL/min. However, large intravenous doses (up to 320 mg or more of furosemide) may be required, which increases the risk of inducing ototoxicity.[91] There is suggestive evidence that bumetanide may be substantially less ototoxic than the other loop diuretics and, therefore, may be the preferred agent in this setting (see p. 100).[92,93]

The thiazide-type diuretics are usually ineffective when given alone to patients with a GFR below 20 to 25 mL/min[94] unless very high doses are used (20 to 150 mg of metolazone, equivalent to 200 to 1500 mg of hydrochlorothiazide).[95] The thiazides may, however, potentiate the diuresis produced by a loop diuretic[96,97] since they may have enough activity to prevent the distal tubule from reabsorbing some or most of the extra sodium chloride delivered out of the loop of Henle.[98] On the other hand, the use of potassium-sparing diuretics (amiloride, spironolactone, and triamterene) should generally be avoided in renal failure because they can cause clinically significant hyperkalemia.

Renal disease usually does not have an important effect on the use of antihypertensive agents. The drug dosage is typically determined by the blood pressure response, not by any pharmacokinetic characteristic of the drug. One exception is the use of an intravenous infusion of nitroprusside to treat a hypertensive emergency. The metabolism of nitroprusside to thiocyanate can present a risk if infusions are prolonged beyond 48 h.[41] Thiocyanate toxicity, which can lead to nausea, vomiting, myoclonic jerks, and seizures, can be alleviated by dialysis since thiocyanate is a relatively small molecule that is easily dialyzed.

REFERENCES

1. Anderson, R. J., R. W. Schrier, and J. G. Gambertoglio: *Clinical Use of Drugs in Patients with Kidney and Liver Disease*, Saunders, Philadelphia, 1981.
2. Bennett, W. M., G. R. Morrison, T. A. Golper, J. Pulliam, M. Wolfson and I. Singer: Drug prescribing in renal failure: Dosing guidelines for adults, *Am. J. Kid. Dis.*, 3:155, 1983.
3. Knepshield, J. H., and J. F. Winchester: Hemodialysis and hemoperfusion for drugs and poisons, *Trans. Am. Soc. Artif. Intern. Org.*, 28:666, 1982.
4. Aronson, J. K.: Clinical pharmacokinetics of digoxin, *Clin. Pharmacokinet.*, 5:137, 1980.
5. Reece, P. A., I. Cozamanis, and R. Zacest: Kinetics of hydralazine and its main metabolites in slow and fast acetylators, *Clin. Pharmacol. Therap.*, 28:769, 1980.
6. Gugler, R., D. W. Shoeman, D. H. Huffman, J. B. Cohlmia, and D. L. Azarnoff: Pharmacokinetics of drugs in patients with nephrotic syndrome, *J. Clin. Invest.*, 55:1182, 1975.
7. Reidenberg, M. M.: The binding of drugs to plasma proteins, and the interpretation of measurements of plasma concentrations of drugs in patients with poor renal function, *Am. J. Med.*, 62:466, 1977.

8. McNamara, P. J., D. Lalka, and M. Gibaldi: Endogenous accumulation products and serum protein binding in uremia, *J. Lab. Clin. Med.*, 98:730, 1981.

9. Gulyassy, P. F., A. T. Bottini, L. A. Stanfel, E. A. Jarrard, and T. A. Depner: Isolation and chemical identification of inhibitors of plasma ligand binding, *Kidney Int.*, 30:391, 1986.

10. Letteri, S. M., H. Mellk, S. Louis, H. Kutt, P. Durante, and A. Glanzko: Diphenylhydantoin metabolism in uremia, *N. Engl. J. Med.*, 285:648, 1971.

11. Szeto, H. H., C. E. Inturrisi, R. Houde, and M. Reidenberg: Accumulation of normeperidine, an active metabolite of meperidine, in patients with renal failure or cancer, *Ann. Intern. Med.*, 86:738, 1977.

12. Gillis, A. M., and R. E. Kates: Clinical pharmacokinetics of antiarrhythmic agents, *Clin. Pharmacokinet.*, 9:375, 1984.

13. Van Scoy, R. E., and W. R. Wilson: Antimicrobial agents in patients with renal insufficiency, *Mayo. Clin. Proc.*, 58:246, 1983.

14. Pechere, J., and R. Dugal: Clinical pharmacokinetics of aminoglycoside antibiotics, *Clin. Pharmacokinet.*, 4:170, 1979.

15. Tartaglione, T. A., and R. E. Polk: Review of the new second generation cephalosporins: Cefonidic, ceforanide and ccfuroxime, *Drug Intell. Clin. Pharm.*, 19:188, 1985.

16. Balant, L, P. Dayer, and R. Auckenthalaer: Clinical pharmacokinetics of the third generation cephalosporins, *Clin. Pharmacokinet.*, 10:101, 1985.

17. Wright, A. J., and C. J. Wilkowske: The penicillins, *Mayo Clin. Proc.*, 58:21, 1983.

18. Eliopoulos, G. M., and R. C. Moellering: Azlocillin, mezlocillin and piperacillin: New broad spectrum penicillins, *Ann. Intern. Med.*, 97:755, 1982.

19. Daneshmend, T. K., and D. W. Warnock: Clinical pharmacokinetics of systemic antifungal drugs, *Clin. Pharmacokinet.*, 8:17, 1983.

20. Holdiness, M. R.: Clinical pharmacokinetics of the antituberculous drugs, *Clin. Pharmacokinet.*, 9:511, 1984.

21. Gnann, J. W., N. H. Barton, and R. J. Whitley: Acyclovir: Mechanisms of action, pharmacokinetics, safety and clinical applications, *Pharmacotherapy*, 3:275, 1983.

22. Wu, M. J., T. S. Ing, S. Soung, J. T. Daugirdas, J. E. Hano, and V. C. Gandhi: Amantadine hydrochloride pharmacokinetics in patients with impaired renal function, *Clin. Nephrol.*, 17:19, 1982.

23. Fillastre, J. P., A. Leroy, C. Baudoin, G. Humbert, E. A. Swabb, C. Vertucci, and M. Godin: Pharmacokinetics of aztreonam in patients with chronic renal failure, *Clin. Pharmacokinet.*, 10:91, 1985.

24. Ambrose, P. J.: Clinical pharmacokinetics of chloramphenicol and chloramphenicol succinate, *Clin. Pharmacokinet.*, 9:222, 1984.

25. Houghton, G. W., M. J. Dennis, and R. Gabriel: Pharmacokinetics of metronidazole in patients with varying degrees of renal failure, *Br. J. Clin. Pharm.*, 19:203, 1985.

26. Patel, R., and P. G. Welling: Clinical pharmacokinetics of co-trimoxazole (trimethoprim-sulphamethoxazole), *Clin. Pharmacokinet.*, 5:403, 1980.

27. Moellering, R. C., D. J. Krogstad, and D. J. Greenblatt: Vancomycin therapy in patients with impaired renal function: A nomogram for dosage, *Ann. Intern. Med.*, 94:343, 1981.

28. Heany, D., and G. Eknoyan: Minocycline and doxycycline kinetics in chronic renal failure, *Clin. Pharmacol. Therap.*, 24:233, 1978.

29. Gillis, A. M., and R. E. Kates: Clinical pharmacokinetics of antiarrhythmic agents, *Clin. Pharmacokinet.*, 9:375, 1984.

30. Singh, B. N., W. R. Thoden, and A. Ward: Acebutolol: A review of its pharmacological properties and therapeutic efficacy in hypertension, angina pectoris and arrhythmia, *Drugs*, 29:531, 1985.

31. Kirch, W., and E. R. Gorg: Clinical pharmacokinetics of atenolol—A review, *Europ. J. Drug Metab. Pharmacokinet.*, 7:81, 1982.

32. Carter, B. L.: Labetalol, *Drug Intell. Clin. Pharm.*, 17:704, 1983.

33. Regardh, C. G., and G. Johnsson: Clinical pharmacokinetics of metoprolol, *Clin. Pharmacokinet.*, 5:557, 1980.

34. Lant, A.: Diuretics: Clinical pharmacology and therapeutic use, *Drugs*, 29:162, 1985.

35. McAllister, R. G., S. R. Hamann, and R. A. Blouin: Pharmacokinetics of calcium-entry blockers, *Am. J. Cardiol.*, 55:30B, 1985.

36. Duchin, K. L., A. M. Pierides, A. Heald, S. M. Singhvi, and A. J. Rommel: Elimination kinetics of captopril in patients with renal failure, *Kidney Int.*, 25:942, 1984.

37. Houston, M. C.: Clonidine hydrochloride: Review of pharmacological and clinical aspects, *Prog. Cardiovasc. Dis.*, 23:337, 1981.

38. Holmes, B., R. N. Brogden, R. C. Heel, T. M. Speight, and G. S. Avery: Guanabenz: A review of its pharmacodynamic properties and therapeutic efficacy in hypertension, *Drugs*, 26:212, 1983.

39. Reece, P. A., I. Cozamanis, and R. Zacest: Kinetics of hydralazine and its main metabolites in slow and fast accetylators, *Clin. Pharmacol. Therap.*, 28:769, 1980.

40. Myhre, F., H. E. Rugstad, and T. Hansen: Clinical

pharmacokinetics of methyldopa, *Clin. Pharmacokinet.,* 7:221, 1982.

41. Cohn, J. N., and L. P. Buke: Nitroprusside, *Ann. Intern. Med.,* 91:752, 1979.

42. Stanaszek, W. F., D. Kellerman, R. N. Brogden, and J. A. Romakiewicz: Prazosin update. A review of its pharmacological properties and therapeutic use in hypertension and congestive heart failure, *Drugs,* 25:339, 1983.

43. Zoster, T. T., G. E. Johnson, and G. A. Dever: Excretion and metabolism of reserpine in renal failure, *Clin. Pharmacol. Therap.,* 14:325, 1973.

44. Aronson, J. K.: Clinical pharmacokinetics of digoxin, *Clin. Pharmacokinet.,* 5:137, 1980.

45. Vohringer, H. F., and N. Rietbrock: Digitalis therapy in renal failure with special regard to digitoxin, *Int. J. Clin. Pharmacol. Therap. Toxicol.,* 19:175, 1981.

46. Affrime, M. B., and D. T. Lowenthal: Analgesics, sedatives and sedative-hypnotics, in R. Anderson and R. Schrier (eds.), *Clinical Use of Drugs in Patients with Liver and Kidney Disease,* Saunders, Philadelphia, 1981, p. 199.

47. Greenblatt, D. J., M. Divoll, D. R. Abernathy, H. R. Ochs, and R. I. Shader: Clinical pharmacokinetics of the newer benzodiazepines, *Clin. Pharmacokinet.,* 8:233, 1983.

48. Forsman, A., and R. Ohman: Pharmacokinetic studies on haloperodol in man, *Curr. Therap. Res.,* 20:319, 1976.

49. Lydiard, R. B., and A. J. Gelenberg: Hazards and adverse effects of lithium, *Ann. Rev. Med.,* 33:327, 1982.

50. McAllister, C. J., E. B. Scowden, and W. J. Stone: Toxic psychosis induced by phenothiazine administration in patients with chronic renal failure, *Clin. Nephrol.,* 10:191, 1978.

51. Amsterdam, J., D. Brunswick, and J. Mendels: The clinical application of tricyclic antidepressant pharmacokinetics and plasma levels, *Am. J. Psychiat.,* 137:653, 1980.

52. Forrest, J. A., J. A. Clements, and L. F. Prescott: Clinical pharmacokinetics of paracetamol, *Clin. Pharmacokinet.,* 7:93, 1982.

53. Levy, G.: Pharmacokinetics of salicylate in man, *Drug Metab. Rev.,* 9:13, 1979.

54. Barnes, J. N., A. J. Williams, M. J. Tomson, P. A. Toseland, and F. J. Goodwin: Dihydrocodeine in renal failure: Further evidence for an important role of the kidney in the handling of opioid drugs, *Br. Med. J.,* 290:740, 1985.

55. Szeto, H. H., C. E. Inturrisi, R. Houde, and M. Reidenberg: Accumulation of normeperidine, an active metabolite of meperidine, in patients with renal failure or cancer, *Ann. Intern. Med.,* 86:738, 1977.

56. Don, H. G., R. A. Dieppa, and P. Taylor: Narcotic analgesics in anuric patients, *Anesthesiology,* 42:745, 1976.

57. Payne, J. P.: The clinical pharmacology of pentazocine, *Drugs,* 5:1, 1973.

58. Estes, J. W.: Clinical pharmacokinetics of heparin, *Clin. Pharmacokinet.,* 5:204, 1980.

59. Kelly, J. G., and K. O'Malley: Clinical pharmacokinetics of oral anticoagulants, *Clin. Pharmacokinet.,* 4:1, 1979.

60. Balant, L.: Clinical pharmacokinetics of sulfonylurea hypoglycemic drugs, *Clin. Pharmacokinet.,* 6:215, 1981.

61. Lebovitz, H. E.: Glipizide: A second generation sulfonylurea hypoglycemic agent. *Pharmacotherapy,* 5:63, 1985.

62. Feldman, J. M.: Glyburide: A second generation sulfonylurea hypoglycemic agent, *Pharmacotherapy,* 5:43, 1985.

63. Rabkin, R., N. M. Simon, and S. Steinger: Effect of renal disease on renal uptake and excretion of insulin in man, *N. Engl. J. Med.,* 282:182, 1970.

64. Bach, J. F., and M. Dardenne: The metabolism of azathioprine in renal failure, *Transplantation,* 12:253, 1971.

65. Crooke, S. T., and A. W. Prestakayo: Bleomycin pharmacokinetics in patients with varying renal function, *Canc. Res. Proc.,* 18:286, 1977.

66. Ehrsson, H., M. Hassan, M. Ehrnebo, and M. Beran: Busulfan kinetics, *Clin. Pharmacol. Therap.,* 34:86, 1983.

67. Balis, F. M., J. S. Holdenberg, and W. A. Bleyer: Clinical pharmacokinetics of commonly used anticancer drugs, *Clin. Pharmacokinet.,* 8:202, 1983.

68. Blachey, J. D., and J. B. Hill: Renal and electrolyte disturbances associated with cisplatin, *Ann. Intern. Med.,* 95:628, 1981.

69. Grochow, L. B., and M. Colvin: Clinical pharmacokinetics of cyclophosphamide, *Clin. Pharmacokinet.,* 4:380, 1979.

70. Follath, F., M. Wenk, S. Vozeh, G. Thiel, F. Brunner, R. Loertscher, M. Lemaire, K. Nussbaumer, W. Niederberger, and A. Wood: Intravenous cyclosporine kinetics in renal failure, *Clin. Pharmacol. Therap.,* 34:638, 1983.

71. Jolivet, J., K. H. Cowan, G. A. Curt, N. J. Clendeninn, and B. A. Chabner: The pharmacology and clinical use of methotrexate, *N. Engl. J. Med.,* 309:1094, 1983.

72. Owellen, R. J., M. A. Roat, and F. O. Hains: Pharmacokinetics of vinblastine and vincristine in humans, *Cancer Res.,* 37:2603, 1977.

73. Hande, K. R., R. M. Noone, and W. J. Stone: Severe allopurinol toxicity: Description and guidelines for

prevention in patients with renal insufficiency, *Am. J. Med.*, 76:47, 1984.

74. Verbeeck, R. K., J. L. Blackburn, and G. R. Loewen: Clinical pharmacokinetics of non-steroidal anti-inflammatory drugs, *Clin. Pharmacokinet.*, 8:297, 1983.

75. Cunningham, R. F., Z. H. Israili, and P. G. Dayton: Clinical pharmacokinetics of probenecid, *Clin. Pharmacokinet.*, 6:135, 1981.

76. Eadie, M. J.: Anticonvulsant drugs: An update, *Drugs*, 27:328, 1984.

77. Conner, C. S.: Atracrurium and vercuronium: Two unique neuromuscular blocking agents, *Drug Intell. Clin. Pharm.*, 18:714, 1984.

78. Ramzam, M. I., C. A. Sharks, and E. J. Triggs: Gallamine disposition in surgical patients with chronic renal failure., *Br. J. Clin. Pharmacol.*, 12:141, 1981.

79. Ramzam, M. I., A. A. Somogyi, J. S. Walker, C. A. Shanks, and E. J. Triggs: Clinical pharmacokinetics of the nondepolarizing muscle relaxants, *Clin. Pharmacokinet.*, 6:25, 1981.

80. Miller, R. D., R. S. Maheo, and L. Z. Benet: The pharmacokinetics of *d*-tubocurarine with and without renal failure, *J. Pharmacol. Exp. Therap.*, 202:1, 1977.

81. Somogyi, A., and R. Gugler: Clinical pharmacokinetics of cimetidine, *Clin. Pharmacokinet.*, 8:463, 1983.

82. Gugler, R.: Clinical pharmacokinetics of hypolipidemic drugs, *Clin. Pharmacokinet.*, 3:425, 1978.

83. Kampmann, J. P., and J. M. Hansen: Clinical pharmacokinetics of antithyroid drugs, *Clin. Pharmacokinet.*, 6:401, 1981.

84. Lehmann, C. R., J. D. Heironimus, C. B. Collins, T. J. O'Neil, W. P. Pierson, J. T. Crose, A. P. Melikan, and G. J. Wright: Metoclopramide kinetics in patients with impaired renal function and clearance by hemodialysis, *Clin. Pharmacol. Therap.*, 37:284, 1985.

85. Gaginells, T. S., and J. H. Bauman: Ranitidine hydrochloride, *Drug. Intell. Clin. Pharm.*, 17:873, 1983.

86. Ogilvie, R. I.: Clinical pharmacokinetics of theophylline, *Clin. Pharmacokinet.*, 3:267, 1978.

87. Cockroft, D. W., and M. H. Gault: Prediction of creatinine clearance from serum creatinine, *Nephron*, 16:13, 1976.

88. Mitchell, J. R., S. H. Cavanaugh, L. Arias, and J. A. Oates: Guanethidine and related agents. III. Antagonism by drugs which inhibit the norepinephrine pump in man, *J. Clin. Invest.*, 49:1596, 1970.

89. Briant, R. H., J. L. Reid, and C. T. Dollery: Interaction between clonidine and desipramine in man, *Br. Med. J.*, 1:522, 1973.

90. Graves, S. W., B. Brown, and R. Valdes, Jr.: An endogenous digoxin-like substance in patients with renal impairment, *Ann. Intern. Med.*, 99:604, 1983.

91. Gallagher, K. L., and J. K. Jones: Furosemide-induced ototoxicity, *Ann. Intern. Med.*, 91:744, 1979.

92. Brown, R. D.: Comparative acute cochlear toxicity of intravenous bumetanide and furosemide in the purebred beagle, *J. Clin. Pharmacol.*, 21:620, 1981.

93. Feig, P. U.: Cellular mechanism of action of loop diuretics: Implications for drug effectiveness and adverse effects, *Am. J. Cardiol.*, 57:14A, 1986.

94. Reubi, F. C., and P. T. Cottier: Effects of reduced glomerular filtration rate on response to chlorothiazide and mercurial diuretics, *Circulation*, 23:200, 1961.

95. Dargie, H. J., M. E. M. Allison, A. C. Kennedy, and M. J. B. Gray: High dosage metolazone in chronic renal failure, *Br. Med. J.*, 4:196, 1972.

96. Wollam, G. L., R. C. Tarazi, E. L. Bravo, and H. P. Dustan: Diuretic potency of hydrochlorothiazide and furosemide therapy in patients with azotemia, *Am. J. Med.*, 72:929, 1982.

97. Oster, J. R., M. Epstein, and S. Smoller: Combined therapy with thiazide type and loop diuretic agents for resistant sodium retention, *Ann. Intern. Med.*, 99:405, 1983.

98. Hropot, M., N. Fowler, B. Karlmark, and G. Giebisch: Tubular action of diuretics: Distal effects on electrolyte transport and acidification, *Kidney Int.*, 28:477, 1985.

INDEX

INDEX

Note: Page numbers in *italic* indicate tables.